Teacher's Manual

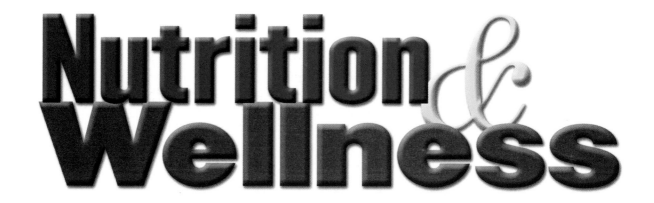

Nutrition & Wellness

SECOND EDITION

by
ROBERTA LARSON DUYFF
MS, RD, FADA, CFCS

CONSULTING AUTHOR
Doris Hasler
MS, CFCS

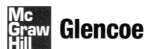 **Glencoe**

New York, New York   Columbus, Ohio   Chicago, Illinois   Peoria, Illinois   Woodland Hills, California

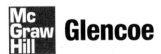

Glencoe

Send all inquiries to:
Glencoe/McGraw-Hill
3008 W. Willow Knolls Drive
Peoria, Illinois 61614-1083

ISBN 0-07-846337-8 (Teacher Annotated Edition)
ISBN 0-07-846332-7 (Student Edition)

Printed in the United States of America

1 2 3 4 5 6 7 8 9 10 071 07 06 05 04 03

Welcome to
Nutrition & Wellness

The second edition of *Nutrition & Wellness* builds on the strengths of this popular textbook program. *Nutrition & Wellness* is the ideal choice for courses that emphasize nutrition, wellness, and fitness. You'll also find concise information on food preparation, food safety, and food science. It's all here for you in a unique, highly motivating program!

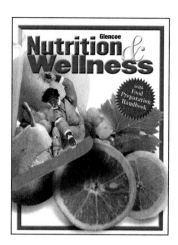

Updated information. This edition includes the latest Dietary Guidelines and Dietary Reference Intakes. New TIME Global Nutrition & Wellness features provide a fascinating look at food customs around the world.

Positive approach. *Nutrition & Wellness* emphasizes enjoyment of food and fitness and promotes personal choice.

Practical focus. *Nutrition & Wellness* helps students learn to eat for health in any situation—at home or on the go.

Food Preparation Handbook. *Nutrition & Wellness* features a Food Preparation Handbook bound into the back of the book. The Handbook gives you maximum flexibility in teaching food preparation skills and food science principles.

Standards and skills. The *Nutrition & Wellness* text meets the Family and Consumer Sciences Education National Standards for Nutrition and Wellness. Active learning, decision making, critical thinking, and problem solving are emphasized. The program also reinforces communication, management, and leadership skills, as well as academic skills.

Program Components

Nutrition & Wellness provides a complete package of program components.

Student Edition. A 576-page, full color textbook with the latest information on nutrition, wellness, and fitness.

Teacher Annotated Edition. Includes activities, teaching tips, and answer keys.

Student Workbook. Provides study guides and activity sheets to maximize learning.

Student Workbook Teacher Annotated Edition. Has answers conveniently printed on each page.

Teacher Resource Guide. Supplies essential teaching tips, lesson plans, and tests.

Effective Instruction CD-ROM. Lets you customize lesson plans and tests to suit your needs.

Transparency Package. Ready-to-use color transparencies to enliven your presentations and enhance learning.

Student Motivation Kit. Provides a wealth of time-saving reproducible resources including recipes, science experiments, and a culinary tour of the world.

Using the Student Edition

The Student Edition of *Nutrition & Wellness* is designed to be not only informative and educationally sound, but appealing and motivating.

Teen-friendly writing style. The text is written in a light, enthusiastic style to interest and motivate teens. The reading level is appropriate for beginning high school students. To aid learning, content is logically organized and color headings clearly identify major topics and subtopics.

Visual appeal. The text's many colorful photographs, drawings, charts, and features add interest and capture students' attention, besides contributing educational value. Special "infographic" pages (such as page 60) combine visual and verbal techniques to concisely explain topics.

Organization

The *Nutrition & Wellness* text is divided into six units, plus the unique Food Preparation Handbook. Each unit has a distinctive theme.

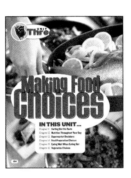

Unit 3: Making Food Choices encourages everyday application of nutrition principles. Students learn how to evaluate nutrition information, plan meals and snacks, shop for food, choose nutrition-wise cooking methods, and make healthful choices when eating out.

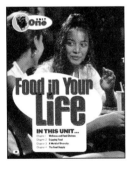

Unit 1: Food in Your Life introduces students to the study of nutrition and wellness. Topics include influences on food choices, etiquette and enjoyment, cultural diversity, and the food supply.

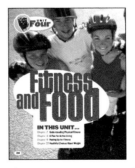

Unit 4: Fitness and Food focuses on physical activity as it relates to nutrition and wellness. Students learn what physical fitness means, how to take part in physical activity safely and sensibly, and the facts about sports nutrition. The chapter on "Healthful Choices About Weight"—prepared in consultation with a USDA expert on teen weight issues—focuses on positive self-image and discourages inappropriate dieting.

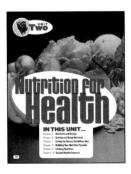

Unit 2: Nutrition for Health provides an in-depth look at nutrition principles including nutrient sources and functions, the Dietary Guidelines, the Food Guide Pyramid, and special nutrition needs.

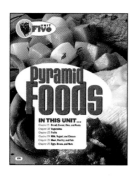

Unit 5: Pyramid Foods looks in turn at each type of food in the Pyramid food groups—from breads to nuts—with emphasis on nutrition, selection, storage, and basic preparation.

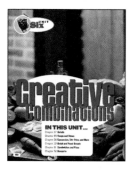

Unit 6: Creative Combinations teaches students about preparing dishes such as salads, soups, stir-fries, quick breads, pizza, and desserts. The emphasis is on preparing these foods in new, "light" ways—as well as how to fit traditional favorites into a healthful eating plan.

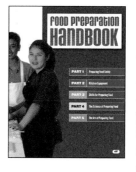

The Food Preparation Handbook presents basic information about food safety, equipment, and food preparation skills. It also extends learning to the science and art of preparing food. The material is divided into short sections that can be used individually, together, or in conjunction with related chapters. See pages TM–7 and TM–8 for more information.

Chapter Opening Pages

The opening pages of each chapter are designed to facilitate learning while also capturing interest.

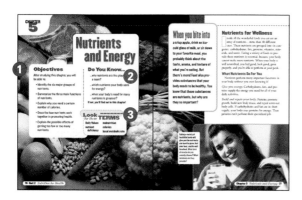

❶ *Objectives* establish specific learner outcomes. The text, review questions, activities, and supplemental materials support these objectives.

❷ *"Do You Know..."* sparks students' interest by posing intriguing questions. Students will find the answers as they read the chapter.

❸ *Look for These Terms* identifies key terms introduced in the chapter.

Chapter Enhancements

Within chapters, teaching and learning are enhanced by these special items:

Vocabulary terms from the "Look for These Terms" list are highlighted in bold type the first time they are used in the chapter. Definitions are italicized for easy identification. These terms and definitions are also included in the Glossary at the back of the book.

Captions include questions or activities for interactive learning.

Check This Out! articles provide interesting sidelights on related topics, with "It's Your Turn!" activities for follow-up.

Tips provide practical suggestions for boosting nutrition, saving time and money, making tasks easier, and other management strategies.

InfoLinks point the reader to related topics in other parts of the text.

PROGRAM OVERVIEW

Chapter Review & Activities

The Chapter Review & Activities pages at the end of each chapter assess student mastery of chapter objectives. Components include:

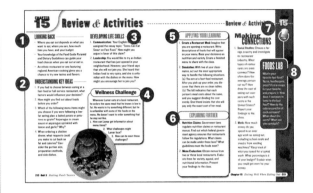

❶ Looking Back—a summary of the chapter's main points.

❷ Understanding Key Ideas—questions to assess mastery of basic concepts.

❸ Developing Life Skills—thought-provoking

questions that help students develop the key skills of critical thinking, creative thinking, communication, leadership, and management.

❹ Wellness Challenge—a scenario that involves overcoming challenges and finding solutions to practical problems.

❺ Applying Your Learning—activities that involve practical application of knowledge and skills learned in the chapter.

❻ Exploring Further—investigations of related topics that can be used as extension, enrichment, or extra-credit assignments.

❼ Making Connections—activities that relate food and nutrition topics to math, science, language arts, social studies, and careers.

❽ Foods Lab—a short, simple activity that gives students the opportunity to work with food in the classroom lab or at home.

Answers to review questions are found on pages TM–32 to TM–63 of this Teacher's Manual.

Special Feature Pages

Each chapter includes at least one of the following special pages:

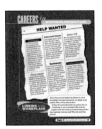

Careers pages each highlight a different career area related to nutrition and wellness. Within each area, specific careers are described in "want ads" that emphasize the skills, aptitudes, and education needed for success. "Linking to the Workplace" activities extend learning.

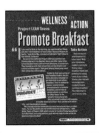

Wellness in Action articles showcase ways in which real-life teens have helped promote nutrition and wellness through action-oriented, teen-powered projects at the

school, community, state, or national level. Each article concludes with a "Take Action" idea for the reader to carry out.

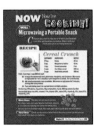

Now You're Cooking! pages provide quick, easy, economical, and nutritious recipes to help students learn and practice basic food preparation skills. Each includes a skill focus, customary and metric measurements, and information about calories and nutrients. "More Ideas" suggests variations to encourage creativity and improvisation. "Your Ideas" provides an activity to extend learning, whether or not students prepare the recipe. The recipes are supported by the *Foods Lab Activities* booklet in the **Student Motivation Kit.**

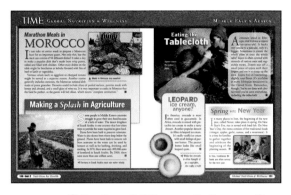

TIME **Global Nutrition & Wellness**

Introduce students to food customs from around the world! These high-interest features, produced in partnership with TIME Learning Ventures, are found at the end of each text unit.

Each four-page feature highlights a different part of the world. Short, interesting tidbits are followed by an in-depth article explaining regional food customs. Photos of the people and foods of the region bring the information to life.

You may use the TIME Global Nutrition & Wellness features individually at the end of each unit or collectively as a unit in themselves—perhaps in conjunction with Chapter 3, "A World of Diversity." The TIME Global Nutrition & Wellness features are extended by 160 pages of information and activities in the *Global Foods Tour* booklet, which is found in the **Student Motivation Kit**.

Food Preparation Handbook

The Food Preparation Handbook, which begins on page 436, provides a convenient, flexible way to teach knowledge and skills related to food preparation. The Handbook is divided into five parts:

Part 1: Preparing Food Safely stresses prevention of foodborne illness and kitchen accidents.

Part 2: Kitchen Equipment illustrates and describes kitchen tools, cookware, appliances, and work centers.

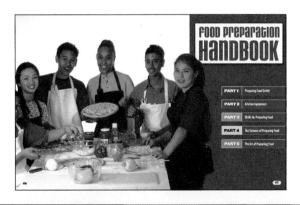

Part 3: Skills for Preparing Food presents basic "how-tos" for following recipes, measuring, cutting, mixing, microwaving, conventional cooking, and managing time in the kitchen.

Part 4: The Science of Preparing Food makes the science behind food preparation come alive. With everyday examples, clear explanations, and colorful illustrations, students will learn the fascinating answers to questions such as "Why does cut fruit turn brown?" and "What makes meringue fluffy?" Highlighted "Science Concepts" briefly explain relevant scientific terms such as solution, enzyme, and emulsion.

Part 5: The Art of Preparing Food helps students learn about making meals appealing, enjoying food preparation as a creative hobby, and entertaining guests.

The five parts of the Food Preparation Handbook are subdivided into brief sections. Each section is one to six pages long and covers a specific topic, letting you choose which sections to teach and when.

You can use the Food Preparation Handbook in several ways:

On its own. All or some of any Handbook Part can be taught as a self-contained learning unit.

With chapters. Individual sections of the Handbook can supplement specific text chapters. For more information, see the planning guide on pages TM–16 and TM–17.

As a reference. Encourage students to use the Handbook on their own as a reference.

Like the text chapters, the Food Preparation Handbook is complete with objectives, vocabulary terms, and Review & Activities pages. Supplemental materials for the Food Preparation Handbook are provided in the ***Student Workbook*** and the ***Teacher Resource Guide***.

Using the Teacher Annotated Edition

Teacher's Manual

The Teacher's Manual at the front of the ***Teacher Annotated Edition*** provides charts to help you plan your course and identify appropriate teaching strategies. A list of references, including Internet, multimedia, and print resources, begins on page TM–24. Answers to the review questions for each chapter and Handbook Part begin on page TM–32.

Annotations

The ***Teacher Annotated Edition*** also provides teaching suggestions in the form of annotations printed on most pages of the text. Types of annotations include:

Activity—a learning activity for students.

Critical Thinking—questions aimed at helping students learn to critique, analyze, and interpret information.

Discuss—other types of questions for class or small group discussion.

Emphasize—important points you may want to stress.

More About—background information related to the text material.

Teaching with Visuals—teaching suggestions relating to photos, drawings, and charts.

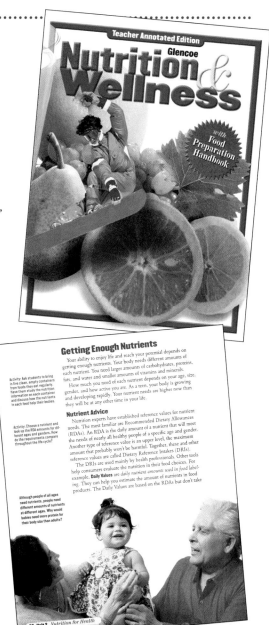

Using the Supplements

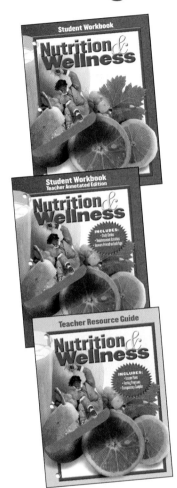

Student Workbook

The *Student Workbook* emphasizes reinforcement and application of chapter concepts. For each chapter and Handbook Part, the Student Workbook provides:

• A visual study guide—in "graphic organizer" format—to help students organize and remember important points from the text. Students can fill in the study guide based on their text reading, then use it for review.

• Two to three activities that support the text's learning objectives. These activity worksheets help students apply chapter information while also building thinking skills.

The *Student Workbook Teacher Annotated Edition* provides answers conveniently printed on each study guide and activity page.

Teacher Resource Guide

This essential component presents:

Teaching Tips to help you plan your course.

Lesson Plans with a variety of activity ideas to help you focus attention, teach concepts, assess learning, and close the lesson.

Tests with objective and essay questions to assess student comprehension.

Sample Transparencies with accompanying teaching suggestions.

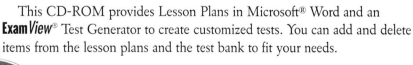

Effective Instruction CD-ROM

This CD-ROM provides Lesson Plans in Microsoft® Word and an **Exam*View*®** Test Generator to create customized tests. You can add and delete items from the lesson plans and the test bank to fit your needs.

Transparency Package

This set of 48 full-color transparencies will enliven your teaching and learning program. The vibrant transparencies can be used to introduce topics, reinforce concepts, generate discussion, or develop thinking skills. Teaching strategies are included for each transparency.

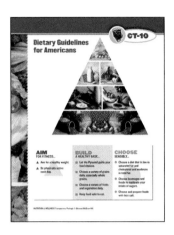

Student Motivation Kit

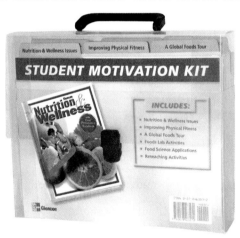

The **Student Motivation Kit** is a collection of reproducible resources for classroom use. The Kit contains six individual booklets that provide information and learning tools. They can be used to supplement the text or as stand-alone units of study. The booklets include:

Nutrition & Wellness Issues. Articles cover topics ranging from biotechnology to health claims on foods, with follow-up questions that promote thinking skills, communication, leadership, and management. Also provides group projects such as conducting a panel discussion and creating a pamphlet.

Improving Physical Fitness. Reproducible articles, diagrams, and charts help students assess their level of fitness, start a fitness program, and safely participate in physical activity.

A Global Foods Tour. Take your students on an imaginary tour of the world to learn about foods and food customs. Students will "visit" 11 world regions, stopping at 25 "ports of call" within the regions. The booklet provides maps, activity sheets, projects, and other resources for teaching about foods of the world, as well as material relating to awareness of global food supply issues.

Foods Lab Activities. Recipes from the "Now You're Cooking!" text pages are provided in convenient reproducible form with a related worksheet on the back of each page. Additional activity sheets help students practice basic food preparation and menu planning skills.

Food Science Applications. Students can explore scientific principles related to food preparation through hands-on Investigation Activities. A teaching guide and answer key are provided for each activity.

Reteaching Activities. These activities provide extra guidance focusing on main ideas. An activity is provided for each chapter and Handbook Part.

FACS National Standards Correlation

The following chart shows how the *Nutrition & Wellness* textbook meets the standards and competencies for the Nutrition and Wellness area of study as outlined in the Family and Consumer Sciences Education National Standards.

Nutrition and Wellness—Comprehensive Standard 14.0

Demonstrate nutrition and wellness practices that enhance individual and family well being.

Content Standard 14.1

Analyze factors that influence nutrition and wellness practices across the life span.

COMPETENCIES	TEXT CHAPTERS
14.1.1 Examine physical, emotional, social, psychological, and spiritual components of individual and family wellness.	Chapter 1: Wellness and Food Choices
14.1.2 Compare the impact of psychological, cultural, and social influences on food choices and other nutrition practices.	Chapter 1: Wellness and Food Choices Chapter 3: A World of Diversity
14.1.3 Examine the governmental, economic, and technological influences on food choices and practices.	Chapter 1: Wellness and Food Choices Chapter 3: A World of Diversity Chapter 4: The Food Supply Chapter 13: Supermarket Decisions
14.1.4 Investigate the impact of global and local events and conditions on food choices and practices.	Chapter 1: Wellness and Food Choices Chapter 3: A World of Diversity Chapter 4: The Food Supply
14.1.5 Examine legislation and regulations related to nutrition and wellness issues.	Chapter 4: The Food Supply

Content Standard 14.2

Evaluate the nutritional needs of individuals and families in relation to health and wellness across the life span.

COMPETENCIES	TEXT CHAPTERS
14.2.1 Assess the effect of nutrients on health, appearance, and peak performance.	Chapter 1: Wellness and Food Choices Chapter 5: Nutrients and Energy Chapter 6: Getting and Using Nutrients
14.2.2 Research the relationship of nutrition and wellness to individual and family health throughout the life span.	Chapter 1: Wellness and Food Choices Chapter 9: Lifelong Nutrition

COURSE PLANNING TOOLS

COMPETENCIES	TEXT CHAPTERS
14.2.3 Assess the impact of food and diet fads, food addictions, and eating disorders on wellness.	Chapter 10: Special Health Concerns Chapter 11: Sorting Out the Facts Chapter 20: Healthful Choices About Weight
14.2.4 Appraise sources of food and nutrition information, including food labels, related to health and wellness.	Chapter 11: Sorting Out the Facts Chapter 13: Supermarket Decisions Chapter 15: Eating Well When Eating Out

Content Standard 14.3

Demonstrate ability to acquire, handle, and use foods to meet nutrition and wellness needs of individuals and families across the life span.

COMPETENCIES	TEXT CHAPTERS
14.3.1 Apply various dietary guidelines in planning to meet nutrition and wellness needs.	Chapter 7: Eating the Dietary Guidelines Way Chapter 8: Building Your Nutrition Pyramid Chapter 9: Lifelong Nutrition Chapter 12: Nutrition Throughout Your Day
14.3.2 Design strategies that meet the health and nutrition requirements of individuals and families with special needs.	Chapter 10: Special Health Concerns Chapter 13: Supermarket Decisions Chapter 14: Food Preparation Choices Chapter 15: Eating Well When Eating Out Chapter 16: Vegetarian Choices
14.3.3 Demonstrate ability to select, store, prepare, and serve nutritious and aesthetically pleasing foods.	Chapter 2: Enjoying Food Chapter 12: Nutrition Throughout Your Day Chapter 13: Supermarket Decisions Chapter 14: Food Preparation Choices Unit 5: Pyramid Foods (Chapters 21-26) Unit 6: Creative Combinations (Chapters 27-32) Food Preparation Handbook

Content Standard 14.4

Evaluate factors that affect food safety, from production through consumption.

COMPETENCIES	TEXT CHAPTERS
14.4.1 Determine conditions and practices that promote safe food handling.	Food Preparation Handbook Part I: Preparing Food Safely

COMPETENCIES	TEXT CHAPTERS
14.4.2 Appraise safety and sanitation practices throughout the food chain.	Chapter 4: The Food Supply Chapter 13: Supermarket Decisions Chapter 15: Eating Well When Eating Out Food Preparation Handbook Part 1: Preparing Food Safely
14.4.3 Determine how changes in national and international food production and distribution systems impact the food supply.	Chapter 4: The Food Supply
14.4.4 Appraise federal, state, and local inspection and labeling systems that protect the health of individuals and the public.	Chapter 4: The Food Supply Chapter 13: Supermarket Decisions
14.4.5 Monitor foodborne illness as a health issue for individuals and families.	Food Preparation Handbook Part 1: Preparing Food Safely
14.4.6 Review public dialogue about food safety and sanitation.	Food Preparation Handbook Part 1: Preparing Food Safely

Content Standard 14.5

Evaluate the impact of science and technology on food composition, safety, and other issues.

COMPETENCIES	TEXT CHAPTERS
14.5.1 Determine how scientific and technical advances impact the nutrient content, availability, and safety of foods.	Chapter 4: The Food Supply
14.5.2 Assess how the scientific and technical advances in food processing, storage, product development, and distribution impact nutrition and wellness.	Chapter 4: The Food Supply Food Preparation Handbook Part 4: The Science of Preparing Food
14.5.3 Determine the impact of technological advances on selection, preparation, and home storage of food.	Chapter 4: The Food Supply Food Preparation Handbook Part 1: Preparing Food Safely Food Preparation Handbook Part 4: The Science of Preparing Food
14.5.4 Assess the effects of food science and technology on meeting nutritional needs.	Chapter 4: The Food Supply Chapter 5: Nutrients and Energy Food Preparation Handbook Part 4: The Science of Preparing Food

Suggested Course Options

The following chart shows how *Nutrition & Wellness* can be adapted for use in a variety of courses. Options are given for several different types of courses with varying term lengths and emphases.

To use the chart, find the heading for the desired type of course. Read down the column to see the suggested number of days to spend on each portion of the *Nutrition & Wellness* text. An asterisk (*) indicates that the chapter or part can be skipped or summarized. These options can easily be adapted to meet your particular needs.

Number of Days Per Chapter For...

		Sports Nutrition/ Food & Fitness 18 weeks	Food Science 18 weeks	Nutrition & Consumer Choices 18 weeks	Nutrition, Consumer & Food Prep 18 weeks	Nutrition, Consumer & Food Prep 36 weeks	Your Course	Your Course
Ch. 1	Wellness & Food Choices	4	*	4	2	4		
Ch. 2	Enjoying Food	*	*	2	1	2		
Ch. 3	A World of Diversity	*	*	2	2	4		
Ch. 4	The Food Supply	*	5	3	2	4		
Ch. 5	Nutrients & Energy	4	4	4	2	4		
Ch. 6	Getting & Using Nutrients	4	4	4	3	4		
Ch. 7	Eating the Dietary Guidelines Way	4	*	4	2	4		
Ch. 8	Building Your Nutrition Pyramid	4	*	4	2	4		
Ch. 9	Lifelong Nutrition	4	4	5	3	5		
Ch. 10	Special Health Concerns	4	2	5	2	5		
Ch. 11	Sorting Out the Facts	4	*	3	2	3		
Ch. 12	Nutrition Throughout Your Day	4	*	5	2	5		
Ch. 13	Supermarket Decisions	5	*	5	2	5		
Ch. 14	Food Preparation Choices	3	4	3	2	4		
Ch. 15	Eating Well When Eating Out	2	*	4	2	4		
Ch. 16	Vegetarian Choices	2	*	2	1	2		

	Sports Nutrition/ Food & Fitness 18 weeks	Food Science 18 weeks	Nutrition & Consumer Choices 18 weeks	Nutrition, Consumer & Food Prep 18 weeks	Nutrition, Consumer & Food Prep 36 weeks	Your Course	Your Course
Ch. 17 Understanding Physical Fitness	6	*	2	1	3		
Ch. 18 A Plan for Active Living	6	*	2	1	4		
Ch. 19 Fueling Up for Fitness	6	*	2	2	3		
Ch. 20 Healthful Choices About Weight	6	*	3	2	5		
Ch. 21 Bread, Cereal, Rice, & Pasta	2	2	2	2	4		
Ch. 22 Vegetables	2	2	2	2	4		
Ch. 23 Fruits	2	2	2	2	4		
Ch. 24 Milk, Yogurt, & Cheese	2	2	2	2	4		
Ch. 25 Meat, Poultry, & Fish	3	3	3	3	4		
Ch. 26 Eggs, Beans, & Nuts	2	2	2	2	4		
Ch. 27 Salads	*	2	*	2	4		
Ch. 28 Soups & Stews	*	2	*	2	4		
Ch. 29 Casseroles, Stir-Fries, & More	*	2	*	2	4		
Ch. 30 Quick & Yeast Breads	*	3	*	3	4		
Ch. 31 Sandwiches & Pizza	*	2	*	2	4		
Ch. 32 Desserts	*	3	*	3	4		
TIME Global Nutrition & Wellness Features	*	*	4	4	12		
Handbook Part 1 Preparing Food Safely	2	10	2	5	10		
Handbook Part 2 Kitchen Equipment	1	4	1	2	5		
Handbook Part 3 Skills for Preparing Food	2	6	2	6	12		
Handbook Part 4 The Science of Preparing Food	*	20	*	5	10		
Handbook Part 5 The Art of Preparing Food	*	*	*	3	5		
TOTALS	90	90	90	90	180		

Food Preparation Handbook Planning Guide

The Food Preparation Handbook, which begins on page 436, provides a convenient, flexible way to teach knowledge and skills related to food preparation. Its five parts are subdivided into brief sections. Each section is one to six pages long and covers a specific topic, letting you choose which sections to teach and when.

One option for using the Handbook is to supplement text chapters with related Handbook sections. For each Handbook section, the following chart identifies chapters that particularly lend themselves to this approach. You may find this chart useful in planning your course and deciding when to teach the Handbook sections.

If you prefer, you may choose to use an entire Handbook part (or selected sections) as a stand-alone learning unit, or to let students use the Handbook as a reference. For more information, see pages TM–7 and TM–8 in this Teacher's Manual.

Handbook Part 1: Preparing Food Safely

HANDBOOK SECTIONS	RELATED CHAPTERS
Section 1-1: What Is Foodborne Illness?	**Chapter 4:** The Food Supply
Section 1-2: Shop Safely & Store Food Right!	**Chapter 13:** Supermarket Decisions
Section 1-3: Keep It Clean!	**Chapter 14:** Food Preparation Choices Any foods lab activity
Section 1-4: Control Temperatures!	**Chapter 14:** Food Preparation Choices **Chapter 25:** Meat, Poultry, and Fish Any foods lab activity
Section 1-5: Prevent Accidents!	**Chapter 14:** Food Preparation Choices Any foods lab activity

Handbook Part 2: Kitchen Equipment

HANDBOOK SECTIONS	RELATED CHAPTERS
Section 2-1: Kitchen Tools	**Chapter 14:** Food Preparation Choices Any foods lab activity
Section 2-2: Cookware	**Chapter 14:** Food Preparation Choices Any foods lab activity
Section 2-3: Appliances	**Chapter 14:** Food Preparation Choices Any foods lab activity
Section 2-4: Organizing the Kitchen	**Chapter 14:** Food Preparation Choices Any foods lab activity

Handbook Part 3: Skills for Preparing Food

HANDBOOK SECTIONS	RELATED CHAPTERS
Section 3-1: Recipe and Math Skills	**Chapter 14:** Food Preparation Choices Any foods lab activity
Section 3-2: Measuring Skills	**Chapter 14:** Food Preparation Choices Any foods lab activity
Section 3-3: Cutting Skills	**Chapter 14:** Food Preparation Choices Any foods lab activity
Section 3-4: Mixing Skills	**Chapter 14:** Food Preparation Choices Any foods lab activity
Section 3-5: Microwave Skills	**Chapter 14:** Food Preparation Choices Any foods lab activity
Section 3-6: More Cooking Skills	**Chapter 14:** Food Preparation Choices Any foods lab activity
Section 3-7: Management Skills	**Chapter 14:** Food Preparation Choices Any foods lab activity

Handbook Part 4: The Science of Preparing Food

HANDBOOK SECTIONS	RELATED CHAPTERS
Section 4-1: Food Science: An Introduction	**Chapter 4:** The Food Supply
Section 4-2: The Science of Heat and Cooking	**Chapter 14:** Food Preparation Choices
Section 4-3: The Science of Grain Products	**Chapter 21:** Bread, Cereal, Rice, and Pasta
Section 4-4: The Science of Vegetables and Fruits	**Chapter 22:** Vegetables **Chapter 23:** Fruits
Section 4-5: The Science of Dairy Foods	**Chapter 24:** Milk, Yogurt, and Cheese
Section 4-6: The Science of Meat, Poultry, and Fish	**Chapter 25:** Meat, Poultry, and Fish
Section 4-7: The Science of Eggs	**Chapter 26:** Eggs, Beans, and Nuts
Section 4-8: The Science of Salads	**Chapter 27:** Salads
Section 4-9: The Science of Thickened Foods	**Chapter 28:** Soups and Stews **Chapter 29:** Casseroles, Stir-Fries, and More
Section 4-10: The Science of Baking	**Chapter 30:** Quick and Yeast Breads **Chapter 32:** Desserts

Handbook Part 5: The Art of Preparing Food

HANDBOOK SECTIONS	RELATED CHAPTERS
Section 5-1: Meals with Appeal	**Chapter 2:** Enjoying Food
Section 5-2: Creative Cooking	**Chapter 2:** Enjoying Food **Chapter 3:** A World of Diversity **Chapter 14:** Food Preparation Choices **Unit 6:** Creative Combinations (Chapters 27-32)
Section 5-3: Easy Entertaining	**Chapter 2:** Enjoying Food

Tips for Teaching Nutrition

As a food and nutrition teacher, you want to not only provide students with accurate information, but frame it with positive, sensible messages to promote good health. The following suggestions can help you do so.

A Positive Approach to Nutrition

Students may come to you believing that most nutrition advice begins with "you can't" or "you shouldn't." Help them see nutrition in a positive light by aligning your words and actions with these philosophies:

Eating is one of life's greatest pleasures. Most people choose foods for taste and the pleasure of eating as their first priority. Help students understand that this is a valid choice. Emphasize the pleasure of eating good-tasting foods in an enjoyable environment.

A healthful eating style balances food choices over time. Remind students to apply nutritional standards to food intake over a day or several days, not to individual foods.

All foods can fit into a healthful eating style. Stay away from terms such as "junk food" and "foods to avoid." Even "healthful foods" implies that other foods are not healthful. Use messages such as "Eat all kinds of foods, but use the Pyramid to guide how much." Instead of "diet," with its restrictive connotation, you might refer to an eating style, eating plan, or strategy for food choices.

Physical activity is an important part of a healthful lifestyle. Promote the enjoyment of active living rather than "exercise" or "working out."

Tailoring the Message to Teens

Adolescents have special nutritional and developmental needs. Keep these in mind as you plan teaching strategies.

Key nutrients. Teens need adequate energy (calories) for growth and have increased needs for calcium, zinc, and iron. When students plan and analyze menus, for example, pay special attention to these nutrients.

Room for improvement. In general, teens don't eat enough fruits and vegetables, and female teens don't get enough foods from the milk group. Encourage your students to enjoy these foods more often.

Physical activity. Adolescents are relatively active at ages 12 to 14. Look for ways to encourage students to keep up their activity level through the later teen years.

Weight issues. Among 9- to 15-year-olds, about 50% of females and 23% of males see themselves as overweight. In actuality, about 11% of adolescents may be at risk for obesity. Dieting to lose weight is not recommended for teens. Restricting food intake is risky at a time when teens need varied and balanced food choices for growth and energy.

Making decisions. As they take on more responsibility in their lives, teens need to practice making their own choices. Provide such opportunities while serving as a positive role model for healthful living.

Adapted from material by Elaine McLaughlin, MS, RD, Food and Nutrition Service, USDA.

Assessment Strategies

STRATEGIES	ADVANTAGES	DISADVANTAGES

Objective Measures
Multiple choice
Matching
Item sets
True/false
	Reliable, easy to validate
	Objective, if designed effectively
	Low cost, efficient
	Automated administration
	Lends to equating
		Measures cognitive knowledge
		  effectively
		Limited on other measures
		Not a good measure of overall
		  performance

Written Measures
Essays
Restricted response
Written simulations
Case analysis
Problem-solving exercises
	Face validity (real life)
	In-depth assessment
	Measures writing skills and higher
	  level skills
	Reasonable developmental costs
	  and time
		Subjective scoring
		Time consuming and expensive
		  to score
		Limited breadth
		Difficult to equate
		Moderate reliability

Oral Measures
Oral examinations
Interviews
	Measures communications and
	  interpersonal skills
	In-depth assessment with varied
	  stimulus materials
	Learner involvement
		Costly and time consuming
		Limited reliability
		Narrow sample of content
		Scoring difficult, need
		  multiple raters

Simulated Activities In-basket Computer simulations	Moderate reliability Performance-based measure	Costly and time consuming Difficult to score, administer, and develop

Portfolio and Product Analysis
Work samples
Projects
Work diaries and logs
Achievement records
	Provides information not normally
	  available
	Learner involvement
	Face validity (real life)
	Easy to collect information
		Costly to administer
		Labor and paper intensive
		Difficult to validate or equate
		Biased toward best samples or
		  outstanding qualities

Performance Measures Demonstrations Presentations Performances Production work Observation	Job-related Relatively easy to administer In-depth assessment Face validity	Rater training required Hard to equate Subjective scoring Time consuming if breadth is needed
Performance Records References Performance rating forms Parental rating	Efficient Low cost Easy to administer	Low reliability Subjective Hard to equate Rater judgment
Self-evaluation	Learner involvement and empowerment Learner responsibility Measures dimensions not available otherwise	May be biased or unrealistic

Meeting Special Needs

SUBJECT	DESCRIPTION	SOURCES OF INFORMATION
Limited English Proficiency (LEP)	Certain students speak English as a second language, or not at all. Customs and behavior of people in the majority culture may be confusing for some of these students. Cultural values may inhibit some students from full participation in the classroom.	*Teaching English as a Second Language* *Mainstreaming and the Minority Child*
Behaviorally Disordered	Children with behavior disorders deviate from standards or expectations of behavior and impair the functioning of others and themselves. These children may also be gifted or learning disabled.	*Exceptional Children* *Journal of Special Education*
Visually Impaired	Children who are visually disabled have partial or total loss of sight. Individuals with visual impairments are not significantly different from their sighted peers in ability range or personality. However, blindness may affect cognitive, motor, and social development.	*Journal of Visual Impairment and Blindness* *Education of Visually Handicapped* *American Foundation for the Blind*
Hearing Impaired	Children who are hearing impaired have partial or total loss of hearing. Individuals with hearing impairments are not significantly different from their peers in ability range or personality. However, the chronic condition of deafness may affect cognitive, motor, social, and speech development.	*American Annals of the Deaf* *Journal of Speech and Hearing Research* *Sign Language Studies*
Physically Challenged	Children who are physically disabled fall into two categories—those with orthopedic impairments (use of one or more limbs severely restricted) and those with other health impairments.	*The Source Book for the Disabled* *Teaching Exceptional Children*
Gifted	Although no formal definition exists, these students can be described as having above average ability, task commitment, and creativity. They rank in the top five percent of their classes. They usually finish work more quickly than other students, and are capable of divergent thinking.	*Journal for the Education of the Gifted* *Gifted Children Quarterly* *Gifted Creative/Talented*
Learning Disabled	All learning disabled students have a problem in one or more areas, such as academic learning, language, perception, social-emotional adjustment, memory, or ability to pay attention.	*Journal of Learning Disabilities* *Learning Disability Quarterly*

TIPS FOR INSTRUCTION

- Remember that students' ability to speak English does not reflect their academic ability.
- Try to incorporate students' cultural experiences into your instruction. The help of a bilingual aide may be effective.
- Include information about different cultures in your curriculum to help build students' self-image.
- Avoid cultural stereotypes.
- Encourage students to share their cultures in the classroom.

- Work for long-term improvement; do not expect immediate success.
- Talk with students about their strengths and weaknesses, and clearly outline objectives and tell how you will help them obtain their goals.
- Structure schedules, rules, room arrangement, and safety for a conducive learning environment.
- Model appropriate behavior for students and reinforce proper behavior.
- Adjust group requirements for individual needs.

- Modify assignments as needed to help students become more independent.
- Teach classmates how to serve as guides for the visually impaired; pair students so sighted peers can assist in cooperative learning work.
- Tape lectures and reading assignments for the visually impaired.
- For the benefit of the visually impaired, encourage students to use their sense of touch; provide tactile models whenever possible.
- Verbally describe people and events as they occur in the classroom for the visually impaired.
- Limit unnecessary noise in the classroom.

- Provide favorable seating arrangements so hearing-impaired students can see speakers and read their lips (or interpreters can assist); avoid visual distractions.
- Write out all instructions on paper or on the board; overhead projectors enable you to maintain eye contact while writing.
- Avoid standing with your back to the window or light source.

- With the student, determine when you should offer aid.
- Help other students and adults understand physically disabled students.
- Learn about special devices or procedures and if any special safety precautions are needed.
- Allow students to participate in all activities including field trips, special events, and projects.

- Emphasize concepts, theories, relationships, ideas, and generalizations.
- Let students express themselves in a variety of ways including drawing, creative writing, or acting.
- Make arrangements for students to work on independent projects.
- Utilize public services and resources, such as agencies providing free and inexpensive materials, community services and programs, and people in the community with specific expertise.
- Make arrangements for students to take selected subjects early.

- Establish conditions and create an environment that leads to success.
- Provide assistance and direction; clearly define rules, assignments, and duties.
- Allow for pair interaction during class time; utilize peer helpers.
- Practice skills frequently.
- Distribute outlines of material presented in class.
- Maintain student interest with games.
- Allow extra time to complete tests and assignments.

Eight Ways of Learning

TYPE	DESCRIPTION	LIKES TO...
Verbal/Linguistic Learner	Intelligence is related to words and language, written and spoken.	read, write, tell stories, play word games, and tell jokes and riddles.
Logical/Mathematical Learner	Intelligence deals with inductive and deductive thinking and reasoning, numbers, and abstractions.	perform experiments, solve puzzles, work with numbers, ask questions, and explore patterns and relationships.
Visual/Spatial Learner	Intelligence relies on the sense of sight and being able to visualize an object, including the ability to create mental images.	draw, build, design, and create things, daydream, do jigsaw puzzles and mazes, watch videos, look at photos, and draw maps and charts.
Naturalistic Learner	Intelligence has to do with observing, understanding, and organizing patterns in the natural environment.	spend time outdoors and work with plants, animals, and other parts of the natural environment; good at identifying plants and animals and at hearing and seeing connections to nature.
Musical/Rhythmic Learner	Intelligence is based on recognition of tonal patterns, including various environmental sounds, and on a sensitivity to rhythm and beats.	sing and hum, listen to music, play an instrument, move body when music is playing, and make up songs.
Bodily/Kinesthetic Learner	Intelligence is related to physical movement and the brain's motor cortex, which controls bodily motion.	learn by hands-on methods, demonstrate skill in crafts, tinker, perform, display physical endurance, and challenge self physically.
Interpersonal Learner	Intelligence operates primarily through person-to-person relationships and communication.	have lots of friends, talk to people, join groups, play cooperative games, solve problems as part of a group, and volunteer help when others need it.
Intrapersonal Learner	Intelligence is related to inner states of being, self-reflection, metacognition, and awareness of spiritual realities.	work alone, pursue own interests, daydream, keep a personal diary or journal, and think about starting own business.

IS GOOD AT...	LEARNS BEST BY...	FAMOUS LEARNERS
memorizing names, dates, places, and trivia; spelling; using descriptive language; and creating imaginary worlds.	saying, hearing, and seeing words.	Maya Angelou—poet Abraham Lincoln—U.S. President and statesman Jerry Seinfeld—comedian Mary Hatwood Futrell—international teacher, leader, orator
math, reasoning, logic, problem solving, computing numbers, moving from concrete to abstract, thinking conceptually.	categorizing, classifying, and working with abstract patterns and relationships.	Stephen Hawking—physicist Albert Einstein—theoretical physicist Marilyn Burns—math educator Alexa Canady—neurosurgeon
understanding the use of space and how to get around in it, thinking in three-dimensional terms, and imagining things in clear visual images.	visualizing, dreaming, using the mind's eye, and working with colors and pictures.	Pablo Picasso—artist Maria Martinez—Pueblo Indian famous for black pottery Faith Ringgold—painter, quilter, and writer I. M. Pei—architect
measuring, charting, mapping, observing plants and animals, keeping journals, collecting, classifying, participating in outdoor activities.	visualizing, hands-on activities, bringing outdoors into the classroom, relating home/classroom to the natural world.	George Washington Carver—agricultural chemist Rachael Carson—scientific writer Charles Darwin—evolutionist John James Audubon—conservationist
remembering melodies; keeping time; mimicking beat and rhythm; noticing pitches, rhythms, and background and environmental sounds.	rhythm, melody, and music.	Henry Mancini—composer Marian Anderson—contralto Midori—violinist Paul McCartney—singer, songwriter, musician
physical activities such as sports, dancing, acting, and crafts.	touching, moving, interacting with space, and processing knowledge through bodily sensations.	Marcel Marceau—mime Jackie Joyner-Kersey—Olympic gold medalist in track and field Katherine Dunham—modern dancer Dr. Christiaan Barnard—cardiac surgeon
understanding people and their feelings, leading others, organizing, communicating, manipulating, mediating conflicts.	sharing, comparing, relating, cooperating, and interviewing.	Jimmy Carter—U.S. President and statesman Eleanor Roosevelt—former First Lady Lee Iacocca—president of Chrysler Corporation Mother Teresa—winner of Nobel Peace Prize
understanding self, focusing inward on feelings/dreams, following instincts, pursuing interests, and being original.	working alone, doing individualized projects, engaging in self-paced instruction.	Marva Collins—educator Maria Montessori—educator and physician Sigmund Freud—psychotherapist Anne Sexton—poet

REFERENCES

Internet Disclaimer

The Internet listings provided are a source of extended information related to *Nutrition & Wellness*. We have made every effort to recommend sites that are informative and accurate. However, these sites are not under the control of Glencoe/McGraw-Hill, and therefore Glencoe/McGraw-Hill makes no representation concerning the content of these sites. We strongly encourage teachers to preview Internet sites before students use them. Many sites contain links to other sites, and following such links may eventually lead to exposure to inappropriate material. Internet sites are sometimes "under construction" and may not always be available. Sites may also move or have been discontinued completely by the time you or your students attempt to access them.

WEB SITES

The following is a small sampling of Internet resources related to food, nutrition, and wellness. For additional web sites of interest, see the "Organizations" section.

La Casa de Comida (The House of Food)
Student-created site featuring a recipe database, food science experiments, and information on food safety, nutrition, digestion, eating disorders, ecology, and more.
http://library.thinkquest.org/15873

Cooking Light
A searchable database of lower-fat and lower-calorie recipes, plus menu ideas, cooking tips, and fitness information.
www.cookinglight.com

Culinary.net
Recipes, food and nutrition information, and a gateway to food associations and companies.
www.culinary.net

Epicurious
Cooking tips, a searchable recipe database, and a dictionary of culinary terms. From the publisher of *Bon Appetit* and *Gourmet* magazines.
www.epicurious.com

Federal Resources for Educational Excellence (FREE)
Teaching and learning resources from numerous federal agencies.
www.ed.gov/free

FDA Kids' Home Page
Information on food safety and other health topics geared toward kids and teens.
www.fda.gov/oc/opacom/kids

Fight BAC!

Information, games, and curriculum resources from the Partnership for Food Safety Education.
www.fightbac.org

FoodSafety.gov

Gateway to government food safety information.
www.foodsafety.gov

Gateway to Educational Materials (GEM)

A database of more than 17,000 education resources. Sponsored by the U.S. Department of Education.
http://thegateway.org

Girl Power—Bodywise

Advice for girls ages 9 to 14, on nutrition, fitness, and eating disorders, from the U.S. Department of Health and Human Services.
www.girlpower.gov/girlarea/bodywise

Healthfinder

Gateway to reliable health information resources selected by the U.S. Department of Health and Human Services.
www.healthfinder.gov

The Healthy Refrigerator

Heart-healthy recipes and tips, nutrition information, and facts on heart disease.
www.healthyfridge.org

Homeplate

Non-judgmental articles about healthful and disordered eating. Sponsored by the Boston College Eating Awareness Team.
www.bc.edu/bc_org/svp/uhs/eating

iEmily.com

Health and wellness site aimed at teen girls. Includes articles, columns, recipes, and interactive forums.
www.iemily.com

KidsHealth.org for Teens

Information from medical experts, plus games and animations. Sponsored by the Nemours Foundation.
http://kidshealth.org/teen

Nutrient Data Laboratory

Searchable, downloadable database of USDA nutrient values for thousands of foods.
www.nal.usda.gov/fnic/foodcomp

Nutrition.gov

A guide to nutrition and health information on federal government Web sites.
www.nutrition.gov

Powerful Bones, Powerful Girls

Articles, quizzes, and games that encourage young girls to eat a calcium-rich diet and stay active. Part of the National Bone Health Campaign.
www.cdc.gov/powerfulbones

Quackwatch

A guide to health fraud, quackery, and intelligent decisions.
www.quackwatch.com

The Recipe Link

Searchable recipe database, menus, message boards, information on hunger relief, and links to food-related sites.
www.recipelink.com

RecipeSource

Wide-ranging recipe database, including many ethnic cuisines. Can be searched by keyword and browsed by region or type of dish.
www.recipesource.com

Shape Up America!

A national initiative, founded by C. Everett Koop, to promote healthy weight and increased physical activity.
www.shapeup.org

Team Nutrition
Nutrition education information for schools, students, parents, and communities. Developed by USDA's Food and Nutrition Service.
www.fns.usda.gov/tn

Tufts University Nutrition Navigator
A ratings guide to nutrition web sites.
http://navigator.tufts.edu

ORGANIZATIONS

Besides the organizations listed here, many food industry organizations and companies provide food and nutrition information. Internet links can help you locate those resources.

American Alliance for Health, Physical Education, Recreation, and Dance
1900 Association Drive
Reston, VA 20191-1598
(703) 476-3400
www.aahperd.org

American Association of Family and Consumer Sciences
1555 King Street
Alexandria, VA 22314
(703) 706-4600
www.aafcs.org

American Council on Exercise
5820 Oberlin Drive, Suite 102
San Diego, CA 92121-3787
www.acefitness.org

American Council on Science and Health
1995 Broadway, Second Floor
New York, NY 10023-5860
(212) 362-7044
www.acsh.org

American Dietetic Association
216 West Jackson Boulevard
Chicago, IL 60606-6995
(312) 899-4718
www.eatright.org

The Body Positive
2550 9th St., Suite 204B
Berkeley, CA 94710
(510) 548-0101
email: info@thebodypositive.org
www.thebodypositive.org

Cooperative Extension Service
(Look in your phone book under the name of your county or under United States Government, Agriculture Department)
www.reeusda.gov

FDA Center for Food Safety and Applied Nutrition
200 C Street SW
Washington, DC 20204
www.cfsan.fda.gov

FDA Consumer Information Office
5600 Fishers Lane
Rockville, MD 20857
(301) 827-7130
1-888-463-6332
www.fda.gov

FDA Office of Biotechnology
200 C Street SW
Washington, DC 20204
(202) 205-4144

International Center for Sports Nutrition
502 S. 44th. Street, Suite 3012
Omaha, NE 68105-1065
(402) 559-5505

International Food Additives Council
5775 Peachtree-Dunwoody Road, Suite 500-G
Atlanta, GA 30342
(404) 252-3663

International Food Information Council
1100 Connecticut Avenue NW, Suite 430
Washington D.C. 20036
(202) 296-6540
email: foodinfo@ific.health.org
http://ific.org

**National Association of Anorexia Nervosa
  and Associated Disorders**
P.O. Box 7
Highland Park, IL 60035
(847) 831-3438
email: info@anad.org
www.anad.org

National Council Against Health Fraud
119 Foster Street
Peabody, MA 01960
(978) 532-9383
www.ncahf.org

National Eating Disorders Association
603 Stewart St., Suite 803
Seattle, WA 98101
(206) 382-3587
email: info@nationaleatingdisorders.org
www.nationaleatingdisorders.org

National Health Information Center
P.O. Box 1133
Washington, DC 20013-1133
(301) 565-4167
1-800-336-4797
www.health.gov/nhic

National Institutes of Health
9000 Rockville Pike
Bethesda, MD 20892
(301) 496-4000
www.nih.gov/health

**National Student Campaign Against Hunger
  and Homelessness**
233 N. Pleasant Ave.
Amherst, MA 01002
(413) 253-6417
email: nscah@aol.com
www.pirg.org/nscahh

North American Vegetarian Society
P.O. Box 72
Dolgeville, NY 13329
(518) 568-7970
www.navs-online.org

**President's Council on Physical Fitness and
  Sports**
200 Independence Ave. SW
Washington, DC 20201
(202) 690-9000
www.fitness.gov

**USDA Center for Nutrition Policy and
  Promotion**
3101 Park Center Drive, Room 1034
Alexandria, VA 22102-1594
(703) 305-7600
www.usda.gov/cnpp

**USDA Food and Nutrition Information
  Center**
National Agricultural Library, Room 105
10301 Baltimore Avenue
Beltsville, MD 20705-2351
(301) 504-5719
email: fnic@nal.usda.gov
www.nal.usda.gov/fnic

REFERENCES

USDA Food Safety and Inspection Service
1400 Independence Ave. SW
Washington, DC 20250
(202) 720-2791
www.fsis.usda.gov

USDA Meat and Poultry Hotline
1-800-535-4555

U.S. Department of Health and Human Services
200 Independence Avenue SW
Washington, DC 20201
(202) 619-0257
www.hhs.gov

U.S. Environmental Protection Agency
Public Information Center
401 M St., SW
Washington, DC 20460
(202) 260-5922
www.epa.gov

Vegetarian Resource Group
P.O. Box 1463, Dept. IN
Baltimore, MD 21203
(410) 366-VEGE
email: vrg@vrg.org
www.vrg.org

MULTIMEDIA

CD-ROMs Available from Glencoe/McGraw-Hill

An Introduction to Food Science
Basic Food Preparation
Eating Healthy: What's a Serving?
Exploring the World of Work: An Interactive Career Planner
Food Safety: What You Don't Know Can Hurt You
Job Readiness Skills Series
Nutrition & Menu Planner
Nutrition and Physical Activity: On Your Own Explorations

Videos Available from Glencoe/McGraw-Hill

Nutrition, Health, and Wellness
ABCNews InterActive: Making Responsible Decisions
ABCNews InterActive: Nutrition & Wellness
Eating Healthy: What's a Serving?
Food Sensitivities: Allergy and Intolerance
Investigating Food Additives
The Exercise and Nutrition Connection
The New Nutrition Pyramid
Nutrition for Active Fitness
Read the Food Label

Eating Disorders
Anorexia: Thin Obsession
Bulimia: The Vicious Cycle
When Food Is the Enemy: Eating Disorders

Weight Management
Controlling Weight Sensibly
Diet and Weight Management
Fad Diets: The Weight Loss Merry-Go-Round

Vegetarian Nutrition

Exploring Vegetarianism: A Healthy Alternative
Vegetarianism

Food Preparation

The After-School Cookbook
Cooking for One or Two
Cooking with Convenience Foods
Cooking with Healthy Seasonings
Ecology in the Kitchen
Herbs and Spices
Low Fat Cooking
Planning a Dinner Party
Quickbreads
Setting the Table
Table Settings: Banquets to Barbecues
Timing & Organization in Food Preparation

Food Safety

Food Safety: What You Don't Know Can Hurt You
Safe and Sanitary Dishwashing
Safety in the Kitchen

Food Science

An Introduction to Food Science
Food Science Experiments Video
Overview of Biotechnology

Historical and Cultural Foods

Foods from Other Lands
The History of American Cuisine
Overview of Cuisine

Careers

Workforce 2000 Video Library

Glencoe/McGraw-Hill
P.O. Box 543
Blacklick, OH 43004-9902
1-800-334-7344
www.glencoe.com

Other Multimedia Sources

Cambridge Educational
P.O. Box 931
Monmouth Junction, NJ 08852-0931
(609) 419-8000
email: custserve@cambridgeeducational.com
www.cambridgeeducational.com

Guidance Associates
100 South Bedford Road, Suite 120
Mount Kisco, NY 10549
(914) 666-4100
email: info@guidanceassociates.com
www.guidanceassociates.com

Learning Seed
330 Telser Road
Lake Zurich, IL 60047
(847) 540-8855
email: learnseed@aol.com
www.learningseed.com

Pennsylvania State University
Students Serving It Safe
CD-ROM, Macintosh and Windows
(814) 863-3826
email: ssis@psu.edu
http://nutr88.hhdev.psu.edu/adow/
    ssis_mainmenu.html

Sunburst Communications
101 Castleton Street
Suite 201
Pleasantville, NY 10570
(914) 747-3310
www.sunburst.com

USDA Food and Nutrition Service
yourSelf Nutrition Education Kit
Includes teacher's guide, videocassette, duplication masters, poster, and 30 copies each of *yourSelf* magazine and student activity guide.
www.fns.usda.gov/tn/Resources/yourself.html

BOOKS

Nutrition, Health, and Wellness

Berg, Frances M. *Children and Teens Afraid to Eat: Helping Youth in Today's Weight-Obsessed World*. Healthy Weight Journal, 2000.

Breier, Davida Gypsy, ed. *Vegan & Vegetarian FAQ: Answers to Your Frequently Asked Questions*. Vegetarian Resource Group, 2001.

Coleman, Ellen, and Suzanne Nelson Steen. *Ultimate Sports Nutrition*. 2nd ed. Bull Publishing, 2000.

Duyff, Roberta Larson. *American Dietetic Association Complete Food and Nutrition Guide*. 2nd ed. John Wiley & Sons, 2002.

Havala, Suzanne. *Being Vegetarian for Dummies*. John Wiley & Sons, 2001.

Katz, David L., and Maura Gonzalez. *The Way to Eat: Why We Eat the Way We Do, and What You Can Do About It*. Sourcebooks, 2002.

Kowtaluk, Helen. *Discovering Food and Nutrition*. 6th ed. Glencoe/McGraw-Hill, 2001.

Kowtaluk, Helen, and Alice Orphanos Kopan. *Food for Today*. 8th ed. Glencoe/McGraw-Hill, 2004.

Margen, Sheldon, and the Editors of the University of California, Berkeley Wellness Letter. *Wellness Encyclopedia of Food and Nutrition*. Rebus, 2002.

Merki, Mary Bronson, and Don Merki. *Glencoe Health: A Guide to Wellness*. 8th ed. Glencoe/McGraw-Hill, 2003.

Pennington, Jean A. T. *Bowes & Church's Food Values of Portions Commonly Used*. 17th ed. Lippincott Williams & Wilkins, 1998.

Food Preparation

AAFCS Nutrition, Health and Food Management Division. *Food: A Handbook of Terminology, Purchasing and Preparation*. 10th ed. American Association of Family and Consumer Sciences, 2001.

Carter, John Mack (ed.) *Good Housekeeping Illustrated Cookbook*. Rev. ed. Hearst Books, 2001.

Herbst, Sharon Tyler. *The New Food Lover's Companion*. 3rd ed. Barrons Educational Series, 2001.

Johnson & Wales University. *Culinary Essentials*. Glencoe/McGraw-Hill, 2002.

Miller, Bryan. *Cooking for Dummies*. 2nd ed. John Wiley & Sons, 2000.

Rombauer, Irma S.; Marion Rombauer Becker; and Ethan Becker. *Joy of Cooking*. Scribner, 1997.

Food Safety

McSwane, David; Nancy Rue; and Richard Linton. *Essentials of Food Safety & Sanitation*. 2nd ed. Prentice Hall, 2002.

Scott, Elizabeth, and Paul Sockett. *How to Prevent Food Poisoning: A Practical Guide to Safe Cooking, Eating, and Food Handling*. John Wiley & Sons, 1998.

Food Science

Barham, Peter. *The Science of Cooking.* Springer Verlag, 2001.

Mehas, Kay Yockey, and Sharon Lesley Rodgers. *Food Science: The Biochemistry of Food and Nutrition.* 4th ed. Glencoe/McGraw-Hill, 2002.

Wolke, Robert L. *What Einstein Told His Cook: Kitchen Science Explained.* W. W. Norton, 2002.

Historical and Cultural Foods

Davidson, Alan. *The Oxford Companion to Food.* Oxford University Press, 1999.

Duyff, Roberta Larson. *Food Folklore: Tales and Truths About What We Eat.* John Wiley & Sons, 1999. (ADA Nutrition Now Series)

Kittler, Pamela Goyan, and Kathryn P. Sucher. *Food and Culture: A Nutrition Handbook.* 3rd ed. Wadsworth Publishing, 2000.

Careers

Kelly-Plate, Joan, and Ruth Volz-Patton. *Exploring Careers.* 3rd ed. Glencoe/McGraw-Hill, 2000.

Kimbrell, Grady, and Ben S. Vineyard. *Succeeding in the World of Work.* 7th ed. Glencoe/McGraw-Hill, 2003.

Ryan, Jerry, and Roberta Ryan. *Preparing for Career Success.* Glencoe/McGraw-Hill, 2000.

PERIODICALS

Consumer Reports on Health
101 Truman Avenue
Yonkers, NY 10703
www.consumerreports.org

Environmental Nutrition
52 Riverside Drive, Suite 15-A
New York, NY 10024-6599
www.environmentalnutrition.com

FDA Consumer
P.O. Box 371954
Pittsburgh, PA 15250-7954
(202) 512-1800
www.fda.gov

Food & Fitness Advisor
P.O. Box 420235
Palm Coast, FL 32142-0235

Mayo Clinic Health Letter
P.O. Box 53889
Boulder, CO 80322-3889
www.mayoclinic.org/publications

Tufts University Health & Nutrition Letter
10 High Street, Suite 706
Boston, MA 01220
www.healthletter.tufts.edu

University of California, Berkeley Wellness Letter
P.O. Box 420148
Palm Coast, FL 32142
www.wellnessletter.com

ANSWERS TO REVIEW QUESTIONS

CHAPTER 1

UNDERSTANDING KEY IDEAS

1. Reaching for your personal overall best level of health; physical, mental/emotional, social.

2. Any four: following a varied and healthful eating plan; drinking enough fluids; getting plenty of physical activity; eating breakfast every morning; getting about eight hours of sleep every night; practicing good hygiene; taking safety precautions such as wearing a seat belt; getting regular medical and dental checkups; avoiding tobacco, alcohol, and harmful drugs; and keeping informed about nutrition and wellness.

3. People with good mental and emotional health often have better physical health. Mental and emotional health helps you cope with change; face problems; handle anger, frustration, and disappointment in an acceptable way; and work toward goals. With emotional well-being comes sensitivity to others, open-mindedness, self-esteem, and self-confidence.

4. The person can praise and accept others; enjoys friends of both genders; is helpful and considerate; can accept rules and be responsible; handles conflict in a constructive way; communicates well; and handles peer pressure without compromising values.

5. Eating well promotes health, energy, and growth; food provides nutrients that nourish your body.

6. Where you live affects what food is available, which in turn can affect your food choices. Other influences include the people around you, your culture, your resources, advertising, your knowledge of food and nutrition, and your age, attitudes, emotions, health, and goals.

7. Set realistic goals that match your abilities and needs.

DEVELOPING LIFE SKILLS

Answers may vary.

1. Answers should include the following steps: Identify the decision. Collect information and identify your resources. Identify the possible choices. Weigh the possible choices. Choose the best option. Take action. Evaluate your decision.

2. Parents and medical professionals have a responsibility for the health of others. In many other situations, wellness is an individual responsibility. The desire for change has to come from within. A leadership role might involve educating others about ways to improve health and wellness, setting a good example by your own actions, and encouraging those who are taking steps to improve their wellness. In these ways peer pressure can be a positive influence.

WELLNESS CHALLENGE

Answers may vary.

1. Jamie could say no to running for club president. She could try to rearrange her work schedule. Tracking how she spends her free time might help her find more time for family, friends, and fun. Setting goals and priorities might help her manage her time.

2. Jamie eats breakfast and lunch every day; she gets physical activity by marching in the band; the Spanish club keeps her involved socially. To improve her nutrition, she might pack nutritious food to eat before going to work.

CHAPTER 2

UNDERSTANDING KEY IDEAS

1. Hunger signals that your body needs food energy and nutrients. The sensation goes away when you've had enough to eat.

2. When you have a good appetite, you're more likely to eat the variety of foods you need for good health.

3. Examples may include: Emotional—eating to relieve stress or boredom, showing love by preparing a meal for someone, craving comfort food when sad. Social—sharing a meal and conversation with family or friends.

4. You might enjoy food less. The papillae on the tongue contain the taste buds. If they were burned you might not be able to experience the full flavor of food, and flavor contributes to eating enjoyment.

5. Eating with others can add to the enjoyment of food. A family meal can be a relaxing way to spend time together and communicate with one another.

6. Etiquette shows respect and consideration for others, helps others feel at ease and valued, and makes mealtimes more pleasant and relaxed. Examples will vary.

7. Discreetly attract the server's attention and politely explain the problem.

DEVELOPING LIFE SKILLS

Answers may vary.

1. Pleasant talk helps people relax and enjoy one another's company. Examples of appropriate topics: talking about the day's activities, sharing enjoyable memories, and discussing books, movies, sports, or current events (if not too controversial or upsetting). Inappropriate topics include any that might stir up conflict, upset or embarrass people, or cause people to lose their appetite; these would make the meal less pleasant for everyone.

2. If students need examples to get started, suggest a decorative houseplant, a colander filled with fresh fruit, or a pitcher filled with colorful rolled-up napkins.

3. Family members might rearrange activities so they can eat together more often. They might increase the time available for eating together by saving time in meal preparation. They might set aside time for special family meals on days when their schedules are more free.

WELLNESS CHALLENGE

Answers may vary.

1. Yes; without a good appetite Nana Rose might not eat enough nutritious food for good health.

2. Older adults often have a less keen sense of taste. Also, Nana Rose might miss favorite foods that she used to prepare when she lived on her own.

3. To help stimulate Nana Rose's appetite, they might think of ways to make meals look and taste more appealing, such as paying attention to the color combinations on the plate. They might ask Nana Rose what some of her favorite foods are, how she likes them prepared, and whether she'd like to help with meal preparation (if she doesn't already). They could make sure that mealtimes are enjoyable family gatherings with pleasant surroundings.

CHAPTER 3
UNDERSTANDING KEY IDEAS

1. Through ethnic food traditions, religious customs, and cultural holidays.

2. Climate, geography, commerce, immigration, and travel. Cuisines feature plentiful foods more than scarce foods.

3. Regional foods develop where climate and geography are good for producing certain foods, and may also reflect the ethnic diversity of the region.

4. Possible examples: Tomatoes, peanuts, cocoa beans, and potatoes all originated in the Americas; tomatoes became identified with Italian sauce, peanuts with African cuisine, cocoa beans with Swiss chocolate, and potatoes with Ireland.

5. It adds variety to your food choices; many cuisines feature plenty of grain products, vegetables, and fruits.

6. Possible examples: try foods at regional or ethnic festivals, visit food markets when you travel, buy regional or ethnic foods when shopping, get ethnic or regional cookbooks, watch TV cooking shows, try an ethnic restaurant, ask friends to teach you how to prepare ethnic dishes, use the Internet.

DEVELOPING LIFE SKILLS

Answers may vary.

1. In some ways modern travel and communication make different parts of the world more alike, but they also allow cultural traditions to reach more people, which might help them be maintained. Students should give reasons to support their predictions.

2. Possible experiences: serving cultural foods at meals and snacks, reading stories about foods, demonstrating how foods are made. Children who are encouraged to eat a variety of foods will be more likely to do so as adults. Variety in foods means getting different nutrients. Children will also learn about a variety of cultures.

WELLNESS CHALLENGE

Answers may vary.

1. They might create posters that show how the foods offered fit into the Food Guide Pyramid (see Chapter 8) or that list the nutrients found in the foods.

2. The types of food offered; the preparation, storage, service, and cleanup; the physical setup, such as constructing a booth; and a budget for purchasing food and supplies.

3. They might ask for help from student volunteers, parents, the school food service manager, the foods and nutrition teacher, or a foreign language or social studies teacher.

CHAPTER 4

UNDERSTANDING KEY IDEAS

1. December, when they are out of season. The demand is higher than the supply, and production and transportation costs increase.

2. Hydroponics, food preservation methods, and packaging.

3. Frozen beans have a longer shelf life and about the same amount of nutrients as fresh beans.

4. Substances added to foods during processing to make them safer, more appealing, or more nutritious. Any three: to preserve food, increase nutritional value, enhance flavor and appearance, or give special qualities to food.

5. Fortified foods contain added nutrients that are not naturally present. Enriched foods contain added nutrients to restore those lost in processing.

6. It sets regulations and standards for food safety and provides consumer information.

7. Climate or geography, lack of modern transportation, lack of cooking fuel, natural disasters, and wars and political conflicts can all contribute to a low food supply in a region.

DEVELOPING LIFE SKILLS

Answers may vary.

1. Encourage students to be creative in their responses.

2. When the supply increases and the demand does not, the price goes down. Therefore, wheat farmers might not make enough money on their crops to cover their costs or stay in business. Consumers will probably pay less for wheat products.

WELLNESS CHALLENGE

Answers may vary.

I. They could research additives through government organizations and/or reliable Internet sources.

2. The information may be difficult to obtain or understand. They may not agree even after collecting information.

3. They could write or call a food company or extension agent for more information. They could discuss the pros and cons and try to reach a compromise.

CHAPTER 5

UNDERSTANDING KEY IDEAS

I. Carbohydrates, fats, proteins, vitamins, minerals, and water. The body cannot make most nutrients, so you must get them from food. The nutrients perform different tasks and all work together to promote good health. If you eat too little of a particular nutrient, the other nutrients may not be able to do their jobs.

2. Supply energy, build and repair your body, and keep your body's system running smoothly.

3. Too much of certain vitamins can cause serious harm to the body.

4. Shortage of a nutrient. If it continues, a nutrient deficiency may result in poor health or lack of energy.

5. He might not have enough energy for physical activities or body processes, because most teen males require at least 2,800 calories a day.

6. Mouth: saliva breaks down food chemically and chewing breaks it down physically; stomach: gastric juices further break down food chemically; small intestines: digestive juices fully break down food.

7. The amount of energy used for body functions.

DEVELOPING LIFE SKILLS

Answers may vary.

I. Because nutrition discoveries are still being made, it is impossible to say whether any product provides all the nutrients you need. Also, the product may not provide the right balance of nutrients or the right amounts for individual needs.

2. Health experts needed a way to communicate information about the amount of nutrients in food products in a way that consumers would find easy to use.

WELLNESS CHALLENGE

Answers may vary.

I. Shanika needs enough fuel from the foods she eats to provide energy for her training sessions and for the charity walk.

2. Shanika could learn more about eating the right kinds and amounts of food for physical activity. She could track the number of calories she consumes each day and compare it to the recommended number for her age, gender, and activity level. She could also train for the charity event by walking several times a week, gradually increasing her time and distance.

CHAPTER 6

UNDERSTANDING KEY IDEAS

I. Your body uses carbohydrates for energy. It can also use proteins for energy, but mainly uses proteins for growth, repair, and to fight disease. Vitamins don't supply energy or build body tissue, but they help regulate those processes and many others.

2. Fiber is a plant material that can't be digested; it helps your digestive system work properly and may help protect against heart disease and cancer.

3. Fat supplies energy, promotes healthy skin and normal growth, and carries fat-soluble vitamins.

4. An eating plan high in saturated fat (butter) tends to increase blood cholesterol level more than unsaturated fat (oil); a high blood cholesterol level increases risk of heart problems.

5. Eat a variety of plant-based foods, including legumes, seeds, and nuts.

6. It is water-soluble and cannot be stored by the body.

7. Regulating body processes; becoming part of body tissues such as bones, teeth, and blood. Possible examples: calcium regulates heartbeat and builds bone. Examples will vary but should be consistent with the chart on page 97.

8. Water performs many life-supporting functions such as carrying nutrients, eliminating wastes, and regulating body temperature. You could live only a few days without water.

9. A doctor might prescribe supplements for people who are elderly, pregnant or nursing, taking certain medications, recovering from illness, or following special diets.

DEVELOPING LIFE SKILLS

Answers may vary.

I. No. Fat is an essential nutrient, so it should not be eliminated from the diet (which would be almost impossible because fat is found in many foods). Students should say they would be skeptical of other statements in the article, since it does not appear to be a reliable source of information. (Note: Chapter 20 explains that the best way to lose weight is with a combination of physical activity and balanced food choices.)

2. Tell the friend that taking extra amounts of vitamin supplements can be harmful and that vitamins don't supply energy. Approaches will vary but should reflect tact and consideration.

WELLNESS CHALLENGE

Answers may vary.

I. She can eat enough foods rich in bone-building minerals—calcium, phosphorus, and magnesium—and perform regular weight-bearing physical activity.

2. If she pays attention to bone-building food choices and physical activity for several weeks, these actions can become a habit. She could: identify specific goals for being active and create an action plan as described in Chapter I; create a motivational poster for herself; enlist a friend or family member to keep her motivated; continue to read about bone health.

CHAPTER 7

UNDERSTANDING KEY IDEAS

I. Helps ensure a healthful eating plan that provides all the necessary nutrients, while limiting those that increase the risk for health problems.

2. Being overweight with too much body fat increases chances of heart disease, some cancers, and diabetes. Being underweight can lead to illness, feeling tired, or not growing properly.

3. Possible examples: Eat several servings of whole-grain cereals and breads a day; drink fruit or vegetable juice with meals; eat legumes (cooked dry beans) several times a week; eat new-to-you foods; add colorful foods like yellow, deep green, orange, and red fruits and veggies.

4. A condition that increases the chances of having health problems. Examples include eating too much cholesterol or fat, especially saturated fat.

5. Fat provides more calories per gram than carbohydrate. The extra calories from any foods, including high-fat foods, are stored as body fat if not used. Ways to eat less fat include choosing foods with little or no fat, eating legumes one or more times a week, eating fish several times a week, and buying lean meat and poultry.

6. Taste food first, then season lightly with salt only if needed; flavor foods with herbs, spices, citrus peel, vinegar, or lemon; and eat fewer salty snacks.

DEVELOPING LIFE SKILLS

Answers may vary.

1. Following the guidelines helps teens get the nourishment they need for wellness now and reduce risks for some health problems later in life. Possible challenges: most teens do not make food purchases for the household; influence of peer pressure and advertising.

2. Guidelines may differ depending on local food habits. For instance, where vegetarianism is common, a guideline for eating plenty of fruits and vegetables may be unnecessary. Guidelines may be similar because nutrient needs are similar for people of the same age and gender, no matter where they live.

WELLNESS CHALLENGE

Answers may vary.

1. They could survey students to find out why they do or don't participate in physical education class and what sports or activities they enjoy.

2. Challenges might include identifying physical activity options that interest teens and finding a creative and effective way to get the physical activity message to teens. Solutions will vary.

CHAPTER 8

UNDERSTANDING KEY IDEAS

1. The groups from which you should eat the most servings are larger blocks in the Pyramid. If you follow Pyramid recommendations for the number of servings from each food group, you will eat a variety of foods including plenty of grain products, vegetables, and fruits.

2. Foods within each group provide similar nutrients. If an eating plan doesn't include enough foods from each group, it might not provide enough of some nutrients either.

3. On average, 9 servings. Example of food choices: a slice of toast, 2 ounces of ready-to-eat cereal, a sandwich, a bagel, and a cup of cooked pasta.

4. About ½ serving from Meat, Poultry, Fish, Dry Beans, Eggs, and Nuts Group (1 egg + ½ oz. ham = 1 ½ oz. meat); ½ serving from Vegetables Group; ½ serving from Milk, Yogurt, and Cheese Group.

DEVELOPING LIFE SKILLS

Answers may vary.

1. Sample answer: bean and cheese burrito with lettuce and tomato; rice; fruit cup. Encourage students to be creative in planning their menus.

2. Create a meal planning checklist to be sure recommended food groups servings are provided; keep a record of recent menus to avoid repeating specific foods too often; plan several weeks of menus at one time.

3. Students who feel the Pyramid conveys information clearly might say that it visually conveys the message of how to choose a healthful eating plan: 1) variety—shows different food groups and includes food choices to match your lifestyle and preferences; 2) balance—uses the pyramid shape to illustrate which food groups should be eaten in larger and smaller amounts; and 3) moderation—places fats, oils, and sweets in the small space at the tip. Students who feel it is not a good communication tool should suggest specific improvements.

WELLNESS CHALLENGE

Answers may vary.

1. Malcolm might explain that variety will provide Dan with different nutrients and flavors. He might show Dan easy ways to make other foods.

2. Dan might be unwilling to change or unsure of how to get started.

3. Malcolm might bring a lunch for Dan to motivate him to try new foods. Malcolm could explain how quickly and easily he made the lunch. Malcolm might challenge Dan to be creative and eat something different at least once during the week. Malcolm and Dan might make a meal plan for Dan and a list of the ingredients he will need to buy in advance. Malcolm could help Dan choose foods that will be easy to make.

CHAPTER 9

UNDERSTANDING KEY IDEAS

1. Both fetus and mother depend on her food choices for nourishment. Folate, iron, and calcium.

2. At two months, babies can eat mother's milk or formula. By about eight months, most can eat strained meats, fruits, vegetables, juice, toast, and teething biscuits.

3. Yes. Their stomachs are small, so they may not be able to eat enough at meals to satisfy their nutrient and energy needs.

4. During the teen years. Energy and nutrient needs are higher during periods of rapid growth.

5. The 11-year old probably needs fewer servings from the fruit, vegetable, and bread groups of the Pyramid, but more servings from the milk group (see charts on pages 84, 119, and 131).

DEVELOPING LIFE SKILLS

Answers may vary.

1. Carolina could introduce new foods in small amounts without pressuring Luis and set an example by eating the foods herself. She could prepare foods that are colorful and cut into interesting shapes. She might use calming music to help make mealtime more pleasant.

2. Possible solutions: agree with family members to eat dinner together on the weekend; coordinate weekday schedule with other family members; consider cutting back or rescheduling after-school clubs; write scheduled family meal on calendar or in weekly planning book; turn down activities that would interfere with a scheduled family meal.

Answers may vary.

1. They might invite their grandfather to join in family meals with them. They might ask him to help them with some simple tasks as they prepare the meals, showing him how to use kitchen equipment in the process. If Grandpa does not live nearby, Cassie and Brian might need to find someone else who could help him, such as one of his neighbors.

2. Possible challenges: scheduling time for meals with Grandpa; arranging transportation for visits; overcoming his possible lack of confidence in his own cooking skills; planning menus that fit his skills and food budget; overcoming possible physical obstacles, such as poor eyesight; finding or creating more opportunities for Grandpa to eat with other people.

3. They might organize a meal and transportation schedule that involves other family members and friends. They could emphasize the fun of cooking and take any kitchen mishaps in stride while Grandpa is learning to cook. They might suggest and shop for simple, inexpensive meals and print menus and recipes in large type. The teens might investigate Meals on Wheels and other senior nutrition programs in the community.

CHAPTER 10
UNDERSTANDING KEY IDEAS

1. Follow an eating plan that has plenty of grain products, vegetables, and fruits and that overall is low in fat and cholesterol.

2. Behavior related to food, eating, and weight that is extremely unhealthy and often related to emotional problems.

3. Eating very large amounts of food at one time; exercising frequently or more intensely than normal; disappearing after eating, often to the bathroom; using diet pills or laxatives.

4. Small, frequent meals that include plenty of fluids and are attractively served.

5. Food intolerance means having trouble digesting or handling a component of food. Food allergy is a sensitivity that involves the body's immune system.

6. Grilled tuna steak because it has less saturated fat.

7. Ask if it should be taken with food or on an empty stomach. Food and medicines can interact. Some medicines are better absorbed with food. Food may destroy the benefits of some medicines.

DEVELOPING LIFE SKILLS

Answers may vary.

1. Yes. The teen years are a time for establishing lifelong healthy habits. Good nutrition today increases your chances for long-term health.

2. Students should recognize that they do have a responsibility to talk to someone because their friend's health may be in serious danger. If the friend says there's no problem, it doesn't necessarily mean that's true—a person with an eating disorder usually doesn't believe that he or she needs assistance or is in any danger. Discuss appropriate people to talk to—medical professionals, a social worker, or the school nurse or counselor.

3. Restaurant: read menus carefully and choose foods with care; ask about ingredients and preparation methods before ordering. At someone's home: let the host know in advance about what foods you cannot eat so he or she can plan and prepare an appropriate menu.

WELLNESS CHALLENGE

Answers may vary.

I. Menu might include hearty soups made with fresh vegetables and grain products in forms that don't require a lot of chewing, such as diced cooked carrots, rice, or egg pastina. Menu could also include plain or flavored yogurt, gelatin, oatmeal, finely mashed beans, and soft fruits such as bananas. Beverages might include juice and water.

2. Possible challenges: extra time it will take to prepare some of these items; Kyle's sister might have a poor appetite; she might become bored with her semi-liquid eating plan.

3. Make a large batch of soup several days before the scheduled surgery and freeze it; serve small, frequent meals if appetite is poor; vary the flavors in the menu to prevent boredom.

CHAPTER 11

UNDERSTANDING KEY IDEAS

I. A degree from a reputable university, medical training in food and nutrition, or the letters *CFCS* or *RD* after the person's name.

2. Remember that the purpose of advertising is to sell a product or service. It's your job to get the facts and make the best choices for your health and budget.

3. Taking such products could produce harmful side effects and may delay reliable health care.

4. No. The fact that it discounts physicians' advice, as well as the words *breakthrough* and *miracle*, are clues to quackery.

5. Research needs to be repeated before it can be considered reliable, and news reports often oversimplify research results. Information to look for: who did the research, what are the researcher's qualifications, who paid for the study, how was the study designed, have other scientists reviewed it, and do the results apply only to certain people.

DEVELOPING LIFE SKILLS

Answers may vary.

I. Students should recognize that qualified experts can sometimes have differences of opinion; this does not mean that either of the two articles is unreliable.

2. Possible methods: school newspaper article, posters, family discussion about TV news reports. Possible main points: don't change food choices based on a single report; reports are often oversimplified; find out who was involved in research, what methods were used, and whether research has been verified; sometimes study results don't apply to everyone.

WELLNESS CHALLENGE

Answers may vary.

I. Segments might cover energy bars, fat-free snacks, or herbal supplements, for example.

2. Foods and nutrition teacher, health teacher, a local dietitian, or school nurse could offer expert advice. Students could discuss healthful lifestyle or play the roles of quacks.

3. They might do their own infomercials, offer fake testimonials with an expert to discuss them, or have students act as audience members on the talk show. They could research current news and then hold a debate or have a local expert speak on the subject.

CHAPTER 12

UNDERSTANDING KEY IDEAS

1. Any three: after the night's fast, you need food to replenish your energy supply; it helps you feel renewed and mentally alert throughout the day; breakfast eaters are more alert in the middle of the morning, concentrate better, think faster, get more done at school or work, and score better on tests than those who skip or skimp on breakfast.

2. Includes foods you like; supplies one-fourth to one-third of the nutrients you need each day; consists of foods from several food groups of the Food Guide Pyramid, such as a vitamin C–rich fruit or vegetable and a calcium-rich dairy food.

3. By choosing nutrient-dense foods; by picking mostly lean or lower-fat foods from the five food groups; by choosing snacks to fill in food-group gaps.

4. Milk, juice, water. Milk and juice offer food-group servings, and water is a nutrient.

5. People of different ages need different amounts of food and nutrients. Small children may want simpler foods and may not enjoy as great a variety of foods as others in the family.

6. You need to know that you have the necessary equipment or that you can provide a substitute. Other resources: time, energy, money, kitchen skills.

DEVELOPING LIFE SKILLS

Answers may vary.

1. Possible examples: spending more on convenience foods when time is short; using skills to perform a task by hand if a special tool, such as a garlic press, is not available; spending money on equipment, such as a bread machine, to save time and personal energy. Trade-offs are key because management involves making the best use of what you have.

2. Possible answers: two forks in place of tongs, two knives in place of pastry blender, fork in place of wire whisk, strainer in place of sifter.

WELLNESS CHALLENGE

Answers may vary.

1. It allows people to consider their own resources, such as their cooking skills, budget, and time. Also, it will help ensure that people's favorite foods are included in the menu.

2. By including a variety of foods from the five food groups for nutritional balance; by balancing different types of dishes, such as cold salads, hot side dishes, and desserts; and by providing foods suitable for people of various ages.

3. She could make a chart that lists categorizes such as appetizers, salads, and so on, with the desired number of blank spaces in each category. When people call, Keisha might ask them to suggest two or three things they would like to bring. She could use her chart to decide which of the suggestions would be a better fit with other items on the menu. She could fill in any gaps in the menu with foods that she or her family makes or buys.

CHAPTER 13

UNDERSTANDING KEY IDEAS

1. Consumers help run a food cooperative, but not a warehouse store.

2. Helps you buy what you need without overspending; reduces the possibility that you will forget items; saves you from making another trip to the store or a substitution to a recipe.

3. Food labels would help you compare nutrients and calories per serving, size of the cans, ingredients, and preparation directions and choose the one that best meets your needs.

4. Using unit prices to compare brands and sizes; using coupons; buying store brands if they are cheaper than name brands; using a frequent customer card.

5. Check the date on the package; put meat in a plastic bag to prevent juices from leaking onto other foods; take milk and meat home and refrigerate them as soon as possible.

6. Return a food item to its proper place if you decide you don't want to buy it; take your cart out of the checkout lane if you have forgotten something, rather than making customers in line behind you wait for your return; wait to open packages until you are outside the store.

DEVELOPING LIFE SKILLS

1. Students' choices will vary. Supermarket: might have higher prices than warehouse store; could overcome by using other money-saving strategies, such as coupons. Warehouse store: food may be sold in bigger quantities (could overcome by sharing with family members or another elderly person); need to bag own groceries (might need to bring someone to assist).

2. Possible answers: They might review how much they have spent on food in the past by examining receipts, check registers, and credit card statements; they might use the library or Internet to research typical consumer spending on food. Families with lower incomes must usually spend a larger percentage of their income on food than families with higher incomes. Other factors include geographic location and the number, ages, and activities of family members.

WELLNESS CHALLENGE

Answers may vary.

1. By making other teens aware of the problems some people face when shopping and recruiting volunteers; by talking to store managers about their idea; by contacting community groups to see if their program might be made part of an already existing program.

2. Helping teens first learn how to be savvy shoppers before they can help others; promoting the program to older adults.

3. Could hold training sessions for teen volunteers. Could promote the program by placing posters, announcements, or pamphlets in places where older adults are likely to see them (for example, retirement community newsletters or clubhouses, the local library).

CHAPTER 14
UNDERSTANDING KEY IDEAS

1. Scratch cooking: use unprepared foods; you can control what's in the dish and how it's made; usually takes more time, energy, and kitchen skills, but often costs less. Speed-scratch cooking: use partly prepared foods or ready-to-eat foods; can assemble a meal quickly and with less effort; usually costs more; you have less control over the ingredients.

2. Choices of moist heat methods include steaming, simmering, stewing, and microwaving. Fastest methods would be steaming and microwaving. None add fat. Choices of frying methods include stir-frying, sautéing, and deep-fat frying. All of these methods are fast. Stir-frying and sautéing would add some fat, and deep-fat frying would add more fat.

3. Compare recipes and consider whether the directions are clear, skills needed, equipment needed, if you have ingredients on hand or the time and money to shop for them, if you have time and energy to prepare the recipe, and how the dish fits into your eating plan.

4. Use less butter or margarine when preparing them; make substitutions such as evaporated fat-free milk for cream; remove the fat from the surface.

5. Add grated cheese; add calcium-fortified tofu.

DEVELOPING LIFE SKILLS

Answers may vary.

1. Packaging of many convenience foods can be wasteful and end up in landfills. Students could suggest recycling or buying in bulk.

2. If Jake doesn't understand the recipe terms, he might not prepare the recipe correctly and it might not turn out well. He might not have the time or skills to prepare a complex recipe. He could look for a simpler recipe or learn more before trying to prepare the recipe.

WELLNESS CHALLENGE

Answers may vary.

1. She might plan to use speed-scratch cooking as much as possible, plus foods that require minimal preparation (such as precooked ham that just needs to be heated). Some dishes might be prepared the day before and refrigerated. She could plan what tasks each committee member will do ahead of time and on the day of the buffet so that they work efficiently.

2. Preparing the meal in the time available; food safety concerns; whether committee members have the cooking skills and equipment needed; cost of partly prepared or ready-to-eat foods.

3. She could take an inventory of the equipment available in the school or that committee members could bring from home. She could have committee members help her select cooking methods and recipes that use available equipment, allow quick or advance preparation, and could be prepared and served safely. She might ask a foods teacher to help her hold a training session for committee members. She could investigate the costs of convenience foods and look for the most economical options.

CHAPTER 15
UNDERSTANDING KEY IDEAS

1. Amount of money you want to spend (meals at full-service restaurants usually cost more than fast food); amount of time you have available (fast food is quicker); how much service you want (full-service restaurant offers more); whether you want food cooked to order (some fast food restaurants won't cook to order); menu choices offered (varies).

2. Look for a chart with calorie and nutrient amounts for menu items; ask the server what a dish contains, how it's prepared, and the size of the portion; check the menu for descriptions, specific nutrition information, or health claims.

3. Baked potato because you can probably ask for sour cream or butter to be omitted or served on the side; potatoes au gratin have butter and cheese baked in. Asparagus with lemon and garlic because cream sauce is higher in fat.

4. Order baked chicken rather than fried; order smaller rather than larger portion; order lighter side dishes such as plain baked potato or request to have gravy served on the side.

Answers may vary.

1. The essay could begin with a paragraph that introduces the topic and grabs the attention of the reader. Successive paragraphs could support the topic with specific points. These might include: the wide variety of foods available at many fast-food restaurants, including broiled or baked foods, soups, salads, juices, and milk; strategies for making smart choices, such as using calorie and nutrition charts, asking to have higher-fat toppings served on the side, and choosing smaller portions of higher-fat items; and the fact that any foods can fit into a healthful eating plan, as long as you keep balance and moderation in mind. The last paragraph could summarize the points made and end with a strong closing statement.

2. You might tell her that she can ask the server to recommend mild dishes and explain what they are before she orders. You could point out that she might like the taste of Indian food, but she won't know if she doesn't try it. You might offer to go to another restaurant afterwards if she doesn't find any foods she wants to try at the Indian restaurant.

WELLNESS CHALLENGE

Answers may vary.

1. He could ask the server questions about the ingredients and preparation of foods, ask the server for a recommendation, and check the menu for descriptions and nutrition information.

2. The menu might not have any other low-fat choices, or the choices might not sound appealing. The server and menu might not be able to provide the information Lamar wants.

3. Lamar might decide he's willing to give a new food a try even if he's uncertain about it. He might ask whether a menu item could be modified to be lower in fat, or whether something that's not on the menu could be prepared. He might ask whether another server or the cook or chef could answer his questions. He might decide to stick with his usual choice but try other restaurants more often.

CHAPTER 16
UNDERSTANDING KEY IDEAS

1. Lacto-ovo-vegetarian. Lacto-vegetarian would include dairy foods, whereas a vegan eating plan would be limited to plant-based foods.

2. Possible answers: soy burgers instead of hamburgers; stir-fry with tofu instead of chicken, beef, or fish.

3. Without careful planning, a vegan might not get enough food energy, protein, calcium, vitamin D, vitamin B_{12}, iron, or zinc. A vegan can avoid nutritional gaps by using the Pyramid as a guideline, choosing beans and nuts from the meat and beans group, and choosing calcium-fortified soy products in place of dairy foods. Fortified cereal also provides important nutrients including vitamins B_{12} and D. Vegans might need more Pyramid servings to provide enough food energy.

4. Any two: Use the Food Guide Pyramid by choosing nonmeat protein sources; modify traditional recipes with nutrient-rich substitutions for meat, poultry, and fish; try vegetarian dishes from around the world by preparing them from recipes or going to ethnic restaurants.

DEVELOPING LIFE SKILLS

Answers may vary.

1. The vegetarian could explain in advance what foods he or she does and doesn't eat. The nonvegetarian could ask questions to improve understanding, let the vegetarian know what foods are planned, and ask whether they will be suitable. Both could show respect for the other's eating style.

2. An eating plan that excludes meat, poultry, and fish is not automatically healthful. Unless it is carefully planned, it may lack variety and therefore nutrients, or it may include too many high-fat foods or sweets.

WELLNESS CHALLENGE

Answers may vary.

1. Answers should address the importance of working together to identify and agree on solutions.

2. Nina might prepare her own meals but eat them with the family. With some foods, such as spaghetti sauce, meat could be cooked separately and added after Nina takes her helping. Nina and her parents could look for vegetarian recipes that the whole family would enjoy.

CHAPTER 17
UNDERSTANDING KEY IDEAS

1. How well your heart and lungs can keep up with your activity. Improving it enables your body to use oxygen more efficiently, so you can be more active without tiring.

2. It offers the benefits of many components of physical fitness, including muscular strength and endurance, flexibility, coordination and balance, and cardiorespiratory endurance.

3. Physical activity helps you look your best, so you feel better about yourself. It also helps you to manage stress by giving you stamina so that you're more energetic and ready to face challenges. It improves your mood, making it easier to concentrate and think positively. It helps you to sleep soundly so that you feel refreshed.

4. Do several short sessions of physical activity during the day adding up to 30 minutes; make everyday activity count for physical activity; do 15 to 20 minutes of more intense activity at least three times a week.

5. Too much physical activity can cause injury and make a person feel too tired for other tasks. In females, too much activity can cause problems with the reproductive cycle.

DEVELOPING LIFE SKILLS

Answers may vary.

1. Physical activity gives you more endurance and energy. It also helps you sleep better so that you feel more refreshed when you wake up.

2. Teens might offer to walk, bike, swim, or play tennis with their parents, grandparents, or other adults in their family. They could organize team sports that everyone might enjoy such as volleyball, basketball, or softball. It is important because people of all ages need to stay physically active. Anyone who engages in physical activity reaps the benefits.

WELLNESS CHALLENGE

Answers may vary.

1. Indoor sports in the school gymnasium when it's not in use; community recreation options such as skating rinks; dressing for the weather and sledding or ice skating; helping older adults shovel snow.

2. She might suggest specific physical activities when she and her friends are making after-school or weekend plans. She could remind her friends of how much they enjoy physical activities at other times of the year. She might point out that she plans to stay in shape through the winter to be better prepared for other activities in the spring.

CHAPTER 18

UNDERSTANDING KEY IDEAS

1. Lack of time could be overcome by making everyday living more active. For example, the teen might walk or ride a bicycle somewhere rather than ride in a car.

2. Determine how active you are now; set challenging but realistic fitness goals; choose physical activities that offer benefits to match your goals; put your plan into action; make health and safety a priority; identify obstacles and ways to overcome them if necessary; check your progress; and adjust your goals if necessary.

3. Possible answers: running, walking, hiking, swimming, mowing the lawn.

4. F.I.T. stands for frequency, intensity, and time. Increasing these factors gradually can help you improve your level of fitness.

5. Warming up prepares your muscles for a workout and increases your heart rate gradually. Cooling down increases flexibility and may help prevent stiffness and soreness.

6. Change your strategies, overcome challenges, reconsider your original goal, and allow yourself more time to achieve your goal.

DEVELOPING LIFE SKILLS

Answers may vary.

1. Elena might be assuming that all activities require the same skills. While coordination is important, field hockey requires muscular strength and endurance. Points to consider: Training could help improve the skills she needs; she doesn't need to be the star player to have fun and enjoy the benefits; other teens have similar challenges; trying a sport is the way to find out if it's right for you; if field hockey isn't right for her, she can try something else.

2. Setting a goal that is too high may cause a person to give up because the task is too difficult. It may also lead to injury if the person strains to achieve results. Too low a goal will not provide enough challenge and the person may lose interest. Following the F.I.T. guidelines can help a person set appropriate goals. The talk/sing test is also a good guideline.

WELLNESS CHALLENGE

Answers may vary.

1. They might encourage their friends to join them for team sports, such as basketball, softball, soccer, or volleyball, or they could organize a group hiking trip or nature walk. They might find out about community centers and other places where people can participate in physical activities. In addition, they might encourage active play with children when they baby-sit or volunteer to do active things with scouting groups, church groups, and so on.

2. They might advertise group activities by posting notices on the school bulletin board or in the school newspaper. They might contact the director of recreational activities at their local community center. They will have to set aside some afternoons, evenings, and Saturdays.

CHAPTER 19

UNDERSTANDING KEY IDEAS

1. Increased physical activity causes increased energy and fluid needs. The Food Guide Pyramid still applies.

2. If you don't replace the fluids you lose by sweating, your strength, endurance, and coordination may be affected. You may risk dehydration, which can lead to muscle cramps and heat exhaustion. Best choices: water, juice, and milk. For activities that last more than one hour, sports drinks are a good idea.

3. Spaghetti would be the better choice. Carbohydrates are a good source of energy for working muscles. Also, a spaghetti dinner is easier to digest than a steak sandwich.

4. Without adequate nutrients and perhaps fluids, fasting may cause dehydration and fatigue and may have a negative effect on performance. Over time, it can also affect growth and development. Bulking up too quickly may result in extra body fat instead of more muscle.

5. Possible advice: This type of plan won't improve your performance. It may not provide the balance and variety of foods your body needs for good nutrition. It won't build muscle either; if the extra protein isn't used for energy, it will be stored as fat.

6. Gradually decreasing training and increasing carbohydrate intake several days before an athletic event. It's not recommended for teens because it may affect growth if used repeatedly.

DEVELOPING LIFE SKILLS

Answers may vary.

1. You would need a plan to make sure you get ½ cup (125 mL) of water every 15 minutes. You might carry a water bottle or arrange for people along the trail to give you water.

2. Act as a role model and promote healthier alternatives. Compete in an appropriate weight class and explain why. Point out that fasting, crash dieting, and trying to sweat off the weight could lead to dehydration and fatigue. Try to get the coach's support.

WELLNESS CHALLENGE

Answers may vary.

1. She might tell them that the jump-rope-a-thon will be a vigorous workout, so they will need enough energy from food and fluids before the event if they want to perform successfully. She might explain that they will need to drink plenty of fluids during the event for strength, endurance, and coordination. She might tell them about the risk of dehydration and heat exhaustion.

2. In addition to planning the next morning's breakfast, they might plan to eat a high-carbohydrate meal together three to four hours before the event. They might also agree to bring light snacks, water, and sports drinks to the event and schedule nutrition breaks.

CHAPTER 20

UNDERSTANDING KEY IDEAS

1. Not necessarily. Appropriate weight depends on one's growth pattern and body type. There is no ideal body shape and size.

2. Follow the Food Guide Pyramid guidelines, consume enough calories but not too much, stay physically active, accept the weight that's right for you as your body grows.

3. Stay physically active; eat a moderate amount of foods that contain some fat and sugar; eat nutrient-dense snacks often; choose more than the minimum number of servings from the five food groups; take bigger portions or second helpings; use Nutrition Facts to find nutrient-dense foods with more calories; eat several small meals if necessary; give it time.

4. Students might mention the possible harmful side effects of diet pills, including drowsiness, anxiety, rapid heart rate, dehydration, and addiction. They might also recommend sensible weight-loss strategies, such as following the Food Guide Pyramid guidelines.

5. You will stay the same weight if over time the food energy from your meals and snacks equals the amount of energy your body uses. You will lose weight if over time you take in less food energy than the amount of energy your body uses. You will gain weight if over time you take in more food energy than the amount of energy your body uses.

6. Weight-loss plans, often based on misinformation, that are popular for a short time. Most are not effective in the long run. They don't always provide enough nutrients and food energy, and they may lead to an unhealthful "seesaw" pattern of weight gain and loss.

DEVELOPING LIFE SKILLS

Answers may vary.

I. Often thin individuals are chosen to promote products, model new fashions, appear on magazine covers, and perform on television. This message leads many young people to believe that thinness is key to being desirable and successful. Publishers, promoters, designers, and directors could include persons with varied body shapes.

2. A legitimate weight-loss plan: uses the Food Guide Pyramid as the basis for menu planning, lets you eat foods you enjoy, matches your food budget, fits your lifestyle, includes regular physical activity, and is a plan you can follow for life. In addition to not having the preceding characteristics, a fad diet may identify "good" and "bad" foods; be promoted with phrases like "secret," "breakthrough," or "miracle"; make exaggerated claims; or originate with someone who is not a qualified nutrition expert. Weight-loss plans that involve liquid diets, fasting, or diet pills are unsafe.

WELLNESS CHALLENGE

Answers may vary.

I. Paul may not understand why this diet may be harmful. He may mistakenly think that because grapefruit juice provides nutrients, this type of diet must also be healthful. He may be so determined to lose weight that he is willing to take short-term risks with his health.

2. Tyrone could explain the drawbacks and possible hazards of the grapefruit juice diet. He could educate Paul about appropriate weight, perhaps helping him see that he doesn't really need to lose weight right now. He might reassure Paul that he looks good for the upcoming dance. If Paul still feels his weight is a problem, Tyrone could encourage him to follow the Food Guide Pyramid and get more physical activity. He might suggest a physical activity that they could do together and be a role model for healthful food choices.

CHAPTER 21
UNDERSTANDING KEY IDEAS

I. Complex carbohydrates (and perhaps fiber), B vitamins (including folic acid), and iron.

2. Sample answer: Breakfast—cereal, bagel, frozen waffles. Lunch—pita, tortilla, hamburger bun. Dinner—rice, spaghetti, pizza shells. Snacks—crackers, breadsticks, English muffin.

3. Three. You would need another three to eight servings.

4. Dry cereal—buy plain wheat flakes or cornflakes and add dried fruits, nuts, or other toppings. Cooked cereal—buy instant or quick-cooking varieties.

5. Store fresh pasta in the refrigerator. Store rice in a container in a cool, dry place.

6. Do not rinse rice before or after cooking. It is cooked when the liquid is absorbed and the rice is tender.

DEVELOPING LIFE SKILLS

Answers may vary.

1. Depending on what foods are chosen instead of grain products, the eating plan may be low in complex carbohydrates, calories, fiber, B vitamins, and iron, and possibly high in fat.

2. Preparing daily menus; making lists of grain products and serving sizes; having snacks from this food group on hand; holding family meetings about food choices.

WELLNESS CHALLENGE

Answers may vary.

1. Substitutions might include dry or cooked cereal for breakfast; sandwiches on different kinds of bread, such as whole wheat or pita pockets; grain products such as bulgur or brown rice mixed into hamburger meat or served as side dishes.

2. They might volunteer to go grocery shopping with their aunt and tactfully suggest the substitutions. They might volunteer to prepare some meals themselves. They might introduce unfamiliar grain foods to the family gradually.

CHAPTER 22

UNDERSTANDING KEY IDEAS

1. Sources of carbohydrates, fiber, vitamins, and minerals; low in fat and no cholesterol; students might also say they have phytochemicals.

2. Keep them on hand, try a new one weekly, try preparing them a different way, add one serving per day.

3. Should look fresh, bright, firm, be heavy for their size; shouldn't look abnormally small or large, or be soft or limp.

4. Shake off excess moisture and refrigerate unwashed broccoli promptly in a plastic bag in crisper bin. Don't refrigerate potatoes—keep in a cool, dark, dry place.

5. Any three: Cook with skin, cut in large pieces, use little water, don't overcook, cover the pan; might say to wash before cooking, but not soak.

DEVELOPING LIFE SKILLS

Answers may vary.

1. He might miss out on getting enough nutrients and fiber to promote his health for the long run.

2. Possible methods: Introduce them to a variety of vegetables prepared different ways; let them help prepare vegetables; teach them about how vegetables grow; help them plant seeds and tend garden. Important because vegetables are necessary for good health and they'll likely be more accepting of vegetables throughout life if they start at a young age.

3. Nutritional benefits of each vegetable; preparation suggestions and storage tips; quality of store's produce. Could use posters, brochures, recipe cards, etc.

WELLNESS CHALLENGE

Answers may vary.

1. Getting permission from lot owner, learning the principles of gardening, finding startup money, recruiting students to help, having a source of water, finding a secure place to store supplies and tools.

2. Talk to the lot owner and principal about funding new group and needed resources, contact the local cooperative extension office for advice and technical support, have an informational meeting for interested students.

CHAPTER 23

UNDERSTANDING KEY IDEAS

1. Fresh fruits are a source of carbohydrates, fiber, and some vitamins and minerals. Most fruits have no fat, and they are all cholesterol-free.

2. If you're not going to eat it immediately. Plums, nectarines, apricots, avocados, bananas, peaches. Place the fruit in a loosely closed paper bag at room temperature for a day or two.

3. Whether the fruit juice is fresh or is made from concentrated juices; whether it contains added vitamins and minerals; whether it is 100 percent juice (see if label says "fruit punch," "fruit drink," "juice blend," or "juice cocktail.")

4. Keep edible peels on; wait to wash fruits until ready to use them; cut fruit just before eating; use ripe fruits within a few days of purchase; refrigerate cut fruit in an airtight container.

5. For tart fruit, a small amount of sugar could be added after cooking.

DEVELOPING LIFE SKILLS

Answers may vary.

1. Examples: serve fruit in a hollowed-out watermelon; make fruit kabobs; use toothpicks to make animal shapes out of cubed fruit; place bowl of fruit inside a container related to the party theme, such as an upside-down hat.

2. Possible basis: certain fruits can be expensive, especially out of season; some fruits bruise easily when carried or are messy to eat. You might point out that fruits can be less expensive than many other types of foods, that supermarket sales and in-season fruits offer bargains, and that fruits such as apples and orange sections work well as portable snacks.

WELLNESS CHALLENGE

Answers may vary.

1. Getting enough orders to be able to give each resident a basket; working out the timing so that fruit doesn't spoil; finding individuals to help deliver baskets.

2. Steps might include promoting the idea; recruiting help; finding a place to purchase baskets; pricing fruit; calculating costs; setting a price to charge per basket.

CHAPTER 24

UNDERSTANDING KEY IDEAS

1. Your bones might not get the calcium and other nutrients needed to grow properly.

2. Whole, reduced-fat, low-fat, and fat-free (nonfat) milk, flavored milk, and buttermilk. Forms for convenient storage include nonfat dry milk, UHT milk, evaporated milk, and sweetened condensed milk.

3. Unripened cheeses are not aged; ripened cheeses are. Possible examples: unripened—ricotta, cottage cheese, mozzarella; ripened—brick, Muenster, Cheddar, Gouda, Colby, Parmesan.

4. Students should provide examples of three to four daily servings from the Milk, Yogurt, and Cheese Group.

5. Cover the yogurt container and refrigerate. Pour the opened can of evaporated milk in a pitcher, cover, and refrigerate. Use both within a few days.

6. Use low heat, stir frequently, watch carefully, and heat just until milk begins to steam.

DEVELOPING LIFE SKILLS

Answers may vary.

1. You might explain the important health benefits of milk, including its role in growth and bone building. You might suggest that she try flavored milk or make a fruit smoothie for a different taste. You might tell her that she could also get the bone-building nutrients she needs from yogurt and cheese instead of milk. You could be a good role model by drinking milk and eating dairy foods yourself.

2. Students should recognize that Ryan did not manage his time well, which in turn may have caused the milk to lose quality and perhaps be discarded. Possible alternatives: take the milk home, put it in the refrigerator, and then return to play basketball; ask Guillermo to store the milk in his refrigerator while playing basketball.

WELLNESS CHALLENGE

Answers may vary.

1. Without electricity, they won't have a refrigerator in which to store dairy foods properly. Without proper storage, many dairy foods will spoil quickly.

2. Tracy and her family might bring a cooler with small containers of milk, yogurt, and cheese that they could eat the first day of the trip. They could bring UHT or dry milk, which doesn't need refrigeration until it has been opened or prepared. They might serve canned or bottled cheese sauce over vegetables or other foods. If there is a store near the campground, they might be able to buy fresh dairy products to eat during the middle of their trip. They could also eat extra dairy products before and after the trip to make up for the servings they missed.

CHAPTER 25
UNDERSTANDING KEY IDEAS

1. Protein, B vitamins, iron, and zinc. Protein is needed to help build and repair body tissues and keep them healthy. Vitamins and minerals have specific roles for growth and good health.

2. Possible answers: Meat—veal, pork, lamb; poultry—chicken, turkey, duck, Cornish hen, goose; finfish—catfish, flounder, haddock, perch, red snapper, salmon, tuna.

3. Check the Nutrition Facts panel for fat and cholesterol information, check the meat's appearance for a cut that has less marbling and very little fat around the edges, choose a steak graded "Select," and look for *round* or *loin* in the name.

4. Make sure fresh fish is tightly wrapped and store it in the refrigerator on a plate or in a pan. Wrap chicken tightly in freezer paper or put it in an airtight plastic bag or container and store it in the freezer.

5. 160°F (71°C). Meat, poultry, and fish must be cooked thoroughly to destroy harmful bacteria; you can't always tell by looking whether food has cooked long enough to be safe.

DEVELOPING LIFE SKILLS

Answers may vary.

1. Reasons might include habit, family meal customs, restaurant portions, etc. Possible consequences: eating plan might be lacking in foods from other food groups; might have too much fat and cholesterol in eating plan if meat, poultry, fish, and eggs are the main choices from this group.

2. When buying, need to consider that less tender cuts may require longer cooking; can also buy convenience forms to save time. When storing, consider how soon you will use the item and store in either the refrigerator or freezer accordingly. When preparing, need to allow enough cooking time for the food to reach a safe internal temperature, yet avoid overcooking; also need to manage meal preparation so that all the food is ready at the desired time.

WELLNESS CHALLENGE

Answers may vary.

1. Determining how much beef and poultry to buy; choosing the supplier; planning how to safely transport the food to the county park; deciding how to keep the food safe, how to cook it, and how to keep it at its proper temperature to avoid foodborne illness.

2. She could estimate about 3 ounces (84 g) of beef or boneless poultry per student. She could look for sales in the local supermarket and talk to the meat department manager. She could then compare the cost with that offered by a wholesale supplier. She might talk to the school food services manager for advice and assistance. She could also review food safety guidelines with the students who will be helping with the event.

MAKING CONNECTIONS

1. The steak costs $1.24 per serving and the chicken costs $1.14 per serving. To serve a family of four, you would need to buy 1 pound of sirloin steak ($4.98) or a 2-pound chicken ($4.58).

CHAPTER 26
UNDERSTANDING KEY IDEAS

1. They can help you meet your protein needs and supply many important vitamins and minerals. Legumes are good sources of complex carbohydrates and fiber.

2. Eggs: check the "sell by" date for freshness; make sure eggs are clean and not cracked. Legumes: check the ingredient list and the Nutrition Facts panel to compare amounts of added salt and fat.

3. Refrigerate fresh eggs in their carton. Store legumes and nuts in airtight containers in a cool, dry cabinet. After cooking legumes, refrigerate leftovers and use within three to four days.

4. Eggs are fully cooked when the white and yolk are completely set and no visible liquid egg remains. Overcooking makes eggs shrink and become tough.

5. Put the legumes in a large pot of water and bring to a boil. Turn off the heat and let the legumes soak in the hot water for 1 hour. Drain the water. Cook the legumes in plenty of fresh water for about $1\frac{1}{2}$ to 2 hours or until tender.

DEVELOPING LIFE SKILLS

Answers may vary.

1. Both provide protein and other nutrients. The yolks of shell eggs are a source of fat and cholesterol, whereas egg substitutes are generally low in fat and cholesterol-free. Shell eggs are stored in the refrigerator and last for a shorter time than frozen egg substitutes. Some people might prefer the taste of shell eggs. Other people might prefer egg substitutes to lower their fat and cholesterol intake or if they want to store eggs for longer periods of time.

2. Encourage students to be creative in developing ideas.

WELLNESS CHALLENGE

Answers may vary.

1. Possible items: bean burritos, vegetarian chili, lentil or split pea soup. Legumes are economical and nutritious.

2. They should consider the food preferences of people attending the football games. If the new menu items are unpopular, the class could lose money. The students will also need to find a food supplier who offers the menu items in pre-prepared forms.

3. They might take a poll of the students to determine about how many people might eat these dishes. They might try to find a supplier who is willing to sign a month-to-month or trial contract. To help ensure success, they might advertise the new menu items in the school newspaper or make posters for school bulletin boards. They might also give out small samples of the new items during the school lunch period or the football games.

CHAPTER 27

UNDERSTANDING KEY IDEAS

1. Grain products provide complex carbohydrates, B vitamins, and perhaps fiber; vegetables and fruits provide vitamins A and C, folate, potassium, and fiber; dairy products supply calcium, protein, and riboflavin; meat, poultry, fish, dry beans, eggs, and nuts provide protein, iron, zinc, and B vitamins; and beans add fiber. Iceberg lettuce has relatively few nutrients.

2. Choose crisp salad greens with evenly colored leaves and no wilting, wash greens under cool running water and drain thoroughly, tear salad greens, cut or slice sweet peppers and tomatoes into bite-size pieces, toss ingredients gently, toss salad with dressing just before serving or serve dressing separately, serve salad on a chilled salad plate or in a chilled bowl.

3. Combine three parts oil and one part vinegar or lemon juice and then add herbs. To cut fat and calories, use less oil or use mild balsamic vinegar and skip the oil altogether.

4. You could cook the hard-cooked eggs and chop vegetables such as celery or onions ahead of time. Store the ingredients in separate plastic bags or covered containers in the refrigerator.

5. Choose plenty of fresh vegetables and fruit; add cooked dry beans, hard-cooked eggs, lean meat, turkey, or shrimp; go easy on mixed salads tossed in oil or mixed with mayonnaise; use just a little salad dressing or choose a fat-free variety; make just one trip to the salad bar.

DEVELOPING LIFE SKILLS

Answers may vary.

1. Produce department manager might use posters, leaflets, recipe cards, creative displays of merchandise, etc. To encourage friend, you might give persuasive reasons in conversation or set an example. In both situations, communication methods are chosen according to what is appropriate for the audience, but the methods themselves are very different.

2. Encourage students to be creative in their responses.

WELLNESS CHALLENGE

Answers may vary.

1. The number of people attending; the location of the event; the amount of food needed; the cost of different ingredients; methods of serving the food; the types of foods most people are familiar with; food safety issues.

2. Make posters for each salad to show which Pyramid food groups are represented.

3. Suggestions will vary.

CHAPTER 28

UNDERSTANDING KEY IDEAS

1. Grain products, such as rice, barley, couscous, and pasta, provide B vitamins and iron and are high in complex carbohydrates. Some also add fiber. Dairy foods, such as milk, yogurt, and cheese, provide calcium and protein.

2. Cook the chicken slowly in a pot of liquid. Add onion, celery, carrots, herbs, and spices. Bring it to a boil, lower the heat, and cook gently until the chicken falls from the bones. Allow the broth to cool, strain it, and skim the fat off the top.

3. Possible answers: canned or frozen heat-and-eat soup, dehydrated soup mix, microwavable cup of soup, or canned condensed soup. You could add more flavor by adding your favorite herbs and spices.

4. Divide the stew into several smaller containers—covered plastic bowls or freezer bags—so that they chill quickly, and store them in the freezer.

5. Possible answers: gumbo—okra, onions, and meat or fish; gazpacho—cucumbers, onions, and peppers; West African peanut soup—chicken, peanut butter or peanuts, and spices.

DEVELOPING LIFE SKILLS

Answers may vary.

1. Can use leftovers; can make a large batch and freeze for later meals; can make in a slow cooker to help manage busy schedule; have many convenience forms to choose from.

2. Encourage students to be creative in their responses.

WELLNESS CHALLENGE

Answers may vary.

1. She might first approach an existing student organization, such as FHA or the Student Council. Later she might start a publicity campaign using posters, articles in the school newspaper, and other publicity to attract volunteers. She might give the project a catchy name that would appeal to students.

2. They'll need to decide whether to limit this program to families of students or extend it to the community in general. They'll need to determine what types of situations might make a family eligible to receive the soup. Sensitivity is called for; some families may feel their privacy is being invaded or may prefer not to receive help for other reasons. In the case of health problems, the teens will need to find out about any dietary restrictions that might affect the type of soup they bring or whether soup is appropriate.

3. Money for soup ingredients (could conduct a fundraiser); location and equipment for preparing soup (might ask for permission to use school cafeteria or foods lab, or volunteers could each prepare soup at home); freezer space for storing soup (at school or in homes); transportation for delivering soup (volunteers might have to provide own transportation).

CHAPTER 29

UNDERSTANDING KEY IDEAS

1. Flexibility: you can make mixed dishes with any foods you like; nutrition and appeal: you can use foods from any food group to get good nutrition and variety.

2. Tuna provides protein and other nutrients. Other ingredients might include noodles, macaroni, or bulgur for complex carbohydrates; green beans, broccoli, or bell peppers for fiber and certain vitamins and minerals; and dry milk or grated cheese for calcium.

3. Plan ahead by checking to see what canned, frozen, or leftover foods you could use to start your dish. Precook ingredients such as pasta, rice, meat, poultry, or fish. Assemble the ingredients in a baking dish, and sprinkle on the topping. Bake the casserole for about 30 minutes in a $1\frac{1}{2}$ quart (1.5 L) casserole dish at 350°F (180°C). In an oven, cover the casserole until the last 15 minutes, then remove the cover for browning. In a microwave oven, leave the cover on for the duration of the cooking time. Use the power level and cooking time recommended in the microwave oven owner's manual or cooking guide.

4. Prepare the couscous, stir in leftovers such as cooked vegetables and meat or poultry, and heat. Add broth to uncooked rice, stir in other ingredients such as leftovers, and cover and simmer until the rice is cooked.

5. Cut chicken and carrots into evenly sized pieces. Heat a small amount of oil in the wok. Stir-fry chicken, remove from wok, and place on a clean plate. Stir-fry carrots first and then add snow peas. Put cooked chicken back in the wok, and add seasonings.

DEVELOPING LIFE SKILLS

Answers may vary.

1. Set a good example by helping him store the leftovers; make a game of it; prepare a dish that he'd like from the leftovers and explain what it's made from; have a contest to see who can think of the most creative way to use the leftovers; let him help prepare a dish from the leftovers; explain that by saving leftovers he can help the entire family.

2. Encourage students to be creative in their responses.

WELLNESS CHALLENGE

Answers may vary.

1. Information about mixed dishes from various cultures (library, Internet, other students and their families); number of people expected to attend, amount of budget (others who are planning the dinner); cost and availability of ingredients used in cuisines of various cultures (survey local food stores).

2. The culture each dish represents (they need to ensure a variety); the nutrition and food group variety of the dishes; the cost and availability of ingredients; the difficulty or ease of preparation; whether they will appeal to students.

3. Look for dishes made with economical ingredients such as pasta, rice, legumes, fruits, and vegetables, with smaller amounts of meat, poultry, and fish; balance higher-cost and lower-cost dishes; check supermarket sale flyers for items that could be used in a variety of dishes; ask stores to donate ingredients in exchange for listing them as a sponsor of the event.

CHAPTER 30

UNDERSTANDING KEY IDEAS

1. Flour gives baked products their structure. Liquids moisten the dry ingredients and help bind them together. Fat adds flavor and richness to breads and helps give the desired texture.

2. Yeast breads: yeast. Examples: whole wheat bread, bagels, and breadsticks. Quick breads: baking powder or baking soda. Examples: pancakes, muffins, and biscuits. Flat breads: little or no leavening agent. Examples: tortillas and pita bread.

3. Sift together all dry ingredients, cut fat into the dry ingredients, add the liquid ingredients, and stir just until blended.

4. Mix the dough using the method given in the recipe. Be sure the ingredients are at room temperature and the liquid is warmed to the temperature given in the recipe. Knead the dough until it becomes satiny and elastic and has little bubbles under the surface. Let the dough rise in a warm place until it doubles in size. Punch down the dough by gently pressing your fist in the center. Pull the dough from the sides of the bowl and press down again. Shape the dough into loaves or rolls. Place the dough into a pan or onto a baking sheet and let the dough rise a second time. Bake according to the recipe.

5. Dry bread mix, frozen or refrigerated dough for bread and rolls, brown-and-serve products.

6. Store-bought breads have additives to help preserve them. Store homemade breads in airtight containers, aluminum foil, or plastic bags in a cool, dry place.

DEVELOPING LIFE SKILLS

Answers may vary.

1. Leon might describe the three main categories of bread and how each one is made. To keep the children's attention, he might demonstrate how to make a quick bread, get volunteers to help with some of the steps, and provide bread samples for the children to taste.

2. Factors might include the cost of each appliance; whether the bread machine can be used to make the types of breads the family enjoys; whether family members enjoy making bread by hand; their schedules and the amount of time they have for making bread. The bread machine would save the most time and effort, but might not be as versatile; the electric mixer might have additional uses, but would not streamline the bread-making process as much.

Answers may vary.

1. She might contact other school organizations and ask if they've held a bake sale before. If so, she could ask a student who participated for advice. Community organizations and school faculty are other possible sources of advice.

2. Set a date for the sale and clear it with the school administration; recruit volunteers to make the breads; coordinate the types of breads to ensure a variety; possibly provide recipes and instructions to students who are not experienced bakers; storage to keep the breads fresh and safe; volunteers to staff the sale; determine prices; promote the sale to the student body.

3. As she coordinates the variety of breads that are being prepared, she might make suggestions for including nutrient-dense food-group ingredients. She might provide nutritious recipes. She might plan to make fresh fruit, fruit juices, and milk available.

CHAPTER 31

UNDERSTANDING KEY IDEAS

1. Nutrition: whole grain breads; lean and low-fat sliced cold cuts or deli meats, cheeses, canned tuna, and canned refried beans; fresh vegetables; low-fat or fat-free mayonnaise. Flavor variety: answers might include breads such as whole wheat, multigrain, rye, or oatmeal; spreads such as hummus, chutney, fruit spreads, cranberry sauce, relish, mustard.

2. Start with a crust, add sauce, seasonings, toppings, and cheese. Bake individual English muffin pizzas with precooked toppings in the microwave or toaster oven until the cheese melts. Bake a pizza with a yeast dough crust according to recipe directions.

3. Keep it cold in an insulated bag with a frozen juice can or cold pack tucked inside, or pack a frozen sandwich. Use a fresh sandwich bag or wash insulated lunch bag before packing.

4. Use taco sauce, enchilada sauce, salsa, or pureed fruit instead of tomato sauce. Choose a cheese such as cheddar, feta, Swiss, or Gouda.

5. Toast bread first. Add sliced tomato and low-fat cheese. Heat in the toaster oven or under the broiler to melt the cheese.

6. Any two: ask for whole grain crust; choose vegetable or fruit toppings; if ordering toppings from the meat and beans group, select mostly lower-fat options; ask for lower-fat cheese.

DEVELOPING LIFE SKILLS

Answers may vary.

1. Suggestions might include fruit chutney, pureed fruit, sliced bananas or apples, and raisins.

2. Use plastic containers from yogurt, sour cream, and cream cheese to pack foods. Reuse plastic bags from the grocery store or other stores to carry your lunch. Save used aluminum foil if it can be recycled in your town. Try not to buy sandwich items packaged in one-use containers and wraps such as cheese and crackers. Would show leadership because it would set a good example of taking personal responsibility for protecting the environment.

WELLNESS CHALLENGE

Answers may vary.

1. If students don't like the new pizzas, they may choose not to eat the cafeteria lunch, and therefore they will not benefit from the nutrition guidelines that are being put in place.

2. Conduct a survey, interview selected students, put a ballot box in the cafeteria.

3. Write an article for school newspaper, put information on school web site, make posters, create catchy slogans, give away samples at a special tasting party.

CHAPTER 32

UNDERSTANDING KEY IDEAS

1. Desserts can contribute toward food-group servings to help balance your day's food choices. It's okay to have rich desserts occasionally as long as you follow Pyramid guidelines and don't overdo on calories and fat.

2. Eat a small portion of a rich dessert or share it with a friend; choose or prepare desserts with less fat and less added sugar; shop for alternatives with less fat and fewer calories.

3. Possible answers: fresh fruit such as peaches or berries eaten with milk; mixed fruits combined with spices, chopped nuts, and other ingredients; apples baked with cinnamon, raisins, brown sugar, and butter or margarine; angel food cake topped with sliced or pureed fresh fruit; bananas or grapes frozen and eaten cold; chopped fruit with flavored gelatin.

4. Homemade pudding is made with milk, sugar, and perhaps eggs. Most recipes are thickened with cornstarch. The mixture is cooked gently, then chilled. Custard is a cooked mixture of milk and eggs prepared on the range top or baked in the oven. The eggs thicken the custard and give it a rich flavor. Sweeteners and other flavorings turn it into a dessert.

5. Cookie press: pressed cookies. Square or rectangular pan: bar cookies.

6. Shortened cakes, foam cakes, and chiffon cakes. Shortened cakes include a fat such as butter or shortening and use baking powder or baking soda as the main leavening agent. Foam cakes do not include butter, shortening, or oil and use beaten eggs whites as the main leavening agent. Chiffon cakes include oil (or sometimes another fat) and egg yolks and are leavened with both beaten egg whites and baking powder.

7. Store puddings and custards in the refrigerator. Store cakes and cookies at room temperature in a tightly covered container, a plastic bag, or aluminum foil.

DEVELOPING LIFE SKILLS

Answers may vary.

1. Students may point out that articles about nutrition, dieting, and so on aren't always accurate. Clues to misleading information might include advice to avoid all desserts and the use of phrases such as "bad for you" or "sinful" in relation to desserts.

2. Bar cookies because you simply bake the dough in a pan without having to mold, roll out, refrigerate, or press it; drop cookies because they don't require special shapes. Convenience options include refrigerated or frozen cookie dough and dry mixes.

Answers may vary.

1. If he feels he can't enjoy desserts anymore, he may have trouble sticking to his new diet, which could affect his health.

2. Offer desserts (such as angel food cake with fruit) that are low in fat, cholesterol, and sodium and that his father would enjoy; modify the family's dessert recipes to be lower in fat, cholesterol, and sodium; look for a special cookbook; encourage his father to occasionally enjoy small portions of richer desserts so he doesn't miss out on old favorites.

HANDBOOK PART 1

UNDERSTANDING KEY IDEAS

1. Sickness resulting from eating food that is not safe to eat. Harmful bacteria can multiply to dangerous levels if they have food, moisture, and the right temperatures. If you eat food contaminated with large numbers of harmful microorganisms, foodborne illness may result.

2. Plan your shopping so that you select refrigerated foods last; look at the dates on packages that tell you about a food's freshness; check that refrigerated foods feel cold; place raw meat, poultry, and fish in plastic bags; make sure food packages don't have holes, tears, open corners, or broken safety seals; take the food home right away and store it properly.

3. Before you begin preparing food; after handling raw food; between handling different kinds of food; after using the toilet or changing a diaper; after touching pets; after touching your mouth, nose, hair, or other parts of your body while handling food.

4. Keep raw flounder and its juices away from ready-to-eat foods; use one cutting board for flounder and another for other foods; use a plastic or other nonporous cutting board that is free of cracks and crevices; wash everything that comes in contact with the raw flounder in hot, soapy water before it's used again; don't place cooked or ready-to-eat food on an unwashed plate or cutting board that previously held raw flounder.

5. Place the steak on the lowest refrigerator shelf in a plastic bag; or place the steak in a microwave-safe container, defrost on the "low" or "defrost" setting, and cook it right away.

6. Any five: store leftovers in refrigerator; refrigerate them as soon as possible, without cooling first; divide them into shallow containers; discard leftovers that have sat at room temperature more than 2 hours (1 hour in hot weather); use refrigerated leftovers within 3 to 4 days; for longer storage, freeze; throw out leftovers that have been in the refrigerator more than 4 days.

7. Store knives in a knife block, rack, or special drawer divider; don't soak knives or other sharp utensils in a sink where you may not see them; use a cutting board; clean up broken glass carefully, using a broom and dustpan or a wet paper towel.

DEVELOPING LIFE SKILLS

Answers may vary.

1. Everyone has a responsibility to help prevent foodborne illness. Students should suggest tactful solutions, such as volunteering to help put leftovers away right after a meal.

2. The juices from the raw meat on the plate might contaminate the cooked hamburgers, and Taylor and her friends could get a foodborne illness. Taylor should have washed the plate in hot, soapy water before putting the cooked hamburgers on it or used a different serving plate.

WELLNESS CHALLENGE

Answers may vary.

1. The teens might produce a graphic showing temperatures where bacteria are destroyed, where they multiply, and so on. After determining what kinds of food are going to be sold, they could give the volunteers information about avoiding foodborne illnesses. They might find articles on outbreaks of illness that took place at similar events to share with volunteers.

2. The teens might devise a list of guidelines for the volunteers to follow and assign someone the task of monitoring them throughout the day.

HANDBOOK PART 2

UNDERSTANDING KEY IDEAS

1. Paring knife or peeler for peeling; utility knife or chef's knife and cutting board for chopping; colander for draining water from cooked potatoes; mixing bowl and mixing spoon for combining potatoes with other ingredients.

2. Similarities: All three are types of cookware used for cooking foods on top of the range. All have handles, come in various sizes, and may come with covers. Differences: Saucepans have one long handle. Pots have two small handles and are generally larger than saucepans. Skillets are shallower than pots or saucepans and may have slanted sides.

3. Safe: heat-resistant glass containers, cookware designed for microwave oven use, plastic items labeled microwave-safe, paper plates and towels labeled microwave-safe. Not safe: metal cookware, aluminum foil, pottery with metallic glazes, plastic containers from dairy foods and take-out foods, brown bags, products made of recycled paper, wooden containers, straw baskets or plates, materials containing synthetic fibers.

4. Before using it, read the owner's manual carefully. Use a thermometer to check the temperature in each compartment. Keep the refrigerator between 32° and 40°F (0° and 4°C) and the freezer at 0°F (-18°C) or less. Clean up any spills right away. Regularly wipe the inside of the refrigerator with a solution of baking soda and water. If the freezer is not self-defrosting, defrost it when ¼ to ½ inch (6 to 13 mm) of ice has formed.

5. Areas of the kitchen devoted to specific tasks. If you store items used for each task in or near the work center where you'll use them, you can work more efficiently.

DEVELOPING LIFE SKILLS

Answers may vary.

1. Students might choose a toaster oven or an electric skillet because of their versatility. These appliances serve some of the same functions as a range but use less energy.

2. Brianna might call a family meeting to explain the problems and discuss possible solutions, such as agreeing on a list of refrigerator rules. She might think of a humorous way for family members to remind each other of the rules when needed. She could be a role model by following the rules herself. Brianna might also take more direct action, such as throwing out old leftovers, purchasing a thermometer, and resetting the temperature controls if needed.

Answers may vary.

1. Blender, food processor, pot, saucepan, slow cooker, measuring tools, cutting tools.

2. She may not have all the needed equipment. Her grandfather may not be looking forward to the soft diet.

3. Kim could substitute some equipment. For example, if she doesn't have a slow cooker for making soup, she could use a pot or a saucepan. Kim could discuss her menu plans with her grandfather and find out his preferences so that the meals will appeal to him.

HANDBOOK PART 3

UNDERSTANDING KEY IDEAS

1. You can use it to figure out that 6 tsp. = 30 mL.

2. Do the following calculation: desired yield: 4; original yield: 8; magic number: $4 \div 8 = \frac{1}{2}$. Multiply all ingredient amounts by $\frac{1}{2}$. Write down new amounts, converting to different units as needed. If some amounts can't be reduced exactly, round them off.

3. Similarities: Both use a dry measure or measuring spoon; choose the exact size for the amount you need. Differences: Brown sugar is packed in firmly by pressing with a rubber scraper or the back of a spoon and filled level. White sugar is spooned in lightly and overfilled slightly, then leveled off with a straight-edge spatula or the back of a knife.

4. Beating is a brisk over and over motion using a spoon, wire whisk, or electric or hand mixer. Stirring means to mix ingredients with a circular or figure 8 motion.

5. Thick foods have to be placed farther away from the heat so that they are thoroughly cooked.

6. Arrange dishes in the order they will be washed: glassware, flatware, dinnerware, and cooking utensils. Immerse a few dishes at a time in a pan of hot water with enough detergent to make the water sudsy. Wash dishes with a clean dishcloth or sponge. Rinse in hot water.

DEVELOPING LIFE SKILLS

Answers may vary.

1. Microwave cooking usually requires attention, such as turning and rearranging foods. In some situations, a method such as roasting or using a slow cooker might be a better time management strategy so that other activities can be done while the food is cooking.

2. Recipes are easy to use and understand when they give ingredients and steps in the proper order, use commonly understood terms, include helpful tips and explanations, etc. Examples of poorly written recipes and how they could be improved will vary.

3. Converting would be a slow and perhaps expensive process; the customary system is familiar and comfortable, so people resist changing. Advantages of the metric system: easier to multiply and divide amounts because it's based on multiples of 10; used by most of the world, which aids trade and communication. Disadvantages: using an unfamiliar measurement system might cause confusion and errors; the costs of conversion.

WELLNESS CHALLENGE

Answers may vary.

1. They can rotate assignments so that each team member has a chance to practice a variety of skills.

2. As they prepare the work plans: assign tasks fairly; resolve disagreements peacefully; accept tasks willingly. As they carry out the work plans: be considerate and willing to help others; carry out assigned tasks to the best of their ability.

HANDBOOK PART 4
UNDERSTANDING KEY IDEAS

1. Water is a molecule (hydrogen, oxygen). Proteins are molecules made up of amino acids (carbon, hydrogen, oxygen, nitrogen). Carbohydrates are simple sugars or chains of simple sugars (carbon, hydrogen, oxygen). Fats are made up of one glycerol molecule and three fatty-acid molecules. A fatty acid is a chain of molecules (carbon, oxygen, hydrogen).

2. Conduction: heat passes from molecule to molecule when they bump into one another. Convection: circulation of liquid or air. Radiation: heat travels through space as waves.

3. The starch in the noodles dissolves in the water, turns gluey as it cools, attaches to the noodles, and makes them sticky. Avoid this by using a lot of water.

4. Eggplant, red cabbage, cherries, blueberries, and strawberries. During cooking, flavonoids dissolve in water and leach out of the food into the sauce or cooking liquid.

5. A process in which a liquid changes into a soft semisolid or solid mass. Possible examples: curdled milk; the processing of cheese; cooking an egg; beating egg whites into foam.

6. The process of fermentation. A sugar is broken down into lactic acid.

7. Enzymes are proteins that help chemical reactions by reducing the energy to start the reaction. Fruits such as papayas, pineapples, and figs contain enzymes that can break down muscle fiber or collagen. Enzyme-containing preparations are also sold as meat tenderizers.

8. As an egg white is beaten or an egg is cooked, coagulation occurs. Protein molecules unwind, collide with one another, and it changes from a liquid into a soft semisolid or solid mass.

9. They must form an emulsion, a blend of droplets that don't normally blend with each other. Examples include mayonnaise, salad dressings, gravies, cream soups, and whole milk.

10. A colloidal dispersion; a mixture in which the particles don't dissolve. The particles, called colloids, are distributed, or dispersed, throughout the other substance.

11. Gelatinization. When heated in water, starch molecules loosen, absorb water, and swell. Less liquid remains, causing the liquid to become thick.

12. A stretchy, three-dimensional structure, formed when wheat flour is mixed with water and kneaded. As the yeast produce carbon dioxide, the walls of the gluten stretch, trap the carbon dioxide, and form small holes in the dough. During baking, the gluten becomes solid.

DEVELOPING LIFE SKILLS

Answers may vary.

1. Encourage students to give specific examples, based on their reading, as evidence.

2. To give clear directions to assistants, write scientific articles and reports, give presentations to colleagues at conferences, and understand the articles, reports, and presentations of others.

WELLNESS CHALLENGE

Answers may vary.

1. Sticky spaghetti: not using enough cooking water or not rinsing after cooking. Dull green vegetables: overcooking, causing the chlorophyll in the vegetables to react with acids. Dry, tough chicken: not controlling the heat, causing proteins to shrink.

2. Cook pasta in lots of water, add I Tbsp. oil, and rinse afterwards. Add vegetables to water after it is boiling and keep cooking time to under 7 minutes, or steam vegetables. Avoid overcooking chicken.

HANDBOOK PART 5

Understanding Key Ideas

1. Colors: Add color contrasts with fruits, vegetables, and the hues of other foods; try not to repeat colors on a plate. Textures: Use foods with different textures, such as crispy, chewy, smooth, or chunky; prepare foods in ways that change their texture. Flavors: Use mild foods to balance strong flavors; try not to repeat a food in the meal.

2. Decide whether you need more than one plate per person; avoid overcrowding a plate; use your imagination to arrange food in an attractive way.

3. Cook for the fun of it; take time to notice and appreciate the colors, textures, flavors, and aromas of food; learn new skills; teach new skills; sample many cuisines; create your own recipes; give the gift of food; explore food as a business.

4. Crumble the dried rosemary between your fingers, and add it to the stew toward the end of cooking time. To substitute dried rosemary for fresh, divide the amount called for by three.

5. Salsa—serve with poultry, fish, and meat dishes; on baked potatoes; tossed with cooked rice or cooked pasta; as a dip for raw vegetables. Chutney—serve alongside meat, poultry or fish; as a spread for bread or sandwiches; with cheese as an appetizer. Vinegar—use to add tartness to foods. Pesto—serve with pasta.

6. Choose a theme, a convenient date and time, and the foods to be served. Make a guest list, invite guests a few days or weeks in advance, plan decorations, make lists of tasks to be done, follow your plan, and cross off tasks as you accomplish them.

Developing Life Skills

Answers may vary.

1. Answers should reflect an understanding of the information provided in this section.

2. Shared activities are one of the main ways in which these values are passed on. Examples include preparing a family recipe together, going to a farmer's market together, etc.

Wellness Challenge

Answers may vary.

1. Promotes mental and emotional health by providing musical enjoyment; promotes social well-being as residents meet choir members; refreshments contribute to physical health.

2. Fruits could be selected for color contrasts and be garnished with sprigs of fresh mint. Muffins might be served in a doily-lined basket or other attractive container. Hot cocoa could be served with cinnamon-stick stirrers or cinnamon-dusted marshmallows.

3. They might decorate the room with balloons and streamers, use matching tablecloths and napkins with a holiday design, and use candles or seasonal flowers as centerpieces.

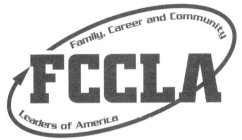

Family, Career and Community Leaders of America, Inc. (FCCLA) is a nonprofit national vocational student organization for young men and women in family and consumer sciences. Involvement in FCCLA offers members the opportunity to expand their leadership potential, explore careers, and develop skills for life.

Through FCCLA, students can participate in a number of programs and competitions to strengthen their skills and leadership abilities. These programs include:

- STAR Events
- Career Connection
- Leaders at Work

STAR EVENTS

STAR Events are competitive events in which FCCLA members are recognized for proficiency and achievement in chapter and individual projects, leadership skills, and occupational preparation.

Depending upon specific event rules and procedures, projects may be carried out by individuals or teams. National *STAR Events* participants are selected by state-established procedures before moving on to nationals. Some event areas include:

- Entrepreneurship
- Illustrated talk
- Job interview

CAREER CONNECTION

Through individual, cooperative, and competitive events, members discover their strengths, target career goals, and initiate a plan for living their chosen way of life. The activity areas offered in the *Career Connection* program include:

- Plug In to Careers
- Sign On to the Career Connection
- Program Career Steps
- Link Up to Jobs
- Access Skills for Career Success
- Integrate Work and Life

LEADERS AT WORK

Leaders at Work is a national program that recognizes FCCLA members who create projects to strengthen their leadership goals on the job. The program emphasizes leadership on the job and helps students identify skills they need to strengthen to become effective leaders. Leadership skill areas include:

- Communication
- Interpersonal
- Management
- Entrepreneurship

Leaders at Work helps students prove they have the skills employers want and provides them with examples to use in job interviews and on college applications. Program participants can also apply to be recognized as an outstanding leader in the targeted career area related to their job. Through this program, students may also receive scholarships.

For more information, contact FCCLA:

http://www.fcclainc.org

email: natlhdqtrs@fcclainc.org

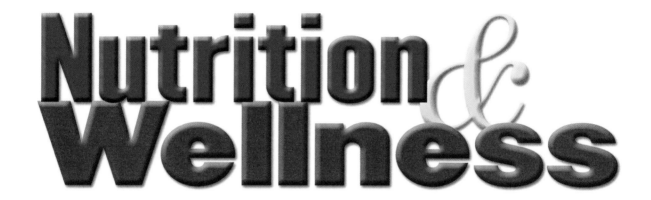

Nutrition & Wellness

SECOND EDITION

by

ROBERTA LARSON DUYFF

MS, RD, FADA, CFCS

CONSULTING AUTHOR
Doris Hasler
MS, CFCS

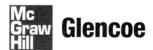

McGraw Hill **Glencoe**

New York, New York   Columbus, Ohio   Chicago, Illinois   Peoria, Illinois   Woodland Hills, California

ABOUT THE AUTHOR

Roberta Larson Duyff is a nationally recognized food and nutrition consultant with over 20 years of professional experience in nutrition, culinary arts, and education. She has authored or contributed to several family and consumer sciences textbook programs, and has also written numerous cookbooks, children's books, magazine and online articles, and consumer books. Among these are *American Dietetic Association Complete Food and Nutrition Guide*, winner of the National Health Information Silver Award. Ms. Duyff is a contributing editor to *Today's Health and Wellness* magazine. She has also developed educational and informational materials for USDA, FDA, the International Food Information Council, and the National Dairy Council, among many others. She frequently addresses consumer and professional groups, both nationally and internationally, on timely food, nutrition, and nutrition education issues. A registered dietitian as well as certified in family and consumer sciences, Ms. Duyff received her bachelor of science degree in home economics education from the University of Illinois and her master of science degree from Cornell University. She is active in numerous professional organizations, including the American Dietetic Association and its Food and Culinary Professionals, the American Association of Family and Consumer Sciences, Consumer Trends Forum International, the Society for Nutrition Education, and the International Association of Culinary Professionals. Ms. Duyff was awarded ADA's First Annual President's Lecture in 1998 and was named AAFCS 1995 National Business Home Economist of the Year. Among the honors her work has received are the ADA President's Circle Award, Nutrition in Action Award, Consumer Education Materials Merit Award, and Family Circle Award for Excellence in Nutrition Education.

ABOUT THE CONSULTING AUTHOR

Doris Hasler has taught foods and nutrition, health, and home nursing on both the high school and college levels. As head of the home economics department at Howe High School in Indianapolis, she was instrumental in revising the foods and nutrition curriculum for the city schools and introducing the class "Food for Athletes." A 50-year member of the American Association of Family and Consumer Sciences, she was recognized in 1995 with the AAFCS Leader Award. The author of two books on family health, Ms. Hasler has a bachelor's degree in education from Ball State University and a master of science degree from Purdue University, and is certified in family and consumer sciences.

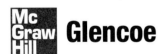

Send all inquiries to:
Glencoe/McGraw-Hill
3008 W. Willow Knolls Drive
Peoria, Illinois 61614-1083

ISBN 0-07-846332-7
Printed in the United States of America
1 2 3 4 5 6 7 8 9 10 071 07 06 05 04 03

CONTRIBUTORS

Betsy A. Hornick, MS, RD, LD
Food and Nutrition Writer and Consultant
Poplar Grove, Illinois

Part 4, The Science of Preparing Food:
Robert G. Brannan, PhD
Research Chef
Pierce Foods
Cincinnati, Ohio

Pat Baird, MA, RD, FADA
Nutrition Consultant and Author
Greenwich, Connecticut

Recipe Development:
Mary K. Sutkus, M Ed
Culinary Consultant and Food Stylist
Florissant, Missouri

TECHNICAL REVIEWERS

Patricia H. Hart, MS, RD
Professor
University of North Florida
Jacksonville, Florida

Kathryn Kolasa, PhD, RD
Professor
East Carolina University
Greenville, North Carolina

Reed Mangels, PhD, RD, LD
Nutrition Advisor
The Vegetarian Resource Group
Amherst, Massachusetts

Jacqueline B. Marcus, MS, RD, LD, CNS, FADA
Food, Nutrition, and Fitness
  Consultant
Northfield, Illinois

Elaine McLaughlin, MS, RD
Nutritionist
Food and Nutrition Service
U.S. Department of Agriculture
Alexandria, Virginia

Kathryn Sucher, ScD, RD
Professor, Director of Dietetic
  Internship
San Jose State University
San Jose, California

Tamara S. Vitale, MS, RD
Clinical Assistant Professor
Utah State University
Logan, Utah

TEACHER REVIEWERS

Marcia M. Bryan, MS, CFCS
Family & Consumer Sciences
  Teacher
Hialeah-Miami Lakes High School
Hialeah, Florida

Linda R. Glosson, PhD
Family & Consumer Sciences
  Teacher
Wylie High School
Wylie, Texas

Kathleen A. Murer Libby, MAT
Family & Consumer Sciences
  Department Chair
Affton Senior High School
St. Louis, Missouri

Lori Robinson, MA
Family & Consumer Sciences
  Educator
Godwin Heights Senior High School
Wyoming, Michigan

Judy Waters Smith, EdD, NBCT
School-to-Career Coordinator
Southeast Raleigh High School
Raleigh, North Carolina

Donna K. Tootle, EdS, ECE
Early Childhood Education Teacher
Tattnall County High School
Reidsville, Georgia

Linda J. Larson Valiga, MEd, CFCS
Family & Consumer Sciences
  Chairperson
School District of Waukesha
Waukesha, Wisconsin

Contents in Brief

Contents

UNIT ONE Food in Your Life

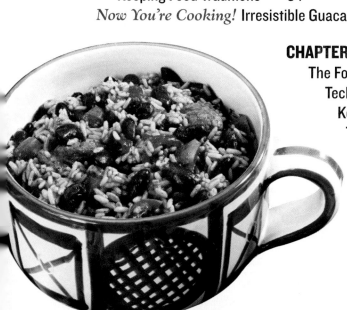

UNIT TWO Nutrition for Health

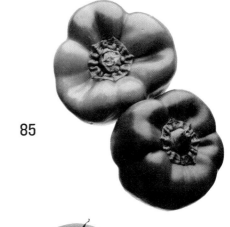
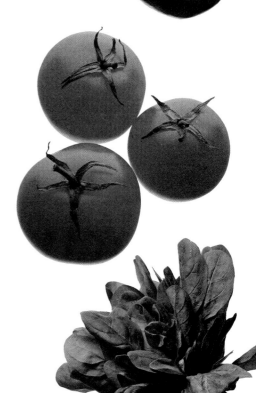

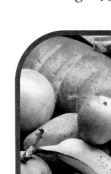

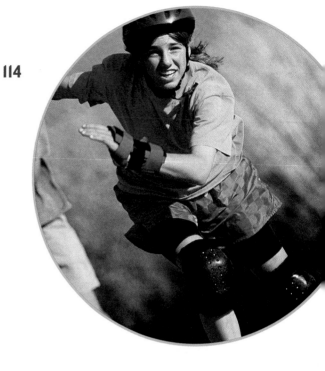

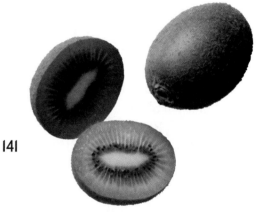

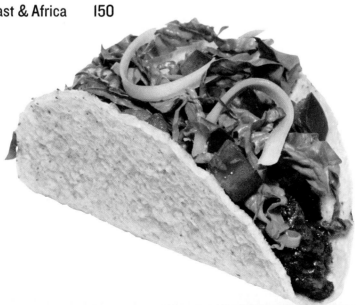

UNIT THREE Making Food Choices

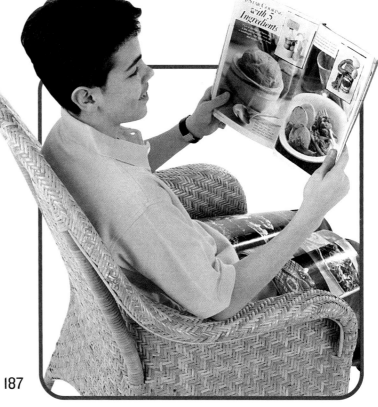

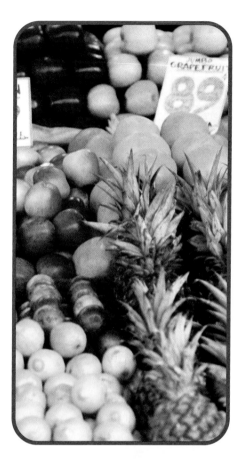

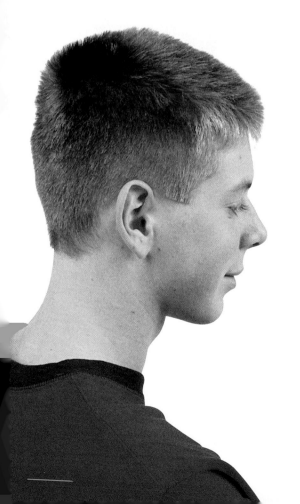

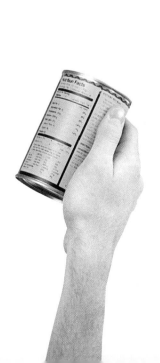

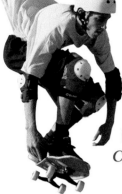

UNIT FOUR Fitness and Food

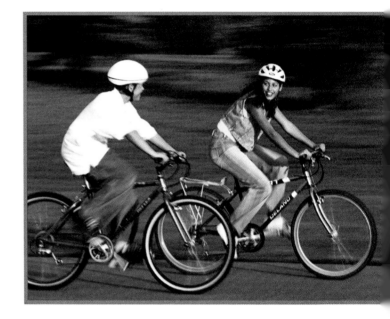

UNIT FIVE Pyramid Foods

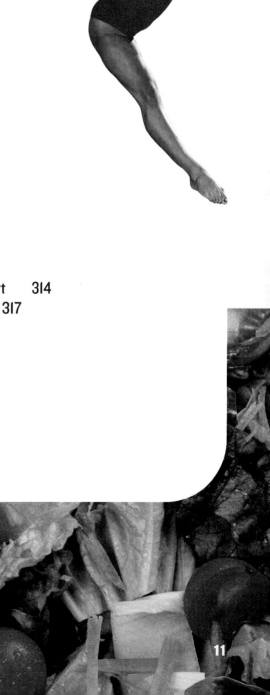

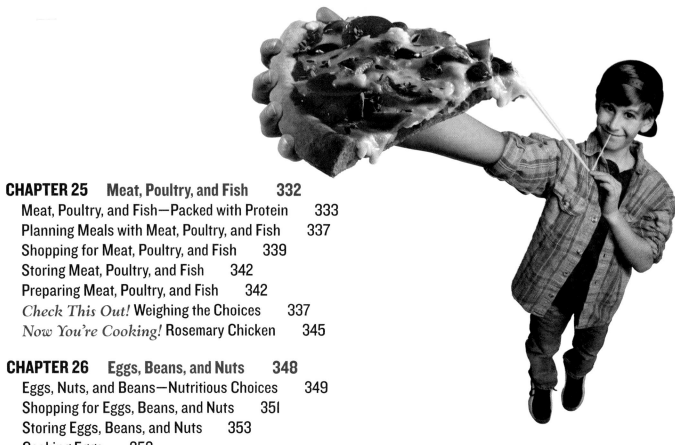

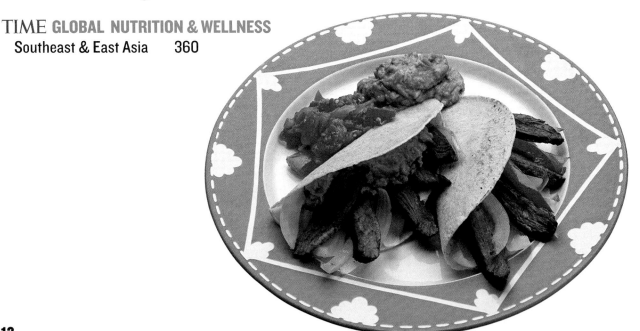

UNIT SIX Creative Combinations

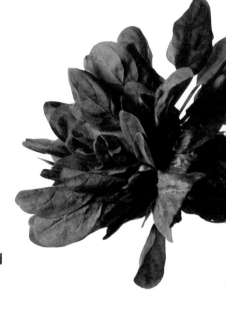

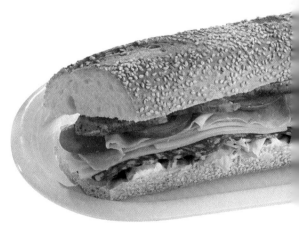

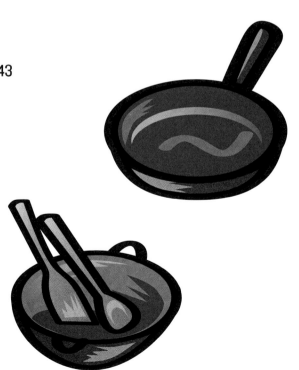

Food Preparation Handbook

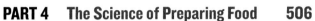

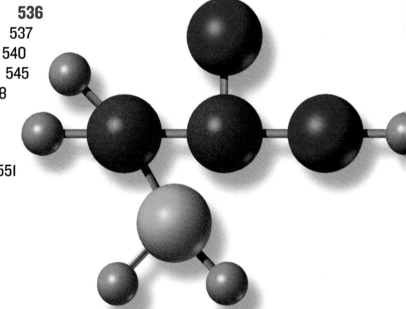

Special Features

WELLNESS *in* ACTION

WHAT ARE TEENS AROUND THE COUNTRY DOING TO PROMOTE WELLNESS? PLENTY! TAKE A LOOK AT THESE REAL-LIFE STORIES...

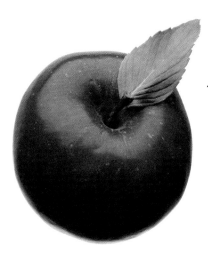

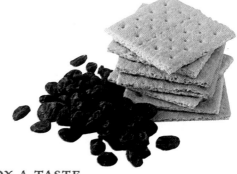

NOW *You're* COOKING!

PRACTICE BASIC COOKING SKILLS—AND ENJOY A TASTE
TREAT—WITH THESE FAST, EASY RECIPES!

Take a culinary trip around the world! Learn about foods and customs as you stop at these ports of call...

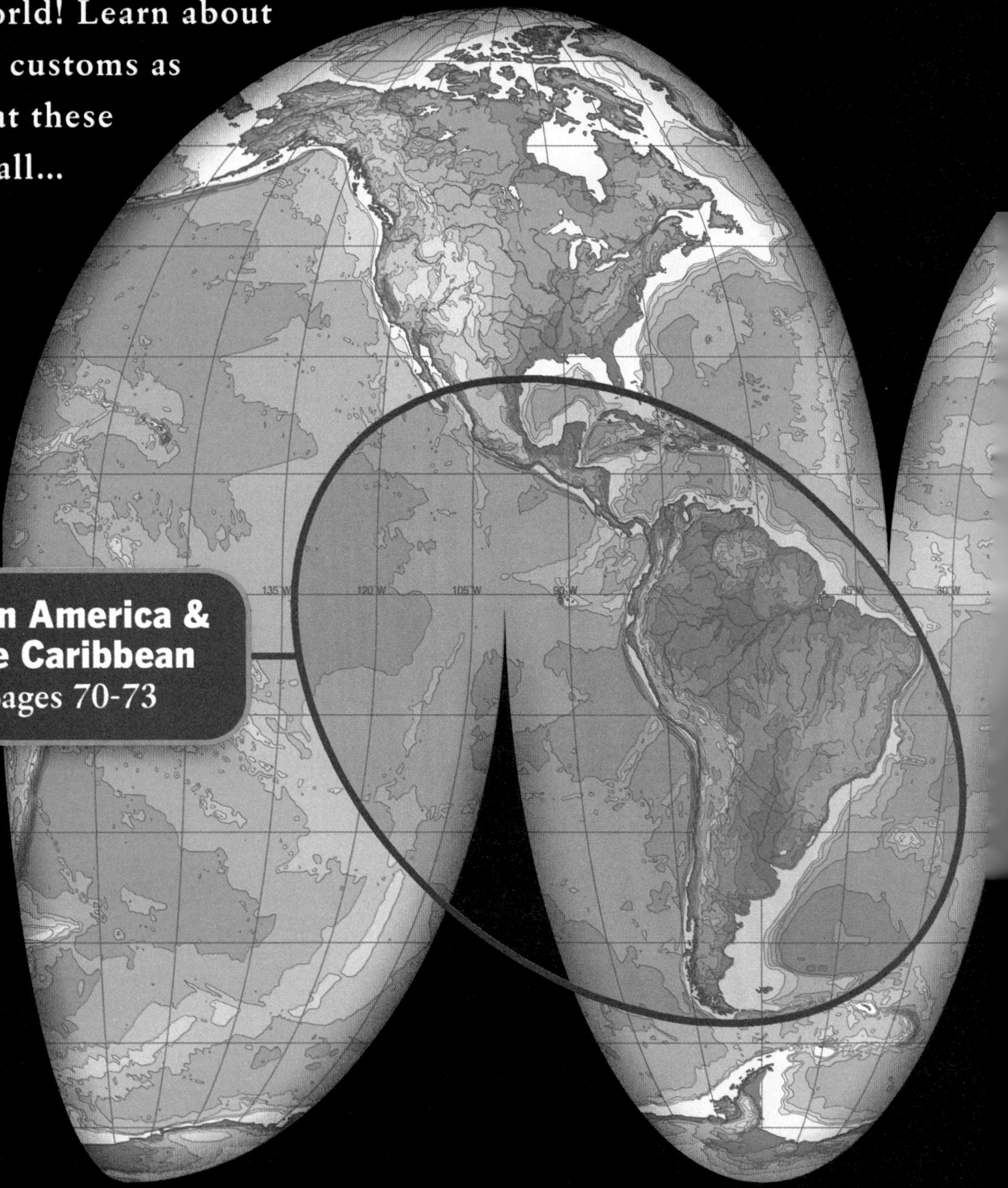

**Latin America &
The Caribbean**
pages 70-73

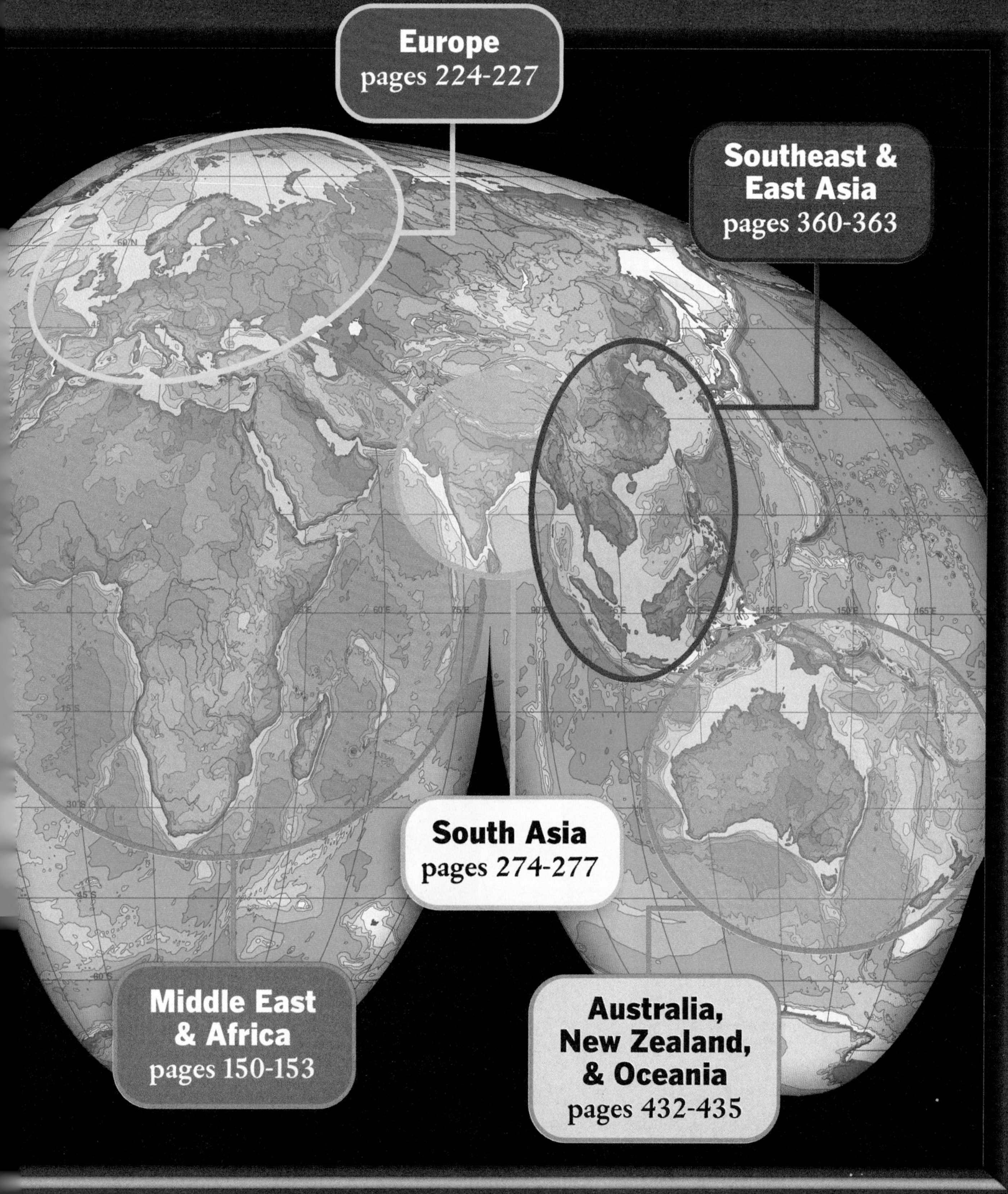

Europe
pages 224-227

Southeast &
East Asia
pages 360-363

South Asia
pages 274-277

Middle East
& Africa
pages 150-153

Australia,
New Zealand,
& Oceania
pages 432-435

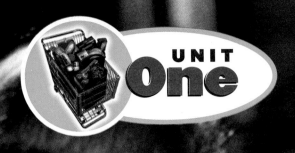

Food in Your Life

IN THIS UNIT...

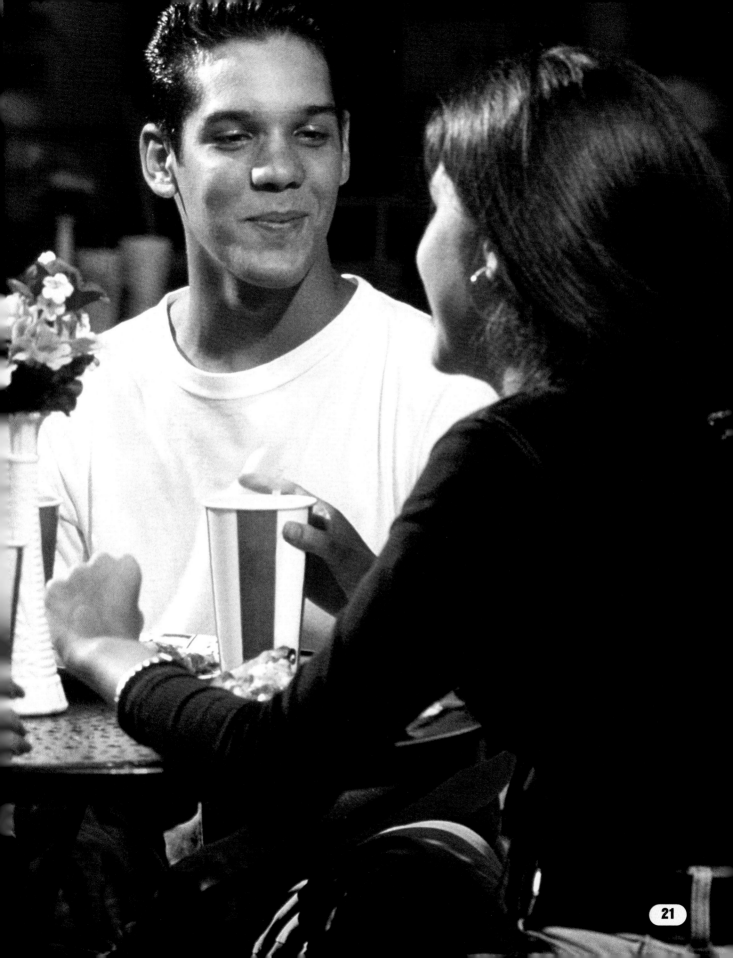

Wellness and Food Choices

Objectives

After studying this chapter, you will be able to:

- Explain three aspects of wellness.

- Discuss how nutrition and physical activity affect wellness.

- Describe the many influences on your food choices.

- Demonstrate how to make decisions and reach goals for wellness.

Do You Know...

...how to handle stress in a healthful way?

...why family foods may be your favorites?

...how to reach your personal goals for wellness?

If not, you'll find out in this chapter!

Look for these TERMS

wellness	culture
lifestyle	resources
nutrition	action plan
nutrients	

Imagine that

someone offered you a deal to help you look your best, save money, give you more energy for schoolwork, sports, and fun, and improve your chances of long life and success. Interested? Actually, it's a deal you can make right now—if you take personal responsibility for your health and well-being. Your good health is up to you!

Wellness: Your Choice for Life!

Wellness means *reaching for your personal overall best level of health.* Practicing wellness means:

- Paying attention to your total health picture: physical health, mental and emotional health, and social health.
- Taking positive steps to improve your current health and help prevent future health problems.
- Recognizing and accepting the responsibility you have for your own health.

Wellness doesn't mean having a perfect body or being free of health problems. Almost no one has that. The key to wellness is accepting and managing your limits and making the most of who you are. Practicing wellness doesn't mean you'll never be sick, either. However, you reduce the chances and get well faster when you make wellness a top priority.

Good Physical Health

Physical health refers to normal functioning of your body systems. A "picture of health" includes bright, clear eyes, firm skin, clean teeth and healthy gums, good muscle tone, and erect posture. Physical health also means having enough energy for daily living, a normal growth rate, resistance to illness, and the ability to relax and sleep well.

The key to wellness is making the most of who you are. Identify three steps you can take that will positively affect your health and well-being.

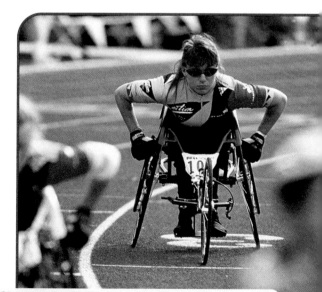

Chapter 1 *Wellness and Food Choices* • **23**

Activity: Record the actions you take in one week to maintain or improve physical health. Evaluate. What are other actions?

Make wellness habits part of your daily routine. If you don't follow these habits regularly, how could you improve? Smart changes are worth the effort!

Taking Action for Physical Health

What can you do to maintain or improve your physical health on your path to wellness? Plenty!

- Follow a varied and healthful eating plan with many different foods, including fruits, vegetables, and whole grains.
- Consume about 8 cups (2 L) of water or other fluids each day, or more if you need it.
- Include plenty of physical activity in your life.
- Eat breakfast each morning.
- Get about eight hours of sleep each night.
- Practice good hygiene.
- Take safety precautions such as wearing your seatbelt.
- Get regular medical and dental checkups.
- Avoid tobacco, alcoholic beverages, and harmful drugs.
- Keep informed about nutrition and wellness.

Mental and Emotional Outlook

Your mental and emotional health includes how you deal with daily life and how you feel about yourself. It affects your overall health more than you may think. People with good mental and emotional health often have better physical health—and they enjoy life!

Mental and emotional health helps you cope with change, face your problems, and handle anger, frustration, and disappointment in an acceptable way. You are able to work toward your goals. With emotional well-being comes a sensitivity to others, open-mindedness, self-esteem, and self-confidence.

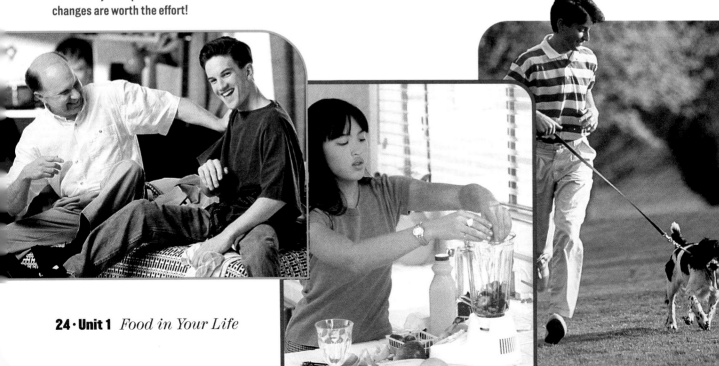

Check This Out!

GREAT STRESS BUSTERS

Stress may get in the way of healthful eating, active living, and other wellness strategies. Learn to handle stress positively!
- Fit physical activity into your daily life.
- Eat smart so that you have the energy to cope with stress.
- Balance school and work responsibilities with time for family, friends, and fun. Don't try to do too much. Learn to say no.
- Admit when you make a mistake, but don't dwell on it. Learn from it and move on.
- Keep a sense of humor.
- Learn how to set goals and priorities and make decisions. That way you manage your life. It doesn't manage you.

It's Your Turn!

Think about specific ways you could put the suggestions given above into practice in your everyday life. How might these ideas help you?

Discuss: How does stress affect food choices, digestion, and nutrition? How does nutrition affect one's ability to manage stress?

Social Well-Being

Social health involves your relationships with others. You have a high level of social health when you:
- Can praise and accept others.
- Enjoy friends of both genders.
- Are helpful and considerate.
- Can accept rules and be responsible.
- Handle conflict in a constructive way.
- Communicate well.
- Handle peer pressure without compromising your values.

Critical Thinking: How does interacting with others contribute to a person's overall wellness?

Tip

You can show you care by preparing a favorite meal for your family, bringing food to a friend, or taking someone out to eat.

Nutrition and Active Living

Does your lifestyle contribute to your wellness? Your **lifestyle** includes *how you live your life and all the things you do.* Two partners for a healthful lifestyle are nutrition and active living.

Nutrition is *how the food you eat affects your body.* For health, energy, and growth, you need to eat a variety of foods in moderate yet adequate amounts. That's because food provides **nutrients,** *chemicals that nourish your body.* Getting the right balance of nutrients helps you look your best, feel your best, and perform well at school and on the job. The food choices you make today will affect your health and quality of life for years to come.

INFOLINK

You'll learn more about nutrients in Chapters 5 and 6.

FIT FOR YOUR FUTURE

Employers look for all three aspects of wellness when they hire someone.

Good physical health
- Ability to work hard, perhaps in physical work.
- Physical energy and stamina to do the job.
- Good hygiene and a neat appearance.

Mental and emotional outlook
- Reliable, responsible attitude toward work, including being on time, following directions, doing your share, and showing respect for the job and workplace.
- Willingness to learn and take initiative.
- Flexibility to adapt as job responsibilities change.

Social well-being
- Friendly, cooperative, respectful, and considerate attitude toward coworkers, customers, and employers.
- Ability to communicate and work well with others.

It's Your Turn!

Imagine that you are an employer with a position to fill. How might you decide whether an applicant has the characteristics listed above? Why would this information be important to you?

Activity: Identify a possible future job. Explain how aspects of wellness would affect job performance.

Active living, with at least 60 minutes of moderately intense physical activity each day, is loaded with wellness benefits. In this book, you'll learn easy, enjoyable ways to eat smart and stay active.

Why You Eat What You Do

Discuss: How does nutritional intake affect health, appearance, and personal life?

Does everyone you know eat and enjoy the same foods? Not likely. You may have favorite foods in common with others, but your overall eating style is unique. Whatever your food choices, keep in mind that any food can be included in an eating plan that promotes wellness.

There are many influences on your food choices. When you know what those influences are, it's easier to make healthful decisions.

People around you. Your family probably has influenced your food preferences and eating habits more than anyone else. You've grown up eating the foods your family likes and learning family food traditions. Your friends influence your food choices, too. Are you a good influence on their choices? Are your food choices affected by peer pressure?

Food choices may be based on family traditions and cultural influences. Ask older friends or family members what food traditions they remember.

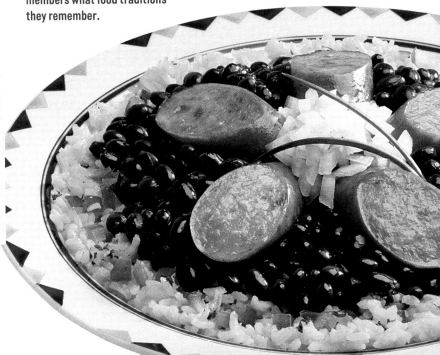

Culture connection. Take a mental trip around the world. Think about the different forms of music or art you hear and see. Like music and art, food is an expression of culture. **Culture** includes *the shared beliefs, values, and behavior of a group of people.* The group might be your local community, your ethnic community, your nation, or your part of the world. Different cultural groups have different food traditions. What are the cultural connections of foods you enjoy? Why can any food be considered a cultural food?

Available food supply. Think of the foods you can buy or grow where you live. What's available in grocery stores, local markets, restaurants, and perhaps your own garden?

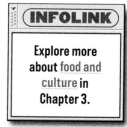

INFOLINK

Explore more about food and culture **in Chapter 3.**

Discuss: List your favorite foods. What cultures do the foods represent?

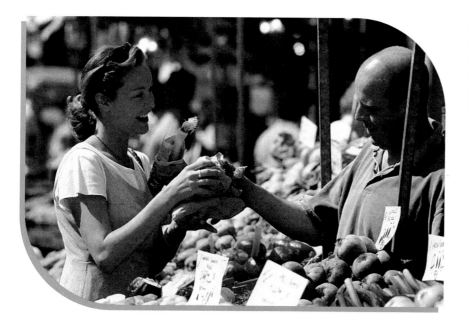

An abundant and varied food supply offers more options for healthful eating. What are some possible health consequences of a limited food supply?

Schedules, energy, budget. The foods you buy and how you prepare them are affected by your resources. **Resources** are *things such as time, money, and personal energy that help you reach a goal or complete a task.* If you're short on money, ground beef might be a better choice than steak. To prepare a quick family meal, you might use foods that are partly or fully prepared.

Advertising and media. How many food advertisements do you read or hear each year? Probably thousands! Ads make you aware of new foods and may provide useful information about nutrition. These same promotions may lead you to buy foods whether or not you really need them.

Discuss: What are major influences on your food choices? List responses on the board. Which is most influential?

Critical Thinking: Find food ads. Determine the methods used to influence people to buy the particular food.

Discuss: What role do media such as television, magazines, newspapers, and the Internet play in your food choices?

INFOLINK

Learn how to find reliable information about nutrition, food, and wellness in Chapter 11.

Discuss: How do your food choices now differ from what they were two years ago? What factors affect the changes?

Knowing about food, nutrition, and wellness. What you know affects the foods you buy, prepare, and eat. The more you know, the more able you are to make food and lifestyle choices that promote wellness.

All about you! Your age, attitudes, emotions, health, and goals all affect what you choose to eat.

Steps to Wellness

Practicing wellness can affect you positively today and into the future. Making responsible decisions and setting realistic goals are important skills to master.

Deciding on Wellness

Each day you make many decisions. Will you eat breakfast? Will you walk to school or get a ride? Will you snack on an apple or a candy bar? Over time, these decisions can impact your health in a major way.

Choose healthful snacks as part of your wellness plan. What other choices can you make today that will benefit your health?

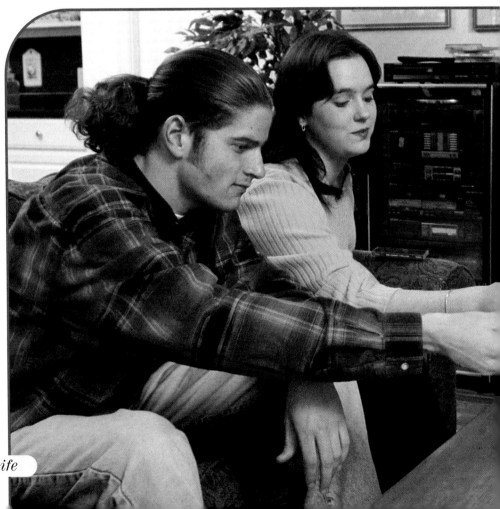

You can follow steps to make sound decisions that match your own goals and values. Using the decision-making steps over and over can help you make choices for your overall wellness—and other aspects of your life.

1. Identify the decision to be made. Some decisions are fairly simple to define. Others are more complex.

2. Collect information and identify your resources. Take time to get facts from reliable sources. Use your critical thinking skills to help you judge what you see, read, and hear. Consider resources such as your time, energy, and budget.

3. Identify the possible choices. When it comes to food and physical activity, you have many options. For example, you can stay active by jogging alone, playing tennis with a friend, or joining a volleyball team.

4. Weigh the possible choices. What are the consequences of each option? What are its pros and cons? Also think about what's important to you and why. When health is a priority, it's easier to make decisions for wellness.

Critical Thinking: Think of a recent decision. Explain how you made it. Apply the seven-step process. Compare the differences, if any, in the final decision.

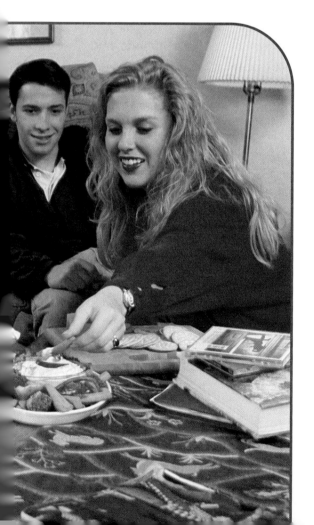

5. Choose the best option. Make your choice based on facts, goals, priorities, and values, not on peer pressure. Your friend's milk shake may not be your best snack choice if you're watching your weight.

6. Take action. Your decision won't benefit you if you don't act on it.

7. Evaluate your decision. Did you get the result you expected? How did your decision affect others? What did you learn? Would you make the same choice again?

Taking Action for Wellness

Activity: Choose a goal to improve your wellness. Use the tips for making an action plan work to help you reach it.

How would you like to feel now—and years from now? An **action plan** is *a step-by-step approach to identifying and reaching your goals.* By making an action plan for wellness, you shape your life and personal success. Here are some tips for making an action plan work for you.

1. Set realistic goals. Match goals to your abilities and needs. You don't need to aim for perfection.

2. Decide on a plan. You probably can reach the same goal in several ways. Use the decision-making process to help you choose the best alternative.

3. Identify small, achievable steps. Write them down. If your goal is to run 5 miles, you can begin with shorter distances and gradually lengthen your runs.

4. Take action. Just do it! A plan that's never acted on can't succeed.

5. Stick with it. Challenges crop up—perhaps you're low on energy or time. Find creative ways to get back on track.

6. Get support. Ask family, friends, and teachers to encourage you. Their support is important. Return the favor by supporting others.

7. Check your progress. Evaluate your efforts. Are your goals realistic? If not, learn from experience. Rethink your plan and try again.

8. Reward yourself. When you reach your goal—or achieve small steps—pat yourself on the back with a trip to the movies or a new CD. Enjoy the satisfaction of taking care of yourself!

Setting and achieving realistic goals builds your self-esteem. Make "can do" goals your focus for success. What realistic goals can you set to achieve wellness and promote your own self-esteem?

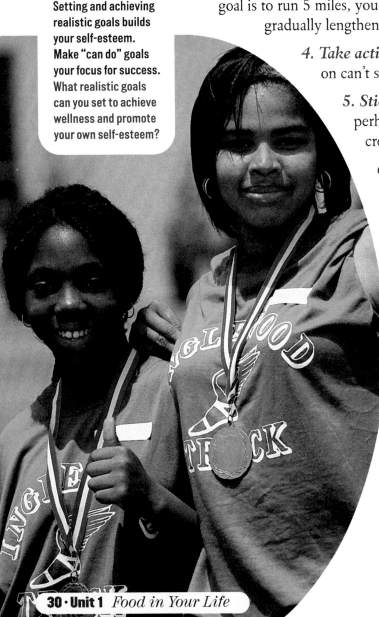

HELP WANTED

Personal TRAINER

Health club seeks energetic personal trainer to plan and supervise individualized fitness programs. Must be physically fit, health conscious, and able to motivate others. Two-year degree preferred. Send resume to Total Health and Fitness Club.

Activities Director

Nursing home needs a creative Activities Director to plan and organize daily activities for individuals with various interests. Associate degree and two years of experience preferred. Good interpersonal skills a must. Send resume to Administrator, Residential Manor.

Community Recreation Director

Large recreation center needs an organized Recreation Director to manage adult and youth programs, supervise staff, oversee facilities, direct programs, and coordinate community events. Excellent leadership skills needed. Degree in recreation management preferred. Send resume to: Human Resources, City of Evergreen.

Teachers

Major metropolitan school district has openings for full-time teachers of Middle School Health and Physical Education and High School Family and Consumer Sciences. Bachelor's degree and current state license required. Also oversee extracurricular activities. Submit resume, transcript, and references to District Superintendent of Instruction.

Weight Reduction Assistant

Successful weight loss clinic seeks Weight Reduction Assistant. Assist clients with weekly assessments. Check vital signs and provide support services. High school diploma and good communication skills required. Nutrition classes a plus. Stop by Center for Healthy Living.

Wellness Specialist

Large manufacturing company seeks a Wellness Specialist to develop and manage employee wellness program. Determine needs of workers and maintain active employee participation. Bachelor's degree and outstanding organizational skills required. Submit resume to Human Resources Director, Chempro, Inc.

LINKING *to the* WORKPLACE

❶ Teaching in Many Jobs: There are many jobs that involve teaching. Research two occupations (outside of a school) in which workers are required to teach others. What do the workers teach? Whom do they teach? What are their other responsibilities?

❷ Managing Multiple Roles: Many workers must fulfill multiple roles on the job, in their family, and in the community. Wellness requires the ability to balance these demands on time and energy. What strategies can help employees manage their multiple roles? What programs and policies do some employers offer that can help?

Review & Activities

LOOKING BACK

- Wellness involves all aspects of your health. Taking responsibility for your own health is also part of wellness.
- Good nutrition and active living are important for promoting wellness.
- Many influences help determine your food preferences and eating habits.
- Making responsible decisions and following an action plan can help you practice wellness.

UNDERSTANDING KEY IDEAS

1. What is meant by "wellness"? What three aspects of health does it include?
2. What actions can help maintain or improve physical health? Name at least four.
3. Why is developing good mental and emotional health important?
4. What are some signs of social well-being?
5. How does nutrition contribute to wellness?
6. How might your decisions about what to eat be influenced by where you live? What else can influence food choices?
7. What should you consider when setting goals for an action plan?

DEVELOPING LIFE SKILLS

1. **Management:** Imagine that you have to make a decision to promote your health, such as how to fit regular physical activity into your daily life. How could you use the seven-step process outlined in this chapter to make the decision?
2. **Leadership:** Practicing wellness involves taking responsibility for your own health. What responsibility, if any, do individuals have for the health of others? How can you take a leadership role when it comes to wellness? Can peer pressure be used to positively influence food choices and other aspects of wellness? Explain your answers.

Wellness Challenge

Lately Jamie's been feeling overwhelmed. She plays the trumpet in the marching band and is treasurer of the Spanish Club. Club members are urging her to run for president. While she eats breakfast and lunch every day, Jamie often doesn't have time to eat dinner before heading to her part-time job. Between her studies, school activities, and work, Jamie often feels she doesn't have the time or energy to keep up with her busy schedule.

1. What strategies might help Jamie reduce or manage stress?
2. What are some ways in which Jamie is currently practicing wellness? What else could she do to build on that foundation?

APPLYING YOUR LEARNING

1. **Wellness Plan:** Create an action plan for wellness. Begin by thinking of a situation (real or imagined) in which you might benefit from a wellness plan. Identify the steps in your plan. Describe how each suggestion given on page 30 applies to the chosen situation.

2. **Identifying Influences:** Think of a meal in which each food illustrates one or more different influences on food choices. (For example, a taco could illustrate the influence of culture.) Create a menu that lists or pictures the foods in your meal and identifies the influences for each one.

EXPLORING FURTHER

1. **Learning About Stress:** Use classroom, library, or Internet resources to find out more about stress. How does stress affect health? What are some common causes of stress? What are possible signs of stress, and what should you do if you notice these signs? Present your findings to the class.

2. **Community Outreach:** Many hospitals offer outreach programs to enhance the wellness of the community. Find out about a community outreach program at a hospital in your area. What classes and services are offered? How might you volunteer to help?

Making CONNECTIONS

1. **Health:** Using what you have learned in health class, explain how healthy habits such as the ones mentioned in this chapter can help increase your resistance to illness.

2. **Language Arts:** Create a poem or short essay to express some of the influences that have had the greatest impact on your own food preferences.

FOODS LAB

Collect two recipes for quick, nutritious breakfast foods. Prepare the foods in class. What was the amount of time needed for preparation? How might you incorporate such recipes into your morning schedule?

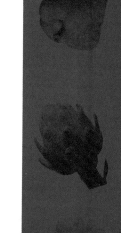

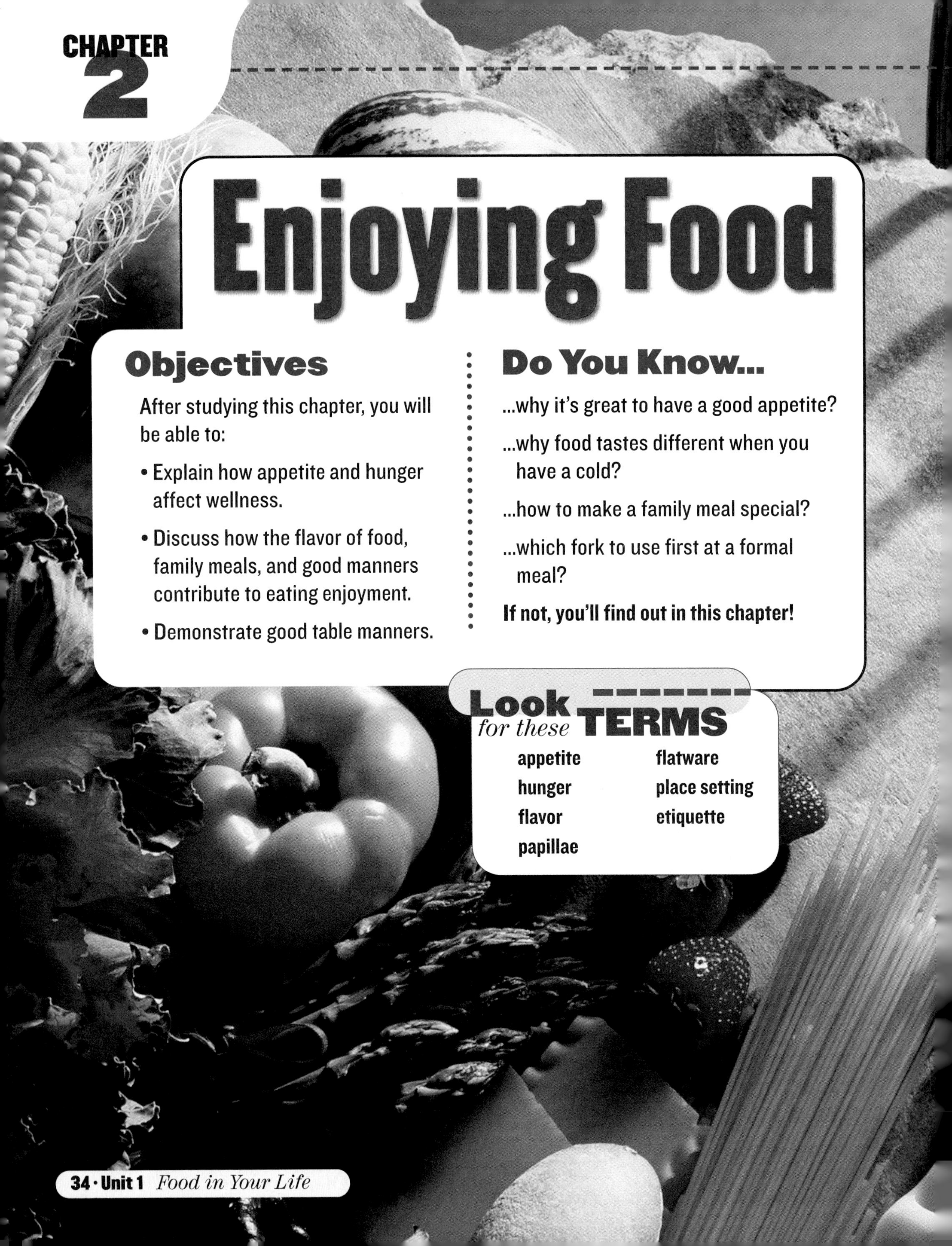

Enjoying Food

Objectives

After studying this chapter, you will be able to:

- Explain how appetite and hunger affect wellness.
- Discuss how the flavor of food, family meals, and good manners contribute to eating enjoyment.
- Demonstrate good table manners.

Do You Know...

...why it's great to have a good appetite?

...why food tastes different when you have a cold?

...how to make a family meal special?

...which fork to use first at a formal meal?

If not, you'll find out in this chapter!

Look *for these* TERMS

appetite
hunger
flavor
papillae

flatware
place setting
etiquette

Food is one of

life's great pleasures! You may relish the taste and aroma of a favorite food. You can enjoy the company of others at special or everyday meals. You may choose a food because it brings back happy memories. Your food choices and the experiences that surround eating can add enjoyment to your everyday life.

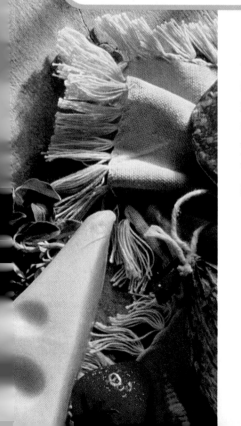

The Appeal of Food

What are your favorite foods? Why are they so appetizing? If you're like most people, great taste topped the list of reasons. Many people choose one food before another because of taste. In an eating plan that promotes wellness, your favorite great-tasting foods fit!

Hunger or Appetite?

"Just looking at that food makes my mouth water!" "I hope it tastes as incredible as it looks!" "The aroma makes me hungry!" Are you really hungry, or is it your appetite?

Your Appetite

The way your senses respond to food does perk up your appetite. Your **appetite**, *a psychological desire to eat,* can be stimulated by the sight or aroma of food as well as its taste. Just seeing your favorite food can make you think you're hungry, even when you aren't. Sound can affect your appetite, too. The sound of popping corn or food sizzling on a grill can perk up your desire to eat.

A good appetite is a sign of wellness and can help you stay well nourished. The reason? When you find food enjoyable and appealing, you're more likely to eat the variety of foods you need for good health.

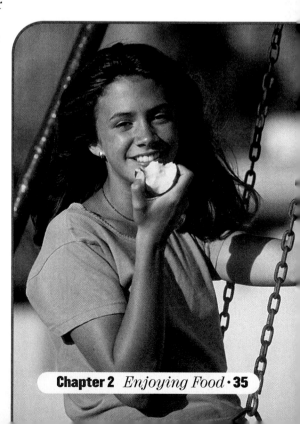

Activity: Make a chart on the board, with the five senses—taste, smell, sight, sound, touch—as headings. Ask student volunteers to fill in the chart with foods that appeal to each of the senses.

What makes certain foods so appealing? What are some foods that trigger your appetite?

Feeling Hungry

When an empty stomach contracts or growls, you're experiencing **hunger**, which is *a physical need to eat.* Hunger pangs signal that your body needs a fresh supply of food energy and nutrients. Fatigue or a light-headed feeling may be signs of hunger.

The sensation of hunger goes away when you've had enough to eat. It takes about 20 minutes for that message to get from your stomach to your brain. Instead of gulping your meal, slow down and enjoy it. That way you're also less likely to overeat.

Food and Your Emotions

Food satisfies more than your physical needs. You may choose foods because of your emotions. Some people eat to relieve stress or boredom, which may lead to overeating. As you learned in Chapter 1, there are more appropriate ways to handle stress.

Food is also used to express positive emotions. Some people show love for their family by preparing a favorite meal. You probably have favorites based on foods you shared with your family at happy times. If you're feeling ill or sad, you may want a food that has special meaning from your childhood. This is known as a comfort food.

Some of your food favorites may remind you of happy times you shared with your family. What are some of your comfort foods?

Activity: Eat slowly the next time you are hungry and time how long it takes for the sensation of hunger to go away. Chart the results.

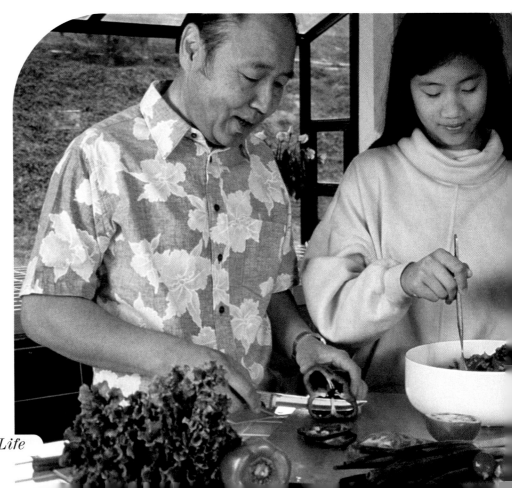

Sensing Food's Flavor

Why do some chilies make your mouth feel fiery hot? Why does ice cream give you a very different experience? It's all in the way your senses help you experience and enjoy food.

When people talk about the taste of food, they often mean flavor. **Flavor** *combines a food's taste, smell, and touch.* People experience flavor somewhat differently. That's one reason why they like different foods. The flavor of spinach or salsa may seem stronger to you than to a friend. Children tend to have a keener sense of taste than adults do—especially older adults.

You experience taste in your mouth, mostly with your tongue. Your tongue is covered with **papillae** (puh-PIH-lee), or *tiny bumps that contain the taste buds.*

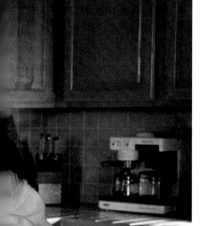

Each papilla has hundreds of taste buds, which distinguish sweet, sour, salty, and bitter tastes. Other nerve endings in your mouth sense the texture and the temperature of food.

When one of your senses is altered, the flavor of food might also be altered. Have you ever noticed that food doesn't taste the same when you have a cold? That's because you can't smell it! To test this, hold your nose and bite into an onion. It'll probably taste more like an apple. Illness and taking medication can dull sensations and detract from the flavor of foods.

Activity: Plan a meal that includes a variety of flavors, such as sweet, tangy, sour, and spicy. Share your meal plans with the class.

Check This Out!

FOR FOOD'S BEST FLAVOR

To get the fullest enjoyment from food, make the most of its flavor with these simple tips.
- Eat fresh foods.
- Prepare food properly. Avoid overcooking. Crisp carrots are more appetizing than limp, brown carrots.
- Serve food at the temperature that brings out the flavor. Hot hamburgers taste better than cold ones.
- Plan interesting meals involving different flavors. Why not serve spicy chicken with a refreshing dip?
- Take time to enjoy the food.

It's Your Turn!

Locate a copy of a restaurant menu or find a menu plan in a magazine or on the Internet. Choose one or more of the dishes and decide how it fits the points covered above.

Tip

Do you like salty foods? If so, it's a preference you learned. Cut back on salt gradually. Your desire for salty foods will decrease. In Chapter 7, you'll learn why you may want to cut back on salt.

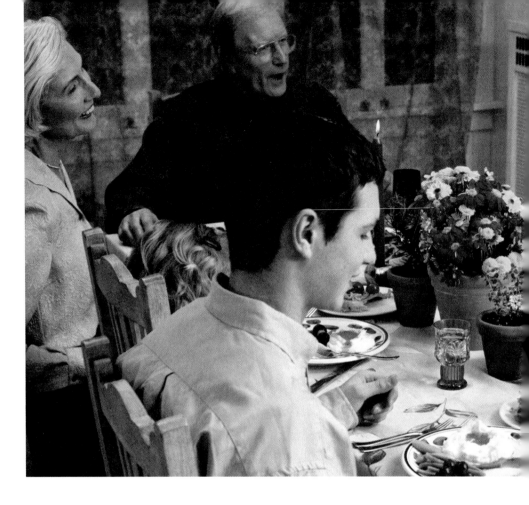

Discuss: How do family eating patterns of today compare to those of the past? What patterns do you predict for the future?

Eating Together

Think of all the wonderful times spent with friends and family. How often do these times include food? Food can help bring people together, and eating with others can add to the enjoyment of food.

INFOLINK

Read how to make meals and snacks appealing **in Part 5 of the Food Preparation Handbook.**

Eating with Your Family

At one time, families almost always ate dinner together. Today, with everyone's busy schedule, sitting down together almost seems like a luxury. You're smart, however, to make time for family meals. Whether it's breakfast, lunch, or dinner, a family meal can be a relaxing chance to spend time together and catch up on the day. Studies show that eating together helps family members follow more healthful eating patterns, too.

Here are some tips to help make the most of family meals at home.

Critical Thinking: Eating together helps family members follow more healthful eating patterns. Do you agree? Why or why not?

- Plan at least one family meal a week when you all can be together. Make it your goal to be home on time.

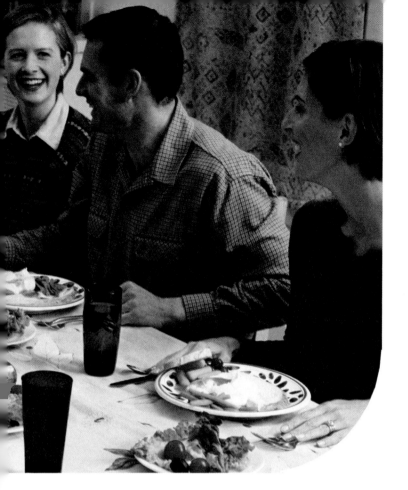

INFOLINK

For tips on planning family meals, check out Chapter 12.

Spending time together is a great way for family members to enjoy a meal. How can you make meal-time more enjoyable when you eat alone?

- Stay at the table until everyone is finished.
- Join in on family conversation. Save unpleasant topics for later.
- Extend your time together by sharing meal preparation and cleanup.

Eating with Your Friends

Pizza parties, slumber parties, school games and dances, snacking at the mall—food seems to go with many things teens like to do. If you're planning meals for friends, think about taste, appeal, nutrition, and fun! Be a trendsetter and serve something different. Try these ideas.

Party foods: popcorn flavored with Parmesan cheese, veggie-topped pizza, potato wedges and salsa, sparkling water mixed with different juices.

Field trip/bus trip snacks: apples, grapes, tangerines, trail mix, granola bars, string cheese and crackers, canned fruit juice.

Mall foods: yogurt-fruit smoothie, bagel with hummus or veggie-cheese spread, oatmeal cookie, hot pretzel.

More About Popcorn: If cooked in oil and topped with butter, popcorn is very high in fat calories. Hot-air popped without toppings has no fat calories. Try low-fat butter sprays or crushed herbs and spices.

Making Meals Pleasant

Eating together is more enjoyable when you make the surroundings pleasant and when your actions show consideration for others.

Your Surroundings

Eating in pleasant surroundings can contribute to positive attitudes about healthful eating. Nice touches include:
- A simple centerpiece, such as a plant, to make the table special.
- Food served in bowls or on plates (not from packages or jars). Have serving spoons and forks ready.
- Pleasing music, not a TV show, so that you can focus on your food and meal companions.
- Pleasant table talk. Listen and add to the conversation yourself.

The Table Setting

A table is set in a specific way to make eating convenient. The illustration below shows where dishes, cups, **flatware** (*the knives, forks, and spoons you eat with*), and napkins go. The *dishes, flatware, glasses, and linens for one person*, or a **place setting**, depend on the menu and the formality of the meal.

Table Manners

In a social setting, your manners are a reflection of you. Another word for manners is **etiquette** (EH-tih-kit)—*polite conduct that shows respect and consideration for others.* Your good manners help

INFOLINK

Read about serving food for special occasions in Part 5 of the Food Preparation Handbook.

Teaching with Visuals: Call on students to set a place at a table, using the photo as their guide.

Allow 20 inches (50 cm) for each place setting so people can sit comfortably. Line up the utensils evenly, about 1 inch (2.5 cm) from the table's edge. Note the placement of the salad plate and salad fork and the cup and saucer. The two glasses allow for a person to have a glass of water and another beverage. If you would not be serving a salad course, which items could you eliminate from this place setting?

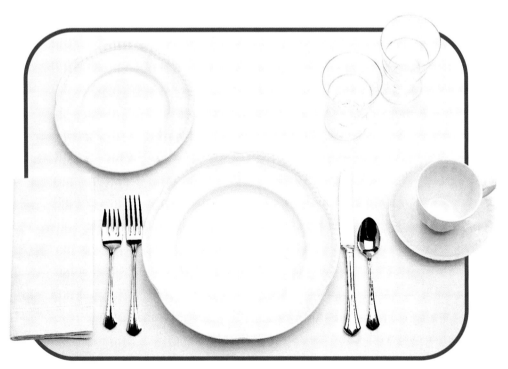

others feel at ease and valued. Being courteous helps you feel good, too. When people practice etiquette, everyone knows what's expected, so mealtime can be relaxed.

Conduct that is considered good manners may vary in different cultures. For example, in southern China, it is polite to lift a bowl close to your mouth so that rice is not spilled.

Following etiquette basics can help you show respect for everyone eating with you—and make meals more pleasant for you. Here are some etiquette basics.

Sitting at the table. Come to the table when the meal is ready—don't make others wait. Sit with good posture. Keep your elbows off the table.

Serving food. Use a serving fork or spoon, not your flatware, to take food from a serving plate or bowl. Ask others to pass food you can't reach. Wait until everyone is served before starting to eat.

Using place-setting items. Unfold your napkin on your lap. If there is more than one spoon or fork, use the one on the outside first. When you're not using the knife, place it across the top of the plate.

Eating. Lift food to your mouth rather than lowering your head toward the plate. Take small bites and eat slowly, chewing with your mouth closed. Let hot food cool before taking a bite rather than blowing on it. Eat everything on the fork or spoon at one time. Use a piece of bread instead of your fingers to push food onto a spoon or fork. Sip beverages rather than gulp them. Drink your beverage when you're done swallowing food.

Handling awkward moments. Remove fruit pits and fish bones from your mouth discreetly, covering your mouth with a napkin. Use a napkin to blot or lightly wipe your mouth if you need to— never for blowing your nose. Cover your mouth if you need to cough or burp. Quietly excuse yourself if you burp. If you spill something, apologize and help clean up. Then forget it so that the accident doesn't remain in the conversation.

Discuss: What are other examples of table etiquette?

Check This Out!

"CHECK, PLEASE!" MANNERS FOR EATING OUT

Good manners and courtesy help you feel comfortable and more confident when you eat out.

Seating tips

- To reserve a table, call ahead. Give your name, the number of guests, and the time you prefer. Arrive on time. Call to cancel the reservation if your group can't go.
- Unless a sign says to seat yourself, wait for the host or hostess to lead you to a table. If you have a preference, perhaps the non-smoking section, ask before you're seated.

Courtesy to the server

- Be patient and considerate, especially when the restaurant is busy.
- Quietly attract the server's attention with a hand motion, a nod, or a smile. If necessary, ask another server to get your server.
- If you receive the wrong order or if it's not prepared properly, politely let the server know.
- Take time to thank the server, especially for handling special requests.

Courtesy to other diners

- Talk quietly so that your conversation won't bother guests at other tables.
- To talk with friends at another table, go to their table. Keep your chat brief.

It's Your Turn!

Divide into groups of three or four. Decide which one of you will be the server in a restaurant. Enact a scene in which some of the above tips come into play. How did you handle any difficult situations?

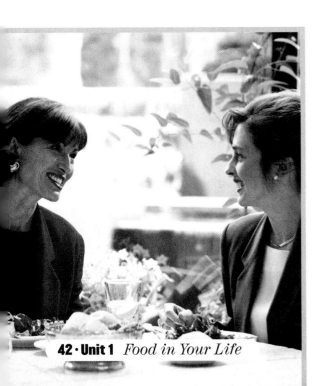

Finishing up. When you're done, place your napkin neatly to the left of your plate. Place your knife and fork parallel across the center of your plate. Offer to clear the table and help with cleanup. If you must leave before others are done, excuse yourself graciously. Thank anyone who prepared the meal—including family members.

In the world of work, using good manners is an important strategy for success. Make them an everyday habit. A business meal may start with introductions. Find out and then demonstrate to the class how to introduce people properly.

Activity: Tipping the server 15-20% of the food bill is a customary part of dining out and shows appreciation for good service. Practice figuring a 15% tip.

Teen "Chefs" Become
Culinary Artists

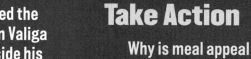

As the sun rose, teens in Waukesha, Wisconsin, added the finishing touches to their culinary creations. Jason Valiga carefully arranged colorful Red Pepper Polenta beside his Proscuitto-Spinach Stuffed Flank Steak. Kerry Liebenthal added a spicy-hot dash of chili powder to her Spanish Rice served with vegetable-filled Fajitas with Pico de Gallo. Don LaPrairie mounded his crunchy Cashew Corn Salsa as the perfect complement to his Texas Beef Tips.

After weeks of training with Mark Lehman, a professional Marriott chef, 11 teens were preparing for their morning competition in the state-wide Wisconsin Restaurant Association Food Show. Each teen developed a unique recipe for beef, giving special attention to the variety of colors, textures, shapes, and flavors of all foods on their menu.

"We like the artistic aspect of preparing a healthful meal!" noted Alexandra Gonzalez. The Waukesha teens proudly returned to their schools with seven top culinary medals—showing how a variety of foods and careful presentation add appeal to any meal!

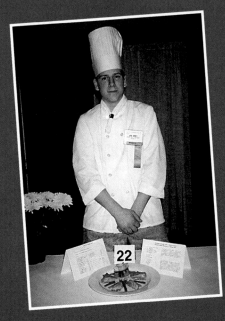

Take Action

Why is meal appeal so important to good nutrition? How can you add creativity and variety to your next meal? Look through the photographs in food magazines. Find several meals that appeal to you and identify what makes them so appetizing. Use the ideas to prepare an appealing meal at home. Take a photograph or draw a picture to show your creativity.

Review & Activities

LOOKING BACK

- Appetite is the psychological desire to eat; hunger is the physical need to eat.
- Flavor helps you experience and enjoy foods.
- Eating with your family and friends can add to the enjoyment of meals.
- Meals are more pleasant when attention is paid to the surroundings, the table setting, and table manners.

UNDERSTANDING KEY IDEAS

1. In what way does hunger help promote physical health?
2. What is the relationship between wellness and appetite?
3. Give examples of ways in which food helps meet emotional and social needs.
4. If you burn your tongue, how might your enjoyment of eating be affected? Why?
5. What are the benefits of eating together as a family?
6. Why is mealtime etiquette important? Give three examples of good manners at the table.
7. Suppose you order a cheeseburger at a restaurant. When your meal arrives, the cheeseburger is cold. What would be the best way to deal with this situation?

DEVELOPING LIFE SKILLS

1. **Communication:** How does pleasant table talk contribute toward making a meal enjoyable? What are some appropriate topics for mealtime conversation? What topics are not appropriate? Why?
2. **Creative Thinking:** Think of ways to make an attractive centerpiece out of items that you already have around the house.
3. **Management:** How might time management help families eat together more often?

Wellness Challenge

About six months ago Rico's great-grandmother, Nana Rose, came to live with his family. Lately Rico has noticed that Nana Rose doesn't seem to be eating as often or as much as usual. When Rico asked her about it, Nana shrugged and said, "Food just doesn't appeal to me anymore. But it's nothing to worry about."

1. Do you think Rico should be concerned? Why or why not?
2. What are some possible explanations for Nana Rose's loss of appetite?
3. What could Rico and other family members do to help?

APPLYING YOUR LEARNING

1. **Simulations:** With other students, act out how you would handle the following situations in a thoughtful manner: (a) Someone spills food on you. (b) You do not care for the taste of a food that is on your plate. (c) At a restaurant, you ask for salad dressing to be served on the side. When the salad arrives, it is drenched in dressing.

2. **Table Setting:** Design a casual or formal table setting for two people. Include dishes, flatware, a tablecloth or place mats, and a centerpiece. You may set an actual table, draw the setting with colored pencils, or make a collage of pictures from catalogs and magazines.

EXPLORING FURTHER

1. **Manners in Other Cultures:** Choose a country or culture outside of North America. Find out what is considered good table manners among the people of that country or culture. (Hint: You might consult travel guidebooks.)

2. **Serving Styles:** Consult etiquette books or other sources to learn about two more styles of serving food: modified English service and formal service. How is the food served? What are the advantages and disadvantages of each method? At what type of occasion might each be used?

Making CONNECTIONS

1. **Science:** Write a brief report about Ivan Petrovich Pavlov's experiments related to stimulation of the appetite.

2. **Career Connections Experience:** Research proper etiquette for a business meal in Japan, including introductions. Compile a list of guidelines, then train a classmate or family member to follow them. Conclude by conducting a simulation of a Japanese business meal. Ask the person you trained to evaluate your skill as an etiquette consultant.

FOODS LAB

Conduct a blind taste test of the following foods: an apple, an orange, broccoli, mustard, and an onion. While blindfolded, try to identify each food by its taste and smell. Then repeat the experiment while holding your nose. Can you identify the foods now? What can you conclude?

A World of Diversity

Objectives

After studying this chapter, you will be able to:

- Analyze how culture and food supply affect food choices.

- Explain how regional foods develop.

- Describe how foods from other cultures can fit into your plan for healthful eating.

- Identify how global food choices are interrelated.

Do You Know...

...why chop suey is really an American dish?

...where tomatoes and potatoes originated?

...what food choices say about cultural influences?

If not, you'll find out in this chapter!

Look for these TERMS

cuisine   regional foods

ethnic foods

When it comes

to food, the world is interconnected! Consider the origins of some of today's breakfast choices. Yogurt was produced in ancient times, perhaps in camel caravans in the Middle East, as milk fermented in pouches. Oranges, which grew in Asia 20 million years ago, were brought to the United States by the Spanish. Hot cocoa was popular in Aztec and Mayan cultures. The flavors of healthful eating reflect a rich worldwide heritage of food and culture.

Different Foods, Different Customs

From country to country and region to region, **cuisine**—*typical foods and ways of cooking associated with a group of people*—differs. For example, in China, squid and sea cucumbers are delicacies!

People around the world eat in different ways, too. Some use just spoons, while others use forks, spoons, and knives, or chopsticks, or fingers. In some places, people pass food in dishes. In others, people reach into a large family bowl of food in the middle of the table. Why are foods and customs so different? Both culture and food supply play a role.

Food and Culture

Culture includes the beliefs, values, and behavior shared by a group of people. The culture you live in is reflected in your everyday life—not only in your clothes and language, but also in your food habits and choices.

Culture influences what foods you eat, when you eat them, and perhaps where, how, and with whom you eat. Cultures have subcultures with their own special food customs. Besides pizza and hamburgers, what foods are associated with American teen culture?

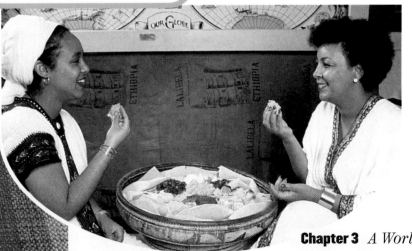

Around the world you'll find a vast variety of food choices and styles of eating. Search the Internet for a favorite food in another country.

Activity: Place pins on a world or U.S. map where students have been. Discuss the type of table, seating, and utensils used.

Activity: Bread is a food in all cultures;it comes in many forms. Find out from which ethnic groups the breads originated and what their ingredients are. Include limpa, pita, gissini, kugel-hopf, matzo, and chapati.

Activity: Make a list of local community events that involve food. Analyze how these events reflect or shape the food customs in your community.

If a religion has food customs, followers of the religion, no matter where in the world they live, will usually adhere to those customs. Research a religion to discover some of its food customs. Try to uncover the reason for those customs.

Ethnic Background

An ethnic group is a race or nationality of people with common cultural characteristics. The *foods and food traditions belonging to an ethnic group* are often called **ethnic foods**. Ethnic food traditions are often passed through many generations. Children learn to enjoy ethnic foods prepared by their families. The foods of many different ethnic groups have shaped American cuisine today.

Religious Customs

Religious customs may include periods of feasting and fasting. They may identify foods that can't be eaten and prescribe ways to prepare and eat other foods. For example, dietary laws of Orthodox Judaism prohibit meat and dairy products at the same meal. Many Christians avoid eating meat during Lent. Islamic laws prohibit eating pork. Sacred writings of Hinduism prohibit beef and recommend avoiding other meats.

Holiday Customs

What foods do you enjoy on Thanksgiving? The Fourth of July? Your birthday? Certain foods are associated with particular celebrations. In most cultures, feasts celebrate important events such as bountiful harvests, national observances, or religious holidays. Families also celebrate personal holidays such as birthdays, graduations, and weddings with foods unique to their family and culture. Food traditions play an important part in life's celebrations.

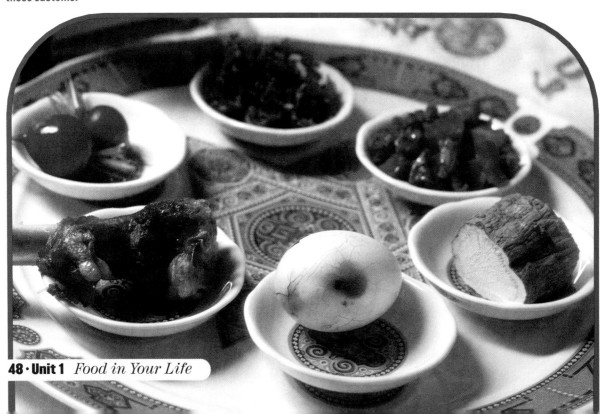

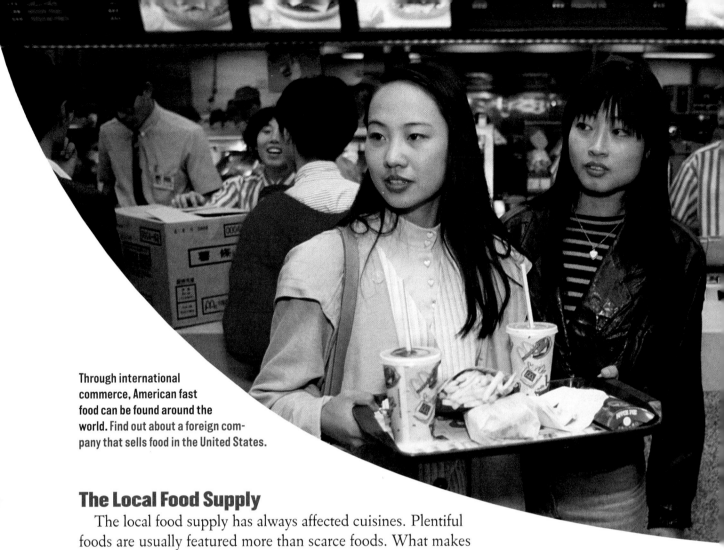

Through international commerce, American fast food can be found around the world. Find out about a foreign company that sells food in the United States.

The Local Food Supply

The local food supply has always affected cuisines. Plentiful foods are usually featured more than scarce foods. What makes food abundant?

Climate and Geography

The cuisine of a particular area depends largely on what can be grown or produced locally. That's why coastal cuisines usually feature seafood, and why fruit is so common in tropical countries. Modern transportation and food preservation techniques, however, are making cuisines less dependent on local climate and geography.

Commerce

Throughout history, food has been exchanged through commerce. For this reason, foods from different places may be surprisingly similar—and foods produced in one place can become part of the cuisine elsewhere. For example, bananas, which originated in Malaysia, are grown today in Central America and imported to the United States, where they top many bowls of breakfast cereal. Politics and trade policies affect commerce and the price of imported food.

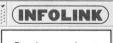

INFOLINK

Read more about the food supply in Chapter 4.

Activity: Find a food in a grocery store that was packaged in a foreign country. Compare and contrast the package label messages with a similar U.S.-packaged food.

INFOLINK

Read more about cuisine around the world in the Global Nutrition & Wellness features. See the list of features on pages 18–19.

Immigration and Travel

When people move to a new place, they often want familiar foods. They find comfort in continuing to enjoy the favorite flavors and preparation methods of their family and culture. They might blend these foods with the local cuisine of their new home.

People often try new foods when they travel and then want to enjoy them back home. That's what European explorers did 500 years ago—they brought foods from the Americas back to Europe.

Foods in North America

Like all countries, the United States and Canada have their own food traditions. They range from everyday foods like hamburgers and hot dogs to holiday favorites like turkey and pumpkin pie. What American food traditions can you think of?

North America's Food Heritage

American cuisine and food traditions began with and include the foods grown, gathered, and hunted by Native Americans. Native Americans helped European settlers survive by teaching them about local foods, including turkey, squash, pumpkin, lima beans, corn, and cranberries.

Each group of newcomers added their influences to American cuisine. For example, German immigrants brought apple strudel; Scandinavians, meatballs; eastern Europeans, many of them Jewish, bagels; the Irish, corned beef and cabbage; and Italians, pasta dishes. French colonists brought delicious casseroles and meat pies to Quebec. Asians brought stir-fry cooking methods. Slaves adapted the bean stews of Africa to create Hoppin' John—ham hocks with black-eyed peas and rice. They prepared sweet potatoes and turnip greens like the yams and greens grown in Africa.

American cuisine continues to change and expand. How are today's immigrants from Latin America, Asia, eastern Europe, and the Middle East, among others, adding variety and flavor to our food heritage?

Activity: Choose a particular group of Native Americans or immigrants. Identify their contributions to American cuisine and find recipes for typical foods. As a class, compile the information and recipes into a book titled "North America's Food Heritage" and display it.

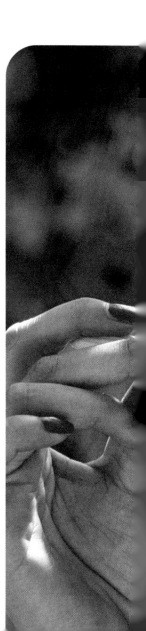

Check This Out!

FOODS THE AMERICAS GAVE THE WORLD

What are *tomatl, mani, mahiz, chilli,* and *papa*? They're the names of foods you may eat every day. *Tomatl* is the Aztec name for tomato. *Mani* is a Quechua (Indian) name for peanut. *Mahiz* is maize or corn in the Arawak language. *Chilli* is the Aztec word for pepper, and *papa* is Incan for potato. Until about 500 years ago, all these foods grew only in the Americas. Then explorers began introducing them to the rest of the world.

The people in the other parts of the world embraced these new foods. That's why residents of Senegal enjoy groundnut stew made with peanuts and Irish stew features potatoes. Cocoa beans from the Americas made the Swiss famous for their chocolate. What about sauce for Italian pasta? That's right, tomatoes from America.

It's Your Turn!

Find out about another food that originated in the Americas and is now popular in other parts of the world. How is it used in these places?

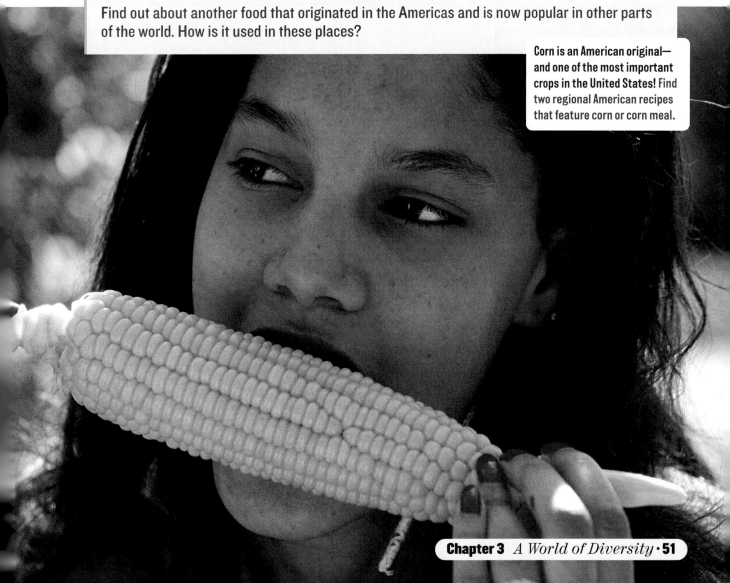

Corn is an American original—and one of the most important crops in the United States! Find two regional American recipes that feature corn or corn meal.

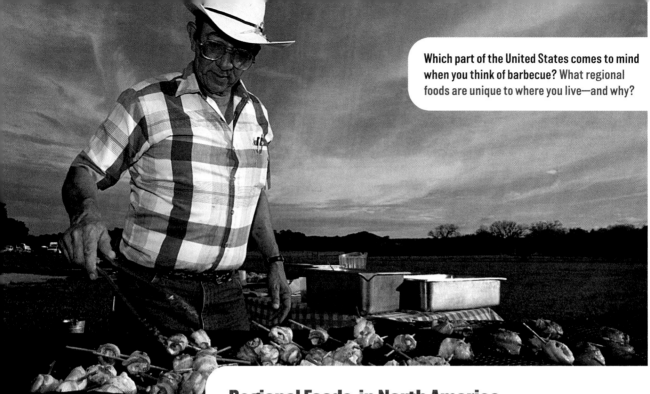

Which part of the United States comes to mind when you think of barbecue? What regional foods are unique to where you live—and why?

Regional Foods in North America

Have you ever tasted Florida key lime pie, fiddlehead soup from New Brunswick, or San Francisco sourdough bread? Each region of the United States and Canada has *foods that are special to the area,* or **regional foods.** They add variety and enjoyment to eating.

Most regional foods develop because the climate and geography are good for producing certain foods. For example, the South is noted for peach desserts and pecan pies. The Southwest, with its cattle ranches, takes pride in barbecued beef. Maple syrup is used to flavor many dishes in New England and eastern Canada. Typical Midwestern fare includes pork and savory corn-on-the-cob. The lakes of Minnesota and central Canada are ideal for growing wild rice. The upper Pacific coast is famous for salmon, crab, and many types of berries. Game such as deer or elk is a feature of Alaskan cuisine. Pineapple, brought to the Hawaiian islands many years ago, is used there to make puddings, pickles, and other dishes.

Some regional cuisines reflect the ethnic diversity of the region. For example, Creole cooking in Louisiana combines the cooking styles of French, Spanish, Native American, and African settlers. Southern cooking—with foods like grits, okra, and catfish—blends traditions of African slaves, European settlers, and Native Americans. On the West Coast and in Hawaii, foods reflect the influence of Asian immigrants. Tamales and enchiladas are favorites in the Southwest, where Mexican heritage is very rich.

Activity: Research these or other regional foods: clam chowder, shoofly pie, tourtiere, jambalaya, hush-puppies, chimichangas, and bierocks. Describe each food, identify the region it is from, and explain its origins.

Your Passport to Nutrition

Nutritious and flavorful foods come from every part of the world. It's fun to give your meals and snacks a passport to healthful eating. You can't beat the benefits! Enjoying your own family food traditions and exploring the flavors of other cultures adds variety to your food choices and enjoyment to your eating, and gives you a chance to share with and learn about others.

Healthful Foods from Many Cultures

Consider the nutrition benefits of including a variety of ethnic foods in your eating style! For example, eating plenty of grain products, vegetables, and fruits is good nutrition advice that's carried out around the world.

- In many Asian cuisines, mixed dishes are made with sliced vegetables.
- Cut-up fruit is a common street snack in Mexico and Central America, and many Middle Eastern cultures feature fruit for dessert.
- Many Mediterranean cuisines feature rice and pasta in an endless variety.
- Hispanic cuisines include the healthful combination of beans with rice, seasoned with different herbs, spices, and vegetables.

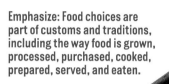

Tip

Enjoy the nutrition benefits of global flavors! Use the Food Guide Pyramid in Chapter 8 to see how ethnic foods fit within a healthful eating plan.

Emphasize: Food choices are part of customs and traditions, including the way food is grown, processed, purchased, cooked, prepared, served, and eaten.

Around the world, people eat many of the same foods, prepared or seasoned differently. In Japan, people eat rice plain or rolled around chopped vegetables or fish. Italians enjoy a rice dish called risotto. Rice and beans are popular in parts of Latin America. Find out how another food, perhaps wheat flour, is used in different cultures around the world.

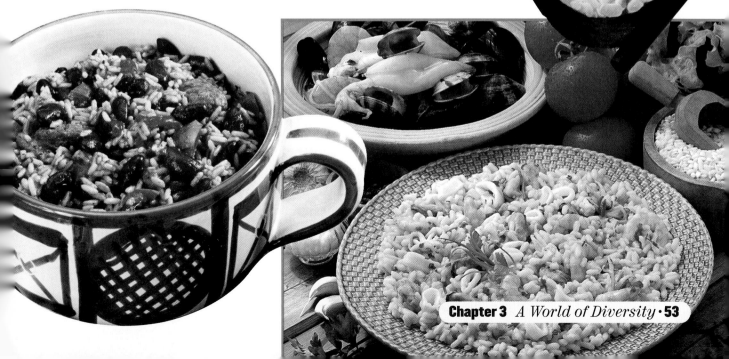

Check This Out!

KEEPING FOOD TRADITIONS

What foods are part of your family tradition? Learn more about them. Besides the nutrition benefits, they're part of who you are—and of what makes you unique.

It's Your Turn!

- Ask a grandparent, parent, or other relative to teach you how to make special family foods.
- Write down family recipes so they're not forgotten.
- Use your family's recipes and food customs when you plan menus for everyday meals and special celebrations.

When eating foods of any culture, make choices for nutrition. When you order Chinese foods, pick stir-fried or steamed dishes. You can combine choices from different ethnic menus, too, for a healthful meal. What choices for nutrition can you make when you order from menus in a Mexican or Italian restaurant?

Exploring the World of Food

Take a flavor trip around the nation and the world! Whether you "travel" within your community or visit other places, you can explore a variety of regional and ethnic foods. Try these ways to add cultural diversity and new flavors to your food choices.

- Try foods at regional or ethnic festivals. Talk with the people who prepared the foods to learn more about the cultural influences.
- If you travel to other places, experiment by tasting new foods. Visit local food markets and places where foods are produced. By learning about food, you learn a lot about a culture.
- Look for regional or ethnic foods in your supermarket or local ethnic food markets. Buy something new for a change of taste.
- Check out an ethnic or regional cookbook from the library. Read about the cuisine and prepare a dish from the cookbook.
- Watch TV cooking shows featuring regional or ethnic cuisine.
- Eat at an ethnic restaurant. Ask the server about foods on the menu. Order something that's new to you.
- Ask friends to teach you how to prepare a traditional family food.
- Search for food sites on the Internet and look up regional and ethnic restaurants and recipes. Visit different countries' web sites and learn about regional foods.

As you learn about food customs, remember to respect the individual food choices of people. Most people eat what they enjoy—not always foods of their own culture. Observe, listen carefully, and ask questions so you don't stereotype people and their foods. For example, you'll learn that many, but not all, Asians eat with chopsticks and that tacos made with fried corn tortillas are an Americanized version of a Mexican food, often called Tex-Mex style. You may learn that chop suey does not exist in China. It's a Chinese-American dish thought to date back to the mid-1800s.

Activity: Select a food recipe to pass down to your relatives. Share the recipe; discuss why it's a favorite.

NOW *You're* COOKING!

(SKILL)
Preparing a Mexican Dish

*G*uacamole (gwah-kah-MOH-lee) can be eaten as a dip, a topping, or a side dish. Avocado, the main ingredient, is a fruit that's a good source of vitamins A and C and some B vitamins. A ripe avocado feels slightly soft when you gently press it. To ripen an unripe avocado, keep it in a paper bag at room temperature for 1 to 2 days.

RECIPE

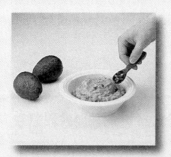

Irresistible Guacamole

CUSTOMARY	INGREDIENTS	METRIC
2 medium	Avocados	2 medium
1 Tbsp.	Finely chopped onion	15 mL
1 tsp.	Minced jalapeño pepper	5 mL
2 tsp.	Lime juice	10 mL

Yield: 4 servings, ¼ cup (50 mL) each

❶ Cut avocados in half and remove the pits. Scoop out the flesh with a spoon and place it in a small bowl. Mash with a fork until slightly chunky.

❷ Add onion, jalapeño pepper, and lime juice. Stir with a fork to mix. Serve immediately.

Per serving: 155 calories, 2 g protein, 6 g carbohydrate, 15 g fat, 21 mg sodium, 3 g fiber

Percent Daily Value: vitamin C 12%, vitamin B_6 12%, folate 14%

More Ideas   For a nice touch of flavor or color:

• Mix chopped tomato or green pepper into your guacamole.

• Stir in chopped fresh cilantro or hot pepper sauce.

Your Ideas   Make a list of foods that you might serve with guacamole. Think about a variety of foods, not just tortilla chips. Consider ways to combine this Mexican dish with foods from the cuisine of other countries. Combining cultural food traditions is called "fusion" cuisine!

LOOKING BACK

- Cuisine and food customs differ from region to region, yet are interconnected.
- American cuisine has developed from many cultures.
- Each region of the United States has foods that are special to the area.
- Eating a variety of foods from different cultures can add flavor and nutrition to your meals.

UNDERSTANDING KEY IDEAS

1. In what ways can culture affect people's food choices and habits?
2. What factors affect whether a food is abundant in a certain area? How does this in turn affect the area's cuisine?
3. What accounts for the fact that different parts of the United States have certain foods associated with them?
4. Give an example of how a food that originated in one part of the world later became identified with another part of the world.
5. What are the nutritional benefits of enjoying foods from other cultures?
6. Give three examples of strategies that could expand the cultural diversity of your food choices.

DEVELOPING LIFE SKILLS

1. **Critical Thinking:** How have modern methods of travel and communication affected cultural and regional food customs? A hundred years from now, will food customs around the world be more distinct from one another, less distinct, or about the same as now? Why?
2. **Leadership:** How can parents, teachers, and caregivers help children experience foods from different cultures? What benefits might tasting experiences have for children?

Wellness Challenge

Southfield High School is sponsoring its first Global Cultures Day. The principal has asked the foods and nutrition classes to participate. After discussing the idea, the students have decided they should provide a variety of foods from different cultures for tasting. They would like to promote good eating habits by pointing out the nutritional benefits of the different kinds of food offered.

1. How might the students communicate their nutrition message to participants at Global Cultures Day?
2. What planning would be needed to include food tasting at the event?
3. Where could the students get advice and support as they carry out their plan?

APPLYING YOUR LEARNING

1. **Celebration Meals:** Choose a type of celebration, such as birthdays, weddings, or a particular national holiday. List as many examples as you can of foods you associate with this celebration. Explain the ways in which you think food contributes to the celebration of the event.

2. **Recipe File:** Collect four to six recipes for regional foods that are typical of your area. Then collect regional recipes for three other parts of the country. Add these to your personal recipe file.

EXPLORING FURTHER

1. **Potatoes Around the World:** Trace the geography and history of the potato. Where did potatoes originate? In what countries are they grown and eaten today? What are some different ways potatoes are prepared in other countries? How did the potato affect history? Make a world map showing what you find out about the potato.

2. **Religious Customs:** Find out about a food or meal that is eaten as part of a religious observance. What significance does this food or meal have for those who eat it? What is the history behind the practice of eating it? Present your findings to the class.

Making CONNECTIONS

1. **Social Studies:** Create a chart or visual display that describes several different types of climate regions. Identify the types of food (if any) that are typically produced in each climate region and why. Relate the information to what you've read in this chapter about the food supply and food choices.

2. **Foreign Languages:** Create a glossary of food-related terms from a non-English-speaking country. Include the spelling, pronunciation, and meaning of the terms. Share your glossary with the class.

FOODS LAB

Chips and dip are standard party fare. Prepare two or three variations of this theme with foods from a variety of cultures. You might choose salsa with corn chips, chutney with *chapati*, and *baba ghanoush* with pita bread. Compare the textures and flavors of your choices.

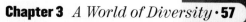

The Food Supply

Objectives

After studying this chapter, you will be able to:

- Trace the steps in bringing food from the farm to the consumer.

- Explain the ways technology increases your food choices.

- Distinguish the roles of industry, government, and consumers in food safety.

- Analyze factors affecting the world food supply.

Do You Know...

...how your after-school snacks get from the farm to your table?

...what you can do to help keep food prices down?

...why frozen vegetables are as nutritious as fresh vegetables?

If not, you'll find out in this chapter!

Look *for these* TERMS

food processing	additive
shelf life	enrichment
irradiation	fortification

Where in the world

did your dinner come from? The foods you prepare in your kitchen may come from local growers as well as from farms all over the country and the world. Together these producers, along with the many other sectors of the food industry, provide you with an abundant, nutritious, and safe food supply.

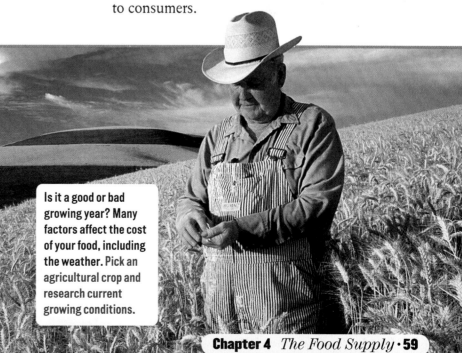

Tip

Shoplifting, damage to packages, and vandalism add to a store's operating costs—and the price of food. Your actions as a responsible consumer can help keep food prices down.

Is it a good or bad growing year? Many factors affect the cost of your food, including the weather. Pick an agricultural crop and research current growing conditions.

The Food Supply Chain

Getting food to your table is a huge, complex business that employs millions of people. Can you think of what steps are involved in the process? Take a look at "Food from Farm to Table" on page 60 and see if you were right.

What Affects the Price of Food?

One week the price of lettuce is 99 cents. The next week it's $1.59. Why the difference? Many factors in food production and distribution affect food prices. Most fall into two basic categories:

Supply and demand. When the supply of a food is higher than consumer demand for it, the price is less. What happens when the demand is higher than the supply? That's right, prices go up. This can happen when weather damages crops, for example.

Production and distribution costs. All the businesses involved in the food supply need to make a profit. If their costs rise—such as the costs of fuel or labor—the increases are passed on to consumers.

HOW DOES FOOD GET
From the Farm to Your Table?

*H*ave you ever stopped to think about all the work that went into processing the glass of milk you're pouring? Do you realize how many people were involved in the steps of taking wheat grain from the field and turning it into a loaf of bread? We often take for granted that we can go to a store and buy any food we want, but how did the food get there?

PROCESSING
Food is taken from farms to processing plants. Examples of processing methods include cleaning, sorting, freezing, and packaging.

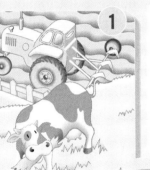

1 PRODUCTION
Farmers grow crops and raise livestock. Product developers work at food companies to research and develop ideas for new food products.

2

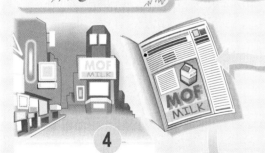

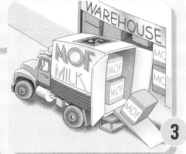

4 MARKETING
Advertising and marketing agencies promote food products to industry buyers and to consumers. Retailers such as stores, restaurants, and schools sell food products to consumers.

CONSUMERS
Consumers like you buy foods to serve and enjoy at the table.

5

3 DISTRIBUTION
Food is shipped from the processing plant to a distributor. Distributors store food in warehouses. Then they sell and transport the food to retailers.

Investigate Further
Find out how your favorite food is grown and processed.

Technology and the Food Supply

Your ancestors relied mostly on foods produced where they lived. That's one reason why regional foods developed. Today you can still enjoy locally grown foods, but an abundant variety of foods available all year long offers you choices for nutrition.

You don't have to live in Hawaii to enjoy pineapple any time you want. You can have fresh fruits and vegetables—from California, Florida, and Mexico, as well as Central America, Asia, and the Mediterranean—in frosty winter months. You can eat seafood whether you live on the coast or far inland. You have all these choices and more because of technological advances in the production, processing, storage, and transportation of food.

Food Production Today

From small local farmers to large operations, farms provide food for your table. Technology helps farmers produce more and better food. Here are just a few examples.

- Hydroponics is a method of growing vegetables indoors in nutrient-rich solution rather than soil. Light, temperature, and humidity are controlled. Scientists expect that hydroponic crops will be grown commercially in space someday.
- Fish farming is a method of growing fish or shellfish in enclosed areas of water. Areas of the ocean are sectioned off for easy harvest and greater yields of seafood. There are also fish farms for freshwater fish.

Who would ever have imagined that you could grow food without soil? Hydroponics is the answer. Find out what foods are grown hydroponically.

Check This Out!

DOWN ON THE FARM

To ensure that their crop yield is high, farmers need to manage pests such as insects, fungus, mold, and rodents. One method is the use of chemical pesticides to protect against pest damage. Farmers need to follow government regulations to make sure the amounts they use are safe. Another approach is *organic farming*. This generally means growing foods using little or no synthetic fertilizers or pesticides. Farmers who use this method find other ways to manage pests. There's no scientific evidence that foods grown this way are more nutritious or safer than others. However, they offer another choice for consumers.

It's Your Turn!

Visit a supermarket in your area to look for organic foods. What did you find? How are organic foods labeled? What does "certified organic" mean?

Activity: Find out what insects help farmers and home gardeners and how. Consider ladybugs, bees, wasps, flies, butterflies, and moths.

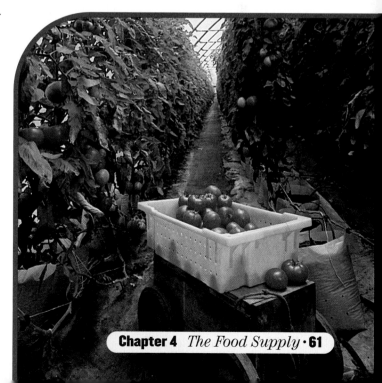

Milk is processed to make other foods such as yogurt, ice cream, and cheese. With still more processing, cheese can be packaged into a convenient shredded form or become part of a frozen pizza. Name two other foods that undergo some kind of processing.

• Greater understanding of genes—the "blueprints" in living cells that carry information about specific traits—has resulted in many developments. Scientists and farmers are using what they know to develop foods with specific desirable qualities. These include plants that are disease-resistant and can withstand severe weather, fruits that ripen on the tree without spoiling fast, and vegetables with more vitamins.

Discuss: How can you buy potatoes besides fresh? What kinds of processing were used? Repeat using another food.

Food Processing Today

As you shop, you see that many foods come in a wide variety of forms. Besides fresh apples, think of all the ways you can buy apples: applesauce, bottled juice, frozen apple pie, frozen juice concentrate, and dried apple slices. All these forms of apples have undergone some kind of processing. **Food processing** includes *methods of preparing and handling food for safety, nutrition, convenience, and appeal.*

Milk is a good example of the many different purposes of processing. Milk that you buy in a carton, jug, or bottle has been processed to make it safe to drink, to add vitamins, to adjust the fat content, and to keep a layer of cream from forming.

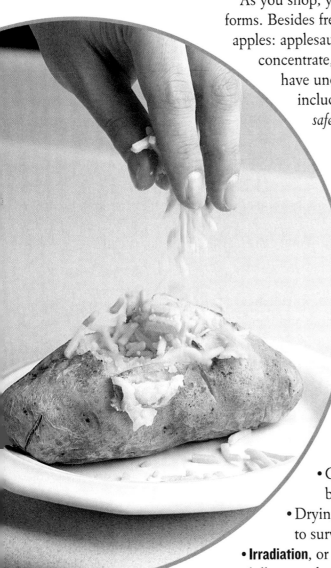

Preservation Methods

Fresh peaches keep for just a few days, but canned and frozen peaches keep for weeks and even months. They have a longer **shelf life**—*the length of time foods stay safe and appealing to eat.* Commercial preservation methods increase the shelf life of many foods and allow you to enjoy them at any time of year.

• Freezing uses cold temperatures to slow down the growth of bacteria that cause spoilage.

• Canning uses high heat to destroy harmful bacteria. The food is sealed in airtight containers.

• Drying food removes moisture that bacteria need to survive.

• **Irradiation**, or *passing food through radiant energy, such as X rays,* kills some forms of disease-causing bacteria without causing nutrient loss. By law, irradiated foods must be labeled.

• Curing uses ingredients such as salt, sugar, spices, and sodium nitrate or nitrite to preserve food. Ham is an example of a cured meat.

Critical Thinking: True or false: Fresh foods have more nutrients than canned or frozen foods. Explain.

Check This Out!

WHAT'S UP IN FOOD PACKAGING?

From the processing plant to your kitchen, food packaging helps food stay safe, helps retain its quality, and provides information about the food inside. The package may double as a cooking or serving utensil, too. Food packaging is updated constantly as technology and consumer needs change.

- *Aseptic packaging*, made of layers of plastics, paperboard, and aluminum foil, lets perishable food keep at room temperature for several months without preservatives. Food is heated quickly to very high temperatures. Then it's packaged in a sterilized container under sterile conditions. Milk, juice, soup, and tofu are some foods that can be packaged this way.
- *Microwave-safe packaging*, made of plastic, paper, or paperboard, offers convenience. You can put the food tray or container directly into the microwave oven—and perhaps into a conventional oven. Read the package directions to find out!
- *Recyclable packaging* helps you reduce waste. On plastic containers, look for the recycling symbol. The lower the number inside the symbol, the more easily the container can be recycled. Aluminum cans, glass containers, and paperboard cartons that are gray inside can be recycled, too.

It's Your Turn!

Check out packaging the next time you shop for food. Look for the same food packaged in different ways. Describe and explain instances in which each type of packaging might be beneficial to you.

Some of these preservation methods cause foods to lose a small amount of their natural nutrients. However, fresh foods, such as fresh vegetables, also lose nutrients between the time they are harvested and when you eat them. In fact, frozen and canned vegetables have about the same amount of nutrients as the fresh version—sometimes slightly more, depending on how you handle them. Whatever form of food you buy, prepare foods carefully to keep their nutritional quality.

Activity: Bring clean food packaging (minus the food). Identify each as aseptic, microwave-safe, and/or recyclable.

Food Additives

Additives are *substances added to foods during processing to make them safer, more appealing, or more nutritious.* Additives are used to:

Preserve. Some additives extend the shelf life of food—for example, by preventing or slowing the growth of mold or bacteria. This reduces food spoilage and waste.

Activity: Read ingredients on packages of foods. Identify the food additives. Do they preserve, enrich, fortify, enhance, etc.?

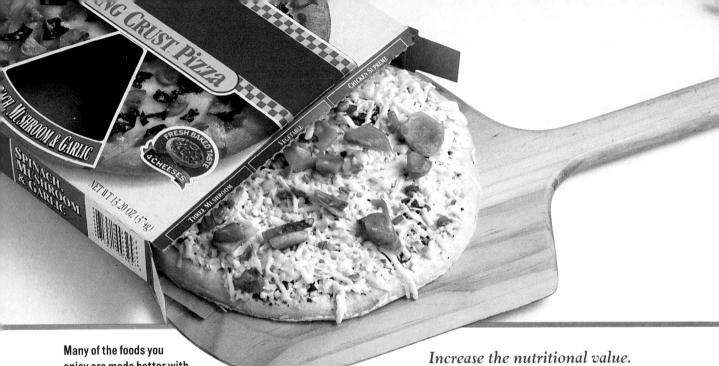

Many of the foods you enjoy are made better with additives. Find out what additives are used in frozen pizza and why they are used.

Emphasize: Some people are allergic to certain foods and food additives. Symptoms include rashes, hives, and difficulty breathing. People with allergies should check food ingredients.

(INFOLINK)

Read more about convenience foods in Chapter 14.

Increase the nutritional value. Some additives enrich or fortify food. **Enrichment** is *adding back nutrients lost in processing.* Grain products are enriched with B vitamins. **Fortification** is *adding nutrients that aren't naturally present.* Milk is fortified with vitamin D.

Enhance the flavor or appearance. Flavorings and colorings add appeal to many prepared or processed foods.

Give special qualities to food. One additive helps make ice cream smooth and thick. Another keeps salt from clumping so that it pours freely.

Food additives and the amounts in which they can be used are carefully tested and controlled. The food industry and government share the responsibility for the safe use of additives. Industry researches an additive's safety. The federal Food and Drug Administration (FDA) evaluates the research results. If an additive is approved, the FDA regulates its safe use.

Some people are sensitive to certain food additives. They can use the ingredient list on packaged foods to identify the additive and avoid foods containing it.

Convenience Foods

For convenience, many packaged foods are partly or fully prepared. Frozen egg rolls, canned chili, dehydrated soups, and sliced, fresh stir-fry vegetables are some of the prepared, packaged foods you might buy.

Keeping Your Food Supply Safe

The government and the food industry share the responsibility for keeping food safe from the farm to the point of purchase. As a consumer, you must stay informed and handle food safely from the time you buy it to when you serve it.

Role of the government. Government agencies set regulations and standards for food safety, including the safe use of pesticides and additives. Agencies watch over the food industry to make sure that regulations are followed. They also provide and set standards for consumer information, such as food labels.

Role of the food industry. Farmers, food manufacturers, stores, and restaurants must comply with government regulations for food safety. In addition, the food industry provides information about food safety to consumers. Many manufacturers have consumer hot lines to which you can report food safety problems.

Activity: Find out how to safely handle the following foods: eggs, chicken, hamburger, and milk. Demonstrate safe handling of each of the foods.

INFOLINK

You can learn more about your role in food safety in Part 1 of the Food Preparation Handbook.

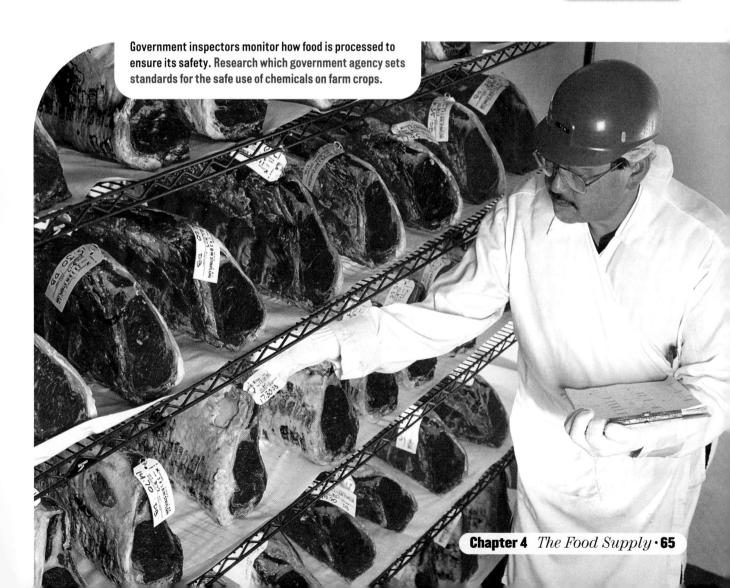

Government inspectors monitor how food is processed to ensure its safety. Research which government agency sets standards for the safe use of chemicals on farm crops.

The World's Food Supply

Not everyone in the world has access to the kind of food supply described in this chapter. In every country, some people go hungry. In some parts of the world, most people go hungry. Feeding the world population is a global problem.

Why does the problem of world hunger exist? The reasons are many and complex. Here are a few.

- The climate or geography in some areas makes it difficult to grow food.
- Lack of modern transportation in some areas means that food can't be distributed to those who need it.
- Lack of fuel may mean that people can't cook enough food.
- Natural disasters, such as droughts or floods, can affect the food supply for years.
- Wars and other political conflicts can destroy farms and disrupt transportation.

What is the solution? Many agencies and organizations are working to help people in need. One approach is to educate people about simple, affordable ways to increase the amount of food they can grow. Another is to search for new food products and new varieties of crops that offer hope for nourishing more people.

More About the Food Supply: Biotechnology uses living organisms to develop new products for food, medicine, fuel, and waste management. For centuries, farmers have replanted seeds from their best crops and bred their best animals.

Feeding the world population is a global problem. Relief centers around the world provide help for those in need. Do research in the library or on the Internet to learn more about the global food problem. What agricultural advances might help feed the world population throughout the 21st century? What is your responsibility?

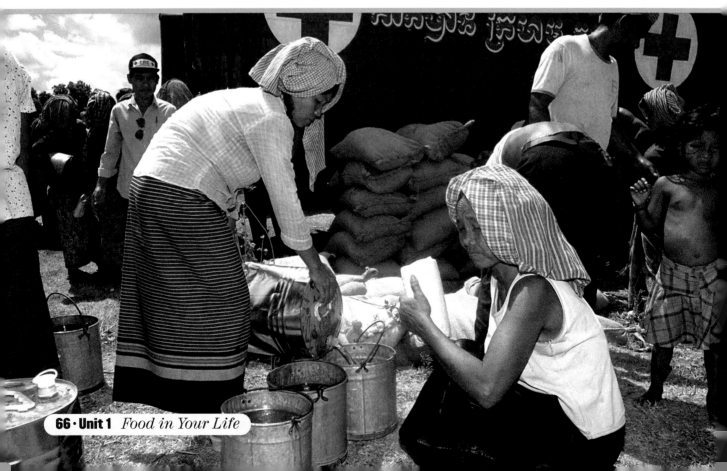

CAREERS *in*

HELP WANTED

Farm Managers

Use your knowledge of business and farming to make management decisions for corporate owner. Monitor operating expenses, make purchasing decisions, and oversee daily operations. Degree in business with a concentration in agriculture required. Minimum 2 years experience. Contact Johnson Land Management.

Crew Leaders

Hire and supervise workers, organize crews, and coordinate daily work activities. Must have proven management ability in labor intensive environment. Short-term contract. Apply in person at Appleton Orchards.

Dairy Processing Equipment Operator

Local dairy processing plant needs equipment operator to oversee milk production. Set up, operate, and maintain equipment. On-the-job training provided for reliable high school graduate. Apply at the Maywood Dairy.

Meatcutter/Department Manager

Large supermarket has opening for meatcutter to manage meat department. Handle ordering, manage and train workers, and assist customers. Apprenticeship training and excellent safety record required. Send resume to Human Resources, National Grocery.

Quality Assurance Manager

Food processing plant seeks Quality Assurance Manager to plan and direct program that ensures nonstop production. Establish standards and direct workers in sanitation and safety programs. Bachelor's degree required. Contact Wholesale Foods, Inc.

Food Technician

Large food processing firm has immediate opening for a production line quality control food technician. Must have a two-year associate degree and be willing to work evenings. Send resume to Lenexa Cannery, Inc.

Food Inspector

USDA has opening for a Food Inspector. Inspect privately owned meat-processing plants for compliance with federal laws. Bachelor's degree or one year of specialized experience in food related occupation required. Apply at USDA Food Safety and Inspection Services.

LINKING *to the* WORKPLACE

❶ Preparation Requirements: Select an occupation listed above. Find out more about the education and training typically needed. What high school classes could help you prepare for this line of work?

❷ Personal Characteristics: Make a list of personal characteristics, such as dependability, that a person working in food production and distribution should have. How do the characteristics you listed compare to your own qualities?

Review & Activities

LOOKING BACK

- Supply and demand, as well as production and distribution costs, affects the price of food.
- Technological developments have led to better and safer ways of producing, processing, and preserving foods.
- The government and food industry are responsible for keeping the food supply safe.
- Feeding the world population is a global problem.

UNDERSTANDING KEY IDEAS

1. When might the cost of strawberries be higher, in December or June? Why?
2. What technological advances have increased the supply of vegetables year-round in colder regions?
3. Why might you buy frozen beans instead of fresh beans?
4. What are additives? Name at least three reasons why food additives are used.
5. Explain the difference between a fortified food and an enriched food.
6. How does the government provide for the safety of the food that you buy?
7. Why is hunger a serious problem in some parts of the world?

DEVELOPING LIFE SKILLS

1. **Creative Thinking:** Imagine you're a bio-engineer who has the ability to design the perfect vegetable—one that is high in nutrition and has the most appealing color, texture, and flavor. What would your ideal vegetable be like?
2. **Critical Thinking:** Predict what would be the impact on wheat farmers if one year they all experienced unusually large yields. Explain your reasoning. What would be the impact on consumers?

Wellness Challenge

Len-Lu and Yu-Kai will be doing the family shopping this week. Len-Lu wants to buy organic foods with no additives because she believes they are safer. Her brother feels that food additives and processing can be beneficial. They both want to be well-informed about the foods they choose.

1. How should Len-Lu and Yu-Kai go about achieving their goal of finding information?
2. What problems might they encounter?
3. How could they find solutions?

APPLYING YOUR LEARNING

1. **Brainstorming:** Divide into groups of two or three students. Pick a food, such as strawberries, and make a list of all the different ways that food can be processed. Trade your list with another group. Look at the list you are given to see if you can think of additional processing for the food.

2. **News Bulletin:** Imagine that you are a reporter on the evening news. Write a brief story about the positive effects of technology on food choices. Present your story to the class.

EXPLORING FURTHER

1. **Government Laws and Policies:** Find out what local, state, and federal agencies are involved in regulating food safety to protect public health. What laws and policies do they enforce? How do they enforce them? Summarize your findings in a report to share with the class.

2. **Put a Trace on It:** Choose a favorite commercial snack. Find out what the major ingredients are and trace these ingredients from the farm to your point of purchase. Where might the ingredients be grown? How are they processed? Where is the snack made? How and where is it shipped? Write a report of your findings.

Making CONNECTIONS

1. **Technology:** Find out what nutrients plants normally get from the soil and how those nutrients are supplied for plants that are grown hydroponically. What are the advantages and disadvantages of hydroponics? Report your findings to your class.

2. **Social Studies:** Find out about a time in history when the supply of a particular type of food was low. What caused the scarcity? What effects did it have on the economy and on people living at the time? How does this relate to what you have learned in this chapter about supply and demand?

FOODS LAB

Conduct an experiment using two slices of bread, one slice without preservatives and one slice with preservatives. Wrap both in plastic and leave them at room temperature. After five days, examine them for spoilage. What conclusions can you draw?

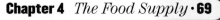

Peru's *Pretty* Potatoes

Through the centuries, thousands of native potato species have been grown in Peru. They come in almost every color of the rainbow. Today's Peruvian farmers mostly produce white potatoes because they are easier to grow. Native potatoes are in danger of dying out. Now, an agricultural group has planted about 1,000 varieties of native potatoes in farming communities. The group hopes to sell these potatoes and turn them into delicious, crunchy potato chips! ■

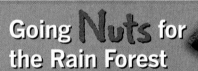

◀ Peru produces a colorful variety of potatoes.

Going Nuts for the Rain Forest

Much of the Amazon rain forest is being destroyed every day. The greatest harm comes from the practice of burning down trees to make room for crops and cattle. Now, some farmers are hoping to save the trees by harvesting what is already growing on them: Brazil nuts. The farmers hope the nuts, as well as other foods of the forest, can be sold for a profit. That might be the successful recipe for helping the Amazon rain forest. ■

THE **bean** POOL

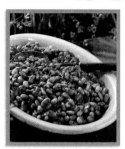

▲ Delicious and healthful pinto beans.

The common bean, a member of the legume family, was first grown by the Incas in Peru some 7,000 years ago. Today, there are hundreds of varieties of beans, which are rich in protein and a food staple in Latin America. People use beans in stews, sauces, chilis, and soups. Many types of beans can be dried so that they will keep for up to a year. That's good news for people who need food during a cold, harsh winter.

Here's a look at **beans** that are eaten in **Latin America**.

BLACK BEANS are about the size of a pea. They are black and oval, and they have a mild, sweet, earthy taste. Black beans are most often used in thick soups. They can also be served with rice. They are the basic bean for many Caribbean, Mexican, and Latin American culinary delights.

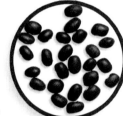

PINTO BEANS are medium-sized ovals in either reddish-brown or beige. They are a favorite for chili, refried beans, and other Mexican dishes.

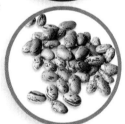

SMALL RED BEANS are dark red in color. They are used in soups, salads, and chili. ■

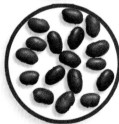

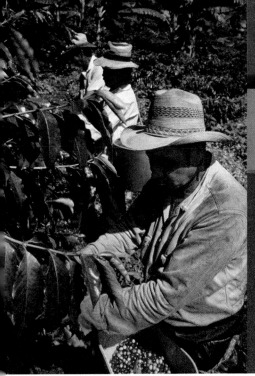

JAVAGIANTS

Coffee grows in places that have rich soil, moderate temperatures, and just enough sunshine and rain. That fits the bill for many Latin American nations where coffee is important to the economy. The top five coffee-producing countries in Latin America are **Brazil**, **Colombia**, **Mexico**, **Guatemala**, and **Peru**. ■

◄ Coffee is the most common crop in Colombia.

MIND YOUR manners

If you visit Latin America, you'll want to keep these dining tips in mind.

In Mexico, when people eat out, the oldest person usually pays for the meal. In most Central American countries, lunch is the main meal of the day. It will probably include black beans, tortillas, meat, vegetables, and fruit. Don't take more than you can eat—it's rude to leave uneaten food on your plate. In Colombia, however, it's polite to leave a small amount of food on your plate when you're finished. It shows you've had enough to eat. When eating in Bolivia, keep your hands on the table, not in your lap. Don't eat with your fingers, no matter what food is served. In Argentina, always cross your knife and fork on your plate when you are finished eating. It's good manners! ■

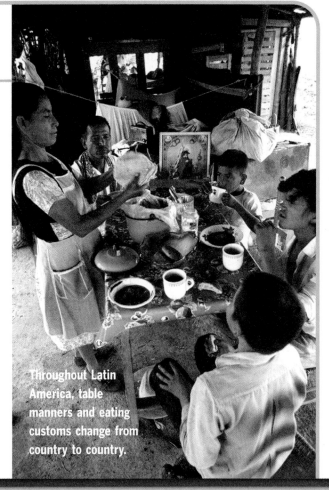

Throughout Latin America, table manners and eating customs change from country to country.

Latin America & The Caribbean

South America is home to nearly half a billion people living in the 16 countries between the steamy rain forests of Colombia and the icy shores of Chile. Many people in the United States lump the continent's cuisines together, but there are differences from nation to nation. Part of the confusion lies in the fact that much of South America shares a similar set of ingredients and a common language. (The same dish or ingredient, however, often has many different names.) Northwestern South America, especially the Andean Mountain nations of Ecuador, Bolivia, and Peru, offers some of the most exotic food in Latin America. Potatoes and the hearty, nutritious grain quinoa (KEEN-wah) were first grown here and still play major roles in the cuisines. Peru is home to some of the spiciest food in South America. The preferred seasoning here is a fiery yellow chili that adds bite to everything from seafood stew to potato salad.

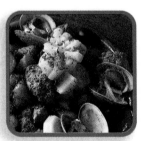

▲ A Brazilian fish stew is pungent with spices.

North central South America—especially Colombia and Venezuela—displays a Spanish influence. Many of the seasonings of the region—cumin, oregano, cinnamon, and anise—came from Spain, as did the ancient Mediterranean flavors of wine and olive oil. Many dishes in northeastern South America, such as tamales (tuh-MAH-leez), feature a combination of sweet and salty flavors, thanks to raisins, prunes, capers, and olives.

Argentina, Chile, Paraguay, and Uruguay make up cattle country. The local residents enjoy luscious beef in the form of asados (ah-SAH-doz), large cuts roasted in front of a campfire. There's more to the region's food than just beef, however. Consider a Paraguayan corn bread that is much like North American corn pudding. Chile, with 2,650 miles of Pacific coastline, is the place for those that crave fish.

Brazil's cuisine is as diverse as its population. Portuguese settlers popularized such European

A cabbage farmer in Ecuador takes pride in his ▶ abundant harvest.

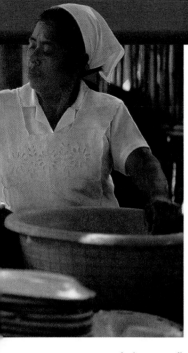

◀ **Fresh, steamy corn tortillas are the wrappings of Mexican tacos.**

ingredients as olives, onions, garlic, and salt cod. The natives of Brazil's rain forests taught the Europeans how to enjoy tropical vegetables and fruits such as cassava root and passion fruit. African slaves contributed okra, yams, peanuts, and palm oil. Their influence lives on in a fish stew flavored with garlic, cilantro, and coconut milk.

Mexico

In Mexico, street food is a celebration of the moment. Just about every street corner in the country has a snack stand of some kind, whether it's selling simply toasted peanuts or pan-seared enchiladas made with local cheese, fresh vegetables, and herbs. Say "street food" in Mexico, and most folks think "tacos." Steak tacos are popular. When street vendors combine seared beef with sweet sautéed onions and stinging chilies, wrap it in corn tortillas, and top it with tangy salsa, they've made a wonderful dish.

Caribbean

The Caribbean is a patchwork of islands, cuisines, and cultures. From Carib Indians to European colonists to African slaves, each group added its own unique flavors to the Caribbean cooks' kettle.

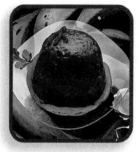

▲ **This plantain dish is called mofongo (muh-FON-go).**

The area's first inhabitants were the Arawaks, fisher-farmers who grew corn and tropical tubers such as cassava root. As seasonings, they used annatto seed (a rust-colored spice with an earthy flavor) and a fiery pepper now known as the Scotch bonnet.

The arrival of the Spanish in the 1500s brought European ingredients including livestock, rice, sugarcane, and oil for frying. Meat pies and rice stews remain popular in the Dominican Republic, Puerto Rico, and Cuba.

Spain, of course, wasn't the only player in the Caribbean. The English fondness for meat pies and fruited cakes survives in Jamaica's limo pies (curried-beef turnovers). French influence can be seen in Martinique's fish soup.

Some of the most important contributions to Caribbean cuisines came from African slaves who brought yams, okra, a nutty-flavored bean called the pigeon pea, and many other influences. Indentured workers from India introduced items such as curry and chutney—especially to Trinidad, where the cuisine still shows an Indian influence. ■

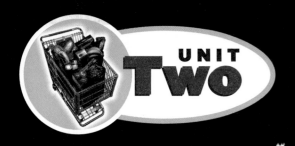

Nutrition for Health

IN THIS UNIT...

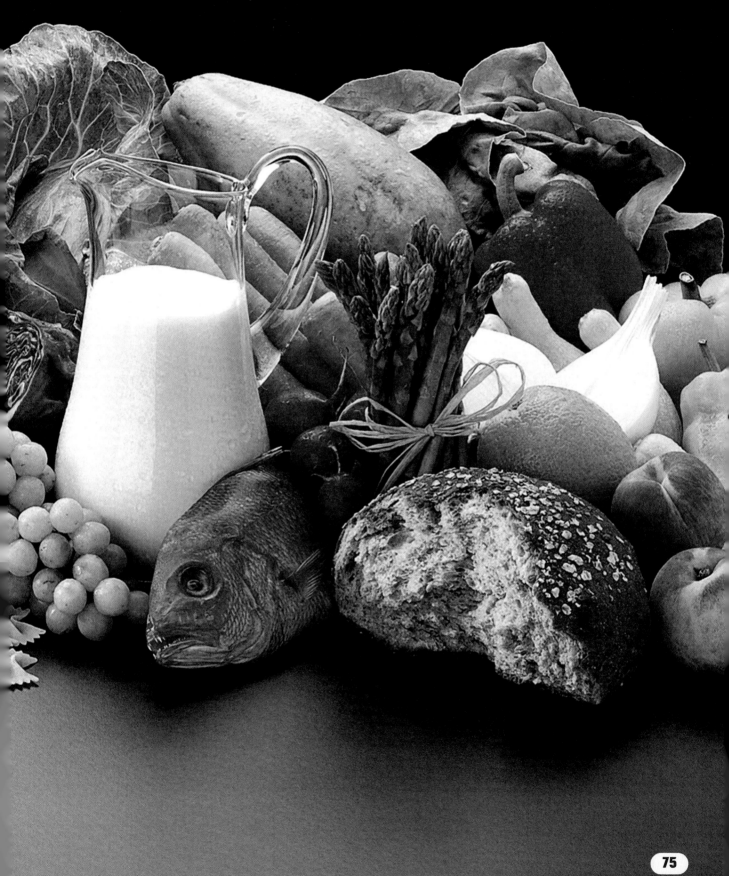

CHAPTER 5

Nutrients and Energy

Objectives

After studying this chapter, you will be able to:

- Identify the six major groups of nutrients.
- Summarize the three main functions of nutrients.
- Explain why you need a certain number of calories.
- Describe how nutrients work together in promoting health.
- Explain the possible effects of getting too few or too many nutrients.

Do You Know...

...why nutrients are like players on a team?

...which nutrients your body uses for energy?

...when your body's need for many nutrients is greatest?

If not, you'll find out in this chapter!

Look *for these* TERMS

Daily Values   malnutrition

nutrient deficiency   calories

basal metabolic rate

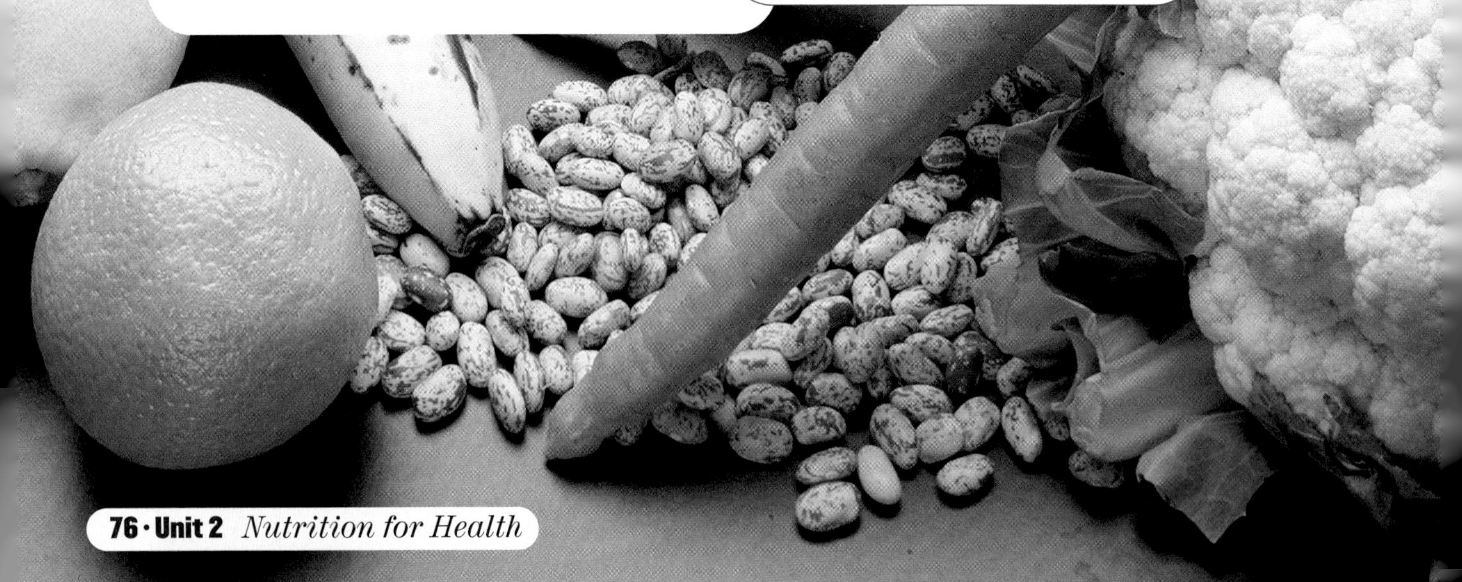

When you bite into a crisp apple, drink an ice-cold glass of milk, or sit down to your favorite meal, you probably think about the taste, aroma, and texture of what you're eating. But there's more! Food also provides substances that your body needs to be healthy. You know that these substances are nutrients, but why are they so important?

Nutrients for Wellness

Inside all the wonderful foods you eat are an array of nutrients—more than 40 different ones. These nutrients are grouped into six categories: carbohydrates, fats, proteins, vitamins, minerals, and water. Eating a variety of foods to provide these nutrients is essential, because your body cannot make most nutrients. When your body is well nourished, you feel good, look good, grow properly, and you're able to perform at your peak.

What Nutrients Do For You

Nutrients perform many important functions in your body without you even knowing it!

Give you energy. Carbohydrates, fats, and proteins supply the energy you need for all of your daily activities.

Build and repair your body. Proteins promote growth, build new body tissue, and repair worn-out body cells. If carbohydrates and fats are in short supply, your body uses proteins for energy. Then proteins can't perform their specialized job.

Activity: Write a paragraph about why it is important that the body sends hunger signals.

Eating a variety of healthful foods will give you the nutrients you need to grow, feel your best, and do well in school. What kind of snacks do you usually choose? What nutrients do they provide?

Keep your body processes going. Vitamins and minerals provide the "spark" that keeps your body's many systems running smoothly. Vitamins and minerals don't provide energy or build body tissue. Instead, they play key roles in regulating these processes. Water is a nutrient because it's essential for life. It aids digestion, helps transport nutrients and wastes, helps regulate body temperature, and does much more.

In order to use the nutrients in the food, your body must process the food. What exactly happens to food and its nutrients when you eat? Look at page 79 to see how your digestive system works.

How Nutrients Work Together

Think of nutrients as players on a team. Just as each player on a soccer team has a specific role, every nutrient has a job to perform in your body. A team reaches peak performance when players work together. When nutrients work together, they promote good health. If one nutrient is missing, other nutrients may not be able to do their jobs. For instance, for activities that last a long time, like long-distance running, fats and carbohydrates must both be available to supply energy. If one nutrient is in short supply, you won't be able to perform your best.

Activity: Describe some activities other than sports that require teamwork. What are some of the requirements of teamwork?

Just as a team relies on each player's contributions, your body needs enough of all the essential nutrients. Think of yourself as the coach. You decide what foods to eat to supply the nutrients your body needs. Record what you eat for five days. Save the record until you have completed Unit 2 and then rate yourself as a "coach."

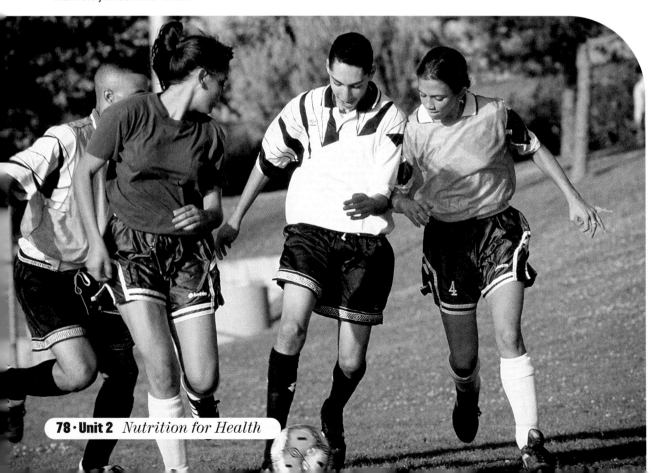

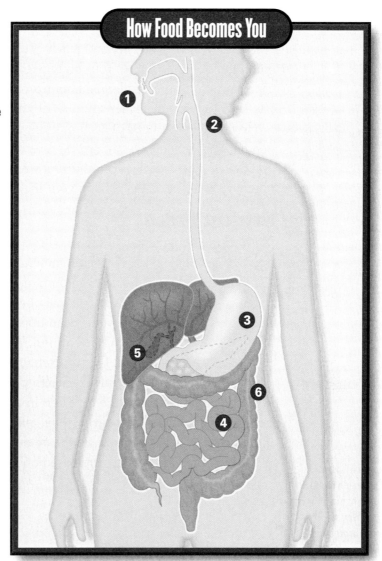

How Food Becomes You

Teaching With Visuals: Have students locate the position of each part of the digestive system as they read about what the parts do. Stress the importance of chemical digestion and absorption.

What happens to food and nutrients when you eat? How is food transformed into the basic fuel your body needs for energy and to build and repair itself?

1 MOUTH Saliva in the mouth starts to break down food chemically. Chewing breaks down food physically.

2 ESOPHAGUS Carries food from the mouth to the stomach in wavelike movements.

3 STOMACH Gastric juices further break down food chemically. Food is churned until it becomes a thick liquid called chyme.

4 SMALL INTESTINE Digestive juices produced in the liver, pancreas, and small intestine fully break down food. The nutrients are absorbed into the bloodstream through the lining of the small intestine.

5 LIVER Nutrients are taken by the portal vein to the liver where they are processed further. They are then transported in the bloodstream to cells throughout the body. When they reach the cells, nutrients carry out their special purposes, such as providing energy.

6 LARGE INTESTINE also called the colon. Waste material, such as fiber, moves into the large intestine. Water, potassium, and sodium are removed from the waste. The rest is eliminated from the body.

As a class, divide into six teams, with each team choosing one part of the digestive system to research more thoroughly. Share your findings with the class.

Getting Enough Nutrients

Your ability to enjoy life and reach your potential depends on getting enough nutrients. Your body needs different amounts of each nutrient. You need larger amounts of carbohydrates, proteins, fats, and water and smaller amounts of vitamins and minerals.

How much you need of each nutrient depends on your age, size, gender, and how active you are. As a teen, your body is growing and developing rapidly. Your nutrient needs are higher now than they will be at any other time in your life.

Nutrient Advice

Nutrition experts have established reference values for nutrient needs. The most familiar are Recommended Dietary Allowances (RDAs). An RDA is the daily amount of a nutrient that will meet the needs of nearly all healthy people of a specific age and gender. Another type of reference value is an upper level, the maximum amount that probably won't be harmful. Together, these and other reference values are called Dietary Reference Intakes (DRIs).

The DRIs are used mainly by health professionals. Other tools help consumers evaluate the nutrition in their food choices. For example, **Daily Values** are *daily nutrient amounts used in food labeling*. They can help you estimate the amount of nutrients in food products. The Daily Values are based on the RDAs but don't take

Activity: Ask students to bring in five clean, empty containers from foods they eat regularly. Have them study the nutrition information on each container and discuss how the nutrients in each food help their bodies.

Activity: Choose a nutrient and look up the RDA amounts for different ages and genders. How do the requirements compare throughout the life cycle?

Although people of all ages need nutrients, people need different amounts of nutrients at different ages. Why would babies need more protein for their body size than adults?

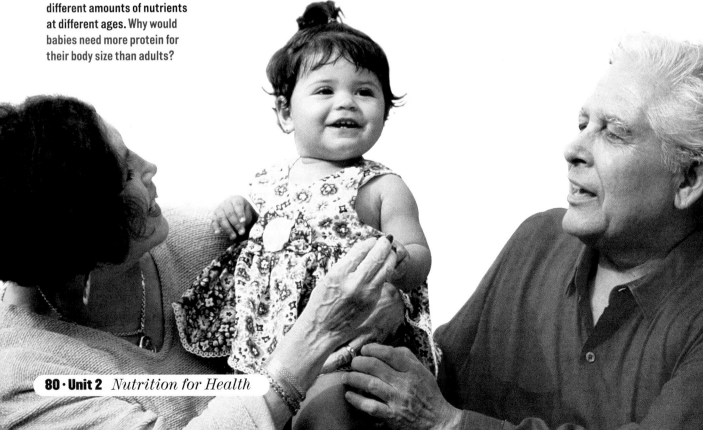

Check This Out!

Nutrients and Technology

One way to find out whether your food choices are meeting your nutrient needs is with the help of a computer. Look in software catalogs or on the Internet for programs designed to analyze your day's food choices. Some programs are low-cost or free.

You'll need to keep a record of everything you eat and drink for several days. Include the specific type of food (was it low-fat or fat-free milk?) and the amount. Remember to record snacks and extras, such as mayonnaise on your sandwich or sugar in your iced tea.

When you have entered all the necessary information, the computer program calculates how much of each nutrient your food choices supplied. It may even compare the totals to your nutrient needs. While it's not necessary to track your food choices in such detail, using nutrient analysis software can be an eye-opening experience!

It's Your Turn!

Find a Web site that lets you enter your food choices and obtain a nutrition analysis. Use it to compare your personal food intake to recommended guidelines. Interpret the results.

Discuss: How can using a food intake analysis program aid you in making better food choices?

---

age or gender into account. As a teen, you may need more than the Daily Value for some nutrients, less for others.

Another consumer tool for making food choices is the Food Guide Pyramid. It offers a practical, easy way to judge whether you are getting enough nutrient-rich foods.

Getting Too Few Nutrients

What happens when your food choices don't supply enough of the nutrients your body needs? If it continues long enough, a **nutrient deficiency,** or *shortage of a nutrient,* may result in poor health or lack of energy. The effects of some nutrient deficiencies take a long time to become apparent. For instance, if you don't get enough calcium when you're young, your bones may break easily when you're older.

A nutrient deficiency is one form of **malnutrition**—*serious health problems caused by a continuing lack of nutrients* or the body's poor absorption or use of nutrients. Malnutrition is often a result of food shortages or poverty. However, even people who have enough to eat can develop malnutrition if they make poor food choices.

> **INFOLINK**
>
> For a list of the Daily Value amounts, see the Appendix at the back of the book.
>
> ---
>
> To see how Daily Values are used on food labels, turn to Chapter 13.
>
> ---
>
> To learn about the Food Guide Pyramid, read Chapter 8.

Check This Out!

FOOD HELP IN YOUR COMMUNITY

In almost every community, there are people who do not have the means to meet the nutritional needs of their families. Fortunately, government, community, religious, and private groups provide food and nutrition information and assistance.

Food stamp program. This government program helps people with limited income to buy food at grocery stores or to buy seeds and plants to grow food. Food stamps work like cash at the store.

Women, Infants, and Children (WIC) program. This government program gives food assistance and nutrition education to pregnant and nursing women, infants, and preschool children who are in need.

Home-delivered meals. Hot or cold meals are delivered to disabled or frail people who can't leave home easily.

Food banks. Individuals, community groups, supermarkets, and restaurants donate to food banks for distribution to people in need.

Community kitchens. Through food donations, the community provides prepared meals at no cost to people in need. In some areas, low-cost meals are served in schools, churches, and other centers, where older adults can gather to eat and be with others. Many community food programs need volunteers. Giving your time has many rewards. As a responsible citizen, you can find an opportunity to volunteer in a local food program.

It's Your Turn!

Research food assistance programs in your area. Determine how students in your school could help. For example, you could hold a canned food drive and donate the food to a community shelter or food bank.

Critical Thinking: Why do you think the WIC program provides nutrition education as well as food assistance?

Getting Too Many Nutrients

Poor nutrition may also result from getting more nutrients than you need. For instance, eating too much fat can increase your chances of heart disease and other serious health problems.

Excess amounts of certain vitamins and minerals can cause serious harm to your body. For example, very large amounts of vitamin A can damage your liver. When you take vitamins and minerals in the form of pills, capsules, liquids, or powders, you run the risk of getting too much.

TIP

Remember, the food choices you make today have long-term effects on your health and quality of life! Smart choices now can help you have an active, enjoyable life for many years to come.

Activity: Design posters to encourage people to donate to a school or community food drive.

Energy and Calories

You need energy for everything you do—from swimming laps to brushing your teeth or thinking about and solving a math problem. You also need energy to power the many processes happening inside your body. The *units used to measure this energy* are called **calories.**

Calories aren't nutrients. They measure the energy you get from carbohydrates, fats, and proteins. Carbohydrates and proteins each provide 4 calories per gram. Fats provide 9 calories per gram—more than twice as much. That's why fatty foods tend to be high in calories. Health experts recommend that 45 to 65 percent of your total calories come from carbohydrates, 20 to 35 percent from fats, and about 10 to 35 percent from proteins.

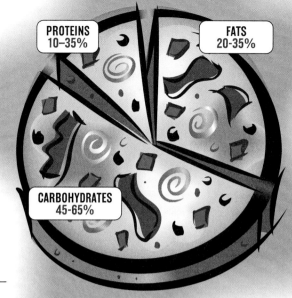

PROTEINS 10–35%

FATS 20-35%

CARBOHYDRATES 45-65%

Energy for Body Processes

The human body uses about 1200 calories or more per day for all the basic living processes. The *amount of energy used for body functions* is called **basal metabolic rate** (BMR).

Some people use more energy for metabolism than others. Teens do because they're growing. Taller and bigger people use more energy than shorter and smaller people. People have different BMRs because of differences in age and body size, the proportion of muscle to fat, genetic makeup, and gender.

The sources of your calories are just as important as the number of calories supplied by your food choices. Why do you think experts say these guidelines apply to your overall food choices rather than a single food or meal?

Activity: Calculate the percentage of calories from carbohydrates, fats, and proteins from your food choices.

Metabolic rates differ depending on many individual factors. Research the effect of exercise on a person's basal metabolic rate.

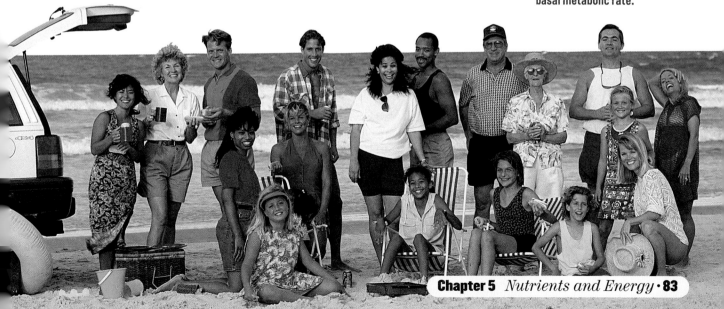

Check This Out!

PHYTOCHEMICALS— A NUTRITION DISCOVERY

One new frontier in nutrition science is the study of *phytochemicals*—natural chemicals found in plants. (*Phyto* means plant.) Plants use phytochemicals as a natural protection from bacteria, fungi, and viruses. The phytochemicals in grain products, vegetables, fruits, and dry beans and peas may have benefits for humans, too!

Phytochemicals aren't fully understood yet. Early research suggests that they may help protect you from health problems such as heart disease and cancer. Until scientists discover more, you're smart to eat a wide variety of foods from plant sources—for their flavor, nutrients, and potential phytochemical benefits!

It's Your Turn!

Find out what nutrition experts are learning about phytochemicals. Contact a registered dietitian for reliable information. Share what you learn with the class.

Energy for Physical Activity

Any physical activity uses energy, or burns calories. The number of calories you burn depends on how active you are. The longer and more intense your activity, the more calories you burn. For example, walking briskly for 15 minutes uses more energy than walking slowly for 15 minutes. Pumping your arms as you walk briskly uses even more energy!

Look at the chart to find the approximate number of calories you may need every day. How many calories did you consume today? That depends on your food choices, how the foods were prepared, and the amount of food you ate.

Discovering More About Nutrients

The study of food and its nutrients is a relatively new science. Even though the knowledge continues to grow, researchers still have a lot to learn. When nutrients were discovered, scientists learned how to prevent deficiency diseases caused by low intakes of certain nutrients. Now people are learning how nutrients can promote wellness, enhance performance, and prevent certain health problems. The details of nutrition advice will continue to evolve as scientists learn more about how nutrients affect our health.

Average Calorie Needs

CATEGORY	APPROXIMATE NUMBER OF CALORIES PER DAY
Children ages 2 to 6 years, most women, and some older adults	1,600
Older children, teen girls, active women, and most men	2,200
Women who are pregnant or breastfeeding	2,200+
Teen boys and active men	2,800

Source: Dietary Guidelines for Americans

Project LEAN Teens

Promote Breakfast

"**I**f you need to think in the morning, you need breakfast! Many kids don't eat breakfast, or lunch either, because life gets so hectic," said Annie Ma, a student at Gabrielino High School in San Gabriel, California.

As part of the California Project LEAN teen nutrition and fitness program in Los Angeles, Annie and other teens in her school became fitness and nutrition advocates, or promoters. They teamed up with their school food service director and a state nutrition expert. Their goal: helping teens jump-start their school day with breakfast.

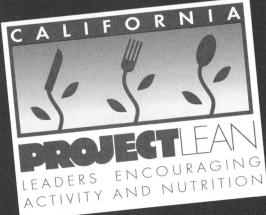

Guided by their own survey of teen breakfast habits, the students planned a campaign to get more kids to eat school breakfast. They worked on menus, created school announcements to promote breakfast, and wrote an advice column on nutrition for other teens. At the school's intercultural fair, they promoted breakfast with samples of freshly-made smoothies—fruit swirled with milk or tofu—and free breakfast passes.

"We're great nutrition advocates at school because we relate to other teens. For us, the adults are real-world resources and partners," added Annie. Teens in Project LEAN (which stands for Leaders Encouraging Activity and Nutrition) are using positive, goal-setting steps to take action for good nutrition at school!

Take Action

How can you promote breakfast to other teens? With your classmates, conduct a survey to find out about breakfast habits and preferences among teens in your school. Create a plan that will encourage more students to eat a nutritious breakfast. Then take steps to carry out your plan.

LOOKING BACK

- Nutrients work together to give you energy, build and repair your body, and keep your body processes running smoothly.

- Your body needs enough of each nutrient to keep you healthy and help you grow.

- Carbohydrates, fats, and proteins provide the energy needed for body processes and physical activity.

- Scientists are still learning about the many health benefits provided by nutrients.

UNDERSTANDING KEY IDEAS

1. What are the six categories of nutrients? Why is it important that your combined food choices provide nutrients from all six categories?

2. What main functions do nutrients perform?

3. Why should you be careful when considering supplements such as vitamin pills?

4. What is a nutrient deficiency? What consequences can it have?

5. What might happen if a male teen took in fewer than 1,600 calories a day for several days? Why?

6. What parts of your body break down food? How does each part perform this task?

7. Define basal metabolic rate.

DEVELOPING LIFE SKILLS

1. **Critical Thinking:** Would you believe an advertisement that claims a certain type of "energy bar" supplies every nutrient the human body needs? Why or why not?

2. **Communication:** How does the development of the Daily Values by health experts relate to communication?

Wellness Challenge

Shanika has signed up for a charity fitness walk. For every mile she walks, she'll earn money for the charity. She's hoping she'll be able to walk at least 10 miles. However, Shanika doesn't usually participate in physical activities that last more than 15 to 30 minutes. She eats less than the recommended number of calories for teen girls. Shanika has three weeks to prepare for the event.

1. How might Shanika's calorie intake affect her preparation for and performance in the walk?

2. What are some steps she might take to make sure that she has enough energy to reach her goal?

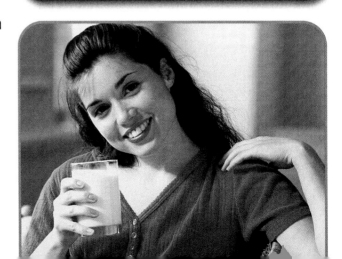

APPLYING YOUR LEARNING

1. **Identifying Nutrient Sources:** Choose one of the nutrients listed in the "Nutritive Value of Foods" chart in the back of the book. Refer to the list of DRIs for teens on page 551 to see how much of this nutrient you may need. Identify a combination of different foods (one serving of each) that would fill your daily needs for the nutrient. What can you conclude?

2. **Simulation:** Imagine that you are the coach of a school sports team. During many after-school practices, the players seem to lack the energy to perform all the drills. Give the team a locker room pep talk that emphasizes the importance of getting enough of all the nutrients to reach peak performance.

EXPLORING FURTHER

1. **Nutrient Deficiencies:** For centuries, sailors who went on long voyages became ill with a disease called scurvy, caused by a nutrient deficiency. Find out more about the history of this disease and how its cure was discovered.

2. **Dehydration:** Learn more about dehydration, a condition in which your body's water level is too low. What are the symptoms? Who is most at risk? How can dehydration be prevented?

Making CONNECTIONS

1. **Social Studies:** A variety of local, state, and federal laws, policies, agencies, and programs are designed to promote nutrition. Use print or Internet resources to find examples. Create a chart summarizing your findings.

2. **Health:** Find out what the thyroid gland has to do with metabolism. Summarize your findings in a brief report.

3. **Math:** Write out formulas for calculating what percentage of calories in a day's food choices come from carbohydrates, fats, and proteins.

FOODS LAB

As part of digestion, saliva breaks down one type of carbohydrate, starch, into another, sugar. Test this by placing a small amount of cornstarch on the tip of your tongue. Mix it with saliva and let it remain there. What change do you notice? How do you explain it?

Getting and Using Nutrients

Objectives

After studying this chapter, you will be able to:

- Summarize basic functions and food sources of carbohydrates, fats, proteins, vitamins, and minerals.

- Explain why water is an essential nutrient.

- Describe when dietary supplements are recommended.

Do You Know...

...what nutrient is your body's best energy source—and what foods provide it?

...how to choose foods from plant sources to meet your protein needs?

...what minerals are especially important in your teen years?

If not, you'll find out in this chapter!

Look for these TERMS

saturated fats

unsaturated fats

cholesterol

amino acids

antioxidants

osteoporosis

dietary supplement

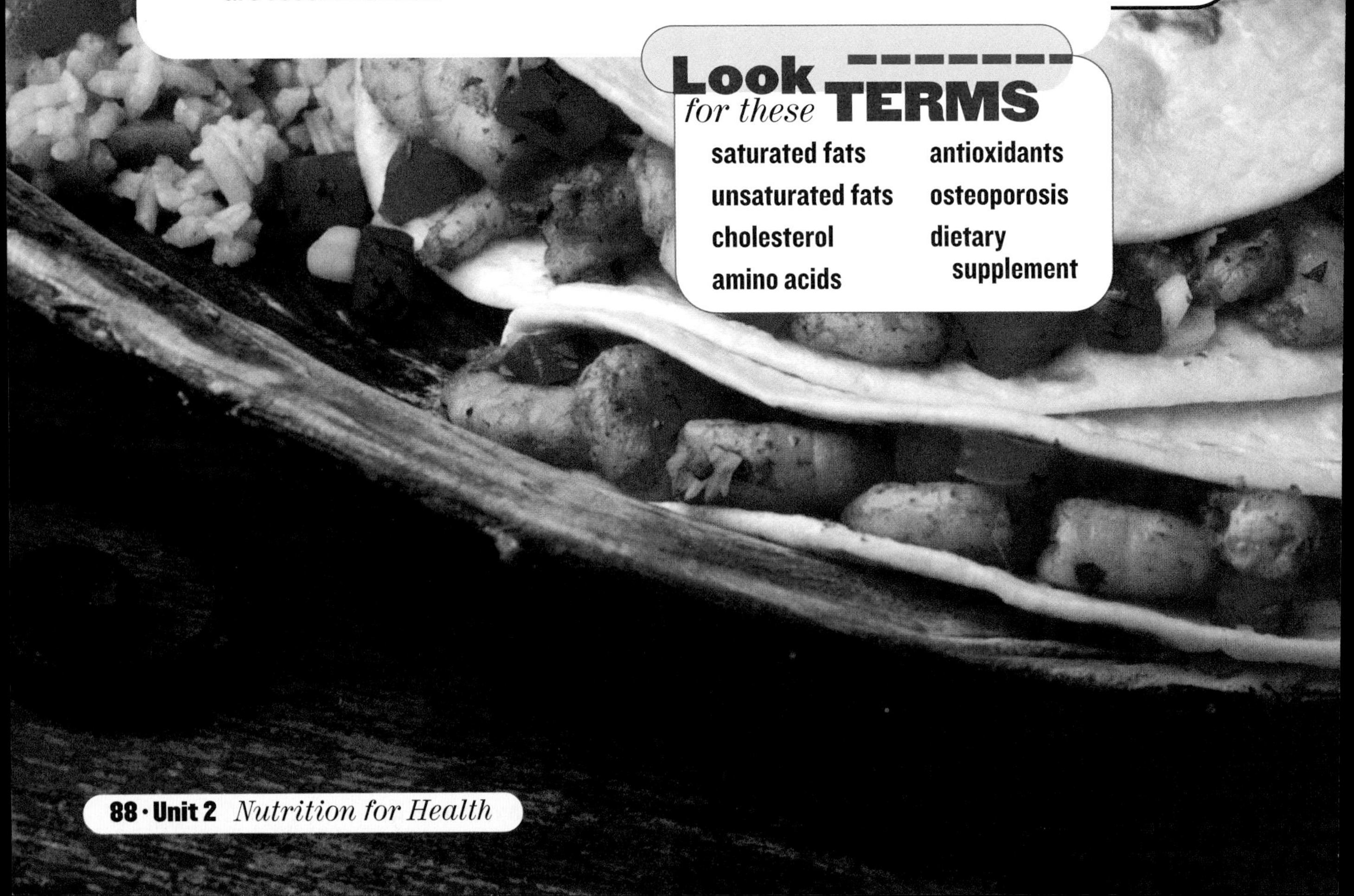

Food nourishes your

body with carbohydrates, fats, proteins, vitamins, minerals, and water. Within these six major categories of nutrients are many specific nutrients—each with a unique job to perform in your body. In this chapter, you'll learn more about the specific nutrients your body needs for energy, health, and growth.

Carbohydrates: Your Main Energy Source

Your body's main source of energy is carbohydrates, which are grouped in two categories: simple and complex. Sugars are simple carbohydrates because they're made of one or two sugar units. Starches are complex carbohydrates because they're made of many sugars, all attached together. During digestion, your body breaks down starches into single sugars, which are taken into your blood to make energy.

If you skip meals or limit foods high in carbohydrates, your body may run short on energy. If you eat more than you need of foods high in carbohydrates, you may get more calories than you need. Eating too many calories from any source may lead to weight gain.

Food Sources of Carbohydrates

Sugars are a natural part of some foods. For example, fruit and milk contain sugars. Foods with natural sugars also carry other important nutrients. Some foods, such as candy, are high in added sugars and have few other nutrients.

Good sources of complex carbohydrates are:
• Grain products, including breads, rice, and pasta.
• Vegetables such as squash, potatoes, and corn.
• Dry beans, peas, and lentils.

Carbohydrates supply your body with energy. Get most of your carbohydrates from complex carbohydrate foods. What happens when you don't eat enough foods that are high in carbohydrates?

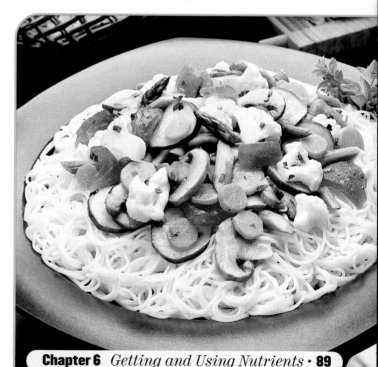

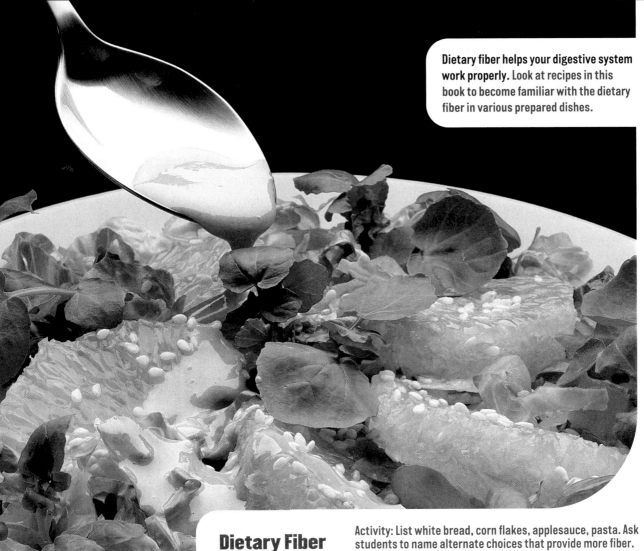

Dietary fiber helps your digestive system work properly. Look at recipes in this book to become familiar with the dietary fiber in various prepared dishes.

Dietary Fiber

Activity: List white bread, corn flakes, applesauce, pasta. Ask students to name alternate choices that provide more fiber.

Many foods high in complex carbohydrates are good fiber sources, too. Dietary fiber is plant material that can't be digested. Fiber helps your digestive tract work properly and may help protect your body from heart disease and cancer.

Fats: Essential to Your Health

Have you ever wondered why your fingers feel slippery after eating foods like potato chips or fried chicken? It's the fat in these foods that you're feeling. Fat is both a food and a nutrient. As a food, it gives your meals flavor and texture. As a nutrient, it supplies energy and has other important roles.

Fat promotes healthy skin and normal growth. It also acts as a partner with certain vitamins, carrying these nutrients to wherever your body needs them. The fat stored in your body acts as a cushion to protect vital organs such as your heart and liver.

Activity: Compare milk with different amounts of fat. How does fat content affect the flavor of the milk?

INFOLINK

To look up the amount of nutrients in specific foods, turn to the Appendix at the back of the book.

Food Sources of Fat

Fats are naturally present in meat, poultry, fish, dairy products, and nuts. Vegetable oil is a liquid form of fat. Butter, margarine, cream, and mayonnaise are almost all fat. These sources of fat are often used as ingredients in foods such as salad dressings, gravy, cakes, cookies, many other baked foods, and ice cream. Foods fried in oil are typically high in fat, too.

Fat in foods is considered either saturated or unsaturated. Most foods with fat contain a mix of the two.

- **Saturated fats** *are hard at room temperature.* Examples include butter, stick margarine, and the fats in meat, poultry, and dairy products.
- **Unsaturated fats** *are liquid at room temperature.* Foods with mostly unsaturated fat are vegetable oils, nuts, olives, and avocados.

What's Cholesterol?

Cholesterol is *a waxy substance that is part of every cell of your body.* Your body can produce all the cholesterol it needs but can also obtain it from food. Cholesterol is found in foods from animal sources: meat, poultry, fish, egg yolks, and dairy products. Foods from plant sources have no cholesterol.

A high level of cholesterol in your blood increases your risk for heart problems. A high-cholesterol diet is one reason why some people have high blood cholesterol. Too much fat, especially saturated fat, increases blood cholesterol even more.

Go easy on high-fat foods. Eating too much fat, especially saturated fat, increases your chances of developing heart disease later in life and can lead to weight gain.

More About Fats: Because fats stay in the stomach longer than other nutrients, they keep you feeling full longer.

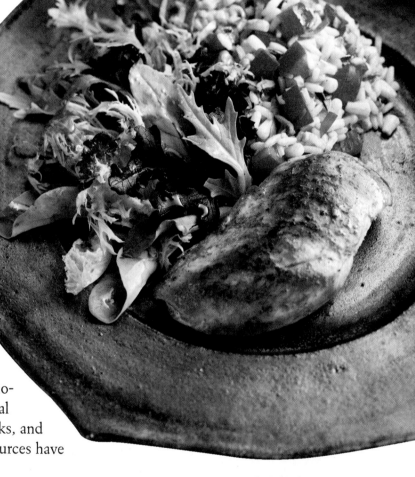

Fat is an essential nutrient that your body needs. For heart health, it's wise to eat foods with saturated fat and cholesterol in moderation. Which food shown here has the most saturated fat?

INFOLINK

You'll learn tips for trimming fat and cholesterol in Chapter 7.

Proteins: Your Body's Building Blocks

More About Proteins: Protein deficiency is a problem in many developing countries. Protein deficiency causes a variety of disorders, including poor growth and intellectual deficits in children and a weakened immune system.

Proteins help your body grow, repair itself, and fight disease. Your body can also use protein to provide energy if needed.

Amino acids are *the many small units that make up protein.* Think of amino acids as the notes in music. The same notes can make up a rock song or classical symphony—they are just arranged differently. The same is true for amino acids in proteins. Your body arranges amino acids to make the different proteins it needs.

Your body makes some amino acids. The ones your body can't make—called essential amino acids—must come from the food you eat.

Every part of your body is made up of protein, including your bones and organs. What role do essential amino acids play in maintaining a healthy body?

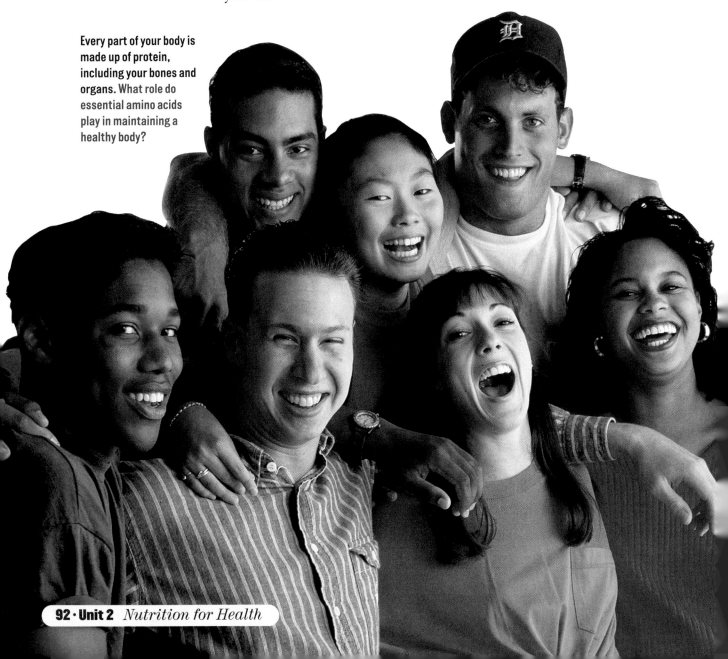

Food Sources of Protein

You can get protein from both animal and plant sources. Foods from animal sources, such as meat, poultry, fish, eggs, and dairy products, have all the essential amino acids. For this reason, they are called complete proteins. Plant sources of proteins include dry beans and peas and nuts. Grain products also have some protein, but not as much. Foods from plants lack one or more essential amino acids, so they're incomplete proteins. However, eating a variety of plant-based foods can provide all the essential amino acids you need.

Most people get plenty of protein from their everyday food choices. When you eat more protein than you need, it's stored as body fat. You don't need to eat extra amounts of protein, even when you're growing. Eating more protein won't build bigger muscles either—only physical activity does that.

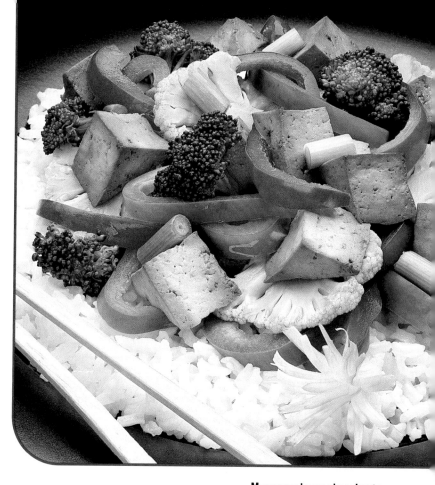

Many people are choosing to have meatless meals, such as this one. Eating a variety of plant-based foods can supply the essential amino acids. Locate a high-protein, meatless recipe you would like to try.

Critical Thinking: Vitamin B_{12} is found naturally only in animal products. Ask: What would you recommend to a friend who eats a strict vegetarian diet?

Vital Vitamins

You need vitamins in only small amounts because they pack a powerful punch! Even though vitamins don't provide energy or build body tissue, they help regulate these processes as well as many others. Vitamins help other nutrients do their jobs. In fact, your body can't produce energy without them. Look at the charts on pages 94 and 95 to see the functions and food sources of some vitamins your body needs.

Vitamins A, C, and E have special roles in your body. They act as **antioxidants**, *helping to protect your body from cell damage that can lead to health problems.* Eat plenty of fruits, vegetables, whole grain breads and cereals, and nuts to get your antioxidants.

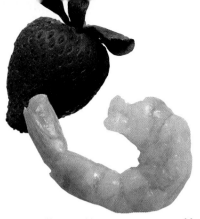

Water-Soluble Vitamins

Vitamin C and the B vitamins dissolve in water. Water-soluble vitamins cannot be stored in your body for later use. That's why it's important to eat regularly a variety of foods that supply these vitamins. Your body gets rid of excess amounts of water-soluble vitamins in your urine. Taking large amounts of these vitamins as supplements can cause your kidneys to work too hard to remove the excess.

Discuss: How could you prepare vegetables to preserve their water-soluble vitamins?

Water-Soluble Vitamins

VITAMIN/FUNCTIONS	FOOD SOURCES
THIAMIN Helps in energy production Maintains healthy nerves	Enriched and whole grain breads and cereals; lean pork; dry beans and peas
RIBOFLAVIN Helps in energy production Helps the body resist infections	Enriched and whole grain breads and cereals; milk products; dry beans and peas; meat; poultry; fish
NIACIN Helps in energy production Needed for a healthy nervous system	Meat; poultry; fish; liver; enriched and whole grain breads and cereals; dry beans and peas; peanuts
VITAMIN B_6 Helps in energy production Needed for a healthy nervous system Helps protect against infection	Poultry; fish; meat; dry beans and peas; whole wheat products; some fruits and vegetables; liver
VITAMIN B_{12} Helps in energy production Helps build red blood cells Needed for a healthy nervous system	Meat; poultry; fish; shellfish; eggs; dairy products Some foods, such as breakfast cereals, are fortified with vitamin B_{12}
FOLATE (FOLIC ACID) Helps build red blood cells May help protect against heart disease Helps to prevent birth defects	Fruits; whole grain products; dark green, leafy vegetables; dry beans and peas; liver Bread, cereal, rice, pasta, flour, and other grain products are fortified with folic acid
VITAMIN C Increases resistance to infection Maintains healthy teeth and gums Helps wounds heal Helps keep blood vessels healthy	Citrus fruits (such as oranges and grapefruits); cantaloupes; tomatoes; green peppers; strawberries; kiwi fruit; mangoes; potatoes; broccoli; cabbage

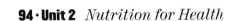

Fat-Soluble Vitamins

As you might have guessed, fat-soluble vitamins dissolve in fat—both in foods and in your body. Fat-soluble vitamins are A, D, E, and K. You store fat-soluble vitamins in body fat and in your liver. When you need them, your body pulls some out of storage. Excess amounts of fat-soluble vitamins can build up to harmful levels in your body.

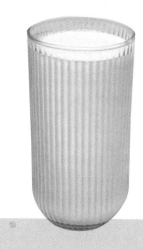

Fat-Soluble Vitamins

VITAMIN/FUNCTIONS	FOOD SOURCES
VITAMIN A Promotes growth and healthy skin and hair Helps eyes adjust to darkness Helps body resist infections	Dairy products; dark green, leafy vegetables (such as spinach); deep yellow orange fruits and vegetables (such as carrots, pumpkin, winter squash, cantaloupe, peaches, apricots)
VITAMIN D Helps build strong bones and teeth Enhances calcium absorption	Fortified milk; egg yolks; fatty fish (such as salmon and mackerel); liver The body can also produce vitamin D from exposure to sunlight
VITAMIN E Helps form red blood cells and muscles Protects other nutrients from damage	Vegetable oils; whole grain breads and cereals; dark green, leafy vegetables; dry beans and peas; nuts and seeds
VITAMIN K Helps blood clot	Dark green, leafy vegetables; wheat bran and wheat germ; some fruits; egg yolks; liver.

Critical Thinking: Ask: Which fat-soluble vitamin can the body produce from exposure to sunlight? Why might relying on this way present problems?

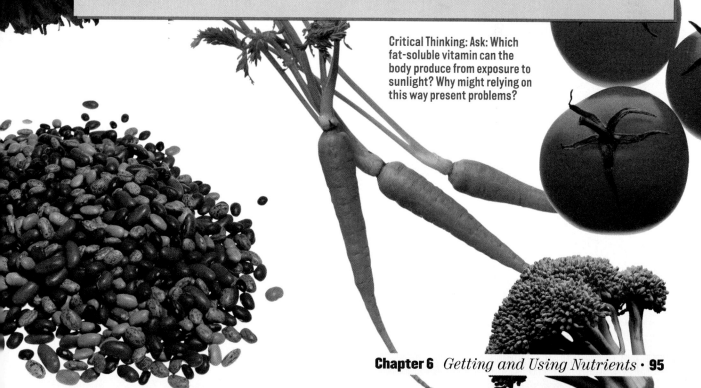

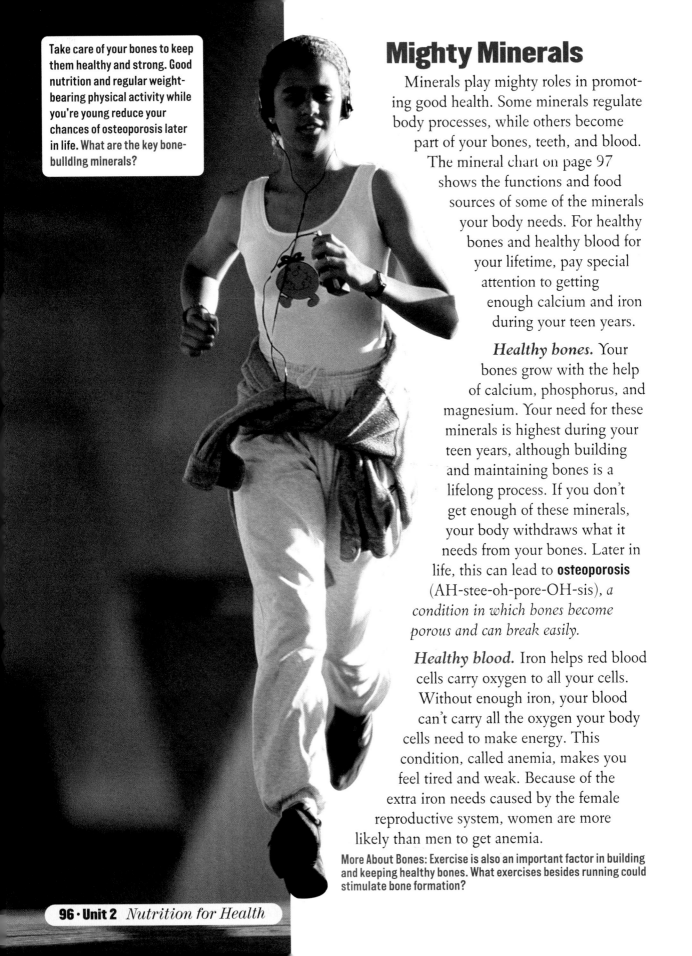

Take care of your bones to keep them healthy and strong. Good nutrition and regular weight-bearing physical activity while you're young reduce your chances of osteoporosis later in life. What are the key bone-building minerals?

Mighty Minerals

Minerals play mighty roles in promoting good health. Some minerals regulate body processes, while others become part of your bones, teeth, and blood. The mineral chart on page 97 shows the functions and food sources of some of the minerals your body needs. For healthy bones and healthy blood for your lifetime, pay special attention to getting enough calcium and iron during your teen years.

Healthy bones. Your bones grow with the help of calcium, phosphorus, and magnesium. Your need for these minerals is highest during your teen years, although building and maintaining bones is a lifelong process. If you don't get enough of these minerals, your body withdraws what it needs from your bones. Later in life, this can lead to **osteoporosis** (AH-stee-oh-pore-OH-sis), *a condition in which bones become porous and can break easily.*

Healthy blood. Iron helps red blood cells carry oxygen to all your cells. Without enough iron, your blood can't carry all the oxygen your body cells need to make energy. This condition, called anemia, makes you feel tired and weak. Because of the extra iron needs caused by the female reproductive system, women are more likely than men to get anemia.

More About Bones: Exercise is also an important factor in building and keeping healthy bones. What exercises besides running could stimulate bone formation?

Minerals

MINERAL/FUNCTIONS	FOOD SOURCES
CALCIUM Builds and renews bones and teeth Regulates heartbeat, muscles, and nerves	Milk; yogurt; cheese; dark green, leafy vegetables; canned fish with edible bones; dry beans; calcium-fortified juices and cereals
PHOSPHORUS Builds and renews bones and teeth Helps in energy production	Milk; yogurt; cheese; meat; poultry; fish; egg yolks; whole grain breads and cereals
MAGNESIUM Builds and renews bone Helps nerves and muscles work properly	Whole grain products; dark green, leafy vegetables; dry beans and peas; nuts and seeds
SODIUM, CHLORIDE, AND POTASSIUM Help maintain the body's balance of fluid Help with muscle and nerve actions	Sodium and chloride: Salt and foods that contain salt. Many ingredients also contain sodium. Potassium: Fruits (such as bananas and oranges); vegetables; meat; poultry; fish; dry beans and peas; dairy products
IRON Helps build and renew hemoglobin to carry oxygen to cells	Meat; poultry; fish; egg yolks; dark green, leafy vegetables; dry beans and peas; enriched grain products; dried fruits
ZINC Helps heal wounds and form blood Helps in growth and maintenance of body tissues	Meat; liver; poultry; fish; dairy products; dry beans and peas; whole grain breads and cereals; eggs
FLUORIDE Helps prevent tooth decay by strengthening teeth	Small amounts are added to the water supply in many communities. Toothpaste also has fluoride, which can be absorbed by brushing teeth.

Water Is a Nutrient, Too!

Water is a vital nutrient! You need a regular supply of water to help your body perform its many life-supporting activities. In fact, while you could live many days without food, you could live only a few days without water. Among its many functions in your body, water carries nutrients, eliminates wastes, and helps regulate body temperature.

Activity: The human body is about 65 percent water by weight. Calculate the amount in pounds for various body weights.

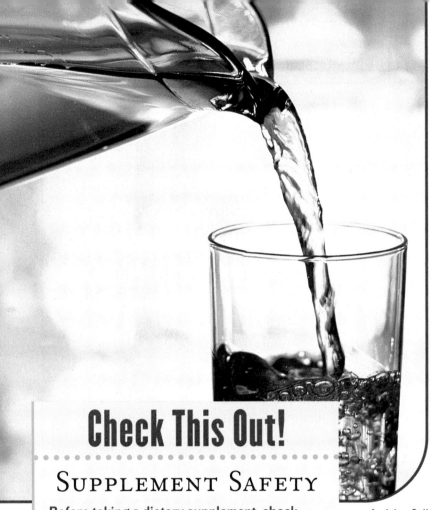

Don't wait until you're thirsty. Make an effort to drink water and other liquids throughout the day so that you get the 2 quarts (2 L) or more of fluid you need. Why aren't soft drinks and coffee or tea the best sources of fluids?

Sources of water. Each day, your body loses about 2 to 3 quarts (2 to 3 L) of water. To help replace it, consume about 2 quarts, or 8 cups, of fluid each day. Choose liquids such as plain water, fruit juices, milk, and soups. Beverages with caffeine—coffee, tea, and some sodas—are not the best sources of water. Caffeine in these drinks makes your body lose some water. Many foods you eat, such as fruits, vegetables, bread, and meat, also supply small amounts of water.

Activity: Collect and analyze the claims of dietary supplement ads. What unrealistic claims are made?

Dietary Supplements

Most people can get all the nutrients they need by eating a variety of nutritious foods. However, under some special circumstances, a dietary supplement may be necessary. A **dietary supplement** *provides extra nutrients in the form of pills, capsules, liquid, or powder.* Supplements may contain vitamins, minerals, fiber, protein, and other substances such as herbs.

A doctor may recommend dietary supplements for elderly people, pregnant or nursing women, people on certain medications, people recovering from illness, or people following special diets or very low-calorie diets.

Check This Out!

SUPPLEMENT SAFETY

Before taking a dietary supplement, check with your doctor to see if you need extra nutrients. When choosing a supplement with vitamins and minerals, look for products that supply no more than 100 percent of the Daily Values. If you take a dietary supplement, always follow the dose on the label, and keep it out of the reach of small children!

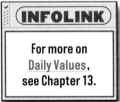

INFOLINK

For more on
Daily Values,
see Chapter 13.

It's Your Turn!

Talk to a nutrition expert. Find out why nutrition experts say "food first"—and why dietary supplements, even one with 100 percent Daily Values, can't replace food. Report your findings to the class.

CAREERS *in*

HELP WANTED

Chemist

Recent chemistry graduate needed for an entry-level position in flavor development. Work in a modern facility and receive a competitive salary plus medical, dental, and life insurance. Excellent training program provided. Send resume to Technical Director, FlavorCorp.

Laboratory Testing Technician

Major food manufacturing company has opening in research and development for a Testing Technician. Work in laboratory setting testing materials and recording results for quality control studies. Applicants should be detail oriented and have a two-year technical degree. Submit resume to Human Resources Director, Cisco Foods.

Food Scientist

Well-known food company is seeking a Food Scientist with a bachelor's degree in food science or related field. Will develop new cereal products from concept through commercial sales. Prefer 3+ years of industry experience. Excellent salary and benefits package. Send resume to Technical Recruiters.

Research Dietitian

National food processing company seeks Registered Dietitian to conduct laboratory experiments. Assist in determining nutritional value of new and existing products and present findings in written reports. Bachelor's degree and research experience required. Masters preferred. Submit resume and salary requirements to Human Resources Director, Baker Corporation.

Food Science Technician

Entry-level position open for a Food Science Technician to assist in quality control and testing proportions of ingredients. Two-year degree required. Excellent training program. Strong computer skills needed. Send resume to Human Resources, AP Industries.

Fish Production Technician

Government owned fish farm has entry-level position for fish production technician. Assist with monitoring tanks and ponds, feeding fish, and maintaining equipment. High school diploma required. Advancement opportunities for person willing to pursue advanced education and training. Apply in person at Valley Hatchery.

LINKING *to the* WORKPLACE

❶ **Writing a Résumé:** Imagine that you are qualified for one of the jobs advertised above. Prepare a résumé that would lead an employer to want to interview you. Be sure to use a standard résumé format.

❷ **Identifying Scientists' Roles:** Explain how the following scientists could be involved in the production of yogurt and ice cream: a microbiologist; a chemist; a computer scientist; an agricultural scientist.

Review & Activities

LOOKING BACK

- Carbohydrates, fats, proteins, vitamins, minerals, and water each have specific functions to perform in your body.
- Each nutrient is supplied by many different foods, including some that are especially good sources.
- Dietary supplements, used appropriately, can provide extra nutrients for people in special circumstances.

UNDERSTANDING KEY IDEAS

1. Compare and contrast the ways your body uses carbohydrates, proteins, and vitamins.
2. What is fiber? What is its role in good health?
3. Why is fat essential to health?
4. Why might it be better to use vegetable oil for cooking rather than butter?
5. If you don't eat foods from animal sources, how might you obtain enough protein with all the essential amino acids?
6. Why is it important to eat foods containing vitamin C regularly?
7. What are two basic types of functions that minerals can perform? Give a specific example of each.
8. Why is water considered an essential nutrient?
9. In what circumstances might a doctor prescribe dietary supplements?

DEVELOPING LIFE SKILLS

1. **Critical Thinking:** Suppose you read an article that says, "The best way to lose weight is to cut fat completely out of your diet." Would you accept this statement as true? Why or why not? How might this influence your opinion of other information in the article?

2. **Leadership:** A friend tells you he has begun taking extra doses of a multivitamin supplement to give him extra energy. You realize he must not be well informed about nutrition or he wouldn't have made this decision. What would you want to tell your friend? How might you approach the subject without offending him?

Wellness Challenge

Recently, Dana has been reading about osteoporosis. She's learned that developing healthy habits now, as a teen, can help make her bones strong so she'll be less likely to have osteoporosis later. Right now she's feeling very motivated to do all she can for a lifetime of healthy bones. However, Dana also wonders whether she might lose interest after a time and forget about paying attention to bone health. She wants to make sure that doesn't happen.

1. What steps can Dana take to help build strong bones for a lifetime?
2. What suggestions do you have for helping Dana continue to build strong bones?

APPLYING YOUR LEARNING

1. **Food Source Collage:** Make a collage or other visual display showing a variety of foods that are good sources of each major category of nutrient.

2. **Getting Enough Fluids:** For three days, keep track of the amount and type of liquids you drink. How much of your liquid intake was from sources such as plain water, fruit juice, and milk? From coffee, tea, and soda? Create a chart or graphic to illustrate your personal record. Include information about the nutrients that juice and milk supply. If you are not drinking enough fluids, how might you increase your intake?

EXPLORING FURTHER

1. **Fiber:** Learn more about the role of fiber in your eating plan. What is the difference between the two main types of fiber, soluble and insoluble? What foods provide each type? How can fiber help protect you from disease? How much fiber do you need each day?

2. **Antioxidants:** Find out more about antioxidant vitamins. What are antioxidants? How do they work? In what foods are they found? How might they promote your health?

Making CONNECTIONS

1. **Science:** Some people believe that taking vitamin C can prevent or cure the common cold. Use reliable sources to learn the facts. What scientific studies have been done to test this theory? What methods were used? What were the results? Present your findings to the class.

2. **Health:** Learn more about osteoporosis. Besides not getting enough of certain minerals, what are some risk factors for osteoporosis? What actions can you take now to prevent it? Write a brief report on your findings.

FOODS LAB

Take a small piece of butter or margarine and rub it on a piece of paper. Label the spot left by the butter or margarine. Repeat this process with samples of other foods. Which foods left a permanent clear spot? How does this compare to the spot left by the butter or margarine? What can you conclude?

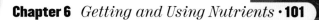

CHAPTER 7

Eating the Dietary Guidelines Way

Objectives

After studying this chapter, you will be able to:

- Explain the purpose of the Dietary Guidelines for Americans.

- Apply the Dietary Guidelines to your food decisions.

- Demonstrate ways to add food variety to your eating plan.

- Determine ways to eat less fat, saturated fat, cholesterol, added sugars, and sodium.

Do You Know...

...how to increase your chances of staying healthy as you get older?

...how to choose snacks with less fat and added sugars?

...how to flavor your veggies without adding salt?

If not, you'll find out in this chapter!

Look for these TERMS

Dietary Guidelines for Americans
eating plan   risk factor
diet

Nutrients are

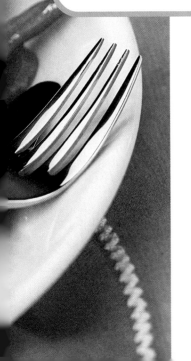

wrapped up in tasty food packages. Besides being enjoyable, your food choices also have a major effect on your health! In Chapter 6 you learned about nutrients: what they do, where they're found, and what you need for energy, growth, and health. The Dietary Guidelines put those facts into advice about healthful eating—for your teen years and for your lifetime!

Dietary Guidelines and You

The **Dietary Guidelines for Americans** provide *advice about food choices for all healthy people age two and over.* The guidelines can aid you, your family, and your friends in making food choices for wellness. Follow them to help you meet your nutrient needs, to reduce your chances of getting certain diseases, and to live a healthful, active life.

An **eating plan,** also called a **diet,** includes *everything you eat or drink.* The Dietary Guidelines offer recommendations for your eating plan. Follow these recommendations to get the nutrients and food energy you need for wellness during your active, growing teen years. Following the guidelines now may also provide benefits as you get older—your chances for developing some health problems may go down.

Keep Trim, Keep Active

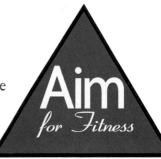

Staying at your appropriate weight and being active throughout life—these are two basics for fitness! This advice helps you be more productive, enjoy life, and be your best in all you do. Active living helps you use food energy, too. That's one way to keep your body weight at an appropriate level.

Making food choices for good health can benefit you now and when you are older. Research physical activity programs in your community. Combine your list with your classmates' lists and distribute them to your school activity center, community centers, and retirement homes.

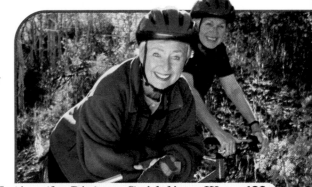

Activity: Analyze your own food choices and then rewrite the guidelines in the order in which you need to improve.

Dietary Guidelines for Americans

AIM
FOR FITNESS...

▲ Aim for a healthy weight.

▲ Be physically active each day.

BUILD
A HEALTHY BASE...

■ Let the Pyramid guide your food choices.

■ Choose a variety of grains daily, especially whole grains.

■ Choose a variety of fruits and vegetables daily.

■ Keep food safe to eat.

CHOOSE
SENSIBLY...

● Choose a diet that is low in saturated fat and cholesterol and moderate in total fat.

● Choose beverages and foods to moderate your intake of sugars.

● Choose and prepare foods with less salt.

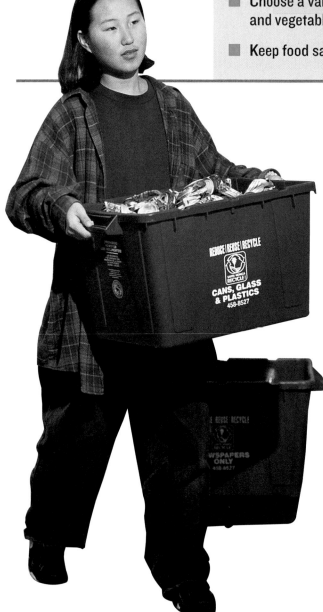

While you are a teen, your body is growing rapidly. You will be putting on weight as your body develops and as you grow taller. Weight gain needs to be looked at in relation to your overall growth and physical development. Keep in mind that your body is changing from that of a child to that of an adult.

As you get older, being overweight with too much extra body fat increases your chances for heart disease, high blood pressure, cancer, arthritis, and other health problems. Keeping an appropriate weight throughout life is wise.

Keep in mind that physical activity doesn't mean just exercising or playing sports. List ways you could be active physically and help your family or community at the same time.

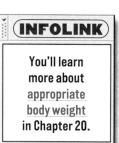

INFOLINK

You'll learn more about appropriate body weight in Chapter 20.

ACTIONS!

When your overall food choices provide more calories than your body uses, the extra calories get stored as body fat. On the flip side, if your body uses more calories than you eat, you may be underweight. For the weight that's right for you, balance how much you eat with how many calories your body uses. And stay active!

To be active:
- Enjoy at least 60 minutes of moderately intense physical activity each day.
- Look for active ways to have fun, such as dancing or in-line skating.
- Move more in your daily life. Use stairs. Walk with your friends.

Vary Your Food Choices

Variety is important! The reason? No single food or type of food provides all the nutrients you need in the right amounts for a day. Enjoy many different foods for all the nutrients and healthful substances they provide. Besides, eating a variety of food means you get to enjoy different flavors, textures, colors, and aromas—and have more fun!

ACTIONS!

The Food Guide Pyramid, an easy-to-use guide, helps you choose the right amount of food with enough variety. You'll learn about this guide in Chapter 8. In the meantime, follow these tips.

For enough food variety:
- Get a firm foundation: plenty of grains, veggies, and fruits. Fit in low-fat dairy foods and protein-rich foods, such as beans and lean meats. Go easy on less-nutritious, higher-calorie foods.
- Try new-to-you foods often. Have you ever tasted snow peas, kohlrabi, papaya, garbanzo beans, or pumpernickel bread?

Check This Out!

WEIGHING HEALTH RISKS

Being overweight with too much extra body fat increases the work load on the heart, lungs, and body frame. In time, that increases the chances of heart disease, some cancers, and diabetes.

Being underweight has health risks also. An underweight person doesn't have much body fat as an energy reserve and may not have many protective nutrients stored up. He or she may be more prone to infection and other illnesses and may feel tired. Being significantly underweight keeps some people from growing properly.

Figuring your Body Mass Index, described in Chapter 20, helps you see if you need to be concerned about your body weight.

It's Your Turn!

Make suggestions for how an underweight person could get more calories while still following the Dietary Guidelines.

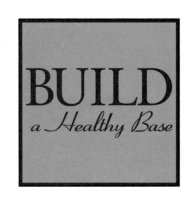

BUILD
a Healthy Base

Go for Grains, Fruits, and Veggies!

How many grain products, veggies, dry beans and peas, and fruits do you eat on a typical day? Like most people, you may not eat enough of these plant-based foods.

Consider the nutritional benefits! Most of your calories—in fact, 45 to 65 percent—should come from carbohydrates. Plant-based foods can supply complex carbohydrates, as well as many vitamins (including vitamins A and C), minerals, and fiber. These foods are also cholesterol-free and naturally low in fats and calories. Make grain products, vegetables, and fruits the main part of your meals. They help protect you from heart disease, cancer, and other health problems.

ACTIONS!

Keep fruits, vegetables, and grain products on hand. Fresh fruits and vegetables make tasty snacks.

Here's a quick hint for healthful eating: Fill three-quarters of your plate with grain products, vegetables, and fruit. The small area remaining is just the right amount for a serving of meat, poultry, or fish. Plan a meal of other food choices in the same proportions. Try to include a milk product, too!

For more grain products:
- Make grain products such as rice or pasta the star of your meals. Flavor with veggies, dry beans and peas, and a little meat.
- Eat several servings of whole-grain cereals and breads each day. Try different kinds of bread for wholesome variety.
- Add rice, pasta, barley, and other grain products to soups.

For more fruits and veggies:
- Enjoy fruit or veggies as a snack. Have fruit for dessert.
- Drink fruit or vegetable juice with your meals or as a snack.
- Eat dry beans several times a week—perhaps in chili, burritos, rice and beans, and bean soup. Refried beans are also enjoyable.
- Think color. Eat a variety of yellow, deep green, orange, and red fruits and veggies! That way you'll be sure to get different nutrients.

Keep Food Safe

Safe food is healthful food. It's free of harmful bacteria and other contaminants that cause foodborne illness.

ACTIONS!

Remember these four words to keep your food safe enough to eat: clean, separate, cook, and chill. You'll learn more about food safety in Part 1 of the Food Preparation Handbook (pages 438–461).

- Keep clean. Take time for washing your hands before and after you handle food. Keep counters and cutting boards clean. Use hot, soapy water.
- Separate raw, cooked, and ready-to-eat foods while you shop, store, and prepare them.
- Cook foods to a safe temperature to destroy possibly harmful bacteria.
- Chill foods that spoil easily as soon as possible after buying or preparing them.

Eat Less Fat and Cholesterol

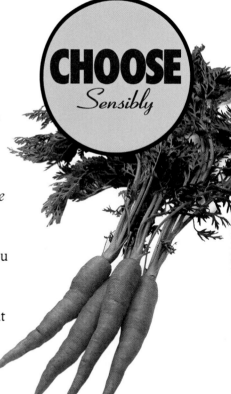

Fat is an essential nutrient. Like most people, though, you may consume more than you need. A high-fat eating plan is often high in calories. Remember, fat provides more calories per gram than carbohydrate or protein. Eating too much fat, especially saturated fat, and too much cholesterol are **risk factors**, or *conditions that increase your chances of having health problems such as heart disease and cancer.* For wellness, follow an eating plan that's low in saturated fat and cholesterol and moderate in total fat.

Your upper limit of fat intake depends on how many calories you need. No more than 20 to 35 percent of the calories you take in over several days should come from fat. Keep saturated fat as low as you can while still eating in a healthful way. Cutting back on fat

re About Fats: The 2000 Dietary Guidelines recommend
more than 30% of calories from fat with no more than
% from saturated fat. The 20-35% figure given here
mes from Dietary Reference Intakes released in 2002.

How Much Fat Is Enough?

IF YOU CONSUME PER DAY ...	1700 calories	2200 calories	2800 calories
TOTAL FAT IN YOUR FOOD CHOICES SHOULD BE NO MORE THAN ...	38-66 grams	49-86 grams	62-109 grams

usually lowers cholesterol intake, too. Limit cholesterol from food to 300 milligrams or less a day. Labels on packaged foods will inform you about their fat content.

ACTIONS!

Try these ways to trim fat and cholesterol but not flavor.
- Go easy on high-fat foods. Choose mostly foods prepared with little or no fat. Cut down on fried foods.
- Make your dairy food choices mostly reduced-fat, low-fat, and fat-free.
- Eat a meal featuring cooked dry beans or peas one or more times a week.
- Enjoy fish several times a week.
- Buy lean meat and poultry. Remove skin from chicken and turkey. Trim away fat you see on meat.
- For less cholesterol, eat egg yolks and whole eggs in moderation or use egg substitutes.

Enjoy Sugar—in Moderation

Many foods that you enjoy have sugars in one form or another. Sugars are naturally present in fruit and milk, which are good sources of other nutrients, too. Foods such as candy, soft drinks, and jelly usually have a lot of added sugar but not many other nutrients.

Why are you smart to eat just small amounts of foods with added sugars? These foods provide extra calories but may be limited in nutrients. Eating a lot of sugary foods may replace nutrient-rich foods in meals or snacks. Sugars are also among the foods that promote tooth decay.

If you would like something sweet, choose fruit. It supplies natural sugars plus other nutrients. Visit a supermarket and find a fruit you have never tried. Research its origin and nutrients.

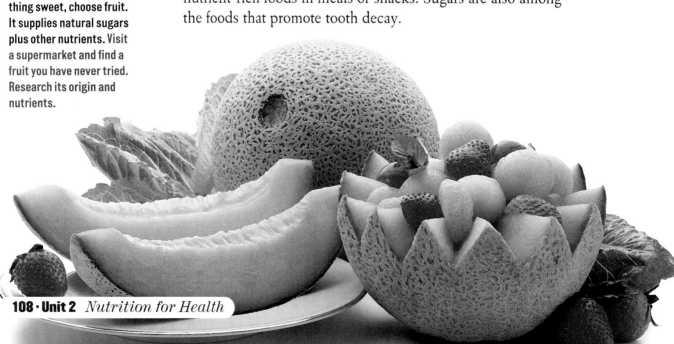

ACTIONS!

In your overall food choices, go easy on added sugars. Here's how.

- Limit soft drinks, fruit ades, candy, and other sweets that have few nutrients. Don't let them crowd out foods that help keep you healthy, such as milk and fruit.
- Check food labels to look for added sugars with names such as *corn sweetener, fructose, honey, maltose, molasses, sugar,* and *syrup.* Any ingredient name ending in "ose" is a sugar.

Control Salt and Sodium

Sodium is an essential nutrient that helps control body fluids. However, most people consume more sodium than they need. Some people are sensitive to sodium. For them, too much sodium can contribute to high blood pressure, which may lead to a heart attack or stroke. As people get older, they may become more sodium sensitive without knowing it. Now is a great time to develop a taste for less salt and to enjoy foods' natural flavors.

ACTIONS!

Most sodium comes from processed foods. Table salt also has sodium. Moderation is a good safeguard. These tips will help you.

- Taste before you salt! Food may have plenty of flavor already. If it needs more, one or two quick shakes of the salt shaker will do.
- Flavor foods with herbs, spices, citrus peel, vinegar, or lemon.
- Ask the cooks in your family to use less salt when preparing food.
- Go easy on salty snacks such as chips.
- Use food labels to find processed foods with less salt or sodium.

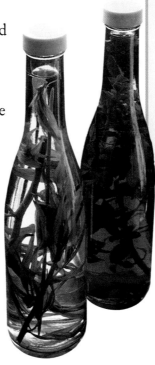

Check This Out!

A UNIVERSAL GUIDELINE

Here's another important principle to follow: eating should be a pleasure. Sometimes we get so concerned with following all the rules that we forget eating can be fun.

- "Enjoy your food." —the first dietary guideline in the United Kingdom
- "A happy family is one whose members eat together, enjoy treasured family tastes, and good home cooking." —Thailand
- "Happy eating makes for happy family life." —Japan
- "Food + Joy = Health." —National Nutrition Council of Norway
- "Eating is one of life's greatest pleasures." —introduction to Dietary Guidelines for Americans

It's Your Turn!

Using one of the above slogans, design a poster or web page that informs people about the pleasure of eating.

Activity: Conduct a blind taste test comparing a salty snack and a low-salt version. Write an evaluation.

HEALTHFUL EATING:
It's All About You!

Following the Dietary Guidelines helps you make food and lifestyle choices for wellness. That gives you the best chance for doing all the things in life you want to do.

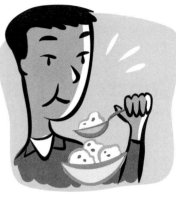

Be sensible! Enjoy all foods, just don't overdo it.

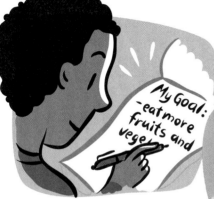

Be realistic! Make small changes over time in what you eat and the level of activity you do. Small steps work better than giant leaps.

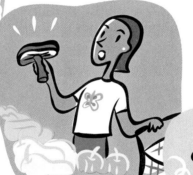

Be adventurous! Expand your tastes to enjoy a variety of foods.

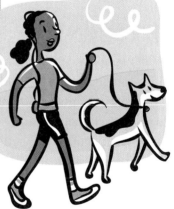

Be active! Walk the dog, don't just watch the dog walk.

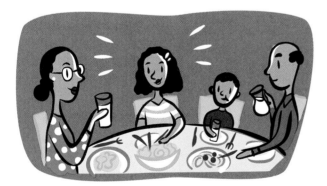

Be flexible! Go ahead and balance what you eat and the physical activity you do over several days. No need to worry about just one meal or one day.

Investigate Further

What steps can you take right away to improve your eating plan?

Source: The Dietary Guidelines Alliance

NOW You're COOKING!

SKILL
Making a Nutritious Snack

*F*resh apples with this yogurt dip are a quick, tasty fat-free snack. If you slice apples ahead, toss them with lemon or orange juice so they won't turn brown. Many other fresh fruits—such as strawberries, cantaloupe, and pineapple—make wonderful dipping fruits, too.

RECIPE

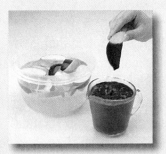

Apples and Fudge-Mint Dip

CUSTOMARY	INGREDIENTS	METRIC
½ cup	Nonfat plain yogurt	125 mL
½ cup	Nonfat hot fudge sauce	125 mL
¼ tsp.	Mint extract	1 mL
2	Medium apples	2

Yield: 4 servings, ¼ (50 mL) cup sauce and ½ apple each

1. In medium bowl, blend together yogurt, fudge sauce, and mint extract until smooth.
2. Slice apples in quarters and remove core. Slice each quarter into 3 pieces.
3. Serve sauce in 4 small cups; arrange apple slices on a separate plate for dipping.

Per Serving: 181 calories, 4 g protein, 33 g carbohydrate, trace fat, 49 mg sodium, 2 g fiber
Percent Daily Value: calcium 10%, phosphorus 10%

More Ideas | When making your dip:
Change the flavor. Try different yogurt flavors or different flavor extracts, such as vanilla. An extract is a concentrated flavoring.

Your Ideas | What other low-fat and low-sugar foods do you think would taste good with this dip? How could you use the fudge-mint sauce in another way? Make your own party or snack recipe with this fudge-mint sauce.

LOOKING BACK

- The Dietary Guidelines for Americans can help you design a healthful eating plan.
- By keeping active, you can achieve or maintain your appropriate weight.
- Eating enough of a variety of foods will help give you the right amount of nutrients and add enjoyment to eating.
- Take action to keep food safe to eat.
- For good health, base your eating plan on the Dietary Guideline recommendations.

UNDERSTANDING KEY IDEAS

1. How can following the Dietary Guidelines for Americans help you lead a long, healthy life?
2. Why is it important to maintain your appropriate weight?
3. What are some ways of increasing the amounts and variety of grain products, fruits, and vegetables that you eat? Give at least three examples.
4. Define risk factor and give an example.
5. How might an eating plan that is high in fat lead to weight gain? How can you cut back on the fat in your eating plan?
6. What are some ways of decreasing the amount of sodium in your eating plan?

DEVELOPING LIFE SKILLS

1. **Critical Thinking:** Why are the Dietary Guidelines for Americans appropriate for teens? What special challenges might you face in following them?
2. **Creative Thinking:** In what ways might dietary guidelines be different in other countries? In what ways might they be the same? Why?

Wellness Challenge

Yolanda and Kelly have noticed that many students in their physical education class make excuses so they don't have to participate. Those who avoid exercise often perform poorly on physical fitness tests. Kelly and Yolanda want to start a fitness campaign to encourage these students and other teens to become physically active.

1. How might Yolanda and Kelly start their campaign?
2. What challenges might they face in keeping their campaign going? How could they overcome those challenges?

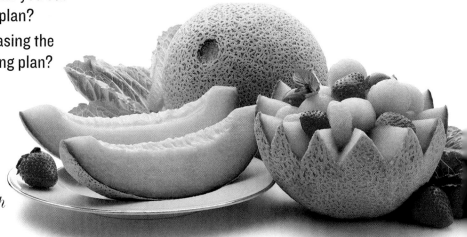

APPLYING YOUR LEARNING

I. **Menu Planning:** Imagine that you are having a party for your friends. You want to provide snacks and beverages that help teens follow the Dietary Guidelines for Americans. Plan tasty snacks based on grains, vegetables, and fruits. What beverages might you offer?

I. **Advice Column:** Write a letter to a health editor at a newspaper describing a problem you have following one of the Dietary Guidelines. Exchange your letter with a classmate. Write a response to your classmate's letter.

EXPLORING FURTHER

I. **Seeking Substitutes:** Some food products use substitutes for sugar or fat. Research these substitutes and select one. Find out how it's used in food and beverages. What are its pros and cons? Are all food items with the substitute low in calories?

2. **Fighting Fat:** Using print or Internet resources, find statistics about the amount of fat and cholesterol in the average American diet. How do these figures compare with those from other countries? How do today's figures compare with those of 10 years ago?

Making CONNECTIONS

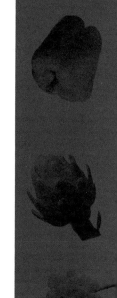

I. **Health:** A can of soda may contain as much as 9 to 12 teaspoons (45 to 60 mL) of sugar. Estimate how much sugar you get from soft drinks in a week. Do you need to cut back? What nutrients would other beverages provide? What changes can you make?

2. **Child Development:** The Dietary Guidelines for Americans are designed for children, too. Also, many people believe that a "sugar habit" or a "salt habit" develops early in life. How can you help children develop a preference for foods with less salt or added sugars? Write a nursery rhyme or design a poster to illustrate your ideas.

FOODS LAB

See how much salt you sprinkle on fries, vegetables, or popcorn. "Salt" a paper plate as if you were salting food. Measure how much salt you added. One quarter teaspoon of salt has 500 milligrams of sodium.

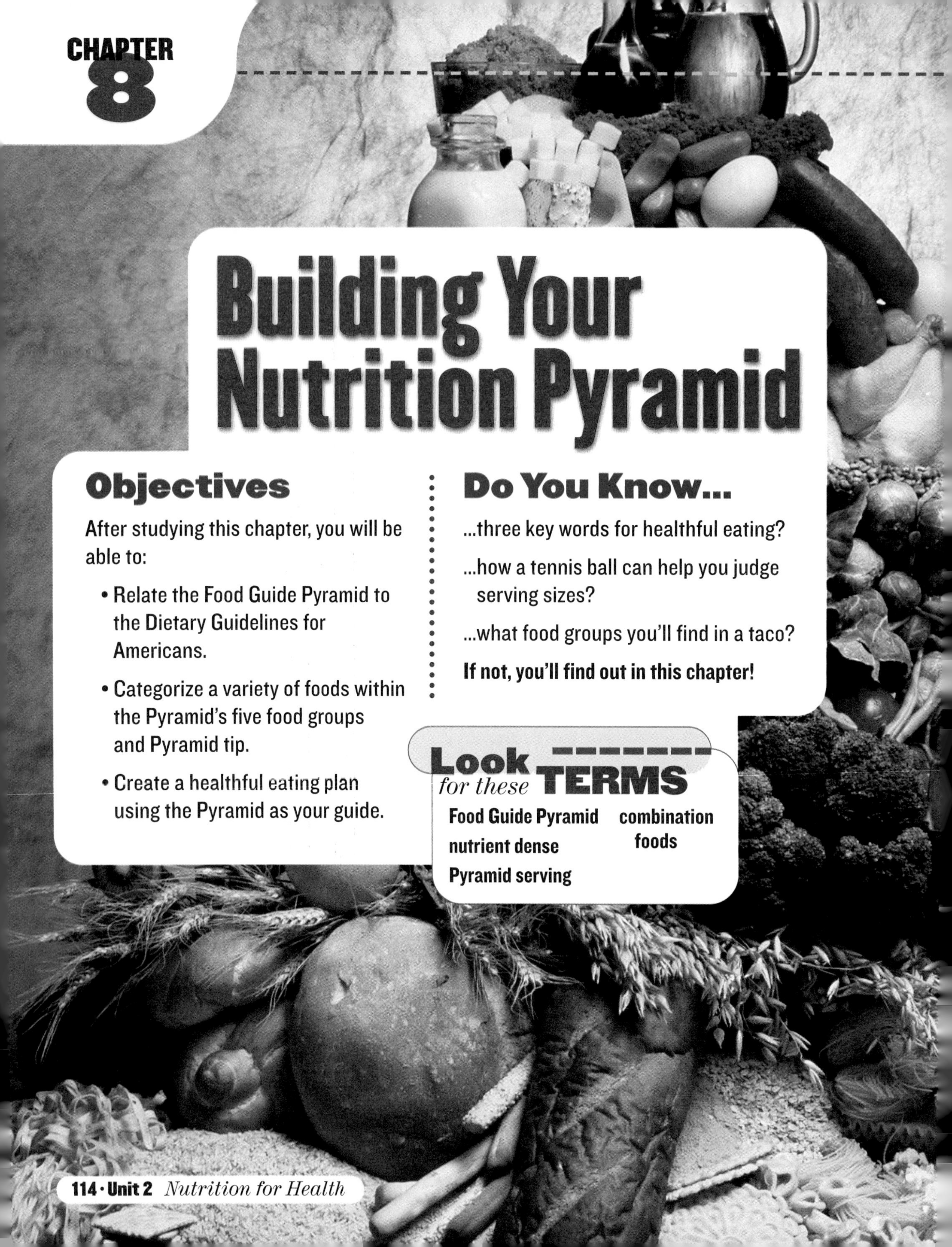

Building Your Nutrition Pyramid

Objectives

After studying this chapter, you will be able to:

- Relate the Food Guide Pyramid to the Dietary Guidelines for Americans.

- Categorize a variety of foods within the Pyramid's five food groups and Pyramid tip.

- Create a healthful eating plan using the Pyramid as your guide.

Do You Know...

...three key words for healthful eating?

...how a tennis ball can help you judge serving sizes?

...what food groups you'll find in a taco?

If not, you'll find out in this chapter!

Look *for these* TERMS

Food Guide Pyramid
nutrient dense
Pyramid serving

combination foods

How can you eat for

wellness? Enjoy the foods you like—as you follow guidelines from the Food Guide Pyramid! The Pyramid is for you and your friends and family. It can help you make wise nutrition choices. Remember, when it comes to smart eating, there are no "good" or "bad" foods— just more and less healthful patterns of eating.

Dietary Guidelines in Action

As your *daily guide for healthful eating*, the **Food Guide Pyramid** is a practical way to follow the Dietary Guidelines for Americans and other expert nutrition advice. The Pyramid is meant for all healthy people age two and over. Use it to make food choices that provide the nutrients and food energy you need.

The Pyramid is simple to use because it's so flexible. Every food you can imagine fits inside— your favorite foods, your family's traditional foods, and foods from cultures other than your own.

Healthful Eating Is...

The Pyramid shows you how to follow the three most basic principles of healthful eating.

Variety. Eat a variety of foods for different nutrients, great flavors, and the fun of eating!

Balance. Eat enough from each of the five food groups to get the nutrients and food energy you need. If you fall short on this goal on one day, make up for it the next day.

Moderation. Eat all kinds of foods, but go easy on amounts to control your calorie intake. That way, you'll get enough variety without overdoing any one food or food group. Limit foods with fat and added sugars.

The Food Guide Pyramid is a guide to help you make sure you get variety in your meals and snacks. Why is variety important?

Discuss: Make a list of food decisions you make each day. Why is it your responsibility to eat healthfully?

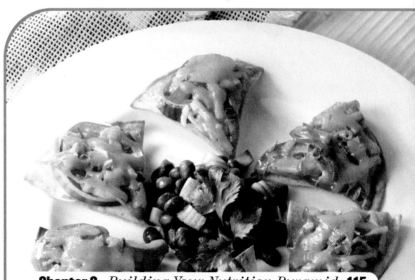

Food Guide Pyramid: Your Guide to Daily Food Choices

Eat Less!
FATS, OILS, AND SWEETS

Key nutrients: carbohydrates, fats

USE SPARINGLY

Eat Enough!
MILK, YOGURT, AND CHEESE GROUP

Key nutrients: protein, calcium and other minerals, B vitamin (riboflavin)

2 TO 3 SERVINGS (3 OR MORE SERVINGS FOR TEENS)

What is a serving? I cup (250 mL) milk or yogurt; I ½ ounces (42 g) natural cheese; 2 ounces (56 g) process cheese

Eat Enough!
MEAT, POULTRY, FISH, DRY BEANS, EGGS, AND NUTS GROUP

Key nutrients: protein, B vitamins (thiamin, niacin), iron, zinc

2 TO 3 SERVINGS—ADDING UP TO 5 TO 7 OUNCES (140 TO 196 g)

What is a serving? 2 to 3 ounces (56 to 84 g) cooked lean meat, poultry, or fish

½ cup (125 mL) cooked dry beans, I egg, or 2 tablespoons (30 mL) peanut butter count as I ounce (28 g) of meat

Eat More!
VEGETABLE GROUP

Key nutrients: carbohydrates; vitamins, especially vitamins A and C and folate; minerals, including potassium; fiber

3 TO 5 SERVINGS

What is a serving? I cup (250 mL) raw leafy vegetables; ½ cup (125 mL) cooked or chopped raw vegetables; ¾ cup (175 mL) vegetable juice

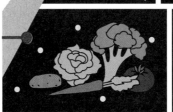
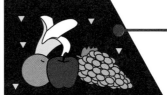
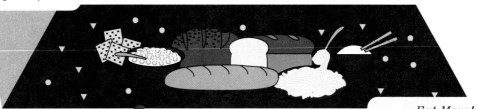

Eat Plenty!
BREAD, CEREAL, RICE, AND PASTA GROUP

Key nutrients: carbohydrates; B vitamins, especially thiamin, niacin, folate; mineals, including iron; fiber

6 TO II SERVINGS

What is a serving? I slice bread; I tortilla; I ounce (28 g) ready-to-eat cereal; ½ cup (125 mL) cooked cereal, rice, or pasta; ½ bagel, burger bun, or English muffin

These symbols show fats, oils, and added sugars in foods:

◻ Fats (naturally occurring and added)

▼ Sugars (added)

Teaching With Visuals: Write down what foods you've eaten today and how many servings they total. How many servings do you still need?

Eat More!
FRUIT GROUP

Key nutrients: carbohydrates; vitamins, especially vitamins A and C and folate; minerals, especially potassium; fiber

2 TO 4 SERVINGS

What is a serving? I medium apple, banana, or orange; ½ cup (125 mL) fruit; ¾ cup (175 mL) fruit juice; ¼ cup (50 mL) dried fruit

All About the Food Guide Pyramid

Discuss: Why is the Pyramid an especially strong symbol for showing the importance of various food groups? How does it help you visualize a good eating plan?

Look closely at the Food Guide Pyramid on page 116. Notice its shape, six parts, and the small symbols inside. What do the Pyramid's visual clues tell you about healthful eating?

The main part is divided into five food groups, the building blocks of healthful eating. The Bread, Cereal, Rice, and Pasta Group is the biggest. You need more servings from this group than any other.

The Pyramid tip is for Fats, Oils, and Sweets. The small symbols inside represent fat and added sugars. These symbols are also scattered within the food groups. Why? That is because some of the foods in these groups also have fat and added sugars.

INFOLINK

For the Dietary Guidelines on the importance of limiting fat and sugar, refer to Chapter 7, pages 107-109.

Why Foods Belong Together

Foods in the five food groups are nutrient packed. They're considered **nutrient dense** because they *contribute a significant amount of several nutrients compared with the food energy, or calories, they contain.* The greater nutrient contribution a food makes in relation to its calories, the higher its nutrient density. Foods in the tip of the Pyramid are not nutrient dense. Their calories come from sugar, fat, or both, but they supply few or no other nutrients.

Foods with similar nutrient content are grouped together. For example, foods in the Milk, Yogurt, and Cheese Group give you plenty of protein for building body cells and calcium for healthy bones. Look for the "Key Nutrients" on page 116.

Within each food group, different foods contain different nutrient amounts. In the Vegetable Group, carrots are a good source of vitamin A, while potatoes with skins are a good source of vitamin C.

Within each group, you'll also find fat-free, low-fat, and higher-fat foods. The chart on page 118 gives some examples.

No single food or food group supplies all the nutrients your body needs. That's why variety is so important! Eating a variety of foods in sufficient amounts from the five food groups provides the nutrient combination essential for your energy, growth, and wellness.

Emphasize: It is important to eat a variety of foods within each food group in order to get all the nutrients you need. No one food in the group supplies them all.

Tip

Calcium-fortified soy milk fits within the Milk, Yogurt, and Cheese Group. Check the label to see how its nutrient content compares to cow's milk.

Teaching With Visuals: Is it possible to eat the right number of servings from each food group and still not have a healthful eating plan? Make up a menu with the lower-fat, lower sugar foods from each food group.

Choices within the Food Groups

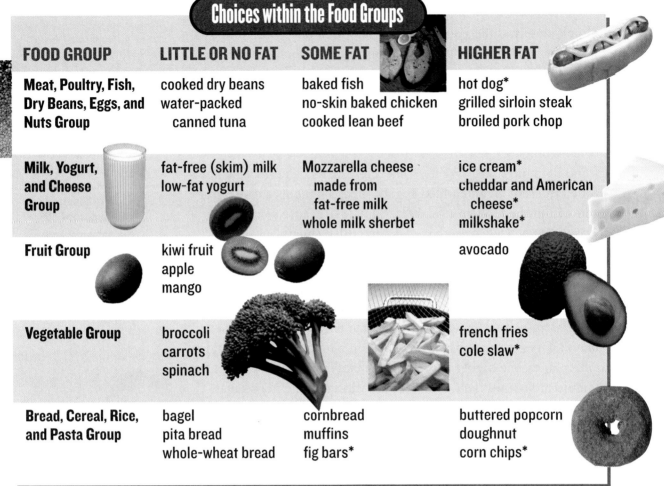

FOOD GROUP	LITTLE OR NO FAT	SOME FAT	HIGHER FAT
Meat, Poultry, Fish, Dry Beans, Eggs, and Nuts Group	cooked dry beans water-packed canned tuna	baked fish no-skin baked chicken cooked lean beef	hot dog* grilled sirloin steak broiled pork chop
Milk, Yogurt, and Cheese Group	fat-free (skim) milk low-fat yogurt	Mozzarella cheese made from fat-free milk whole milk sherbet	ice cream* cheddar and American cheese* milkshake*
Fruit Group	kiwi fruit apple mango		avocado
Vegetable Group	broccoli carrots spinach		french fries cole slaw*
Bread, Cereal, Rice, and Pasta Group	bagel pita bread whole-wheat bread	cornbread muffins fig bars*	buttered popcorn doughnut corn chips*

*Lower-fat versions of these foods are available.

The food groups include foods with varying amounts of fat. Analyze your food choices over two or three days. What changes, if any, do you need to make so that most of your choices are lower-fat ones?

(INFOLINK)

To see how easily you can fit 6 to 11 servings from the Bread, Cereal, Rice, and Pasta Group into your day's eating plan, turn to Chapter 21.

How Many Servings for You?

The Pyramid gives recommended serving ranges. The right amount for you depends on how much food energy you need, based on your age, gender, and physical activity level.

Everyone should have at least the smallest recommended number of servings from each food group daily. With mostly lean and low-fat food choices, that's about 1,700 calories. Are you physically active? Are you growing fast? Then you probably need more servings and more calories. On average, teen girls need about 2,200 calories a day. Teen boys need about 2,800 calories. Keep in mind that this is an average. Individual needs may be lower or higher.

The chart on page 119 shows how your servings might stack up. These are the number of servings you should have if you choose mostly low-fat and lean foods with moderate amounts of fats, oils, and sweets.

Here's a Plan for Pyramid Servings

NUMBER OF DAILY SERVINGS
If you need...

		About 1,700 calories	*About 2,200 calories*	*About 2,800 calories*
EAT ENOUGH	Meat, Poultry, Fish, Beans, Eggs, and Nuts Group	2 (for a total of 5 oz. or 140 g)	2 (for a total of 6 oz. or 168 g)	3 (for a total of 7 oz. or 196 g)
	Milk, Yogurt, and Cheese Group	3 to 4*	3 to 4*	3 to 4*
EAT MORE	Fruit Group	2	3	4
	Vegetable Group	3	4	5
EAT PLENTY	Bread, Cereal, Rice, and Pasta Group	6	9	11

* Children and adults age 24 and over need two to three servings. Teens, as well as women who are pregnant or breast-feeding, need 3 to 4 servings.

There are no serving ranges for the Fats, Oils, and Sweets in the Pyramid tip. Except for fat and added sugars, they don't provide many nutrients. Follow the advice, "Use sparingly." Enjoy just small amounts for the flavor and pleasure they add to your meals and snacks.

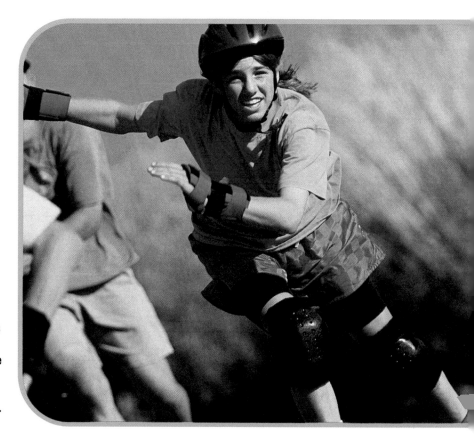

The right number of servings for you depends on several factors, including how active you are. Research which of your daily activities consumes the most calories.

These visual clues will help you understand Pyramid servings. How do your normal helpings compare with Pyramid servings?

Teaching With Visuals: To help internalize the relative sizes of portions, replace the items shown on the chart with similarly sized items from your own lives.

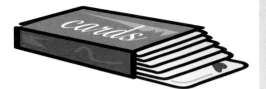

3 oz. (84 g) cooked meat, poultry, or fish = deck of cards

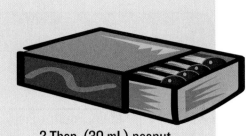

2 Tbsp. (30 mL) peanut butter = matchbox

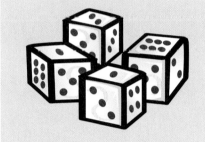

I oz. (28 g) cheese = four dice

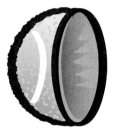

½ cup (125 mL) cooked vegetables = half a tennis ball

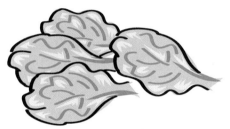

I cup (250 mL) raw leafy greens = four lettuce leaves

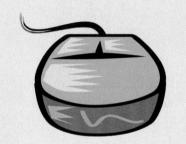

I medium potato = computer mouse

Tip

To add variety to your food choices, try a new food from each food group! You get the nutrient benefits and the fun of a new flavor.

A Pyramid Serving Is . . .

Think about the helpings of food you eat at home and the portions served in restaurants. What amounts of food are served? What about the serving sizes given on food labels? The size of all these portions may differ from Pyramid servings. **Pyramid servings** are *specific measured amounts of food given as serving sizes in the Food Guide Pyramid.*

To use the Pyramid, compare your size helpings to Pyramid servings. You don't need to measure. Just estimate. If your helping is bigger, it counts as more than a serving. For example, if you have a sandwich with two slices of bread, you are getting two servings from the Bread, Cereal, Rice, and Pasta Group. If your serving is smaller, it counts as less than a Pyramid serving.

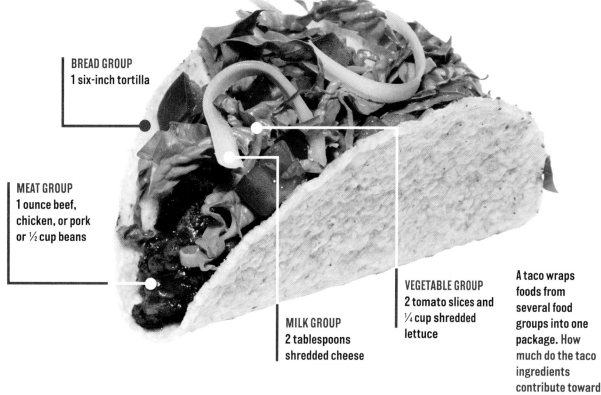

BREAD GROUP
1 six-inch tortilla

MEAT GROUP
1 ounce beef,
chicken, or pork
or ½ cup beans

MILK GROUP
2 tablespoons
shredded cheese

VEGETABLE GROUP
2 tomato slices and
¼ cup shredded
lettuce

A taco wraps foods from several food groups into one package. How much do the taco ingredients contribute toward each food group?

What About Mixed Foods?

How do you estimate serving sizes for a slice of pizza, a veggie omelet, a spring roll, or a chicken Caesar salad? These are **combination foods,** or *mixtures of several ingredients that belong in two or more food groups.* To determine Pyramid serving sizes, estimate the amount of each ingredient and name its food group. Decide if each ingredient provides more, less, or the same amount as one Pyramid serving in that food group.

Wise Choices from the Pyramid

The Food Guide Pyramid can be your action plan! Use it as a planning and decision-making tool to help you meet your goals for healthful eating.

As you make food-group choices, keep these thoughts in mind:

• Enjoy variety within each food group for the different nutrients that different foods provide.
• Choose mostly lean and low-fat foods. Go easy on foods with added sugars.
• Eat enough fruits, vegetables, grain products, and milk products. Some teens come up short on these food groups.
• Eat at least one vitamin A-rich and one vitamin C-rich fruit or vegetable daily! Which ones might you enjoy?
• Try to eat three servings of whole-grain foods each day for dietary fiber.

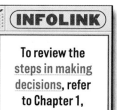

INFOLINK

To review the steps in making decisions, refer to Chapter 1, page 30.

Activity: Choose one of the bulleted suggestions as your "personal goal of the week." Copy the key words from the suggestion on an index card and carry it around as a reminder. Remember that changing one habit at a time is more likely to succeed than trying to change a whole pattern of eating.

Teaching with Visuals: Revise the eating record you started in Chapter 5. Use a different color pen to write in foods that you could add to meet Pyramid needs and cross out foods that put you over the limit.

Putting Your Pyramid Together

If your day's food choices usually come up short on one or more food groups, make changes gradually. Start by adding one more food-group serving to your day's food choices. Once you're in the habit, tackle another simple change, until Pyramid guidelines become your eating pattern for life!

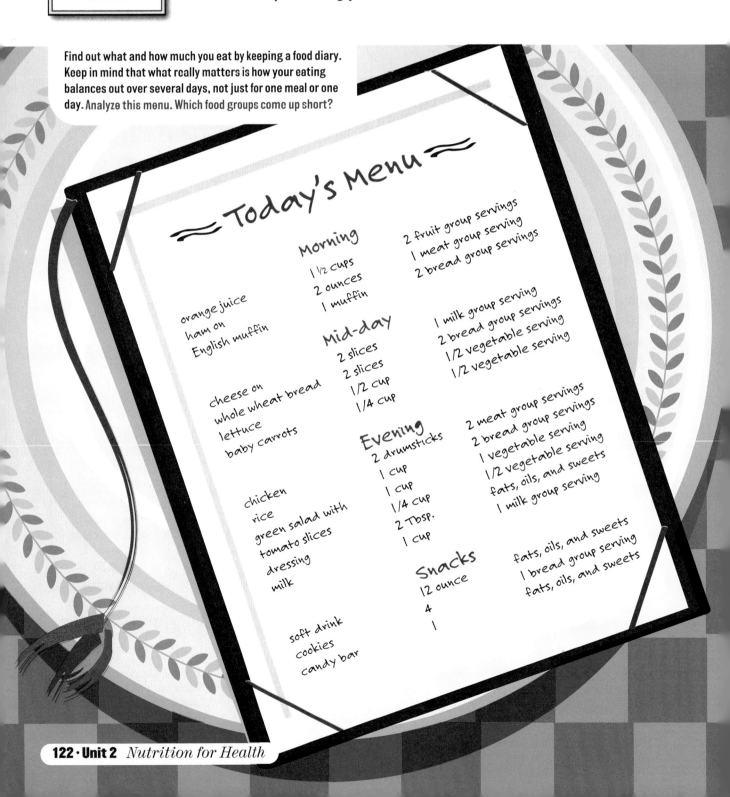

INFOLINK

You'll learn more about foods in the five food groups in Unit Five.

Find out what and how much you eat by keeping a food diary. Keep in mind that what really matters is how your eating balances out over several days, not just for one meal or one day. Analyze this menu. Which food groups come up short?

~Today's Menu~

Morning

orange juice — 1 1/2 cups — 2 fruit group servings
ham on — 2 ounces — 1 meat group serving
English muffin — 1 muffin — 2 bread group servings

Mid-day

cheese on — 2 slices — 1 milk group serving
whole wheat bread — 2 slices — 2 bread group servings
lettuce — 1/2 cup — 1/2 vegetable serving
baby carrots — 1/4 cup — 1/2 vegetable serving

Evening

2 drumsticks — 2 meat group servings
chicken — 1 cup — 2 bread group servings
rice — 1 cup — 1 vegetable serving
green salad with — 1/4 cup — 1/2 vegetable serving
tomato slices — 2 Tbsp. — fats, oils, and sweets
dressing — 1 cup — 1 milk group serving
milk

Snacks

soft drink — 12 ounce — fats, oils, and sweets
cookies — 4 — 1 bread group serving
candy bar — 1 — fats, oils, and sweets

Team Nutrition Features

Teen Artists

"**G**ood Health: It's in the bag!" That's the healthful eating message that Louisiana teen artists want consumers to follow as they choose foods to fill their grocery bags.

As one of six nationally-chosen community art groups, teens from YAYA (Young Aspirations, Young Artists, Inc.) in New Orleans used their graphic talents to create one of six nationally-distributed posters about smart eating for the nation's food stamp program. Student artists from Chicago, Jacksonville, Los Angeles, Poughkeepsie, and the Cañoncito Reservation near Albuquerque designed five other posters. Their nutrition themes: the importance of food variety, fruits and vegetables for health, smart snacking, nutritious food from many cultures, and teaching children about healthful eating.

The posters featuring teens' art were displayed in food stamp program offices across the country. Thousands more have been distributed by USDA's Team Nutrition project, bringing the students' colorful nutrition messages to schools throughout the nation. Teens are making a difference!

Take Action

What message could you spread about healthful eating? Create a slogan to get that message across. Choose a medium for your message—poster, radio announcement, TV commercial, billboard, web page. You decide! Make sketches or write a script to show how you'd use your slogan.

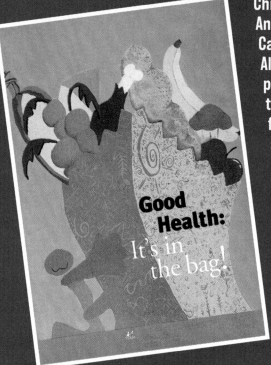

Good Health: It's in the bag!

LOOKING BACK

- The Food Guide Pyramid shows how to follow the basic principles of healthy eating: variety, balance, and moderation.

- The main part of the Food Guide Pyramid is divided into five food groups based on nutrient content. Fats, Oils, and Sweets, which supply few nutrients, are located at the tip of the Pyramid.

- Your age, gender, and level of physical activity determine the number of servings you should get from each food group daily.

UNDERSTANDING KEY IDEAS

1. How does the shape of the Pyramid help you determine how many servings from each food group to eat? How does it help you follow the Dietary Guidelines?

2. Why is it better to get your calories from a combination of foods from the five food groups than from just one or two groups?

3. How many servings of food from the Bread, Cereal, Rice, and Pasta Group should an average female teen eat each day? List the food choices she could make to fulfill this need.

4. What food group servings are provided by one egg scrambled with ¼ cup (50 mL) green peppers and onions, ½ ounce (14 g) ham, and 1 ounce (28 g) process cheese?

DEVELOPING LIFE SKILLS

1. **Creative Thinking:** If you were in charge of fixing dinner for your family tonight, what could you prepare that would provide at least one serving from each food group?

2. **Management:** What management techniques could help you plan meals with variety from the five food groups?

3. **Communication:** How would you rate the Food Guide Pyramid as a communication tool? Does it clearly convey the intended information? Why or why not? What improvements can you suggest?

Wellness Challenge

Dan and Malcom have lunch together almost every day. They both bring bag lunches from home. Malcom makes an effort to prepare something different every day. Dan, on the other hand, always brings a peanut butter and jelly sandwich and a candy bar. He says that his lunches are easy to make and don't require much thought. Malcom is concerned about the lack of variety in Dan's choices.

1. What steps might Malcom take to encourage Dan to vary his lunches?
2. What challenges might Malcom face?
3. How might Malcom go about finding a solution?

APPLYING YOUR LEARNING

1 **Computer Lab:** Using the appendix, choose three foods from each of the five food groups and compare their nutrient density. Make a bar graph to show the nutrients provided by one serving of each food. What nutritional similarities do you see in each food group? Present your findings in class.

2. **Reading Food Labels:** Plan a meal using only packaged or canned foods. Check the Nutrition Facts panel on these foods for the serving sizes. Compare the serving sizes to the recommendations in the Food Guide Pyramid. What conclusions can you draw about packaged food servings?

EXPLORING FURTHER

1. **Then and Now:** Current advice regarding nutrition differs significantly from that of 50 to 60 years ago. What nutrition messages were communicated to Americans around the time of World War II? Why? Trace the progress of dietary recommendations.

2. **Decisions, Decisions:** Find out who plans the school's lunch menu and learn how they use the Pyramid and the Dietary Guidelines in their menu decisions. How do you think the menu portions contribute to your daily serving needs?

Making CONNECTIONS

1. **Math:** As a teen, you need about 1,300 milligrams of calcium daily. Using the Appendix, choose 3 to 4 servings of appealing foods from the Milk, Yogurt, and Cheese Group. How much calcium in grams would you get with these servings? Compare your results with your classmates' to see how calcium varies in different foods.

2. **Language Arts:** Write a rap song or poem on how to use the Food Guide Pyramid to make snack choices. Describe the way that snacks can fit into a healthful eating plan and provide daily servings from the food groups.

FOODS LAB

Find out how big— or small—your helpings really are. Pour a typical serving of breakfast cereal into a bowl, spoon a helping of cooked pasta or rice onto a plate, or pour a glass of milk. Now measure the amounts. How do your helpings compare with the Pyramid serving sizes?

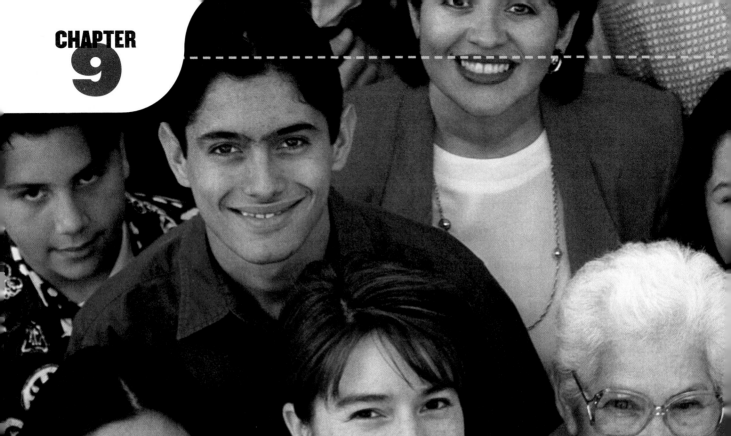

Lifelong Nutrition

Objectives

After studying this chapter, you will be able to:

- Compare nutrition needs throughout the life cycle.

- Prepare a healthful eating plan for different stages in life.

- Explain why good nutrition and active living in the teen years promote lifelong health.

Do You Know...

...how to feed kids when you're baby-sitting?

...why you need so much calcium during your teen years?

...how to help make a meal special for an older relative or friend?

If not, you'll find out in this chapter!

Look *for these* TERMS

life cycle   fetus

prenatal   food jag

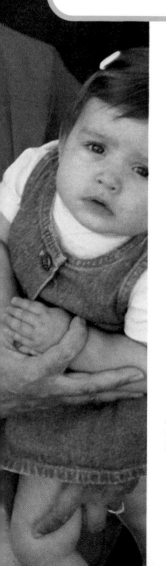

Consider how your

eating plan has changed since you were a baby! You've needed the same nutrients, but the amounts have changed, along with the variety of foods you can enjoy. The guidelines for healthful eating continue through a lifetime.

Nutrition and the Life Cycle

Nutrition throughout your **life cycle**—*from before birth through adulthood*—affects your growth, energy, and health. The Recommended Dietary Allowances—nutrition recommendations developed by experts—reflect different nutrient needs throughout the life cycle. For children, teens, and adults, the Dietary Guidelines and Food Guide Pyramid offer the best advice for healthful eating all throughout life.

Eating for a Healthy Pregnancy

During the **prenatal** period, *between conception and birth*, a single cell develops into a baby. During pregnancy the **fetus,** or *unborn baby*, depends on the mother for nourishment. Good nutrition and health habits, along with proper medical care, are a mother's most important responsibilities. Her baby's health and her own depend on it!

Before and During Pregnancy

Good nutrition before pregnancy helps prepare a woman for a healthy pregnancy. For women who are pregnant or may become pregnant, three nutrients need special attention. Folate, a B vitamin, helps the body make new cells. A deficiency, especially early in pregnancy, may result in birth defects in the spine. As the blood volume for both mother and baby increases, more iron is needed. Calcium builds the baby's bones and teeth and helps renew the calcium in the mother's bones.

Activity: Create a public-service announcement for radio or television explaining why pregnant women need to eat foods high in folate, iron, and calcium.

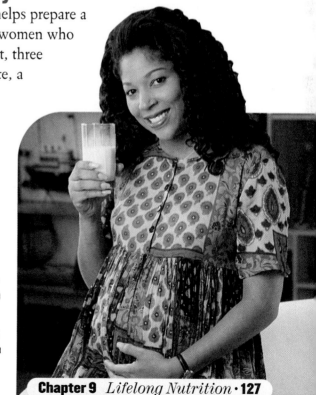

During pregnancy, a woman needs to drink more fluids, at least 8 to 12 cups (2 to 3 L) a day. Why is milk a good choice?

Activity: Prepare a food plan for adding an extra **300** calories a day from nutrient-dense foods to a pregnant woman's eating plan. List the foods, the amounts, and the calories of each. Share your plan with the class.

For times when breast-feeding isn't possible, breast milk can be stored and given to the baby in a bottle. This allows the father to participate in feeding, too. Find out about community resources that give advice on breast-feeding.

During pregnancy, enough servings from the Milk, Yogurt, and Cheese Group (three for adults, four for teens) provide calcium and protein. Foods from the Meat, Poultry, Fish, Dry Beans, Eggs, and Nuts Group provide iron as well as protein. Fruits, vegetables, dry beans, and fortified grain products are essential for folate and other nutrients. Doctors may also prescribe supplements of calcium, iron, or folate to help ensure good health for mother and baby.

A weight gain of 25 to 35 pounds (11 to 16 kg) during pregnancy is normal. Poor nutrition, including too few nutrients or calories, can lead to low birth weight. This means the baby's weight at birth is less than 5 ½ pounds (2.5 kg). Babies with low birth weight are more likely to develop health problems and have difficulty learning. Adding an extra 300 calories a day from nutrient-dense foods to the mother's eating plan provides the food energy that the fetus and mother need. Pregnancy is not the time for a weight-loss program.

Nutrition for Infants

A baby changes rapidly during the first year! The baby may grow in length by 50 percent and triple in weight. The brain and other organs continue to develop. To thrive, a baby needs the right nourishment. At first, all a baby needs is mother's milk or infant formula.

Mother's Milk or Formula?

Breast-feeding is a natural way to feed a baby. Mother's milk provides a balance of nutrients as well as antibodies that build immunity to infection. It's easily digested, prewarmed, germ-free, and economical. A mother who breast-feeds her baby needs to follow Food Guide Pyramid servings to ensure enough milk for her baby and enough nutrients for her own health.

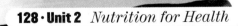

Infant formula that's properly prepared is nutritionally similar to mother's milk. The main ingredient in most formulas is modified nonfat cow's milk. Nutrients are added to the milk. Most doctors advise using an iron-enriched formula. Babies who cannot tolerate cow's milk can drink soy-based formulas or other alternatives.

Plain cow's milk can't substitute for mother's milk or formula. It doesn't contain all the nutrients babies need. Also, until about one year, babies can't digest it properly. After that, whole milk, which contains fats essential for growth, is appropriate, along with solid foods.

Solid Foods for Babies

Infant feeding progresses in steps, following a doctor's advice.

By four to six months: Most babies are physically ready to eat iron-enriched infant cereal and strained fruits and vegetables.

By seven to nine months: Babies are ready to eat strained meat and poultry, unsweetened juice, plain toast, and teething biscuits.

By 10 to 12 months: Babies usually can eat chopped soft foods, unsweetened dry cereals, plain soft bread, and pasta.

After one year: Toddlers start to eat many of the foods other members of their family enjoy.

To make it easier to detect food allergies, introduce new foods one at a time to a baby. A baby will accept new foods better if they are served at the first part of the meal when she or he is hungry. Babies need:
• Food served warm or at room temperature, not hot.
• Calm surroundings.
• Time to chew and swallow.
• The chance to be messy. It's part of learning to eat.
• Someone with them while they're eating.

Check This Out!

BOTTLE-FEEDING BASICS

While they are being bottle-fed, babies need to:
• Be held.
• Be in calm, quiet, and clean surroundings.
• Have their head and back securely supported.
• Surround the nipple with their lips.
• Rest after eating.
It's okay if the baby doesn't finish the bottle, but any formula that's left should be discarded. To avoid tooth decay, a baby shouldn't be put to bed with a bottle.

It's Your Turn!

Research one of the following topics related to bottle-feeding a baby.
• How to warm formula.
• Why formula shouldn't be heated in a microwave oven.
• How to clean bottles and bottle nipples after feeding.
• How to burp a baby.
Share your findings with the class.

Activity: Using a life-size baby doll, practice bottle-feeding basics.

Critical Thinking: Doctors warn parents to discard any unused formula and not put a baby to bed with a bottle. Why are these warnings important for parents to follow?

Healthful Eating for Children

The Food Guide Pyramid helps in planning meals and snacks for kids ages two and up! Children need the same food variety that adults and teens do. The difference is in the amount of food they need. The chart on page 131 shows how to adjust serving sizes and number of servings for preschool-age and school-age children.

Meals and Snacks for Kids

Children need a regular meal schedule. Feeling tired or cranky from hunger affects their appetites. Active, growing children need snacks, too. The reason? Their stomachs are small, but their energy levels are high. They may not be able to eat enough at mealtime to satisfy their food needs.

Children under three or four years may choke on some foods. Avoid small hard foods like nuts, popcorn, pretzels, raw carrot pieces, raisins, seeds, and chips. Avoid hard candy and cough drops, too. Cut meat and poultry into small pieces, and slice grapes in half.

Learning Good Eating Habits

If you have younger brothers or sisters, set a good example by joining the family and eating with them. Positive experiences with food encourage children to become good eaters. It's unwise to reward good behavior with food or withhold a favorite food as discipline. Using food in those ways teaches negative attitudes about eating.

Emphasize: Grapes need to be sliced because if a child swallows a whole grape it could fit perfectly in the throat and cause choking. Hot dogs should be cut lengthwise for the same reason. Name other foods that should be sliced before given to a young child.

Children need positive food experiences. Find a recipe for a snack that would be appealing to a child.

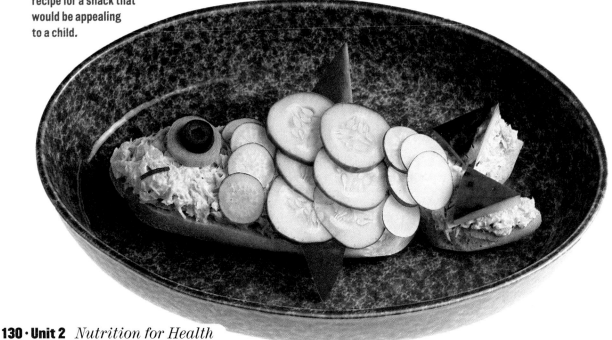

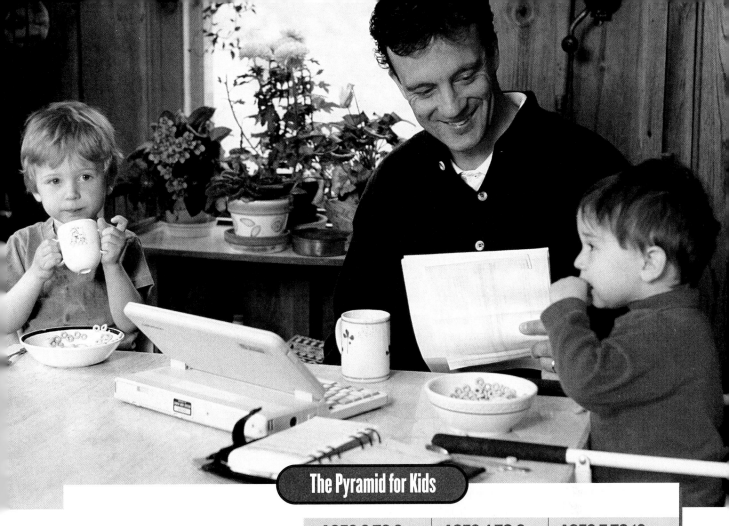

The Pyramid for Kids

A PYRAMID SERVING IS... (Note: Children may prefer servings to be divided into smaller portions. What counts is the total for the day.)	AGES 2 TO 3 About two-thirds of an adult-size Pyramid serving, except for the milk group.	AGES 4 TO 6 The same size as an adult Pyramid serving.	AGES 7 TO 12 The same size as an adult Pyramid serving.
Meat, Poultry, Fish, Dry Beans, Eggs, and Nuts Group	2	2	2 to 3
Milk, Yogurt, and Cheese Group	2 (adult size servings)	2	3 to 4
Fruit Group	2	2	2 to 3
Vegetable Group	3	3	3 to 4
Bread, Cereal, Rice, and Pasta Group	6	6	6 to 9

(Left margin label: NUMBER OF DAILY SERVINGS)

Teaching With Visuals: Cut poster board in the shape of the Pyramid and add pictures of appropriate foods for kids.

Check This Out!

NO-COOK SNACKS—EASY AND SAFE!

When kids get home from school, they often are hungry. If parents are not yet home, children can be responsible for getting their own snacks. It's important they make healthful choices. Making their own snacks also gives kids a chance to develop kitchen skills. Here are some easy and nutritious snacks older children can make on their own.

- Dip tortilla chips or baby carrots in salsa.
- Put apple and cheese slices between graham crackers.
- Mix two fruit juices together.

- Mix fruit with milk, yogurt, or softened ice cream.
- Top bread with peanut butter and banana slices.

It's Your Turn!

Think of a creative snack you could show kids how to make. Write or draw a description of the snack.

Activity: Plan a week's menu of nutritious no-cook snacks. Then create a grocery list of needed items. If possible, prepare one of your snacks.

Sometimes a young child goes on a **food jag,** *wanting just one food for a while.* This is a step toward independence and not a cause for worry. Food jags usually don't last long. If a child acts like a picky eater, don't give up. Continue introducing new foods in small amounts, as you teach children to eat a variety of foods. Also, children:

- Need mealtimes that are pleasant, not pressured. Don't rush a child.
- Like colorful foods and interesting shapes.
- Like small servings. Children can always ask for more.
- Enjoy being involved in food preparation, serving, or table setting.
- Can decide how much they need to eat.

Nutrition for Your Teen Years

Healthful eating and active living top the list as two smart ways to be your personal best. What you eat and how active you are during your teen years also have positive long-term effects.

Eating to Be Your Best

You grow faster during your teen years than at any time since infancy. You're probably very active, too! That's why nutrient and energy needs are as high now as they'll ever be—and why you probably need more Pyramid servings. Go easy on high-fat foods, and choose plenty of nutrient-dense foods that are high in complex "carbs" for more food energy and for their nutrients.

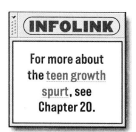

INFOLINK

For more about the teen growth spurt, see Chapter 20.

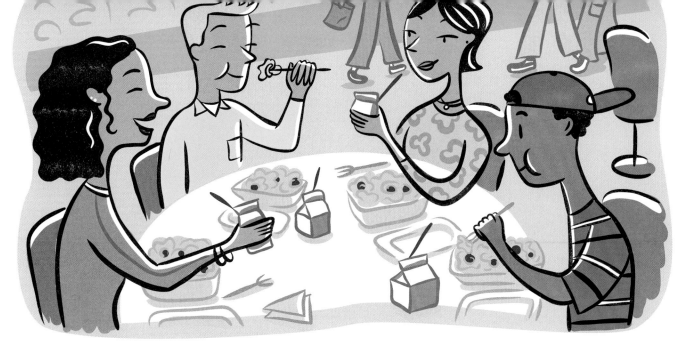

Food for a Teen Lifestyle

Busy with homework, school activities, friends, and maybe a job? Here are some ways to fit healthful eating into your busy schedule.

- *If you have a raging after-school appetite*—tuck portable snacks (fruit, crackers and cheese, raisins, oatmeal cookies) in your school or lunch bag.
- *If your after-school schedule interferes with family meals*—work out a plan with your family. Ask someone to set aside a plate of food for you to eat later. Join family meals whenever you can.
- *If you're still hungry after eating fast*—slow down! Remember, it takes time to feel full.
- *If you don't have time for breakfast or lunch*—make time! You'll feel better and do better at school and after-school activities.
- *If you hang out with friends at a fast-food place*—be a role model. Order juice or milk to drink. Try a salad.

Smart Eating During Adulthood

Good nutrition and active living when you're young can contribute to good health as an adult. Staying fit continues through adulthood. Like you, adults need good nutrition and physical activity!

Because the body is no longer growing, adults' energy needs can be lower. Also, as the years go by, the body uses energy for basal metabolism at a slower rate. Choosing mostly low-fat and lean foods from the Pyramid is the best way for less active adults to keep a healthy weight.

You may need more calories as a teen, but it is best to get more food energy from foods high in complex carbohydrates and less from high-fat foods. Divide into groups of five students and make a list of healthful snack foods you could carry to school. Share your list with the class.

Discuss: Which of the bulleted items describe your lifestyle? What can you do to fit healthful eating into your busy schedule? Give specific examples of solutions.

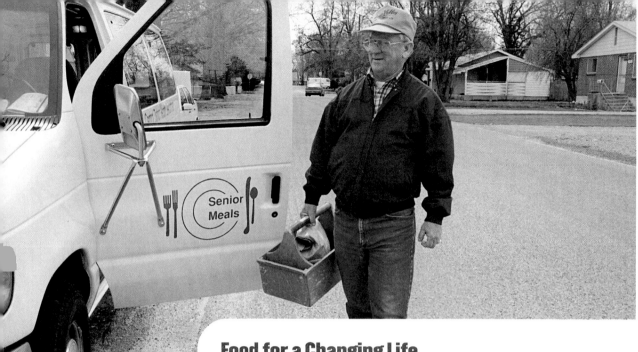

Food for a Changing Life

Because people in the 60-and-up age group aren't all the same, their food needs differ, too. Some older adults are as healthy as ever! Good nutrition and active living earlier in life are part of the reason. On the other hand, many older people can't be as active anymore. Some have health problems that limit food variety or require a special diet.

Lifestyle changes also affect food choices. People who live alone may lose interest in preparing food. A fixed income is a challenge for many older people as food costs go up. If older people can't drive, buying food can be difficult. Remaining independent can be a challenge.

Staying Independent

Most older adults want to remain independent as long as they can. The same techniques used by busy families—such as buying easy-to-prepare foods or cooking ahead and freezing meals—can help. In addition, community services may provide shopping and meal assistance. Health care aides teach new cooking skills to people with physical limits.

You can help make mealtime easier and pleasant for older relatives or friends. Think especially about those who live alone or have health problems. Could you offer your help with food shopping or meal preparation? Could you bring a meal you prepared at home or invite the person to your home? Sharing meals, and your time and attention, with older adults is one way to help make eating a pleasure all through life!

The importance of good nutrition continues through a lifetime. What challenges do some older adults face in meeting their nutritional needs?

Activity: Contact the local or county government to identify community services that provide shopping, meal, and health-care assistance to older adults. Compile the class's findings into a directory.

NOW *You're* COOKING!

(SKILL) Creating a Snack for Kids

*H*ere's an easy snack that kids will enjoy making and eating as much as you will. Try this finger-food recipe and have some fun. What food groups does this snack fit in?

RECIPE

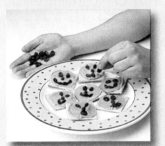

Peanut Butter Faces

CUSTOMARY	INGREDIENTS	METRIC
¼ cup	Peanut butter	50 mL
1 Tbsp.	Honey	15 mL
2	Graham crackers	2
2 Tbsp.	Raisins	30 mL

Yield: 4 servings, ½ cracker with peanut butter, honey, and raisins each

1. In small bowl, stir peanut butter and honey until blended.
2. Cut each graham cracker in half to form a square. Spread 1 Tbsp. (15 mL) of peanut butter mixture in a circle on cracker.
3. Decorate with raisins to make a face.

Per Serving: 143 calories, 4 g protein, 15 g carbohydrate, 8 g fat, 94 mg sodium, 1 g fiberPercent Daily Value: vitamin E 16%, niacin 11%

More Ideas For more kid flavor and fun:

- Create funny faces with chunks of banana, apple slices, grapes (cut in half), or flaked coconut. What other foods could you use that won't be a choking hazard for young children?
- Substitute peach or apricot jam for honey.

Your Ideas Make a list of easy snacks that you can prepare with children's help when you babysit. For more kid-appealing ideas, check out some cookbooks. Then try these ideas with kids!

Review & Activities

LOOKING BACK

- The Dietary Guidelines and Food Guide Pyramid offer advice for healthful eating throughout the life cycle.

- Healthful eating before and during pregnancy will help ensure that the mother and baby get the nutrients they need.

- Infant feeding progresses from mother's milk or formula to various soft foods.

- Children need the same food variety as adults, but serving sizes and the number of servings are different.

- Teens need to pay particular attention to healthful eating because they are still growing and are usually very active.

- Adult food needs depend on the physical activity level, health, and lifestyle.

UNDERSTANDING KEY IDEAS

1. Why should good nutrition be a priority during pregnancy? What three nutrients may need special attention for pregnant women?

2. Compare what babies can eat at two months with what they can eat at eight months.

3. Should you encourage young children to eat food-group snacks? Why or why not?

4. Besides infancy, at what stage in life will you experience the fastest growth? Why is good nutrition so important during periods of rapid growth?

5. How do the nutritional needs of an 11-year-old differ from those of a 40-year-old?

DEVELOPING LIFE SKILLS

1. **Leadership:** On the weekends, Carolina baby-sits her four-year-old neighbor, Luis. Carolina finds mealtimes difficult because Luis won't sit still and he doesn't like meat or vegetables. How can Carolina encourage Luis to try new foods? How can she try to make mealtime more pleasant?

2. **Management:** If you worked after school on most weekdays and participated in some after-school clubs, how would you make sure that you ate dinner with your family at least once or twice a week?

Wellness Challenge

The TV news carried a feature about malnutrition among the elderly. Brian and Cassie thought immediately about their grandfather. Ever since their grandmother died six months ago, Grandpa has been eating poorly and losing weight. Grandma had always done the cooking, and Grandpa seems at a loss to know what to do in the kitchen. Besides, he says that he hates eating alone. Cassie and Brian decide they want to help.

1. What steps might the teens take to get started?
2. What challenges might they face?
3. How could they find solutions?

APPLYING YOUR LEARNING

1. **Snacking Habits:** Draw cartoons or make a list of words that describe your snacking habits. Think of what you eat and when you like to snack. How might you improve your current snacking habits?

2. **Dinner for Two:** Imagine you are going to baby-sit for a three-year-old child. You are planning to make dinner for yourself and the child using six food items from your house. Which items will you choose? Why? How nutritious is your dinner plan? How will you determine how much to make? If possible, carry out your plan using the advice in this chapter.

EXPLORING FURTHER

1. **Meal Assistance:** Find out what community programs are available for older adults who need help with meals. Combine your list with your classmates'. Make flyers that can be distributed in neighborhoods to help inform people of these services.

2. **When I Was Your Age:** Interview your grandparents or older friends of your family to find out what practices they followed for feeding their children. Ask your family how these practices are different from the way you were raised. How are they similar?

Making CONNECTIONS

1. **Child Development:** What are the advantages of breast-feeding for a mother and child? How do breast milk and infant formula compare? Investigate this topic and present your findings to the class in a brief report.

2. **Health:** What would you do if you were baby-sitting and the child began to choke? Find out how to administer the Heimlich maneuver to infants and young children. Learn about cardiopulmonary resuscitation (CPR), too. Contact your local Red Cross to find out where CPR classes are held in your community.

FOODS LAB

Prepare two no-cook snacks: one for a school-age child and one for a teen. Compare their textures, colors, and flavors. Why would the snack that you prepared for the child appeal to him or her? Why might the other snack appeal to a teen? How many servings of which food groups do the snacks supply?

Special Health Concerns

Objectives

After studying this chapter, you will be able to:

- Describe warning signs of an eating disorder.

- Summarize meal and snack time guidelines for helping someone who is sick or recovering from illness.

- Identify which special diets are used for certain health problems.

- Explain how food and medications may affect each other.

Do You Know...

...what steps you might take if a friend shows signs of an eating disorder?

...how to make meals more appealing for a person with a poor appetite?

...that being "sensitive" to milk doesn't mean having to give it up?

If not, you'll find out in this chapter!

Look *for these* TERMS

eating disorder   food allergy

food intolerance   diabetes

lactose intolerance

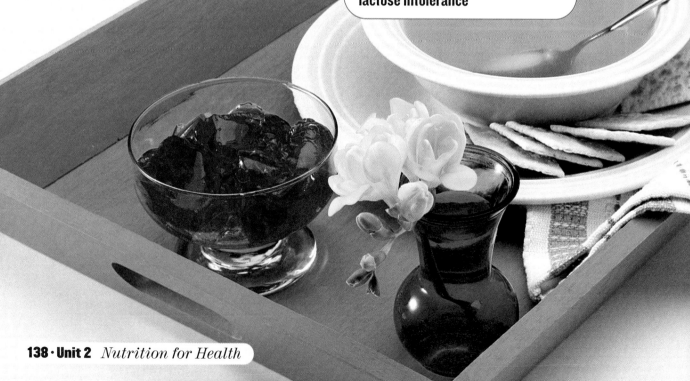

Eating smart is one

way of keeping your good health. Good nutrition is linked to health in another way. It's an important part of recovering from an illness, such as the flu. Wise food choices can even help prevent, treat, or manage many health problems.

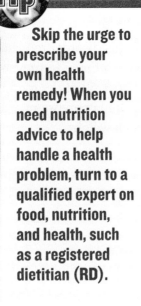

Tip

Skip the urge to prescribe your own health remedy! When you need nutrition advice to help handle a health problem, turn to a qualified expert on food, nutrition, and health, such as a registered dietitian (RD).

Nutrition for Prevention

You can decide now that you want to be as healthy as you can be. No matter what your age, you lower your chances for potential health problems by making good choices. Choose to eat smart now, and you'll have a greater chance of keeping your good health—for a lifetime!

How can your wellness habits, including good nutrition and an active lifestyle, help reduce the risk of health problems? You've probably already learned about some of the ways in other chapters.

• You can reduce your risk of osteoporosis, the condition in which bones break easily. Eat enough dairy foods or other foods with bone-building nutrients—calcium, phosphorus, and vitamin D. Staying active helps strengthen your bones, too.

• By following the Dietary Guidelines, you can help protect yourself against heart disease, high blood pressure, some forms of cancer, and other health problems. Steps to take include eating plenty of grain products, vegetables, and fruits; choosing mostly low-fat and low-cholesterol foods; and staying active.

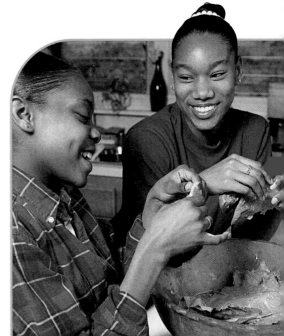

A lifetime of wellness can depend on your food choices now. How could you improve your overall eating plan today?

Activity: Locate research about ways to reduce the risk of heart disease, high blood pressure, or colon cancer. Report your findings to the class.

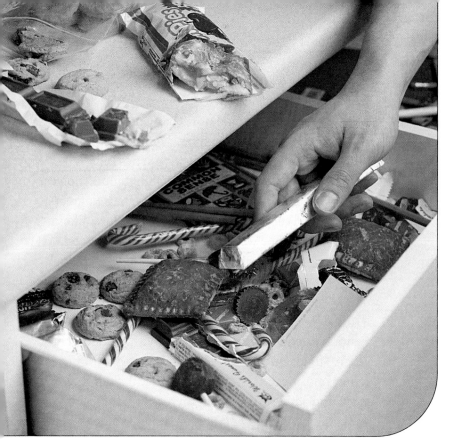

Eating Disorders

The term **eating disorder** describes *behavior related to food, eating, and weight that is extremely unhealthy and often related to emotional problems.* Eating disorders occur mainly in teens and young adults, especially females.

Types of Eating Disorders

There are three main types of eating disorders.

Anorexia nervosa. A person with this disorder ignores feelings of hunger and eats very little or refuses to eat. Victims of anorexia nervosa see themselves as overweight even when they are dangerously underweight.

Bulimia nervosa. A person with this disorder repeatedly binges, or eats very large amounts of food at a time. To prevent weight gain, the person may then purge—get rid of the food by vomiting or taking laxatives. People with bulimia nervosa may also exercise excessively. Often they are a normal weight.

Binge eating disorder. A person with this disorder binges but does not purge or exercise excessively. A person with binge eating disorder may be overweight or may "seesaw" between losing and gaining weight.

Dangers of Eating Disorders

An eating disorder is more than just a problem with eating. It's an emotional illness. If the illness is not treated, it can have long-term effects and cause serious health problems. These problems may include heart and kidney problems, breathing difficulties, and digestive troubles. Eating disorders can even cause death.

Activity: Investigate strategies for prevention, treatment, and management of eating disorders.

Some people with an eating disorder binge on large amounts of sugary foods. If you think a friend or family member might have an eating disorder, encourage him or her to get professional help. Check the medical listings in your local yellow pages. Do any of these professionals treat eating disorders?

Emphasize: Dangers of bulimia include: stomach acids from frequent vomiting can damage the teeth and injure the mouth and throat. Starvation can damage the heart. Overeating can cause the stomach to enlarge. Vomiting can cause the stomach to rupture. Vomiting and using excessive amounts of laxatives can empty the body of nutrients, causing malnutrition.

How to Get Help

The first challenge in dealing with eating disorders is recognizing that a problem exists. People with eating disorders often hide their behavior from others. The box on this page lists some warning signs of eating disorders.

If you think you or someone you know has an eating disorder, don't try to solve the problem alone. Talk to a parent, teacher, counselor, school nurse, or doctor about getting professional help. The sooner treatment begins, the better the chances for full recovery. Treatment may involve medical and dental care along with nutritional and psychological counseling. Support from family and friends helps promote recovery.

Nutrition and Illness

When someone is sick or recovering from an illness or injury, good nutrition can help speed recovery. You can help by providing foods with nutrition in mind. Follow these guidelines.
• Provide plenty of fluids. Soup and juice, as well as water, are usually appealing choices during illness.
• Help the person sit comfortably before bringing food.
• Serve a nutritious meal attractively so that it is more appetizing.
• Be calm and patient if you eat with the person.
• For a sick person with a poor appetite, fix small, frequent meals.
• Use disposable dishes, cups, napkins, and utensils to prevent the spread of illness.

Discuss: What kinds of fluids might appeal to people with the flu, cold, or sore throat?

Check This Out!

WARNING SIGNS OF EATING DISORDERS

If you or someone you know shows any combination of the following, seek help.
• Refusing to eat—or eating tiny amounts.
• Noticeable extreme weight loss or weight that seems to go up and down.
• Exercising frequently and more intensely than normal.
• Eating secretly.
• Disappearing after eating, often to the bathroom.
• Unhealthy teeth and gums.
• Loss of menstrual cycle.
• Use of diet pills or laxatives.

It's Your Turn!

Divide into groups of three or four students. Using the Internet or library resources, find out about support groups that might be available for teens who have an eating disorder.

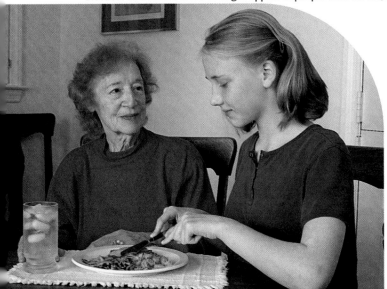

A person who is recovering from an illness may need assistance with meals. Why is paying attention to how food looks when serving a sick person so important?

INFOLINK

For information about preventing foodborne illness, see Part 1 of the Food Preparation Handbook.

Activity: Make a poster that encourages someone with eating disorders to get help from a professional.

Special Diets for Health Problems

Special diets are often part of medical treatment. A person may need to follow a special diet for a short time or a lifetime, depending on the health condition. Only a doctor or other qualified health professional should recommend a special diet. If you're preparing food for someone following a special diet, ask what foods the person can eat. Then be sure to respect the person's needs so that he or she can eat and enjoy the meal.

Food Intolerance

A **food intolerance** *means that the body has trouble digesting or handling a component of food.* For instance, some people cannot digest gluten, a protein found in wheat and some other grains. Symptoms may have many causes, so a medical diagnosis, not a self-diagnosis, of a food intolerance is important.

One of the more common types of food intolerance is lactose intolerance. **Lactose intolerance** is *the inability to adequately digest lactose, the natural sugar found in milk and milk products.* Symptoms may include nausea, stomach pain, gas, and diarrhea.

For those with lactose intolerance, there may be ways to enjoy milk and milk products, and get their nutritional benefits, yet limit the side effects.

• Drink milk with other foods and in small servings of one cup or less.

• Try eating milk products with less lactose, such as hard cheeses (cheddar, American, Swiss) and yogurt.

• Look in the dairy section for milk and milk products that have been specially treated. They're labeled as "lactose-reduced" or "lactose-free." You can also buy tablets and drops that reduce the lactose when they're added to milk.

• Ask your doctor if you can take a supplement that will help your body digest lactose.

Activity: Review the cafeteria and highlight any foods that people with gluten intolerance should avoid. Repeat for lactose intolerance.

Avoiding milk products isn't a smart way to treat lactose intolerance. You may not get enough calcium for healthy, growing bones. What are some effective ways to handle lactose intolerance without coming up short on calcium?

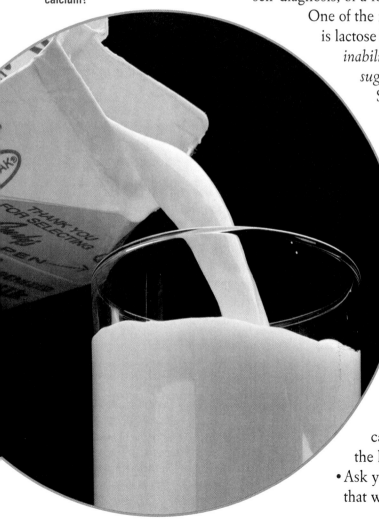

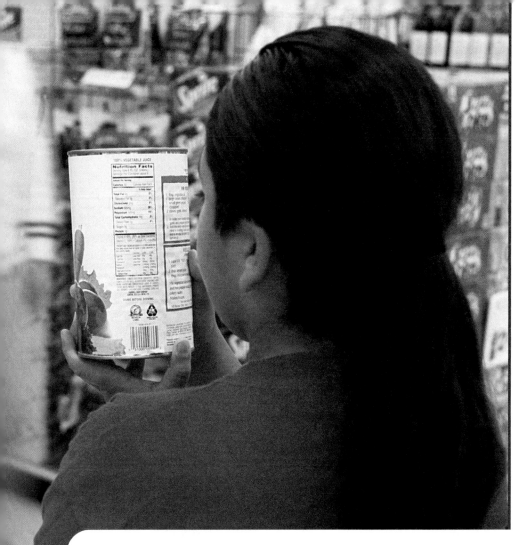

Managing food sensitivities means reading food labels carefully and consistently as a way to identify foods that may cause a reaction. What types of reactions might you experience if you have a food sensitivity?

Teaching with Visuals: Scan the ingredient lists on a variety of foods to identify products that contain the following ingredients that cause allergic reactions: milk, eggs, wheat, peanuts, soy, tree nuts (such as almonds and pecans), fish, and shellfish (such as shrimp and lobster.)

Tip

Avoiding specific foods because of a food allergy or intolerance can be more challenging than it sounds. If you have either of these conditions, pay close attention to the list of ingredients on packaged foods. Talk with a registered dietitian to make sure you're still getting all the nutrients you need.

Food Allergies

A **food allergy** is *a sensitivity to food that involves the body's immune system.* The immune system mistakenly reacts to the food as if it were an illness to fight. The results might include a rash, itching, stomach cramps, breathing problems, headache, nausea, and vomiting. These symptoms usually occur soon after eating even a small amount of the food. For some people, they can be life-threatening.

True food allergies are not common. Still, they affect many people. Foods that most often cause an allergic reaction are milk, eggs, wheat, peanuts, soy, tree nuts (such as almonds and pecans), fish, and shellfish (such as shrimp and lobster).

If you think you have a food allergy, consult a qualified health professional to diagnose and treat it. Special tests can determine which foods may cause the reaction. Food allergies are treated by preventing the reaction. This requires making very careful food choices to avoid foods that cause the allergic reaction.

Food and Diabetes

Diabetes is *a condition in which the body cannot control levels of sugar in the blood properly.* It has to do with insulin, a body chemical that helps sugar in your blood move into your body's cells, where it's used to produce energy. In one type of diabetes, the body doesn't produce enough insulin. In the other type, the body doesn't use the insulin that is produced normally.

Managing diabetes involves eating regular meals and snacks, making careful food choices, and being physically active. Oral medicine or insulin injections may be necessary. Diabetes is a lifelong concern for people who develop it when they're young. As you get older, being overweight increases the chances of developing diabetes—another reason to keep an appropriate weight! For some people, losing weight and active living can be enough to manage blood sugar levels if diabetes develops later in life.

Emphasize: The tendency to develop diabetes can be inherited. Also, the tendency to develop diabetes can be triggered by obesity.

People with diabetes must pay special attention to what they eat. The American Diabetes Association offers guidelines and suitable recipes. Using the library or Internet, learn more about diabetes.

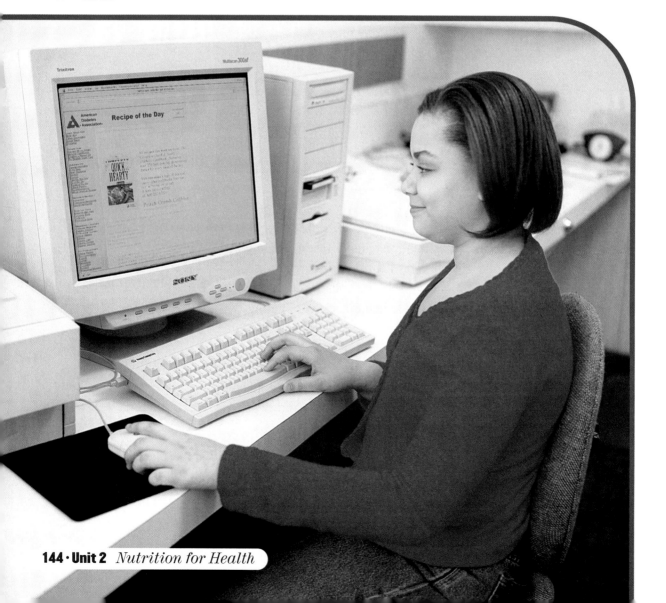

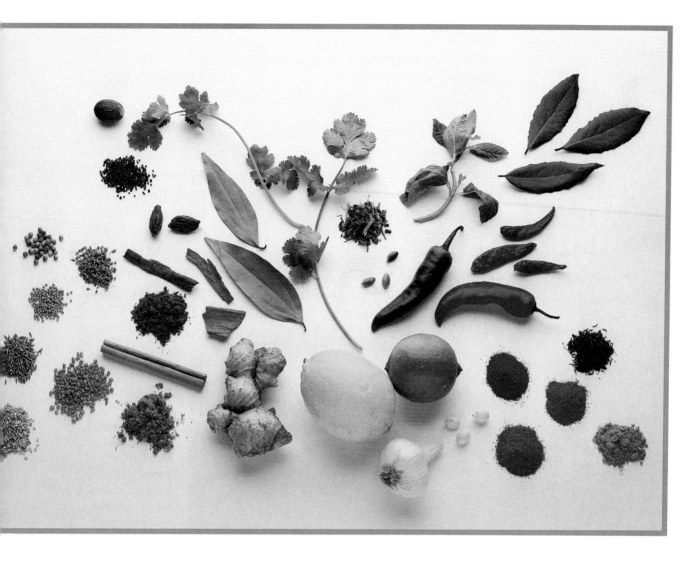

Modified Diets

A modified diet is a special eating plan that helps to keep a medical condition under control. It may involve limiting certain foods or choosing foods for their nutrients or for texture. For instance:

- A low-fat, low-cholesterol diet may help people lower high levels of cholesterol in their blood.
- A low-sodium diet is useful in lowering blood pressure for sodium-sensitive people. This diet is also used in managing kidney disease.
- A high-fiber diet is helpful for treating certain digestive problems, such as constipation. This type of eating plan also may be recommended for people with diabetes or heart disease.
- A soft diet may be recommended for someone having difficulty chewing.

People on a low-sodium diet can enjoy seasoning foods with herbs, spices, or lemon instead of salt or other high-sodium ingredients. Find a recipe that you would enjoy, using herbs as a seasoning.

Activity: Divide into groups of four and develop a one day meal plan for one of the following diets: low-fat, low-cholesterol; low-sodium; high-fiber; and soft diet.

Activity: Choose a diet-related disease or medical condition, such as diabetes or high cholesterol. Find out what treatment strategies are typically used.

Food and Medications

Taking medicine may not seem like a food issue. However, food and medicines can affect each other and your body's chemistry. Food can help or hinder your body's use of medicines. Similarly, some medicines affect how your body uses nutrients.

Tips for Taking Medications

To get the full benefits of both food and medicine, always follow directions for how much medicine to take and when to take it. Some medicines should be taken with food. For example, if you take aspirin for a headache, take it with food to keep your stomach from getting upset. Other medicines are taken on an empty stomach because food may slow the medicine's absorption or action. Some foods cannot be eaten while you are taking certain medications. If you're unsure about how to take a medicine, always check with a doctor or pharmacist.

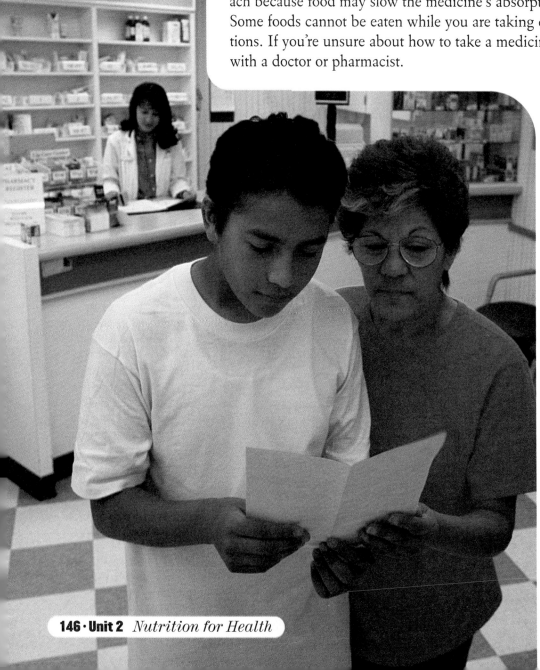

Follow the instructions for taking medicines to get their full benefits. For instance, citrus fruits and juices can destroy penicillin, a medicine often prescribed for an infection. If you are unsure about how and when to take a medicine, whom can you ask for advice?

HELP WANTED

Epidemiologist

U.S. Food and Drug Administration seeks experienced Epidemiologist to investigate foodborne illness outbreaks. Supervise staff and coordinate with other government agencies. Degree in health sciences or related field required. Excellent communication skills a must. Submit federal employment application to Office of Human Resources.

Clinical Dietitian

Licensed Clinical Dietitian needed to manage food service program at small hospital. Oversee menu planning, purchasing, and direction of staff. Bachelor's degree and experience required. Send letter of application to Human Resources Director, Jones County Hospital.

Public Health Educator

Health agency seeks a Public Health Educator to direct health education, wellness, and disease prevention programs in community. Will work with other health specialists and civic groups. Strong people skills needed. Bachelor's degree required. Contact Morton County Public Health Director.

Sanitarian

Environmental Protection Agency has opening for an experienced Sanitarian to organize and conduct training programs in environmental health practices for schools and small groups. Enforce regulations concerned with food processing and serving. Work with other health agencies conducting investigations when needed. Degree in health sciences required. Call EPA.

Dietary Aide

Memorial Hospital has opening for a Dietary Aide. Assist in preparation of patient food trays, deliver and collect trays, and maintain records of special food items. High school diploma required. Evenings and weekends. Apply to the Human Resources Department, Memorial Hospital.

Community Health Nurse

Licensed Practical Nurse needed to work in community nursing program. Visit homes, provide treatments following physician's instructions, evaluate home environment, and assist patient and family as needed. Must be licensed LPN and have own transportation. Send resume to Human Resources, Mt. Carmel Outreach Program.

LINKING *to the* WORKPLACE

❶ **Employment Opportunities:** Conduct research to identify three other health care occupations that are related to nutrition. What are the preparation requirements for each? What are the job responsibilities?

❷ **Maintaining Employment:** Write a story in which a worker in a nutrition-related occupation demonstrates attitudes and habits that will lead to long-term success on the job.

LOOKING BACK

- Good nutrition helps lower the risk for a variety of health problems.
- Eating disorders are characterized by extreme and unhealthy behavior. These emotional illnesses need professional help.
- Good nutrition can help speed recovery for someone who is ill.
- A person who is following a special diet needs to make careful food choices.
- Food can help or hinder your body's use of medicines.

UNDERSTANDING KEY IDEAS

1. How should you eat to lower your chances for heart disease and high blood pressure?
2. What does the term eating disorder mean?
3. Name several warning signs that indicate someone may have bulimia nervosa.
4. What types of meals might you prepare for someone who is sick?
5. What is the difference between a food intolerance and a food allergy?
6. Which would be better for someone with a high cholesterol level—a grilled tuna steak or a grilled sirloin steak? Why?
7. What might you ask the pharmacist regarding a medicine and food? Why?

DEVELOPING LIFE SKILLS

1. **Critical Thinking:** Should teens be concerned with health problems, such as heart disease, that won't develop for many years to come (if at all)? Why or why not?
2. **Leadership:** If you suspected a friend of having an eating disorder, would you have a responsibility to tell someone? Why or why not? What if the friend reassured you there was no problem?
3. **Management:** What steps might a person with a severe food allergy take to avoid that food when eating at a restaurant? When dining at someone else's home?

Wellness Challenge

Next week Kyle's older sister will undergo oral surgery to have her wisdom teeth removed. For a few days after the surgery, she will not be able to chew most solid foods, including fresh, crunchy fruits and vegetables. She's worried about what she'll be able to eat. Kyle would like to help her design a nutritious menu that will speed her recovery.

1. What kind of menu do you think will appeal to Kyle's sister?
2. What challenges might Kyle and his sister face in carrying out their menu plan?
3. How could they go about finding solutions?

APPLYING YOUR LEARNING

1. **Managing an Allergy:** Suni is allergic to wheat. Make a list of foods that she can eat from the Bread, Cereal, Rice, and Pasta Group. Check labels to be sure the food products you listed don't contain wheat, wheat flour, semolina, bran, bulgur, or other wheat products.

2. **Recipe File:** Collect six recipes, two for each meal of the day, for dishes you could prepare for someone who is sick with a cold or the flu. Pick recipes that would appeal to you if you were sick. Add these to your personal recipe file.

EXPLORING FURTHER

1. **Folk Medicine:** People have used plants for their medicinal qualities for centuries. Write a report about plants used in today's medicine and what the plant origins are of aspirin, digitalis, and quinine.

2. **Particular Purchases:** Many processed foods, including some candy bars, cereals, baked goods, and sauces, are made with peanuts, peanut oil, and peanut flour, which poses a problem for people who are allergic to them. At a local store, study food labels. Prepare a handout listing those foods that include peanuts or peanut oil. Share your findings with the class.

Making CONNECTIONS

1. **Health:** Research and report on Type II diabetes. What causes it? Why are more and more children and teens developing it? How is it managed and treated?

2. **Career Connections Experience:** Interview a person with a nutrition-related health concern in order to learn about his or her food needs and preferences. Plan a week's menus that follow the Food Guide Pyramid and accommodate the person's special dietary needs. Prepare a shopping list and present it to the person along with the menus. Ask the person to try them and discuss the results with you.

FOODS LAB

Conduct a blind taste test of two kinds of broth—one regular and one low-sodium. How do your tasters rate each for flavor? How would you enhance the taste and appeal of both kinds of broth?

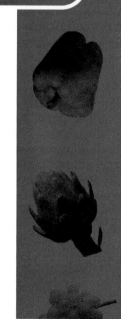

Marathon Meals in
MOROCCO

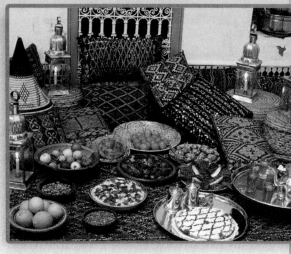

▲ Meals in Morocco are massive!

It can take an entire week to prepare a Moroccan feast for an important guest. Not only that, but the meal can consist of 50 different dishes! It takes a day to make a popular dish that's made from crisp pastry, rolled and filled with chicken. Other main dishes on the table might be brochettes or kebabs flavored with bits of beef or lamb or vegetables.

Various salads such as eggplant or chopped tomato might be served as a separate course. Another course generally includes couscous, the Moroccan national dish made of pasta granules. Desserts could include slices of peeled melons, pastries made with honey and almond, and a small glass of mint tea. It is very important to cooks in Morocco that the food be perfect, so the guests will feel *chban*, which means "complete satisfaction." ■

Making a *Splash* in Agriculture

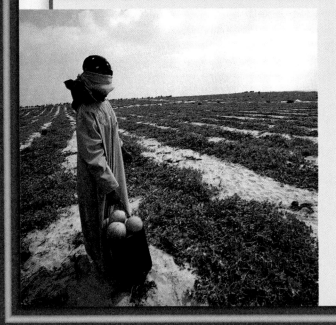

◀ Farmers in Saudi Arabia must use water wisely.

Some people in Middle Eastern countries struggle to grow their own food because of a lack of water. The desert kingdom of Saudi Arabia is one country that has taken steps to provide the water required to grow food.

Dams have been built to preserve rainwater. Water is also drawn from rivers deep below the ground. Plants have been built to remove salt from seawater so the water can be used by farmers as well as for bathing, drinking, and cooking. In 1976, there were only 400,000 acres of farmland in Saudi Arabia. By 2000, there were more than one million acres. ■

Eating the Tablecloth

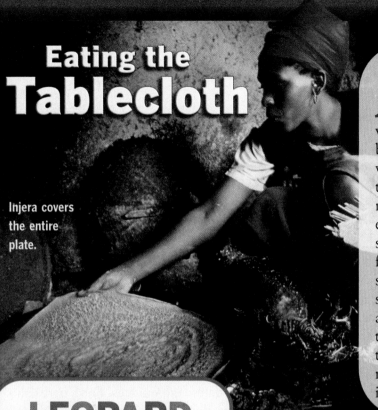

Injera covers the entire plate.

A common bread in Ethiopia and Eritrea is injera (en-JEHR-uh). It looks very similar to a pancake, only it's bigger. Sometimes it covers the whole plate or even the whole table! Injera is often covered with mounds of various meat and vegetable stews. Diners tear off a small piece of injera with their fingers and use it to scoop up the stew. Injera has an interesting, slightly sour flavor. It's available at many Ethiopian restaurants in the United States. Remember, though: You're not done with dinner until you've eaten everything, including the tablecloth! ■

LEOPARD
ice cream, anyone?

In America, avocado is most often used in guacamole. In Africa, avocado is mixed with pistachio ice cream to make a tasty dessert. Another popular dessert in Africa is leopard ice cream. It's really vanilla ice cream with small dollops of peanut butter. The peanut butter looks like small leopard spots. ■

◀ While the avocado is often thought of as a vegetable, it's really a fruit!

Spring INTO New Year

In many places in Iran, the beginning of the new year, called Noruz, takes place in spring. On New Year's Eve, rice is served with fried fish. On New Year's Day, the menu consists of five traditional foods (vinegar, apples, garlic, sumac, and a sweetmeat). It is a time for families to gather together and celebrate the beginning of the planting season. ■

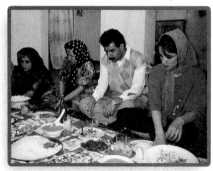

In Iran, traditional ▶ foods are often served for the new year.

Middle East & Africa

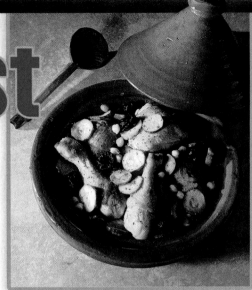

From Morocco to Iran, Middle Eastern cuisine is full of rich flavors and aromas. Kebabs, savory pies made with paper-thin pastry, stuffed vegetables, and pastries filled with nuts and soaked in sweet syrup are common throughout the region. Lamb is a favorite meat; eggplants, zucchini, artichokes, okra, and bell peppers are frequently used vegetables. Meat stews are slow-cooked with dry beans, peas, or lentils, vegetables, and sometimes fruit. Pine nuts, almonds, and pistachios are common pastry fillings. Sweet dishes are perfumed and flavored with orange blossom water or rose water.

Spices and aromatics are very important. In fact, you can tell where you are by the spices and flavorings used in the food.

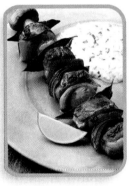

▲ Kebabs are very popular Middle Eastern dishes.

Iran Iran's cuisine is based on long-grain rice. It is mixed with meats, vegetables, fruits, and nuts, or served plain with sauces on the side. Iranians use a variety of gentle spices, especially allspice, cinnamon, and saffron.

The stews of Morocco are called tajines ▲ (TAH-jins). They are cooked in cone-shaped pots.

Meat dishes are often served with fruits such as raisins, dates, and quinces. Fresh herbs and yogurts are almost always on the table. Dried limes provide a special flavor in stews and soups, as do dried sumac berries, which are plum-colored and acidic-flavored.

Syria, Lebanon, Jordan, and Egypt

The cooking styles of Syria, Lebanon, Jordan, and Egypt are similar to one another. City cooking is based on rice, while the country staple is cracked wheat. Syrian and Lebanese specialties include a variety of meat pies, interesting salads, and kibbeh (KIHB-beh), which is ground lamb mixed with bulgur wheat and spices. Pomegranate syrup and tamarind lend a delicate flavor to certain dishes. Mint and flat-leaf parsley are the herbs of choice. The distinctive flavor of Egypt is crushed coriander seed, which is fried with garlic or mixed with cumin. Cardamom and turmeric are also important spices.

◀ Mashed chickpeas (far left) and ground meat mixed with spices (near left) are popular dishes in the Middle East.

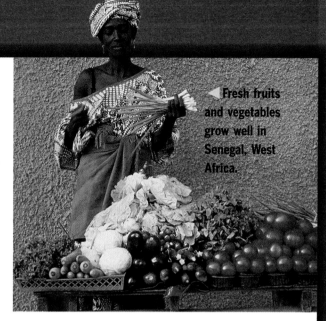

▲ Fresh fruits and vegetables grow well in Senegal, West Africa.

Turkey Turkish cuisine is famous for its kebabs, rice dishes, stuffed vegetables, yogurt dishes, nut sauces, and large variety of savory pies called boreks (BOH-reks). The pies are filled with cheese, spinach, minced meat, or mashed pumpkin. Meat is often flavored with cinnamon and allspice. Dill, mint, and flat-leaf parsley are favorite herbs. Toasted pine nuts and a sprinkling of red paprika mixed with oil are common garnishes.

Africa Algeria, Morocco, and Tunisia make up North Africa. Moroccan cooking is based on a pasta granule called couscous. Spices such as cumin and chiles are used to flavor cold vegetable appetizers and fish dishes.

A blend of flavors—which include cinnamon, ginger, saffron, mint, and cilantro—are a feature of North African foods, which may be very delicate or peppery hot. Harissa (hah-REE-suh), a paste of garlic, chilies, and spices that makes most Tunisian dishes fiery, is added in Morocco with a light touch. North Africa is also famous for its paper-thin pancakes, its savory stews called tajines (TAH-jins), and its steamed dishes.

South of the Sahara Desert lies the largest part of the continent of Africa. In both East and West Africa, starchy root vegetables such as yams and cassava are the main ingredient in a meal. Greens; hot spices, including red pepper and ginger; and chicken stews are popular. Peanuts (which are called groundnuts in Africa) can be found in many dishes.

People in Nigeria and the coastal parts of West Africa like to add hot chilies to their food. Africans in coastal nations eat plenty of fish, which they mix with tomatoes and ginger and fry in peanut oil. West Africans use black-eyed peas and okra to thicken soups and stews.

Even though East Africa is filled with wildlife, people there use very little meat in their cooking. Cattle, sheep, and goats are a sign of wealth. Instead of being eaten, the animals are often traded for other items.

South Africa's cuisine is a result of colonization by the Dutch and British. Workers from Asia brought curries that helped to spice up the plain English and Dutch recipes. In rural areas, however, native Africans' main dishes are starches and stews. The flavors of the African continent are as varied as its nations and its people. ■

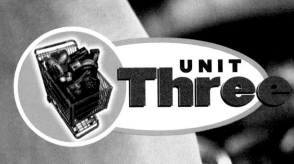

Making Food Choices

IN THIS UNIT...

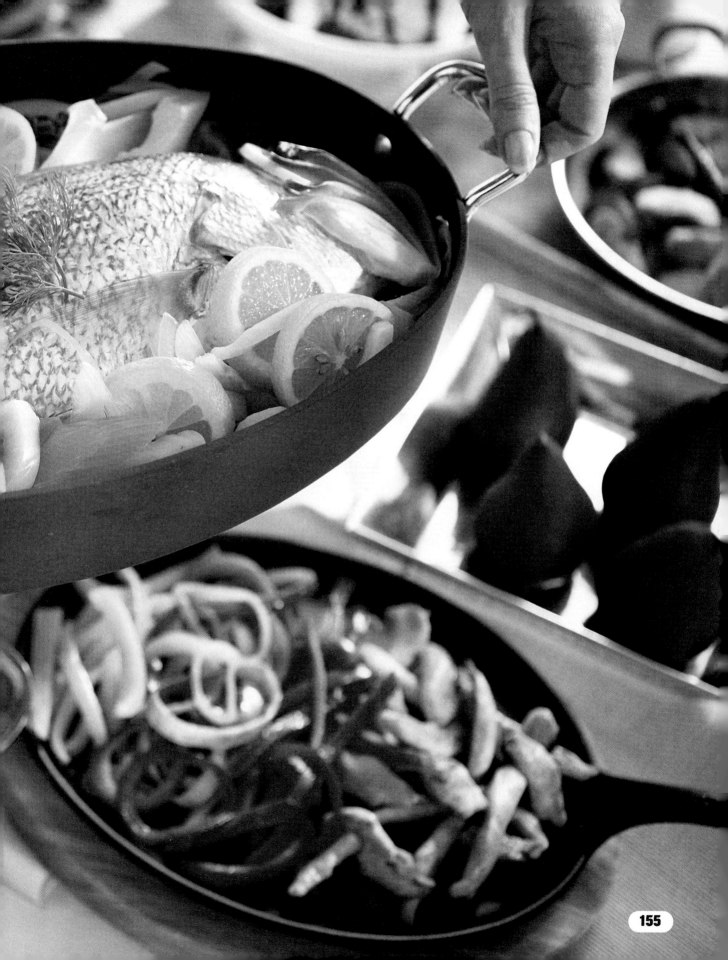

Sorting Out the Facts

Objectives

After studying this chapter, you will be able to:

- Evaluate sources of nutrition information for reliability.
- Recognize false nutrition claims.
- Interpret food and nutrition news.

Do You Know...

...where to get reliable answers to your questions about food and nutrition?

...how to judge nutrition advice in a teen magazine?

...how to surf the Internet for sound food and nutrition information?

If not, you'll find out in this chapter!

Look *for these* **TERMS**

health fraud   quack

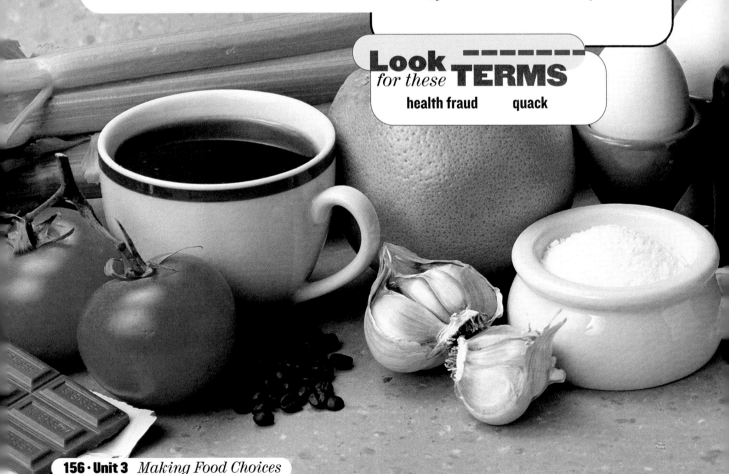

True or false?

The more you know about food and nutrition, the better equipped you are to make smart decisions for your health. Of course this is true. Smart choices for wellness are based on sound, scientifically proven information.

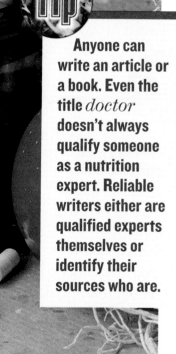

Tip

Anyone can write an article or a book. Even the title *doctor* doesn't always qualify someone as a nutrition expert. Reliable writers either are qualified experts themselves or identify their sources who are.

Finding Nutrition Facts

If you've ever done a report as part of your food, nutrition, or health class, you know that finding information about food and nutrition is quite easy. It's all around you! Radio and television talk shows, magazines devoted to food or fitness, food and health features in newspapers, and best-selling books are filled with advice. You may find leaflets in supermarkets and doctors' offices. The Internet links you to recipes, labeling information, and nutrition resources.

Knowing how to distinguish reliable information from unreliable information, however, is more challenging! As a wise consumer, you need skills to know when you're getting the real and accurate scoop.

Who Are the Experts?

Whether you're getting advice in person, in print, over the airwaves, or on the Internet, make sure it comes from people who are qualified. Professionals with degrees in the fields of food and nutrition from reputable colleges and universities offer information you can trust. Physicians and nurses receive training in nutrition, too.

Develop skills to judge the reliability of information about nutrition, foods, and new food products. Look for articles on food and nutrition in your local newspaper or a teen magazine. Report on what you find.

Critical Thinking: How can you identify nutritional experts on the radio? On television? In magazine/newspaper ads? Billboards?

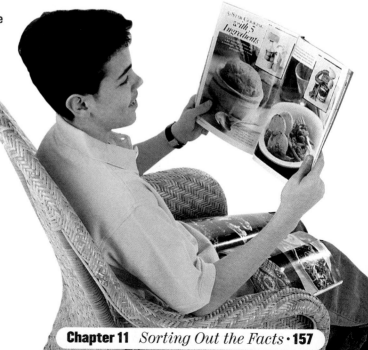

INFOLINK

Learn more about many food and nutrition professionals in the career features in this book. See the Table of Contents for a complete list.

Someone may call himself or herself a "nutritionist" or "nutrition adviser" but may not even have a college degree in nutrition. The real experts indicate their credentials with letters after their names. The letters *CFCS* after a person's name mean that the person is certified in family and consumer sciences. The letters *RD* mean the person is a registered dietitian. These credentials acknowledge the person's expertise and science-based education.

When You Have Questions

When you need to talk or write to someone about your food and nutrition questions, turn to these reliable sources.

At school get advice from family and consumer sciences, or home economics, teachers; health teachers; and the school nurse.

In your community get advice from registered dietitians, your doctor, city or county nutritionists, and cooperative extension specialists from your state university.

National organizations that can help include The American Dietetic Association, the American Association of Family and Consumer Sciences, the Food and Nutrition Information Center of the United States Department of Agriculture, and the Society for Nutrition Education. Using library or Internet research, you can find out how to contact these organizations. If you have trouble locating the information, ask your teacher for guidance.

Registered dietitians are qualified to provide expert advice on nutrition. Find out how people qualify to use the letters *RD* and/or *CFCS* after their names.

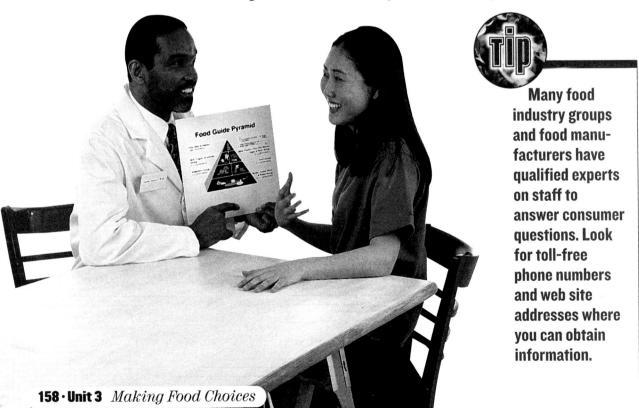

Food Guide Pyramid

Tip

Many food industry groups and food manufacturers have qualified experts on staff to answer consumer questions. Look for toll-free phone numbers and web site addresses where you can obtain information.

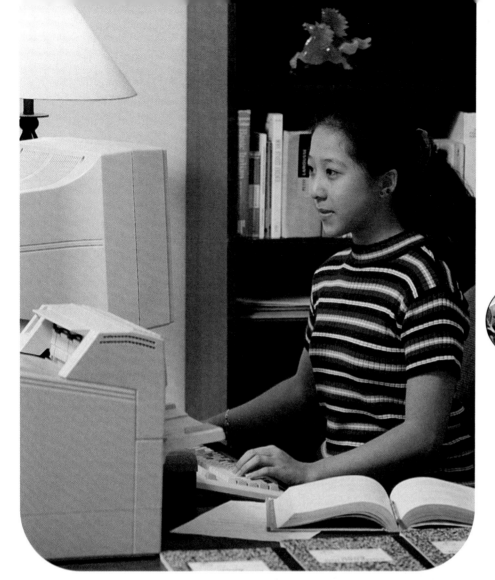

The web sites of organizations such as The American Dietetic Association are full of food and nutrition information. Many reliable web sites are linked to other reliable web sites. Judge information you get on-line carefully. Use a computer to get on-line information about food or nutrition. How can you tell if the information you get is reliable?

Tip

The Internet, like other media, includes both reliable and unreliable information. In general, web sites with the extensions .gov (government), .edu (education), or .org (organization) are reliable. Use your critical thinking skills!

Advertising—What's Behind It?

Advertisements are everywhere! They can be informative, and they're often entertaining. Remember, however, that most advertising has only one real purpose—to get you to buy a product or use a service. It's not the advertiser's job to make sure that you have all the facts and that you make the best choices for your health and your budget. That's your job!

Advertisers use many powerful techniques to influence your buying decisions. They appeal to your emotions—your desire to be popular, more attractive, more athletic. They use well-known celebrities, eye-popping graphics, and catchy music to get your attention. It's okay to enjoy these entertaining aspects of advertising. Just remember—before you make a decision, get the facts!

INFOLINK

Review the steps in making sound decisions that you learned in Chapter 1, page 29.

Emphasize: Advertising, what parents or other family members buy, and peer pressure influence one's nutrition choices. Nutrition choices you make affect you alone. Use the decision-making process to help you make your own decisions.

CAUTION ABOUT HERBAL PRODUCTS

Today, many herbal products are promoted for health benefits. However, there's little scientific evidence yet to support many of these claims. A few herbals, such as chaparral, comfrey, ephedra, lobelia, and yohimbine, are known to be dangerous in large amounts. That's why qualified experts routinely don't recommend most herbal products. A healthful eating plan along with regular physical activity is still the smartest approach to health!

It's Your Turn!

Using library or Internet research, locate an article in which a qualified expert evaluates an herbal product. Share your findings with the class.

Fact or Fallacy?

Everyone wants to be healthy. However, rather than following a sensible lifestyle and eating smart, many people spend several billion dollars annually on products that claim quick and easy fixes. As a wise consumer, you need to know how to spot **health fraud,** or *false and possibly harmful approaches to personal health care.*

Have you ever heard food or nutrition supplements promoted as a "cure," "guarantee," or "miracle food"? That's hype, not fact! **Quacks** are *people who promote products by making false health claims.* At the very least, these products are usually a waste of money and can create false hope. Using a food or supplement as an easy "health fix" may have serious consequences. For example, very high doses of some vitamins, often promoted by quacks, can have harmful side effects. People may use these products as substitutes for good medical care—sometimes with harmful results.

Be cautious of claims that sound too good to be true. Watch out for words like *secret, breakthrough,* and *magical,* which are clues to quackery. Before you believe exaggerated claims or try any "miracle" food products, check with a qualified nutrition expert.

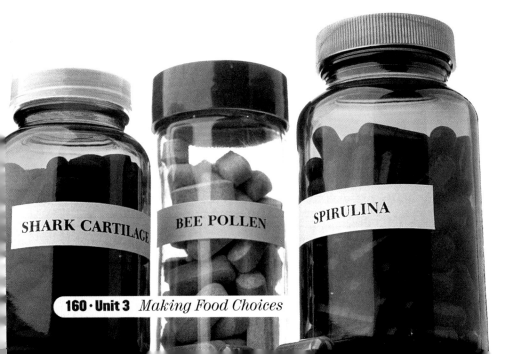

SHARK CARTILAGE

BEE POLLEN

SPIRULINA

Activity: Bring in a newspaper or magazine ad about food and nutrition. Evaluate the ad using the warning signs on the next page. Are the ads reliable?

Bee pollen, shark cartilage, and spirulina are among the supplements often promoted with misleading claims. Where could you get advice you could trust about products or devices touted as health remedies?

It's Myth Information!

Some beliefs about food are not based on facts. Even so, they get passed from person to person. Do a quick poll among your friends to see if they believe any of the common myths here.

Teaching with Visuals: Brainstorm other beliefs about foods, such as, "Eating carrots will improve your eyesight." Find a reliable source to determine whether they are myths or facts. Make a class chart titled, "Myths or Realities About Foods."

INFOLINK

For food myths related to sports, see Chapter 19.

For weight loss myths, see Chapter 20.

Myths About Foods

IT'S A MYTH!	HERE ARE THE FACTS!
"Chocolate and greasy foods cause pimples."	Hormone changes cause acne, not chocolate or greasy foods.
"Sugar makes you 'hyper.'"	Hyperactivity isn't related to eating candy or sweet drinks. Scientists don't yet know all the real reasons for hyperactivity.
"Bread is fattening."	A slice of bread has only about 70 calories. Extra calories come from higher-fat spreads.
"Nutrient supplements can make up for poor eating."	No one supplement provides all the nutrients and other substances that food supplies. Supplements don't supply enough—if any—food energy either.
"You can build muscle by eating more sources of protein."	Only physical activity builds muscles. Extra protein from food can become body fat.

Check This Out!

MORE WARNING SIGNS

Still not sure whether advice about food and nutrition is reliable? Ask yourself these questions.

• *Does the advice discount or ridicule qualified nutrition experts?* If so, the message is probably unreliable. Experts may disagree, but they respect each other's scientific work.

• *Does the advice identify "good" foods and "bad" foods?* No food alone is "good" or "bad"—the overall food choices you make are what counts.

• *Are emotional appeals and testimonials used?* People who aren't experts often use these tactics to influence their audiences.

It's Your Turn!

Write an advertisement for a phony product using the techniques described above. Trade with a classmate and identify the warning signs in each other's "ads."

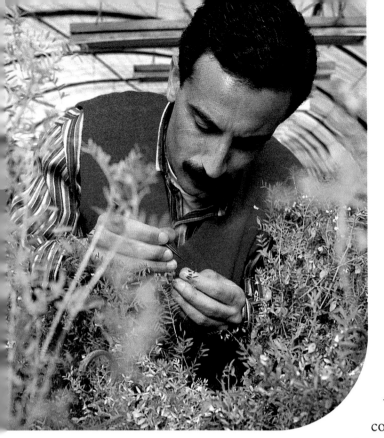

Nutrition scientists do ongoing research to learn more about the special health benefits of plant substances, such as isoflavones in soybeans. Find out about recent and current research on isoflavones.

Food and Nutrition— In the News

Every day scientists learn more about the links between food and health. As promising new research emerges, it gets reported in the news. Sometimes one study seems to contradict a previous study you've heard about. Nutrition news can be confusing!

Should you change your food choices based on a single report? Probably not. Experts know they can't rely on a single study. One study is just one piece in a large puzzle. Sometimes one puzzle piece leads to a change in thinking or raises many new questions. Research needs to be repeated again and again before reliable advice can be given to consumers. Sometimes scientists find that the results of a study cannot be duplicated, perhaps because they were misinterpreted. That means the puzzle piece needs to be discarded or studied in a different way.

Remember, too, that brief news reports often oversimplify research results. Good health is complex. It's related to heredity, gender, age, and many food and lifestyle choices people make.

When you read an article about nutrition research, look for the answers to these questions.
• Who did the research? What are the researcher's qualifications?
• Who paid for the study? Might that have influenced the conclusions?
• How was the study designed? Have other scientists reviewed the methods used?
• Have other studies reached the same conclusions?
• Do the results apply only to a certain group of people? Do they apply to you? For instance, good advice for adults may not be good advice for teens.

No matter where you read or hear nutrition advice—in a book, magazine, or newspaper article; on radio, television, or the Internet—think carefully before you follow it. Use your critical thinking skills. That may be the most important nutrition advice of all!

Teens Create Nutrition
Web Sites

Build a better taco with your computer mouse. Keep your own physical activity log. Get nutrition facts from fast food chains. Download snack recipes. Do all this and more on the Web!

Developed by teens for teens, interactive web site activities are helping students explore healthful eating and living on their own. Computer students from Alexandria and Chantilly, Virginia, turned the Team Nutrition teen magazine *yourSELF* into a fast, personal, and "high-tech" way for teens to get in touch with wellness.

Three teens from Thomas Jefferson High School for Science and Technology—Michael Craig, Daniel Willenson, and Menelik Yilma—are among those who adapted the print material into an interactive computer experience.

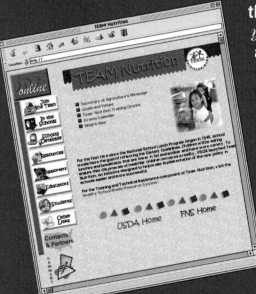

"Information on the World Wide Web is freely available, so a nutrition web site makes a good introduction," they commented. "Because the Internet is interactive, students on our nutrition site input their own data to get personalized results. It's a more exciting way to learn."

Teens around the nation can click into these nutrition activities—anytime, anywhere—on the Team Nutrition web site from the U.S. Department of Agriculture.

Take Action

What can you learn about wellness on the Internet? Plenty! Search using key words such as "nutrition," "milk," or "physical activity." Then create your own directory of informative, teen-friendly web sites on nutrition and wellness. Send it to your friends by e-mail.

LOOKING BACK

- A wise consumer uses critical thinking skills to evaluate food and nutrition information.

- Check the source of food and nutrition information to be sure it's reliable.

- Advertisers use powerful techniques to influence your buying decisions.

- Be alert for false, misleading, or exaggerated food or nutrition claims.

- A single research study is not enough of a basis for changing your food choices.

UNDERSTANDING KEY IDEAS

1. What credentials should you look for when judging the qualifications of a person who is giving nutrition advice?

2. As a consumer, what is your responsibility in regard to advertisements?

3. Why is it unwise, and possibly dangerous, to use food or nutrition supplements to treat an ailment instead of seeking medical care?

4. A magazine article says that everything physicians tell you about vitamin supplements is false. It also states that a new breakthrough miracle supplement will revolutionize the way people eat. Would you consider this information reliable? Why or why not?

5. Why should you treat any news report about nutrition research with caution? What types of information should you look for in the report?

DEVELOPING LIFE SKILLS

1. **Critical Thinking:** Suppose you read two different articles about sugar substitutes. Both articles are written by registered dietitians, and both provide the same basic facts. However, the advice given by the two authors differs. What would you conclude about the reliability of these articles?

2. **Communication:** How could you share guidelines on judging nutrition news with others? If you were to create a poster or web page, what four main points would you emphasize?

Wellness Challenge

Sam-Sook and Tara are on the student staff of their high school's cable television channel. They would like to introduce a new program that encourages students to seek and obtain practical, sound advice about health and nutrition. Tara and Sam have decided to use a talk show format with both funny and serious guests to communicate to the audience.

1. What are some topics that might be addressed on the talk show?

2. Who might Tara and Sam invite to speak and why?

3 What are some creative ways that the teens can present their messages?

APPLYING YOUR LEARNING

1. **Evaluating Articles:** Scan newspapers and magazines for articles about food and nutrition. Bring at least two clippings to class. Be prepared to summarize them for the class, and then determine as a group which articles seem to offer reliable information.

2. **Ask the Experts:** Think of a question about food and nutrition. To get your answer, contact one of the national organizations listed on page 158. Report to the class. What did you find out? What are the credentials of the person who responded?

EXPLORING FURTHER

1. **Consumer Protection:** The United States government has enacted legislation to protect consumers from fraud. Find out about the basic rights of the consumer. If you were the victim of fraud, what steps might you take to obtain justice?

2. **Herbal Supplements:** Using reliable sources, investigate an herbal supplement. What scientific research has been done? What were the results, and how do they relate to the claims made on the product's label or in advertising? What safety concerns exist, if any?

Making CONNECTIONS

1. **Science:** Find out what's involved in a double-blind placebo controlled study. Why would this help provide dependable findings?

2. **Language Arts:** Using language arts books as references, identify techniques used in persuasive writing. Find examples of advertisements that use these techniques. How would you rate their effectiveness? Why? What is the difference between a persuasive ad and a misleading ad? Try writing your own advertisement that is persuasive but not misleading.

FOODS LAB

Find several advertisements that make specific claims about a food product, such as "better tasting" or "ready in 10 minutes." Choose one of the products to prepare and/or taste-test in class. Do you think it fulfills the promises made in its advertising? Why or why not?

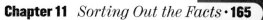

Nutrition Throughout Your Day

Objectives

After studying this chapter, you will be able to:

- Develop breakfast menus that fit your schedule.
- Fit food-group snacks into your eating plan.
- Explain how your resources affect your menu plans.
- Plan menus to meet your family's needs and food preferences.

Do You Know...

...why breakfast can give your day an energy boost?

...how to get the most from your next snack attack?

...how to plan a meal for your family?

If not, you'll find out in this chapter!

Look *for these* TERMS

menu   trade-off

appetizer

Do you eat three

meals a day or six mini-meals? Are you a snacker? There's no single pattern of eating. Even your own pattern may change from day to day. Your lifestyle, schedule, family, culture, and physical needs affect when you eat and how much. For the nutrition you need, use the Food Guide Pyramid for planning meals and snacks!

Breakfast for a Healthy Start

Your morning meal is more important than you may think! Imagine you have a meal or snack at 7 P.M. Breakfast at 7 A.M. the next day will be the first food you eat after 12 hours of fasting. Fasting means going without eating for a long time. The term *breakfast*, in fact, means "break, or end, the fast."

To produce energy, body cells need glucose, which is the form of sugar in your blood that originates from food. As you sleep, your body uses energy for breathing, for keeping your heart pumping, for growing new cells and repairing damaged ones, and for other body processes. By morning, you need breakfast to refresh your energy supply. Those energy-producing nutrients you get at breakfast will help you feel renewed and mentally alert through the day.

Breakfast eaters are usually more alert in the middle of the morning than breakfast skippers. Most breakfast eaters concentrate better, think faster, get more done at school or work, and score better on tests—all great reasons to eat breakfast! Breakfast skippers or skimpers may spend the rest of the day trying to make up for the nutrients they missed in the morning.

How could you help make your morning or evening meal a family get-together? Plan a breakfast menu you could serve this weekend.

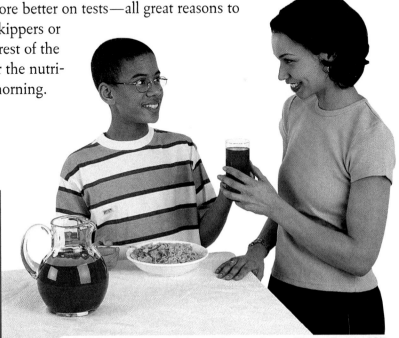

A breakfast bar, plus fruit and milk, can be a nutritious start to your day. Read the label so that you can size up the bar's nutrition content.

What's for Breakfast?

Breakfast can be any food you like. Breakfast refers to when you eat, not what you eat. Cereal, milk, and fruit or a scrambled egg, toast, and juice are two typical breakfast menus. A **menu** is *all foods served at a meal or for the whole day's meals and snacks*. A cheeseburger and tomato juice or a burrito, fruit, and milk make good breakfasts, too.

Breakfast can supply one-fourth to one-third of the nutrients your body needs each day. To reach that goal, pick foods from several food groups of the Food Guide Pyramid. Breakfast is a good time for a vitamin C–rich food such as grapefruit, orange juice, or strawberries and for a calcium-rich dairy food such as milk or yogurt.

Discuss: What did you eat for breakfast today? How does your breakfast fit into the Food Guide Pyramid? Did your breakfast supply one-fourth to one-third of the nutrients your body needs each day? How can you improve your breakfast?

There are no hard-and-fast rules about what you eat for breakfast. What foods do you like to eat for breakfast?

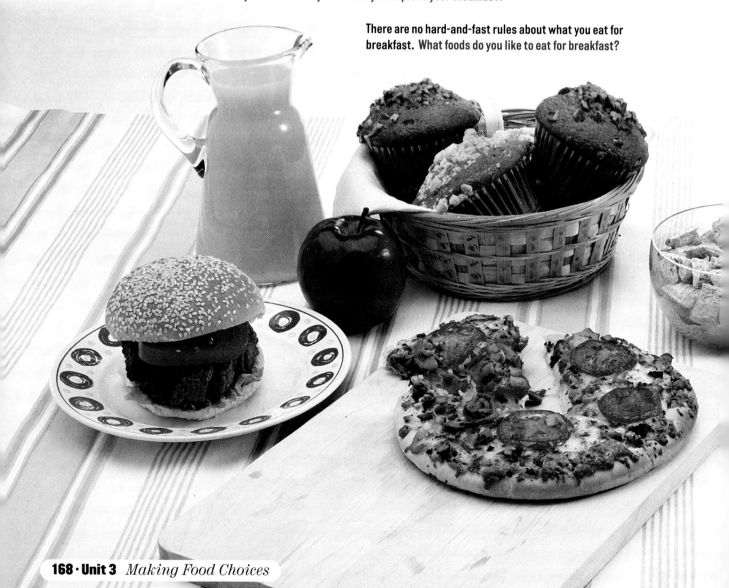

Easy Solutions for Breakfast Skippers

You've probably heard or made excuses for skipping breakfast. However, there are many easy ways to eat smart in the morning.

- *"I'm not hungry when I get up."* Get ready first, then eat breakfast. You could also pack a breakfast to eat later in the morning.
- *"It makes me fat."* Eat breakfast to control your appetite. Breakfast skippers often eat more at lunch or nibble on late-morning snacks.
- *"No time!"* Make breakfast, such as a sandwich, the night before. Take finger food—perhaps whole-wheat crackers, cheese, and grapes—to eat at the bus stop. Wake up a few minutes earlier! On those days when you just run out of time, you may need to stop at a vending machine or convenience store for a nutrient-dense boost.
- *"I don't like breakfast foods."* Enjoy any foods for breakfast that you like—perhaps a pizza slice, a sandwich, or last night's leftovers. Add foods to the family shopping list that you'd eat in the morning.

Activity: List phrases cereal companies use in advertising. Then create catchy phrases to counter excuses for skipping breakfast.

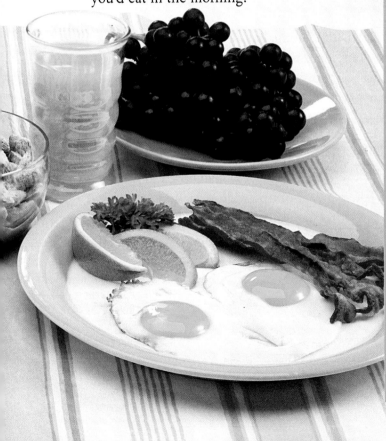

Check This Out!

Breakfast—FAST!

Check your watch! These breakfasts can be prepared in two minutes or less. How do they fit within the Food Guide Pyramid?

- Cereal with yogurt or milk, orange juice.
- Leftover pizza, cranberry juice.
- Toaster waffle with strawberries, instant hot cocoa made with milk.
- Ham and cheese on an English muffin, carrot sticks, grapefruit juice.
- Muffin, string cheese, raisins.
- Blender shake (made with milk and sliced fruit), whole-wheat toast.
- Bagel, yogurt-juice drink.

It's Your Turn!

How fast can you whip together a tasty, nutritious breakfast? Try one of the above breakfasts or some new combinations of your own. What combinations are your favorites?

Activity: Bring in the packaging from your favorite processed snack foods (include those found in the school's vending machines). Analyze the Nutrition Facts panel. Organize the findings in a chart. Identify the most nutritious snacks.

Tip

Hungry for a snack? Remember that people who consume a lot of soft drinks or sugary snacks often come up short on calcium. Reach for milk or yogurt!

Smart Snacking

Smart snacking contributes to smart eating, so snack if you're hungry! Snacks provide extra food energy along with nutrients you may have missed at other times during the day. Growing, active teens need the "refueling" that snacks can provide. Your snack choices deserve as much attention as your breakfast, lunch, and dinner choices.

Snacks in the Pyramid

Make snacks count! Choose nutrient-dense snacks to help you meet Pyramid goals.

- Pick mostly lean or lower-fat snacks from the five food groups. Good choices are fruit, raw veggies, yogurt, milk, pretzels, popcorn, a bagel, and lean deli meat.
- Choose snacks to fill in food-group gaps. For example, snack on string cheese if you're short on servings from the Milk, Yogurt, and Cheese Group. A vitamin C–rich tangerine can make up for the juice you may have missed at breakfast.
- Go easy on higher-fat or high-calorie snacks, such as candy and ice cream. Occasionally these foods are okay—if your overall eating plan follows Pyramid guidelines.
- Time snacks for two to three hours before mealtime. That way, you won't feel like skipping lunch or dinner. Also, a well-chosen snack can help curb your appetite so that you won't overeat at the next meal.
- Use the Nutrition Facts panel on food labels to compare snack choices.
- If you're tempted to snack just because you're bored, tense, or upset, do something else! You could listen to music or call a friend.

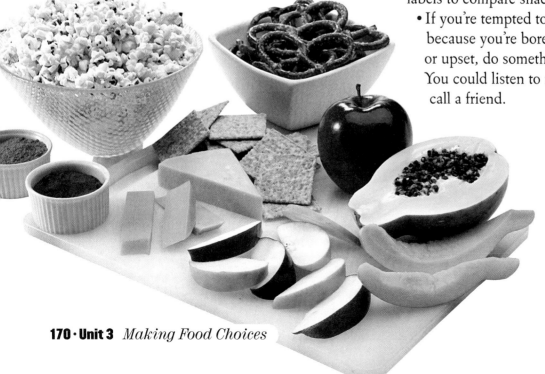

Snacks can fill in the gaps in your Food Guide Pyramid servings. What snacks did you eat yesterday? Did they provide food-group servings?

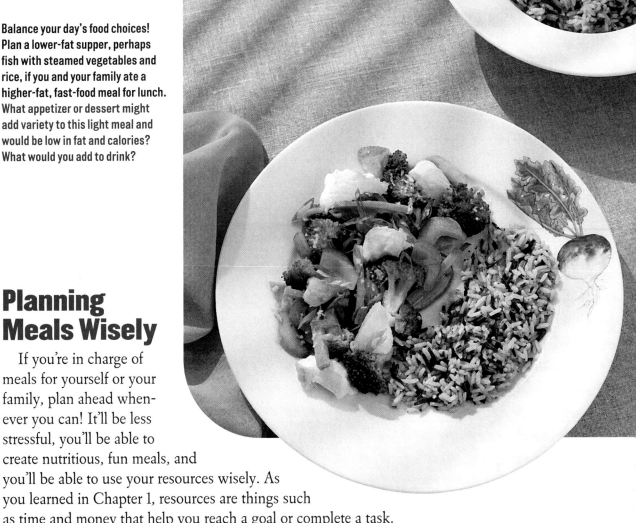

Balance your day's food choices! Plan a lower-fat supper, perhaps fish with steamed vegetables and rice, if you and your family ate a higher-fat, fast-food meal for lunch. What appetizer or dessert might add variety to this light meal and would be low in fat and calories? What would you add to drink?

Planning Meals Wisely

If you're in charge of meals for yourself or your family, plan ahead whenever you can! It'll be less stressful, you'll be able to create nutritious, fun meals, and you'll be able to use your resources wisely. As you learned in Chapter 1, resources are things such as time and money that help you reach a goal or complete a task.

Do you prefer a big meal for breakfast, lunch, or dinner? No matter what time of day, your body uses calories in the same way. The choice is yours. There's no single blueprint for meal planning. If your midday meal is big, you might prefer a light supper and vice versa.

Discuss: People may eat their big meal at noon or midday rather than in the late afternoon or evening. What occasions or factors contribute to which meal is bigger?

Light Meals

A light meal usually supplies about one-third of your nutrients and food energy for the day, with foods from several food groups. Which Pyramid food groups are represented in these meals?
• Grilled chicken salad, carrot bread, kiwi fruit, chocolate milk.
• Bean soup, tossed salad, cheese and crackers, fruit juice.
• Scrambled egg, fresh berries, bagel, hot cocoa.
• Chicken burrito, pepper circles and zucchini sticks, milk.

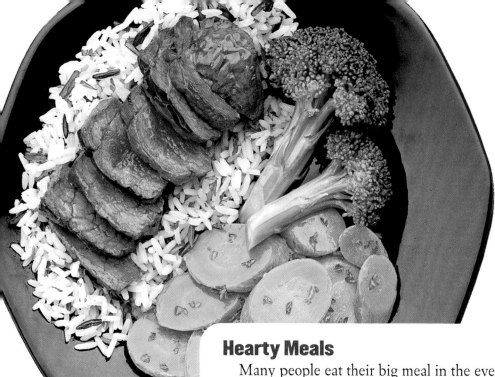

A hearty meal often features foods from the five food groups. Identify the food groups in this meal.

More About the Main Dish: Nutritionists consider the meat dish as the "side dish" rather than the "main dish" and the vegetables and pasta dishes as the "main dish" rather than "side dishes" to reflect the same importance as groups in the Food Pyramid.

Hearty Meals

Many people eat their big meal in the evening with their family. Hearty meals often feature variety from all five food groups and may include the following.

Appetizer. An **appetizer**, *a small portion of food served at the start*, can make a meal special—or can take the edge off hunger until the meal is ready. It could be an easy soup or veggies and dip.

Main dish. Choose your main dish and plan the rest of the meal around it. You might decide on a meat or bean dish or a mixed dish such as shrimp and vegetable stir-fry or a vegetarian bean-rice dish.

Side dishes. Choose vegetables, rice or pasta, salad, and bread as side dishes to complement the flavor, texture, and color of the main dish.

Beverage. Offer a nutritious beverage with the meal. Milk and juice supply food-group servings. Remember, too, that water is a nutrient.

Dessert. End with a dessert if you like. What desserts could add food-group servings to your meal?

INFOLINK

For more about planning meals with appeal, turn to Section 5-1 of the Food Preparation Handbook.

Tip

You can enjoy a higher-fat dessert. Balance it, though, by choosing lower-fat foods for the rest of your meal.

Planning Family Meals

If you've ever planned a family meal, you know there's a lot to think about. Try to create menus that appeal to everyone by considering:

Food preferences. To make a meal special, plan one that includes family and personal favorites. Serve new foods as taste adventures.

Age. Everyone in your family needs the same nutrients, but people of different ages may need different amounts. Teens and active adults may want bigger portions than a younger brother or sister or an older grandparent. Most people enjoy a greater variety of foods as they get older. Small children may like simpler foods.

Schedules. With today's school and work schedules, people in your family may not all be home at mealtime. For days when you can't eat together, plan foods that can be reheated easily.

Special food needs. You may need to plan menus around someone's food allergy or special diet. That might mean planning one menu that everyone can eat—or providing an alternative for the person with a special need.

Check This Out!

KEEPING THE PEACE

Does everyone in your family like the same foods? Probably not, but you can work together to resolve conflicts over food choices. Here are some ideas.

- Look for compromises. Suppose you like green pepper but your sister doesn't. You could make a mixed green salad and serve chopped green pepper on the side.
- Take turns. Use the meat loaf recipe you like best this time and your brother's favorite the next time.
- Try preparing less favorite foods in different ways. If a family member doesn't like cooked spinach, perhaps fresh, raw spinach in a crisp salad might appeal to everyone's tastes.
- Plan assemble-your-own meals occasionally. Arrange ingredients for foods such as sandwiches and salads in serving dishes. Then each person can take the ingredients he or she wants.

It's Your Turn!

What conflict around food choices has come up in your family? Name three ways you might resolve it so that everyone's needs are satisfied.

Everyone in a family needs the same nutrients, just different amounts. Why might these family members have different calorie needs?

INFOLINK

For more about special food needs, see Chapter 10, pages 142–145.

INFOLINK

For timesaving meal strategies, see Chapter 14.

You can find money-saving tips in Chapter 13.

For more on using management skills to plan the preparation of meals, see the Food Preparation Handbook, Section 3-7.

Managing Your Resources

In an ideal world, healthful and delicious meals would be inexpensive or free and ready in an instant—with no pots and pans to clean up! In reality, to plan satisfying, healthful meals, you need to use your resources wisely.

Using resources wisely may require trade-offs. A **trade-off** is *giving up one thing so that you can have something else.* For instance, when you have more time than money, you might make a homemade meal rather than use more costly convenience foods.

Resources to consider include:

Time and energy. If your life is busy, your time and energy may be limited. Plan menus you can prepare quickly. Save time-consuming meals for days when you have time. Remember, shopping for and serving food take time, too.

Money. For most people, money is a limited resource. Learn ways to stretch your food dollars. This includes money spent for foods eaten at home as well as meals and snacks at school, work, or restaurants. Limited money doesn't mean sacrificing nutrition or food appeal.

Kitchen skills. Whether you're a beginner or an expert cook, take into account your food preparation skills as you plan menus.

Kitchen equipment. Plan menus to match the tools, appliances, and cookware you have. If a dish calls for special equipment, consider substituting something else. For example, you can make a stir-fry dish in a regular skillet just as easily as in a wok.

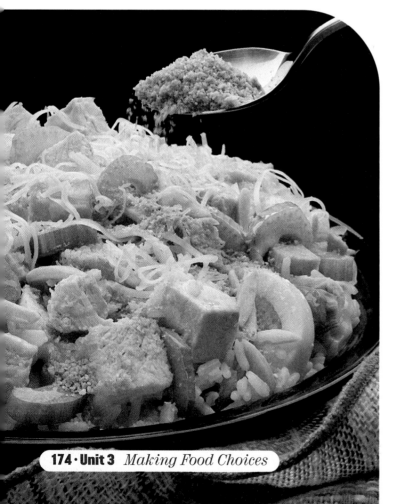

Using leftovers to make a quick meal, like this crunchy chicken salad, saves time and energy. What are some other ways you might use leftover chicken or turkey?

Activity: Divide into three groups. Assign each a school-day lunch: brown bag from home, bought the school cafeteria menu, and purchased from vending machines or other vendor. Compare/contrast the cost and food-group servings of each.

NOW *You're* COOKING!

SKILL
Microwaving a Quick Breakfast

*I*n a rush before your carpool or bus arrives? Here's an easy breakfast. Add a glass of orange juice and some milk, and you'll be out the door in a few minutes!

RECIPE

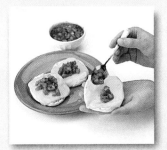

Red-Eye Muffin

CUSTOMARY	INGREDIENTS	METRIC
2	English muffins	2
4 slices	American cheese	4 slices
4 Tbsp.	Drained salsa	60 mL

Yield: 4 servings, ½ muffin with cheese and salsa each

1. Split English muffins with a fork.
2. On microwave-safe plate, place 4 muffin halves. Top with cheese. Microwave on medium power for 10 to 15 seconds or until cheese is melted.
3. Place 1 tablespoon (15 mL) of salsa on top of cheese on each muffin. Serve immediately.

Per Serving: 178 calories, 9 g protein, 14 g carbohydrate, 10 g fat, 641 mg sodium, 0.6 g fiber

Percent Daily Value: vitamin A 12%, riboflavin 11%, calcium 22%, phosphorus 24%

More Ideas

- Instead of salsa, add a spoonful of chili or vegetables that were left over from last night's dinner.
- If you're really hungry, use a whole English muffin and make it into a quick sandwich.
- Are you watching your fat grams? Use low-fat cheese.

Your Ideas
English muffins make a great base for quick open-face breakfast or snack sandwiches. What else could you use to make a breakfast sandwich? What else could you put on top? Look in cookbooks for ideas. Then create your own recipe.

LOOKING BACK

- You can fit a nutritious breakfast into your morning in many easy, quick ways using foods you like.

- Snacks provide extra energy and can help you meet Pyramid goals.

- Meals can be light or hearty any time of day.

- Plan menus for family meals that match everyone's needs and tastes.

- When you plan meals, you may need to make trade-offs to manage your resources.

UNDERSTANDING KEY IDEAS

1. Give three reasons why eating a nutritious breakfast is a smart way to start the day.

2. In general, how would you describe a well-planned breakfast menu?

3. How can you make snacks count nutritionally?

4. What are some nutritious beverage choices? Why?

5. Why do you need to consider the age of family members when you are planning a family meal?

6. Why do you need to consider your kitchen equipment when planning a meal? What other resources should you consider?

DEVELOPING LIFE SKILLS

1. **Management:** Taking time to make a homemade meal rather than spending more on convenience foods—that's one example of making a trade-off when managing resources. What are some others? Why is making trade-offs an important part of good management?

2. **Creative Thinking:** What are some ways that common kitchen items can "pinch-hit" for specialized equipment that you're missing? Try thinking of substitutes for the following: tongs, a pastry blender, a wire whisk, a sifter. (If you're not familiar with these items, refer to Part 2 of the Food Preparation Handbook.)

Wellness Challenge

This year Keisha's family will be hosting Thanksgiving dinner for about 20 relatives of all ages. Keisha's parents have asked her to help by coordinating the menu. In a few days, relatives will begin calling Keisha to ask what food they can bring to the dinner. She's not sure what to tell them. Keisha would like people to bring whatever they want, but she also knows the menu should be well balanced.

1. What are the advantages in letting people choose what to bring?

2. In what ways does the menu need to be well balanced?

3. How might Keisha meet both of her goals for the menu?

APPLYING YOUR LEARNING

1. **Breakfast Menus:** Plan five days of quick and nutritious morning meals. How do your breakfasts rate for food-group servings?

2. **Snacking Record:** For three days, keep a record of what you snack on, where, when, and with whom. Do you notice a pattern in your snacking? How often did you include food-group snacks in your eating plan? How could you improve your snack choices?

3. **Family Meal Menu:** Plan a menu for a midday or evening meal for your own family or another family. Identify the family members by age and whether they are male or female. How does your menu account for family members' needs and preferences?

EXPLORING FURTHER

1. **Meals for One:** Using library or Internet resources, find suggestions aimed at helping single people plan nutritious meals. What challenges do they face? How can they be overcome?

2. **Planning Menus for a Living:** Interview someone who plans meals served to large groups of people, such as a caterer or the school food service director. What do they consider when planning meals? How do they come up with their menus?

Making CONNECTIONS

1. **Language Arts:** Prepare a 15- or 30-second public service announcement that would motivate teens to eat breakfast in the morning. If possible, tape record your announcement and play it for the class.

2. **Social Studies:** Choose a country and find out about a typical hearty meal from that place. At what time of day is it eaten? Who gathers for the meal? Does it follow the pattern of appetizer, main dish, side dishes, beverage, and dessert? If not, how does it differ? How would you rate the typical meal for variety from the five food groups?

FOODS LAB

To compare snack choices, prepare three samples of popcorn: one in a pot with a small amount of oil, one in an air popper, and one bag of microwave popcorn. Compare these methods in terms of taste, cooking time, cost per serving, and fat content per serving.

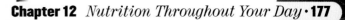

CHAPTER 13

Supermarket Decisions

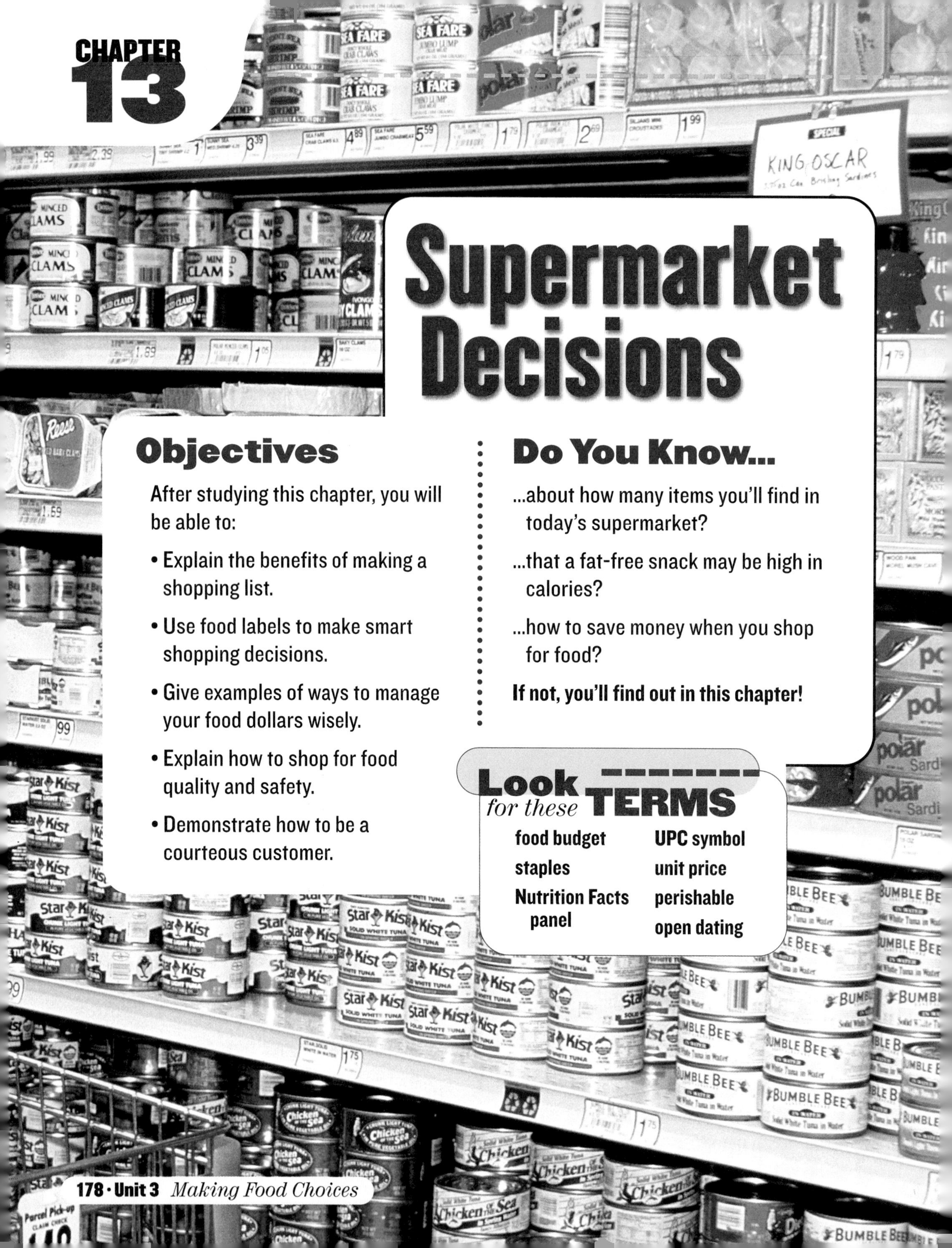

Objectives

After studying this chapter, you will be able to:

- Explain the benefits of making a shopping list.

- Use food labels to make smart shopping decisions.

- Give examples of ways to manage your food dollars wisely.

- Explain how to shop for food quality and safety.

- Demonstrate how to be a courteous customer.

Do You Know...

...about how many items you'll find in today's supermarket?

...that a fat-free snack may be high in calories?

...how to save money when you shop for food?

If not, you'll find out in this chapter!

Look for these TERMS

food budget
staples
Nutrition Facts panel

UPC symbol
unit price
perishable
open dating

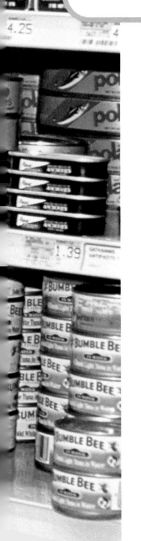

When you shop for

food, what's your first consideration? Many consumers say it's taste. With a few supermarket skills, you can make smart decisions based not just on taste, but on nutrition, price, quality, safety, and convenience as well.

Places to Shop

Where will you shop? Depending on your needs and preferences, you may shop in more than one place.

Supermarkets. With more than 20,000 different items to choose from, supermarkets offer one-stop shopping.

Specialty stores. These may sell foods that you can't find elsewhere, such as ingredients you need for ethnic dishes.

Convenience stores. Often open 24 hours a day, these small stores are handy for a quick stop. Prices may be higher than at a supermarket.

Food cooperatives. Consumers save money by buying food at wholesale prices and sharing in the work of running the co-op.

Farmers' markets. They often sell locally grown foods.

Warehouse stores. Stores with "no frills" may offer savings because they spend less on displays and customer services. Food may be sold in bigger quantities. You may need to bag your own groceries—or even bring your own bags or boxes.

A farmers' market usually sells foods grown on local farms. Seasonal fruits and vegetables often cost less at a farmers' market. What locally grown products are available in your area?

Activity: Examine newspaper inserts from a variety of grocery stores to compare the items that are featured and on sale. What would be the best buys at each store?

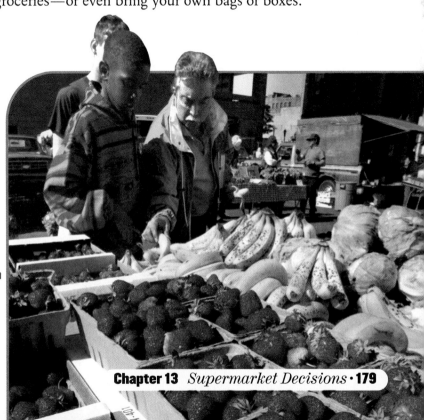

Activity: Plan a menu around grocery store ad specials. Compare your menus with a classmate's.

Discuss: How can making a shopping list help save money and time?

INFOLINK

To review the basics of planning menus, see Chapter 12, page 172.

Tip

Get to know the layout of the store where you shop most often. Then organize your shopping list according to the store's layout. You'll save time because you won't have to go back to find items you missed.

Planning Before You Shop

A successful shopping trip usually starts before you leave home. Planning ahead can save money, time, and effort. Start by determining your **food budget,** *the amount you plan to spend on food.* Plan menus that match your budget. Most stores advertise weekly specials in the newspaper. You might choose the store with the best specials and then plan your menus around the discounted items.

Making Your Shopping List

With a shopping list, you'll be able to buy quickly just what you need without overspending. You'll also avoid an emergency shopping trip to buy what you forgot!

- Check your supply of **staples,** or *foods your family keeps on hand,* such as milk, rice, or flour. List any staples that are running low.
- Check your menu plan. List items you don't have on hand. Include the amount and, if necessary, the form you need. For example, do you want sliced or crushed pineapple?
- If you save coupons, match coupons to foods on your list.

Reading Food Labels

Supermarkets are full of information to help you become a smart shopper. Look at the food label on page 181 to discover all you can learn from a label.

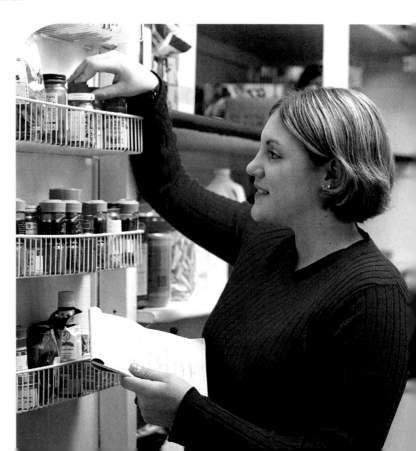

A shopping list will help you save money. You'll buy what you need to prepare planned menus and you'll save time in the store, too. Why is it important to check what foods you have on hand before going to the store?

How Label Terms Help You

FOR NUTRIENTS OR CALORIES, IF YOU WANT:	LOOK FOR THESE WORDS ON THE LABEL:
Plenty or more	Added, contains, enriched, fortified, good source, high, more, provides, rich
Less	Lean, extra lean, fewer, less, low, lower, light, reduced
None	Free, insignificant, no, without

Reading Food Labels

INGREDIENT LIST
Ingredients are listed in order by weight, from greatest to least.

DESCRIPTION
The description identifies the food and sometimes how it's prepared.

FRESHNESS DATE
Some foods, especially perishable foods, are dated.

PREPARATION DIRECTIONS
Some containers provide instructions for conventional and microwave preparation and perhaps a recipe.

NUTRITION INFORMATION
The **Nutrition Facts** panel *shows the calories, nutrients, cholesterol, and fiber in one serving.* (See page 182 to learn more.)

FOOD EXCHANGES
This information helps people with diabetes make careful food choices. It is based on a system called Exchange Lists for Meal Planning developed by the American Diabetes Association and the American Dietetic Association.

FOOD COMPANY AND ADDRESS
The name and address of the manufacturer or distributor is helpful if you have questions or need to report a problem. Check for a company's web site address for consumer information about the product.

UNIVERSAL PRODUCT CODE (UPC)
The **UPC symbol is** *a bar code that is read by a scanner when you check out.* The code contains information about price and is used by stores to track inventory.

AMOUNT
The quantity is listed by volume or by net weight—the weight of food without the container.

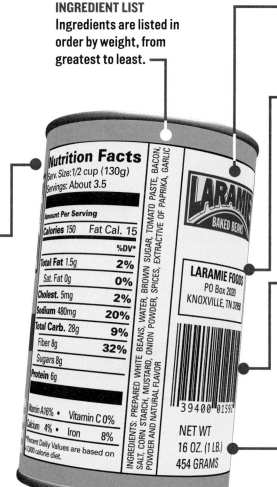

Nutrition Facts
Serv. Size: 1/2 cup (130g)
Servings: About 3.5

Amount Per Serving

Calories 150   Fat Cal. 15

	%DV*
Total Fat 1.5g	2%
Sat. Fat 0g	0%
Cholest. 5mg	2%
Sodium 480mg	20%
Total Carb. 28g	9%
Fiber 8g	32%
Sugars 8g	
Protein 6g	

Vitamin A 16%	•	Vitamin C 0%
Calcium 4%	•	Iron 8%

*Percent Daily Values are based on a 2,000 calorie diet.

INGREDIENTS: PREPARED WHITE BEANS, WATER, BROWN SUGAR, TOMATO PASTE, BACON, SALT, CORN STARCH, MUSTARD, ONION POWDER, SPICES, EXTRACTIVE OF PAPRIKA, GARLIC POWDER AND NATURAL FLAVOR

LARAMIE BAKED BEANS

LARAMIE FOODS
PO Box 2020
KNOXVILLE, TN 37199

39400 01592

NET WT
16 OZ. (1 LB.)
454 GRAMS

Critical Thinking: What kinds of foods would you expect to have freshness dates? Why do you think it's important to pay attention to these dates? What might happen if you didn't?

Checking for Nutrition

Imagine you're buying tomorrow's lunch. Which deli meats have less fat? Which bread has more fiber? Which canned fruit has more vitamin C? How many calories do fat-free cookies have? Use food labels to compare foods and to choose foods that provide nutrients you need.

• Look for nutrient content claims, such as "low-fat" and "more calcium." Use these quick clues for foods with more or less of a nutrient or food substance. These words mean what they say because foods must meet government criteria to be labeled with such terms.

• To get specific nutrition information, check the Nutrition Facts panel. See below.

• Look for health claims. These claims describe benefits that the food, or a nutrient in it, provides. For example, eating vegetables can reduce the risk of cancer, and consuming calcium lowers the chance of osteoporosis. Health claims must be based on scientific evidence.

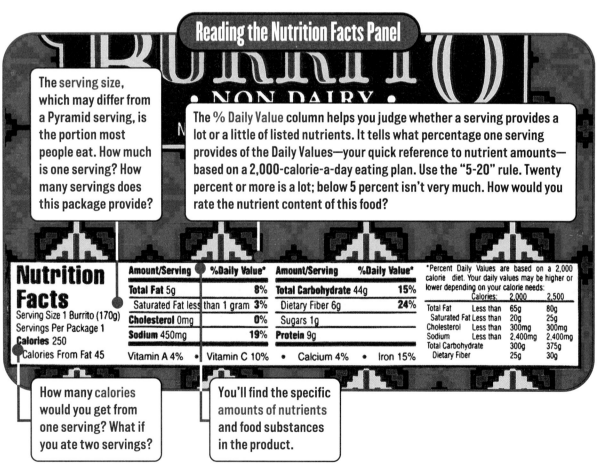

Reading the Nutrition Facts Panel

The serving size, which may differ from a Pyramid serving, is the portion most people eat. How much is one serving? How many servings does this package provide?

The % Daily Value column helps you judge whether a serving provides a lot or a little of listed nutrients. It tells what percentage one serving provides of the Daily Values—your quick reference to nutrient amounts—based on a 2,000-calorie-a-day eating plan. Use the "5-20" rule. Twenty percent or more is a lot; below 5 percent isn't very much. How would you rate the nutrient content of this food?

How many calories would you get from one serving? What if you ate two servings?

You'll find the specific amounts of nutrients and food substances in the product.

Getting Your Money's Worth

To save money, stick to your shopping list and try to avoid shopping for food when you're hungry. You won't be tempted to buy more food than you need. Once you're at the store, you can put your smart shopping skills to work.

Comparing Prices

How much would you want to spend for the same bag of groceries, $30 or $22? The answer is obvious! If you know how to compare prices and shop wisely, you can spend less for the same amount of food or buy more food and stay within your budget. These tools can help you.

Unit price. The **unit price** on the shelf *tells how much an item costs per unit of measurement.* One jar of pasta sauce may cost 8.6 cents per ounce. A larger jar with a higher total price may cost only 7 cents per ounce. Use the unit price to find the most economical brand and size for you.

Coupons. Use the cents-off coupons you find in advertisements, in mailers, and at the store to save on items you'd buy anyway or to try new items. You can save even more when stores double the coupon value.

Store brands. Store brands often cost less than national brands. Check unit prices.

Frequent customer card. Some stores reward their frequent customers with special savings at the checkout counter. Computers read the card, ring up the discount, and may print coupons—just for you.

Tip

If you can, buy foods such as nuts, dried fruit, and pasta from bulk bins. Foods in bulk bins cost less because you don't pay for packaging. You buy only what you need. It's also environmentally friendly since the foods don't require extra packaging materials.

Activity: Provide prices and weights for different brands and sizes of the same type of cereal. Calculate the unit price of each and decide which is the best buy.

What's the unit price on each of these? Which one is the best value for you? Why?

Discuss: Why should you not grocery shop when you're hungry?

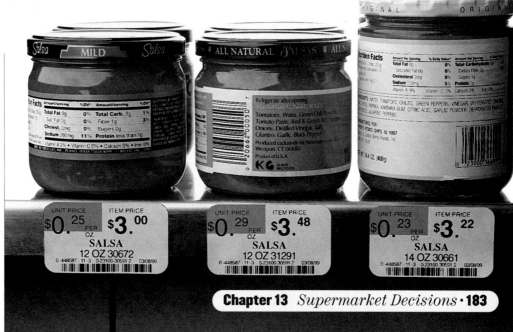

UNIT PRICE	ITEM PRICE
$0.25 PER OZ	$3.00

SALSA
12 OZ 30672

UNIT PRICE	ITEM PRICE
$0.29 PER OZ	$3.48

SALSA
12 OZ 31291

UNIT PRICE	ITEM PRICE
$0.23 PER OZ	$3.22

SALSA
14 OZ 30661

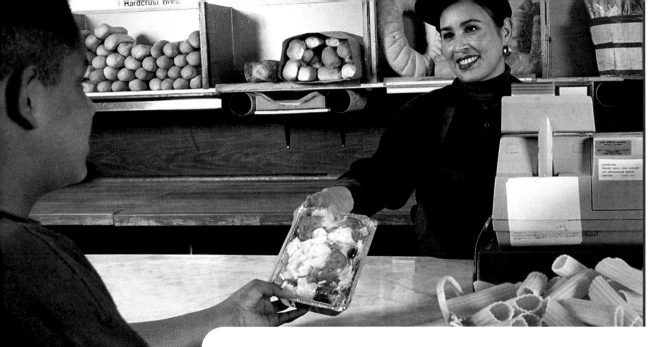

How Much Do You Need?

Do you need a single portion or the large economy size? The bigger container often costs less per unit, but not always. Check the unit price.

Food that spoils before you have a chance to eat it is a waste of money. Buy a large size only if you can store it properly and will use it before it spoils. Buy only the amount you need of **perishable** foods—those that *keep their peak quality for a short time and may spoil quickly*—such as fresh fruits and vegetables.

Choosing the Form

Many foods are sold fresh, frozen, or canned. The nutrient content is often about the same—as long as you store foods properly and use them at their peak. By comparison shopping, you can decide which is the best buy. Keep in mind that the price of fresh fruits and vegetables may be lower or higher at different times of the year.

Canned and frozen foods are sold in different ways, such as whole, sliced, or in chunks. Read the description on the label and choose the form that's right for the dish you plan to prepare. For example, why pay extra for solid-packed tuna if you are making a casserole for which the appearance of the tuna won't matter?

Think about the cost of convenience. The trade-off of convenience is additional cost. A frozen dinner probably costs more than the same meal you make yourself—unless the homemade version requires you to buy more ingredients than you will use.

Food Safety and Quality

To get the most for your food dollar, keep safety and quality in mind. Food bought at its peak contains more nutrients. It keeps longer—and it tastes better!

While You Shop

- Handle fresh fruits and vegetables gently. Bruised fruits and vegetables spoil faster.
- Look for dates on the package. **Open dating** means *the packages are marked with freshness dates that consumers can understand.* A "sell by" date means you can buy food by this date and still store it for a reasonable time. A "best if used by" date tells when food is at its peak quality. Some foods have packing dates. Remember, these dates relate to peak quality, not food safety.
- Look for undamaged containers. Give bulging, rusted, or dented cans or broken containers to a clerk. Check safety seals and buttons, too.
- Choose solidly frozen foods. Ice crystals or discoloration on the package are clues that the food thawed and was refrozen.
- Put meat, poultry, and fish in plastic bags to prevent their juices from leaking onto other foods.
- Fill your cart and grocery bags carefully so that fruits, vegetables, and other soft foods aren't bruised or crushed.

Discuss: When would you buy discounted day-old bakery products? When would you not choose them?

Look carefully to make sure packages aren't damaged. What should you do with any damaged products you find?

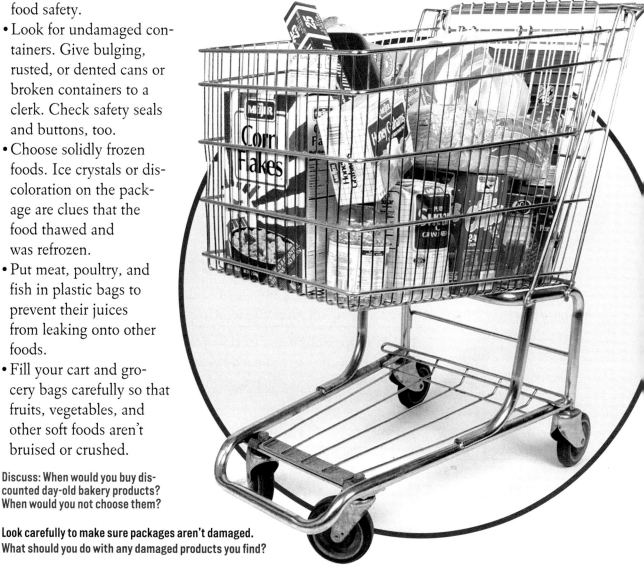

INFOLINK

To learn more about buying and storing specific types of food, refer to the chapters in Unit 5.

Activity: What products are marked with "sell by" dates and "best used by" dates?

Return home after grocery shopping and store perishables in the refrigerator right away. If you had to make a stop on your way home, how could you keep cold foods cold? How could you keep hot items hot on the way home?

Activity: Working in small groups, write a skit that illustrates examples of customer courtesy. Perform your skit for the class.

INFOLINK

To see a Safe Handling Instructions label found on meat and poultry, turn to Chapter 25.

Tip

Consider bringing your own cloth grocery bag or reusing plastic or paper bags. You'll be helping the environment by not using extra resources, and some stores offer small discounts for customers who use their own bags.

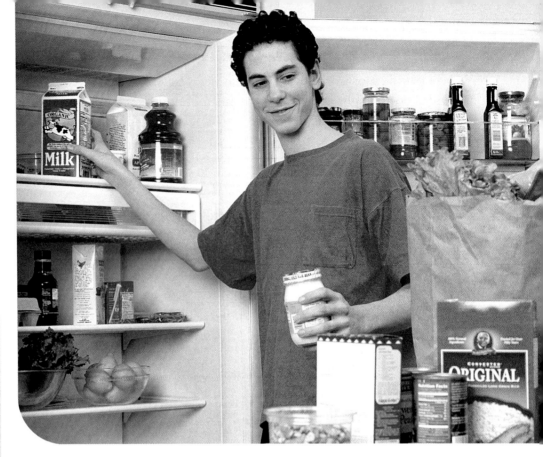

After You Shop

- Take food home and store it right away! Milk, meat, and other perishable foods, as well as hot and cold take-out foods, need to be refrigerated. Save other errands for another time or do them first.
- Follow the safety information found on meat and poultry packages.

Customer Courtesy

You expect courtesy from store employees. Courtesy from customers also makes shopping more pleasant for everyone.

As you shop. Return any food you don't want to its proper place. Politely ask a clerk if you need help. Take a number and wait your turn at the deli, meat, or take-out counter. Don't open packages in the store.

At the checkout counter. Use the express checkout lane only if you have the number of items allowed. Do you need to get something you forgot? Take your cart out of line so that you won't keep others waiting. Have your coupons and money ready.

In the parking lot. Take your shopping cart to the cart return. That way it won't damage someone's car.

Activity: Survey local grocery stores to find out whether any offer discounts to customers who use their own bags.

HELP WANTED

Sales Representative

Dynamic Sales Representative needed to work with retailers to establish promotional programs and advertising. Must be able to maintain current customers and obtain new accounts. Extensive travel. Four-year degree preferred. Salary plus commission. Send resume to Diversified Foods.

Manager

Use your management skills in a supermarket chain to direct sales, customer service, stock, and inventory. We are looking for college graduates with leadership skills to enter our formal training program. Salary, benefits, and opportunities for advancement. Send resume to Quality Food Markets.

Retail Buyer

Retail Buyer needed for convenience store chain. Make buying decisions, negotiate prices, and write contracts. Four-year degree and assistant buyer experience required. Computer skills a plus. Must work in a fast-paced environment. Send resume to Quick Markets.

Cashier

Entry-level openings for cashiers, full- or part-time. Must have good customer service skills and basic math abilities. High school diploma required for full-time. Apply at United Foods.

Inventory Clerk

Dependable Inventory Clerk needed for evening shift. Code products, maintain records, and track merchandise. High school diploma and computer skills required. Competitive hourly wage. Apply at Merchants Superstore.

Assistant Banquet Manager

Large hotel and conference center is looking for a highly motivated individual to join management team. Plan banquets and work with clients to guarantee satisfaction. Candidates should be detail and sales oriented. Salary and bonus plus benefits. Two-year degree preferred. Contact Truman Hotel.

Customer Service Representative

Leading provider of major food brands seeks customer service rep to work directly with retail clients. Assist in processing orders and solving problems. Must have excellent communication skills, computer proficiency, and "can-do" attitude. Associate degree preferred. Contact Worldwide Foods.

LINKING *to the* WORKPLACE

❶ Employment Opportunities: Check "help wanted" ads in a local newspaper or on its Web site. How many employment opportunities in the food industry can you find? Categorize the job openings according to the amount and type of education required.

❷ Workplace Ethics: In any job, workers are expected to demonstrate ethics—standards of professional conduct. Give examples of the ethical behavior that you, as a customer, expect from workers in food sales and retailing.

LOOKING BACK

- Depending on your needs and preferences, you may shop for food in a variety of places.
- Planning ahead before you shop can save you money, time, and effort.
- Read food labels to compare foods and find those that meet your nutrition needs.
- To get your money's worth, compare prices and choose the amount and form of food that meets your needs.
- Keep food quality in mind while you shop. Make food safety a priority while shopping and at home.
- Practice courtesy on your food shopping trips.

UNDERSTANDING KEY IDEAS

1. How does a food cooperative differ from a warehouse store?
2. What are the advantages of making a shopping list?
3. How might you use food labels to choose between two types of canned soup?
4. Give several examples of ways you might save money when shopping for food.
5. What are several steps you might take to help ensure quality and safety when buying perishable foods such as milk and meat?
6. Describe three ways you could be a courteous customer.

DEVELOPING LIFE SKILLS

1. **Critical Thinking:** If you were a retired person on a fixed income, would you choose to do most of your food shopping at a supermarket or a warehouse store? Why? What disadvantage would each choice present, and how might it be overcome?
2. **Management:** A budget is a plan for saving and spending money. When planning a budget, how might a family determine how much to allow for food expenses? What are some reasons why one family might need to spend a larger percentage of their income on food than another family?

Wellness Challenge

Lori and Carlos want to start a teen volunteer program to help older adults shop for groceries. The teens would go to the store with older adults who may need assistance with lifting heavy items, reading the small print on food labels, or reaching items on high or low shelves.

1. How might Carlos and Lori start this program?
2. What challenges might they face?
3. How can they go about finding solutions?

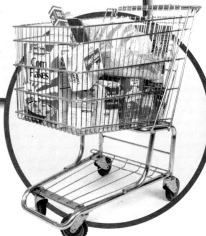

APPLYING YOUR LEARNING

1. **Analyzing Labels:** Obtain the label or other packaging from two foods in the same category, such as two kinds of breakfast cereal. Compare and contrast the nutrition of the two products based on the ingredient list and Nutrition Facts panel. Which product would you be more likely to choose? Why?

2. **Economy Buying:** List several food items your family buys regularly. Decide which items your family might purchase in large economy sizes, and which items it might purchase in regular or small quantities, to get the most for your food dollar. Explain your reasoning.

EXPLORING FURTHER

1. **Label Messages:** Find out what the following label terms mean: *free* (as in "sodium-free"), *reduced* (as in "reduced fat"), *high* (as in "high in vitamin C"), *good source, light,* and *healthy.* Make a chart of your findings.

2. **Online Shopping:** In some areas of the country, people can shop for groceries online. Using the Internet, find out more about this service. Where is it offered? How does it work? What are the advantages and disadvantages? What is the cost?

Making CONNECTIONS

1. **Math:** Explain how to compare unit prices when one is given as cents per ounce and another is given as dollars per pound.

2. **Language Arts:** Write a letter to a food manufacturer giving a suggestion for improving a product or its packaging. Use proper business letter format.

3. **Career Connections Experience:** Research techniques used by food stores to encourage shoppers to buy. Then visit two local food stores to compare and contrast their use of these techniques. Write a report of your findings.

FOODS LAB

Conduct a taste test of four or five kinds of bread, each having at least one whole grain ingredient. Rate the breads for flavor, texture, and appeal. Analyze the Nutrition Facts panels. How do the breads compare nutritionally? Which would you buy and why?

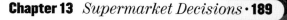

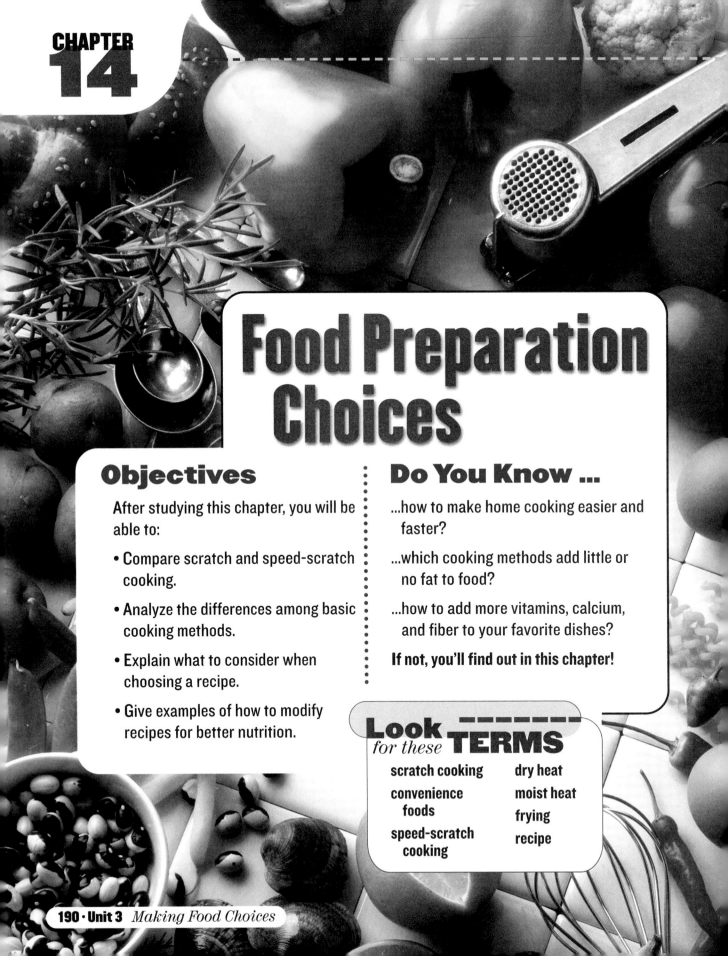

Food Preparation Choices

Objectives

After studying this chapter, you will be able to:

- Compare scratch and speed-scratch cooking.

- Analyze the differences among basic cooking methods.

- Explain what to consider when choosing a recipe.

- Give examples of how to modify recipes for better nutrition.

Do You Know ...

...how to make home cooking easier and faster?

...which cooking methods add little or no fat to food?

...how to add more vitamins, calcium, and fiber to your favorite dishes?

If not, you'll find out in this chapter!

Look for these TERMS

scratch cooking

convenience foods

speed-scratch cooking

dry heat

moist heat

frying

recipe

You've probably

faced choices about how to prepare meals for yourself or your family—or you soon will. No single approach is right every time. You need to weigh the pros and cons of different approaches as you juggle your resources and make decisions. Whatever approach you use, meals that take flavor and nutrition into account get high marks!

Scratch or Convenience Cooking?

Your great-grandmother probably spent hours cooking a family meal. With today's appliances and convenience foods, you can make a meal in 30 minutes, 15 minutes—or even less time.

Like your great-grandmother, you can cook from scratch. **Scratch cooking** is *preparing a homemade dish from unprepared foods.* You control what's in the dish and how it's made. The result is homemade flavor. Scratch cooking often costs less than using **convenience foods**, *partly prepared or ready-to-eat foods.* The trade-off is that scratch cooking usually takes more time, energy, and kitchen skills.

Convenience foods let you assemble a meal quickly with less effort. These foods often cost more since some or all of the preparation is done for you. With ready-to-eat foods, you don't have control over the ingredients. However, information on the label can help you make smart choices.

Speed-scratch cooking *uses partly prepared foods for homemade dishes.* For instance, you might top a store-bought unbaked pizza shell with pre-pared sauce, packaged shredded cheese, and other pizza ingredients. With speed-scratch cooking, you can save time and energy and get a home-cooked taste. It's a chance to be creative as you prepare a healthful meal!

Activity: Describe a meal you could make using speed-scratch cooking.

Using prepackaged pie shells allows you to create homemade desserts in less time than it would take from scratch. What other products are available for speed-scratch cooking?

Discuss: Compare the time needed to make a pizza from scratch with preparing a frozen pizza. What are the advantages of each?

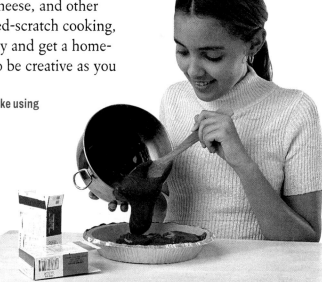

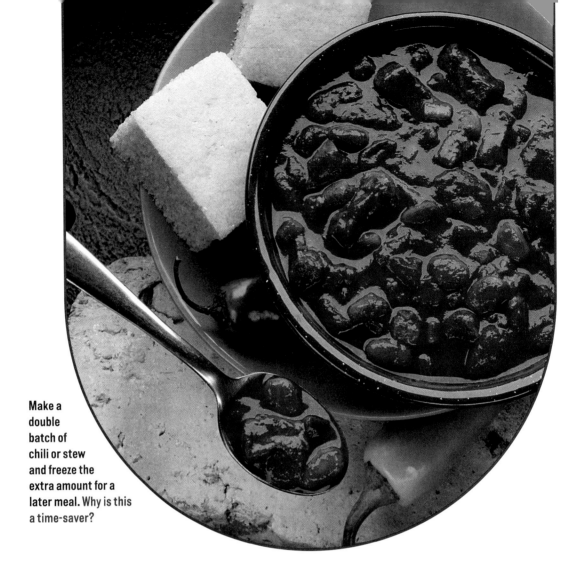

Make a double batch of chili or stew and freeze the extra amount for a later meal. Why is this a time-saver?

Emphasize: Dishes made from preparing double or triple batches can be separated and frozen. Each can be thawed and heated in a microwave oven at a later date for a quick and easy meal.

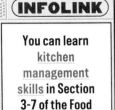

INFOLINK

You can learn kitchen management skills in Section 3-7 of the Food Preparation Handbook.

More Paths to Quick and Easy Meals

There are many ways to prepare nourishing, tasty meals with less time and effort. Besides convenience foods and speed-scratch cooking, try these strategies.

• Do some steps ahead. You might assemble a casserole to freeze, then bake later when you need it.

• "Double batch" by preparing enough for two meals. One night's meat sauce for spaghetti can become a baked potato topper the next night.

• Use timesaving equipment, such as a microwave oven and food processor.

• Learn management skills that can help you work efficiently in the kitchen.

Which Cooking Method?

Activity: List your favorite cooked foods or dishes and how they are cooked. Can any be prepared by another cooking method?

Another important decision is what cooking method to use. Will you fry chicken or bake it? Will you steam vegetables or stir-fry them? With many foods, several methods can give tasty results. Your decision may be based on how much time you have available to prepare the meal. Nutrition enters in, too—some preparation methods add more fat than others.

To compare cooking methods, take a look at the chart on page 194. Notice that cooking methods fall into three categories.

- **Dry heat** means *cooking food uncovered without added liquid.*
- **Moist heat** *involves liquid or steam.*
- **Frying** means *cooking in fat.*

(INFOLINK)

Read more about choosing cooking methods for specific foods in Unit 5.

Find how-to tips for basic cooking methods in Sections 3-5 and 3-6 of the Food Preparation Handbook.

For a list of recipes that teach basic cooking skills, see the Table of Contents.

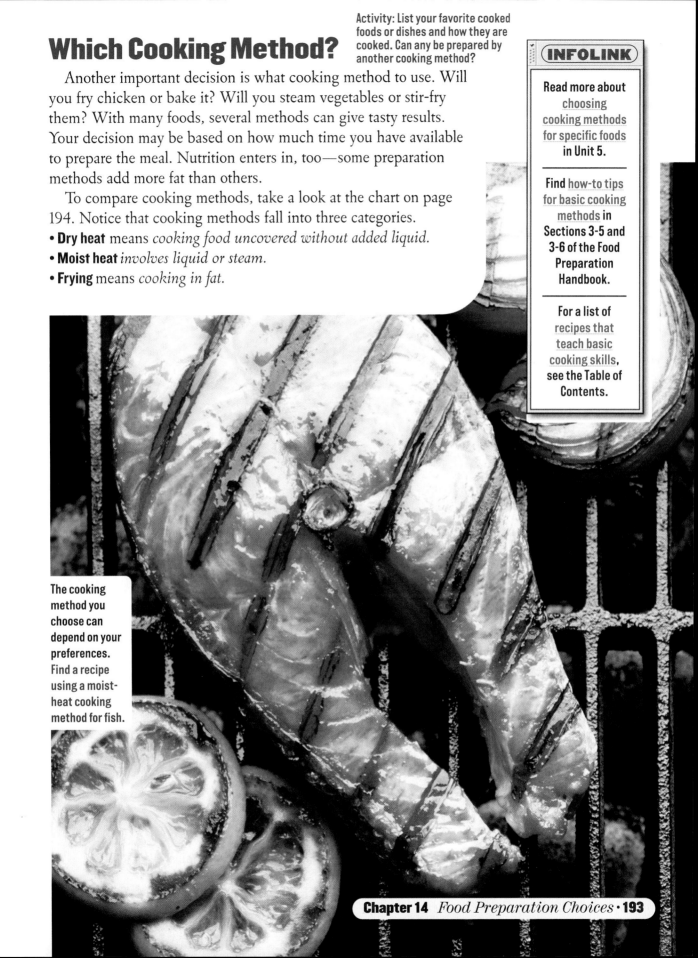

The cooking method you choose can depend on your preferences. Find a recipe using a moist-heat cooking method for fish.

How Do Cooking Methods Compare?

❶ Adds no fat ❷ Adds some fat
❸ Adds more fat

	METHOD	HOW IS FOOD COOKED?	TYPICAL USES	HOW MUCH FAT?	FAST?
DRY HEAT	**Bake/ Roast**	In an oven, uncovered.	Breads, Casseroles, Tender meat, Poultry, Fish, Some vegetables	❶	
	Broil	Under intense, direct heat. Can be done using a range, toaster oven, or countertop broiler.	Tender meat, Poultry, Fish, Some vegetables	❶	✔
	Grill	On a grid over intense, direct heat. Can be done on an outdoor grill or with an indoor grilling appliance.	Tender meat, Poultry, Fish, Some vegetables	❶	✔
	Pan-broil	Uncovered, in a skillet without added fat. Fat from the food is poured off as it collects.	Hamburgers, Bacon	❶	✔
MOIST HEAT	**Boil**	In liquid heated to the boiling point. Bubbles form rapidly and break on the surface.	Pasta	❶	✔
	Steam	In steam that rises from boiling water.	Vegetables, Fish, Rice	❶	✔
	Simmer	In liquid just below the boiling point. Bubbles form slowly and rise gently to the surface.	Vegetables	❶	
	Poach	Gently, covered in simmering liquid, being careful to keep the food's shape.	Fish, Eggs, Fruit	❶	
	Stew	By simmering, usually for a long time. Food is usually cut in small pieces.	Less tender meat, Poultry, Vegetables	❶	
	Braise	Food is browned, then covered and simmered in a little liquid.	Less tender meat, Poultry	❷	
	Microwave	In a microwave oven.	Many foods	❶	✔
FRYING	**Stir-fry**	Quickly, in a small amount of oil over high heat. Food is cut into small pieces and stirred constantly.	Tender meat, Poultry, Fish, Vegetables	❷	✔
	Sauté	In a small amount of fat or oil over low to medium heat, stirring or turning frequently.	Tender meat, Poultry, Fish, Vegetables	❷	✔
	Pan-fry	In a small amount of fat or oil over low to medium heat.	Tender meat, Poultry, Fish, Eggs	❸	✔
	Deep-fat fry	Completely covered in hot fat or oil.	Poultry, Fish, Vegetables	❸	✔

You might organize recipes by type, such as appetizers, main dishes, soups, salads, and desserts. Choose a system that works for you. List the advantages and disadvantages of two ways to organize recipes.

Activity: Look through a variety of cookbooks. Select a recipe you would like to prepare and eat. Explain your choice.

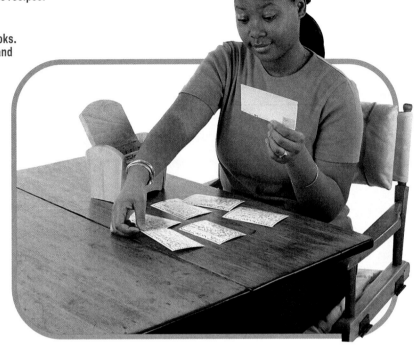

Which Recipe?

As you gain experience with basic cooking methods—such as knowing how to broil meat, steam vegetables, and boil pasta—you'll find you can create a simple, tasty meal without opening a cookbook. Many times, though, you'll want to use a recipe. A **recipe** is like a road map. It's *a list of ingredients and a complete set of instructions for preparing a certain dish.* Use recipes for scratch and speed-scratch cooking.

Recipes can be resources for healthful eating. You can get them from newspapers, magazines, cookbooks, supermarkets, food packages, the Internet, friends, or relatives. Why not start a collection of favorite recipes and new ones you'd like to try? Organize your recipes using small cards, a computer file, a notebook, or file drawer. That way you can find them when you need them.

Choosing Recipes

Before you decide to use a recipe, read it carefully and ask yourself these questions.
- Are the directions clear?
- Do I have the skills I'll need?
- Do I have all the equipment needed?
- Which ingredients do I already have? Do I have the time and money to shop for any ingredients I don't have on hand? If not, can I substitute other ingredients?
- How long will it take to prepare the recipe? Do I have the time and energy?
- How does this dish fit into this meal and my eating plan?

(INFOLINK)

Read more about recipes in the Food Preparation Handbook:
What a recipe tells you and tips for using recipes successfully in **Section 3-1.** Recipe terms and techniques in **Sections 3-2 through 3-6.**

Discuss: If you were choosing among recipes to make chili, how would you decide which one to use?

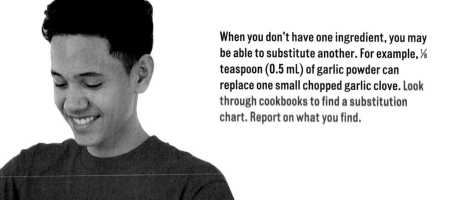

When you don't have one ingredient, you may be able to substitute another. For example, ⅛ teaspoon (0.5 mL) of garlic powder can replace one small chopped garlic clove. Look through cookbooks to find a substitution chart. Report on what you find.

Tip

Write down recipe changes as you make them. If you like the results, you'll be able to use your new version again. If not, your notes can help you decide what to do next time.

Activity: Look in magazines to find a standard recipe along with one that has been revised to make it more nutrition-wise. How were the ingredients changed and how is the dish more nutritious?

Nutrition-Wise Recipe Makeovers

Remember the Dietary Guidelines you learned in Chapter 7? Consider variety, balance, and moderation in your overall eating plan as you choose recipes. If the dish is higher in calories or fat, you can serve it with other foods that have less fat and calories. Another option is to try making changes in the recipe. You can modify many dishes for nutrition—without giving up flavor!

Recipes for many dishes—such as salads, soups, stir-fries, and casseroles—are flexible. They are good choices for experimenting with recipe changes. With baked foods such as bread or cake, the amount and type of ingredients in the recipe are essential to an appealing result. Until you become experienced, you'll be more successful with these baked foods if you follow the recipe exactly.

For more vitamins ...
• Add more vegetables—and a greater variety of vegetables—to casseroles, pasta dishes, and other mixed dishes. Shredded carrots and zucchini taste great in mashed potatoes.

For more calcium ...

- Add dry milk to mashed potatoes, meat loaf, and many mixed dishes.
- Add grated cheese to casseroles and mashed potatoes. Use it as a topper on soups, stews, salads, and vegetables.
- Add calcium-fortified tofu to salads, stir-fries, and other mixed dishes.

For less fat ...

- Use reduced- or low-fat ingredients in your recipes.
- Use smaller amounts of high-fat ingredients such as butter, margarine, salad dressing, and peanut butter.
- Skim fat from soups, stews, pan juices, and gravies. Fat is lighter than water, so it rises to the top.
- Make one or more of the substitutions listed in the chart on page 198.

Adding veggies to dishes increases nutrients. What veggies might you add to one of your favorite dishes?

Check This Out!

THREE Rs OF AN EARTH-FRIENDLY KITCHEN

Using resources wisely is a choice you make in the kitchen. When you prepare food, remember the three Rs:

Reduce. Conserve energy and water in the kitchen. Turn on appliances only when you need them. Open the refrigerator door as short a time as possible. Turn off the faucet when you've drawn enough water. Run the dishwasher when it's full, not half empty. To reduce trash, look for foods sold with less packaging.

Reuse. Use leftovers creatively in other meals. Find ways to use packaging items you might discard. For example, wash out empty jars and use them to store bulk foods or leftovers.

Recycle. Try to buy foods sold in recyclable packaging. Look for the recycling symbol on the package. Use recycling services to cut down on trash.

It's Your Turn!

Think of other ways to use less food, energy, and water and cut down on trash.

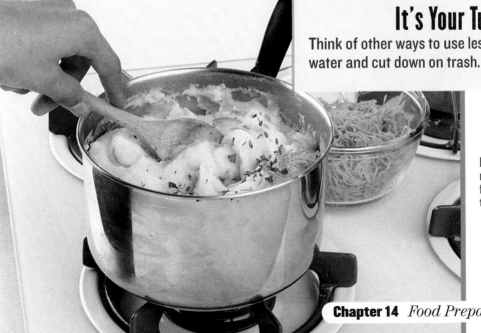

Discuss: How could you modify a recipe for a favorite dish to increase the calcium in it?

Easy Substitutions for Less Fat

These substitutions lower fat and cholesterol without sacrificing flavor.

WHEN RECIPES LIST ...	USE INSTEAD ...
Cream	Evaporated fat-free milk
Sour cream	Plain yogurt, light or nonfat sour cream, or cottage cheese (blended until smooth)
Whole milk	Fat-free, low-fat, or reduced-fat milk
Cheese	Reduced-fat or fat-free cheese
Ground beef or sausage	Lean or extra-lean ground beef, lean ground turkey or chicken, or 95% fat-free sausage
Bacon	Ham, smoked turkey, or Canadian bacon
1 whole egg	2 egg whites or 1/4 cup (50 mL) egg substitute
1 ounce baking chocolate	3 tablespoons (45 mL) cocoa powder plus 1 tablespoon (15 mL) oil

Critical Thinking: Does the chart mean that you should *never* use the ingredients in the left column? (No.)

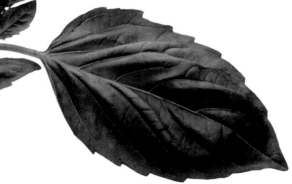

INFOLINK

For more nutrition-wise tips for food preparation, refer to Chapter 7 and Units 5 and 6.

To learn how to change the amount a recipe makes, turn to Section 3-1 of the Food Preparation Handbook.

Read about reducing fat and sugar in baked desserts in Chapter 32.

For more fiber ...
- Use whole-grain pasta and brown rice in recipes.
- Add fiber-rich dry beans and peas to soups and mixed dishes.
  - Mix bran into casseroles.

For less added sugar ...
- Use vanilla, cinnamon, and other spices to bring out the natural sweetness of many foods.

For less sodium ...
- Cut down on the salt in recipes. Use herbs and spices to enhance flavor.
  - Use low-sodium versions of ingredients such as broth, soy sauce, and canned foods.

Teens Cook Off

For Health

Teens from Timberlake High School in Helena, Oklahoma, organized a community beef cook-off as part of the school's Student Body program. This FCCLA (Family, Career and Community Leaders of America) program helps young people learn to eat right, be fit, and make healthy choices. "We're trying to make people in our school and community more health conscious," said Ryan Jenlink, one of the students.

The teens kept healthful eating in mind when they set guidelines for their cook-off. Recipes had to be prepared with leaner cuts of meat. The student body and local journalists chose the winners, ranging from "Jenny's Meatballs" to "Trig-a-Bobs" from the math class.

At the teens' exhibit, cook-off entrants and judges learned low-fat meat preparation tips: "Buy cuts with 'loin' or 'round' in the name. Trim off fat. Broil, grill, or stir-fry meat with fresh ingredients that add flavor but not fat." The teens also spread their message with

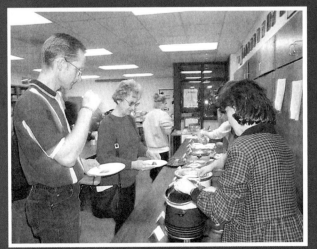

newspaper articles, radio announcements, and exhibits at basketball games and supermarkets. Courtney Cochran, another student, said: "People choose turkey and chicken because they're lean. We show them that today's beef can be lean, too, when they know how to select and prepare it."

Take Action

What healthful food preparation tips could you promote? Plan a recipe contest for your class, school, or community with nutrition guidelines for entries—and make it happen. Offer a health-smart prize to the winners!

LOOKING BACK

- You can cook from scratch or use partly or fully prepared foods, depending on your time, energy, kitchen skills, and the amount of money you want to spend.
- Choose a cooking method based on available time and the nutritional effect.
- Recipes are available from many sources. Always read the recipe carefully before you decide to use it.
- You can modify many recipes to improve nutritional value without giving up flavor.

UNDERSTANDING KEY IDEAS

1. What are the differences between scratch and speed-scratch cooking?

2. Compare several moist heat and frying cooking methods for preparing raw vegetables. Which method would be the fastest? Which method(s) would add the least amount of fat?

3. If you were selecting among various recipes for lasagna, how would you decide which one to use?

4. How can you reduce the amount of fat in soups, stews, pan juices, and gravies?

5. Name two ways you might add more calcium to a salad.

DEVELOPING LIFE SKILLS

1. **Leadership:** What impact does using prepared or convenience foods have on our environment, including landfills? What could you do to change any negative effects?

2. **Critical Thinking:** Jake wants to make an elegant French meal for his parents' wedding anniversary. He has borrowed several cookbooks on French cuisine from the library. However, most of the recipes include unfamiliar terms and many preparation steps. Predict what might happen if Jake prepared one of these challenging recipes. What might be some alternative solutions?

Wellness Challenge

The high school music and art departments plan to hold their annual show on Friday night. Nitara has been chosen to head a committee of six students who will make a buffet dinner.

The students will be preparing the dishes on Friday afternoon. About 70 people are expected to attend. Nitara would like to organize the meal preparation using time-saving techniques.

1. How might Nitara set up the meal preparation for this event?
2. What challenges might she face?
3. How could she find solutions?

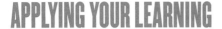

Review & Activities

APPLYING YOUR LEARNING

1. **Personal Food Record:** Food from every food group is sold in ready-to-eat form. Track your eating plan for the next three days. How many of your food choices are convenience products? Compare the cost of each convenience product with that of making the food item from scratch.

2. **Recipe Makeover:** Find a recipe for one of your favorite dishes and change it to boost the nutrient content or lower the fat, cholesterol, sodium, or calories. If possible, prepare the dish and describe your results.

EXPLORING FURTHER

1. **Cooking of Yore:** Using library or Internet resources, obtain a recipe that's at least 100 years old. How is it different from a recipe that you might find in a modern cookbook? Why? Does it provide enough information for you to carry it out? What changes or substitutions might you make and why?

2. **Modified Atmosphere Packaging:** Some convenience foods are preserved with modified atmosphere packaging. Find out more about this method. With what types of food is it used? How is it helpful to consumers? Share your findings in class.

Making CONNECTIONS

1. **Language Arts:** Imagine that you are an advice columnist for the health section of a local weekly newspaper. Your next column will answer readers' questions about ways to cut down on fat in food preparation. Be creative in your answers about cooking methods and recipe makeovers. Share your column with the class.

2. **Science:** Using a science textbook as a reference, learn about the concept of specific heat. What does it refer to? Which has a higher specific heat, air or water? Which requires more heat energy to reach a given temperature? How might this relate to cooking?

FOODS LAB

Prepare three samples of pancakes: one from scratch, one from a mix, and one from a ready-to-pour container. Compare textures and flavors. Which version is most appealing? Why? How do they compare nutritionally? How do they compare in cost per serving?

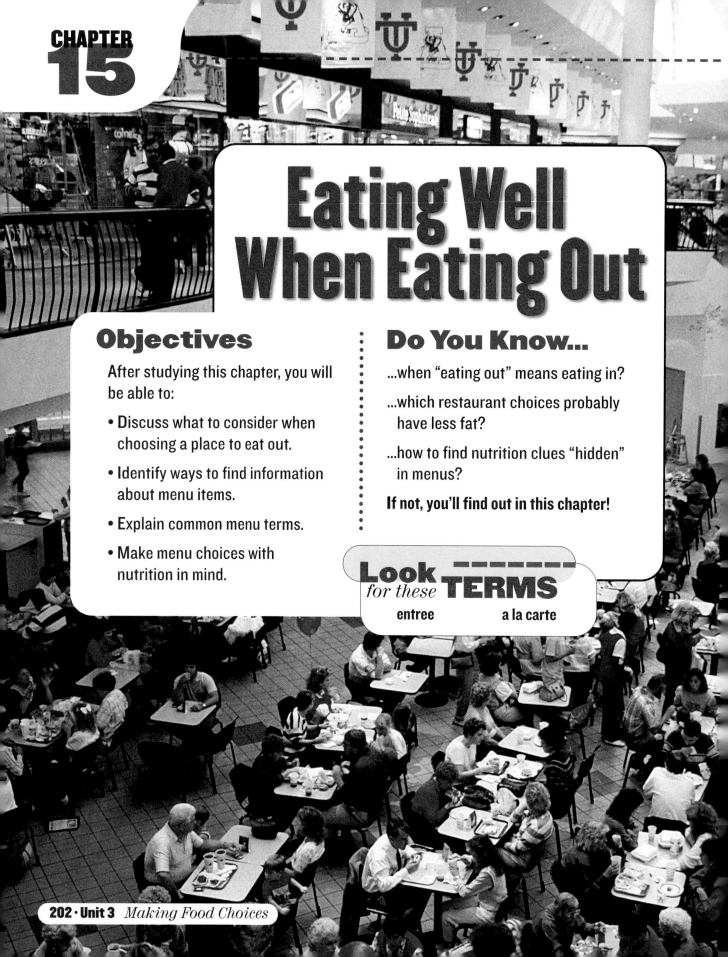

Eating Well When Eating Out

Objectives

After studying this chapter, you will be able to:

- Discuss what to consider when choosing a place to eat out.
- Identify ways to find information about menu items.
- Explain common menu terms.
- Make menu choices with nutrition in mind.

Do You Know...

...when "eating out" means eating in?

...which restaurant choices probably have less fat?

...how to find nutrition clues "hidden" in menus?

If not, you'll find out in this chapter!

Look for these TERMS

entree   a la carte

How many times

have you eaten out in the past week? Remember to count school breakfast or lunch, fast food from the drive-up window, pizza ordered over the phone, and snacks at the mall or from a vending machine. All these foods make up a large portion of your weekly choices. That's why it's wise to pay attention to nutrition when eating out!

Choosing Where to Eat Out

Restaurants and other eating-out options offer almost any kind of food you can think of—and at a wide range of prices. How do you choose where to eat out? Your answer probably varies from day to day. It depends on what you want to eat, where you are, how much time you have, and the amount of money you're willing to spend. What's important is that you make informed decisions.

Weighing Price, Speed, and Service

One basic decision is how much money you want to spend. Remember that the cost of eating out is part of the family's food budget. Meals at restaurants where a server takes your order at the table usually cost more. However, the meal is usually leisurely, and you get food cooked to order.

For quicker service, the options range from fast-food counters to cafeteria lines, self-service buffets, sidewalk vendors, and vending machines. Generally, places that provide food quickly can do so because they offer a limited menu and less personal service. Don't assume, though, that quick always means inexpensive. Look carefully at prices.

Menu options depend on the type of restaurant. Your responsibility is to keep a balanced eating plan in mind. Survey several students to find out how many times they have eaten out in the past week and where.

Activity: How many times in the last week have you eaten from the school cafeteria, restaurants (table service, fast food, take-out), vending machine? Calculate the class totals.

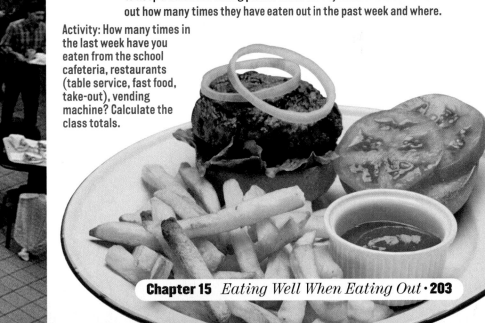

Check This Out!

ORDERING OUT TO EAT IN

Take-out and delivered meals are growing in popularity. People enjoy dining at home without having to prepare the food or do a lot of cleanup in the kitchen. You can get take-out meals from restaurants, delis, and supermarkets. Keep these points in mind.

- Unlike frozen dinners and other packaged foods, take-out foods may not come with nutrition or ingredient information. As a result, it's harder to know just what you're buying and to comparison shop.
- Many take-out foods need to be eaten right away or refrigerated to retain their quality and prevent foodborne illness.

It's Your Turn!

Identify reasons why families might choose to order take-out food rather than eat in a restaurant. Do you think this trend will continue? Why or why not?

Cleanliness Counts

Cleanliness is part of good service—and helps prevent foodborne illness. When choosing a place to eat, look around. Are floors, tables, plates, and utensils clean? If you see any signs that food safety is being neglected, bring your concerns to the attention of the manager.

Where Can You Go for Good Nutrition?

Which is a better choice when it comes to nutrition: a gourmet restaurant or a fast-food counter? Actually, it depends on the individual menu, not the type of restaurant. Before deciding on a restaurant, check the menu. Does it offer a variety of food-group choices? Use your knowledge of the Food Guide Pyramid and the Dietary Guidelines to evaluate whether the menu items fill out your day's nutrition needs.

Do restaurants in your area have limited menus? Then rotate restaurants for balance and variety in your overall choices. Explore the food variety in different types of eating places in your community, including ethnic restaurants. If a restaurant doesn't offer the choices you'd like, make your opinions known. Many restaurants provide comment cards for this purpose.

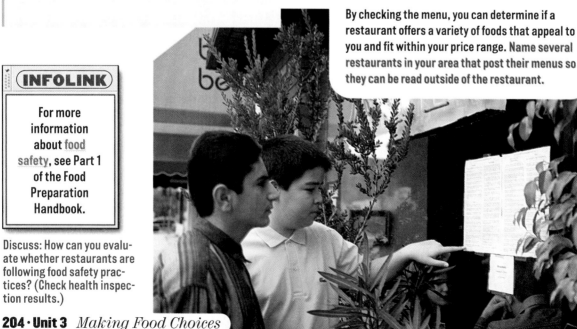

By checking the menu, you can determine if a restaurant offers a variety of foods that appeal to you and fit within your price range. Name several restaurants in your area that post their menus so they can be read outside of the restaurant.

(INFOLINK)

For more information about food safety, see Part 1 of the Food Preparation Handbook.

Discuss: How can you evaluate whether restaurants are following food safety practices? (Check health inspection results.)

Check This Out!

MONEY MATTERS

Eating at a table-service restaurant is different from ordering fast food in many ways—including paying for your food. Here's a guide to help make paying the bill as trouble-free as possible.

- If each person in your group wants to pay separately, ask for separate checks when you order.
- If separate checks aren't possible, let one person pay, then settle up later. Avoid haggling over a bill at the table.
- When someone else is paying for your meal, be thoughtful of the cost. If you're not sure what price range is appropriate, ask the person who is paying, "What are you having?" or "What do you suggest?" Use the cost of the item named as a guideline.
- Check the bill before you pay. If you see a mistake, discuss it quietly with the server.
- In some restaurants, you pay the cashier as you leave. In others, you pay the server at the table. If you're not sure where to pay, ask the server.
- When paying at the table, place your money or credit card with the bill so that it's easy to see. The server takes your payment to the cashier and returns with the change or the credit card slip.
- In most table-service restaurants, tips are the major part of a server's pay. The standard tip for good service is 15 to 20 percent of the bill, not including tax. Leave at least 50 cents for a small order.

It's Your Turn!

Suppose you received a bill for $15.75 plus $1.42 in tax. How much would you leave for a tip if the service was good? Why?

Activity: Work in small groups to simulate ordering and paying the bill at a table-service restaurant using the guidelines here. Decide who will be the server and who will be served.

Making Menu Choices

Your knowledge of the Food Guide Pyramid and Dietary Guidelines can guide your food choices when you eat out or eat in. Before placing your order, consider the other food choices you have made, or expect to make, during the day. For instance, if you are considering a breakfast item that's somewhat high in fat, decide whether you'll be able to have lower-fat meals and snacks the rest of the day. When snacking at the mall, make choices that help fill in your food-group gaps—such as a fruit smoothie for a Fruit Group serving.

INFOLINK

To review the Dietary Guidelines for Americans, see Chapter 7, page 104.

For another look at the Food Guide Pyramid, turn to Chapter 8, page 146.

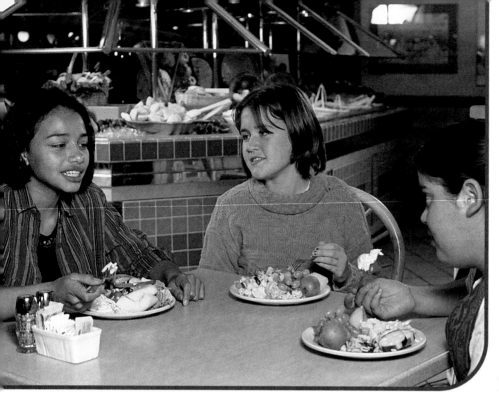

Getting Information

To make healthful choices when eating out, you're wise to know more than just the names of menu items. Fortunately, you have many ways to find out about foods before you order. You can get information:

From signs and leaflets. Many fast-food restaurants provide a chart that lists calories and nutrient amounts for menu items. Use the chart to compare items and the Food Guide Pyramid to make wise choices.

From the server. The server probably can describe what a dish contains, how it's prepared, and the size of the portion. If you have a special concern, such as a food allergy, you need to ask questions.

From the menu. A restaurant's written menu may be a good source of information. See page 207 for some examples.

Boosting Nutrition and Variety

Depending on the choices, meals eaten out may come up short on whole grains, vegetables, fruits, and dairy foods. How can you add these foods—and get the variety and nutrients they provide—when eating out? Start with these ideas.
• Ask for your sandwich on whole grain bread for extra fiber.
• Add lettuce, tomato, and other vegetable toppers to sandwiches.
• Add cheese to a sandwich for more calcium.
• Choose a vegetable or fruit side dish.
• Order milk to drink with your meal.
• Have fresh fruit or low-fat frozen yogurt for a tasty, nutrient-rich dessert.

You don't have to miss out on variety and nutrients when eating out. How could you boost nutrition in the next meal or snack you eat out?

Emphasize: If you have a food allergy and the server is uncertain of the menu item ingredients, ask the server to ask the cook.

NUTRITION ON
The Menu

*L*ooking for a restaurant meal that's low in fat? Want to balance your choices with the day's other meals and snacks? Studying the menu can help you make the selection that's right for you.

NUTRITION INFORMATION

Some menus list specific nutrition information—such as the number of calories and amount of fat and sodium per serving—for some or all of the items.

DESCRIPTION CLUES

If the menu doesn't provide specific nutrition information or claims, it may still offer nutrition clues. Just read the menu and apply your knowledge. A dessert described as "rich and creamy," for instance, is likely to be high in fat.

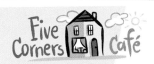

Five Corners Café

for the Hearty Appetite

Fried Chicken
Tender fried chicken served with buttery corn-on-the cob and homemade mashed potatoes.

Smothered Chicken
Char-broiled chicken breast smothered in mild sour cream and sharp cheddar cheese served with mixed spring vegetables and potato of your choice.

Stuffed Pork Chops
A hearty portion of our house favorite. Two roasted pork chops filled with our famous sausage-cornbread stuffing. Served with creamed corn and potatoes au gratin.

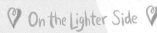
On the Lighter Side

Low-Fat Garlic Chicken Pasta
Linguine topped with fresh steamed vegetables and grilled garlic chicken breast. Served with our house salad.
700 calories, 10 g fat, 500 mg sodium.

Grilled Salmon
Fresh coho salmon served on a bed of herbed rice with steamed vegetables.
410 calories, 12 g fat, 400 mg sodium.

Pasta Primavera
Angel hair pasta tossed in a garlic herb broth and topped with lightly sautéed asparagus, broccoli, baby carrots, and spring pea pods. Accompanied by a mixed green salad and garlic bread.
740 calories, 9 g fat, 200 mg sodium.

NUTRITION CLAIMS

Menu items might have nutrition claims such as "low-fat" or "low-sodium." The same federal laws that apply to such terms on packaged food labels apply to menus.

MENU TERMS

Understanding menu terms can help you figure out what's in the dish or how it's prepared. Which of these terms have you seen on a menu?

- **Au gratin**–topped with bread crumbs or grated cheese.
- **Au jus**–served in the juices from roasting.
- **Florentine**–with spinach.
- **Hollandaise**–sauce made with butter, egg yolks, and other ingredients.
- **Primavera**–with fresh vegetables (for example, pasta primavera).
- **Scalloped**–baked in a cream sauce.

Investigate Further

Obtain copies of restaurant menus in your area to evaluate. Share your menus with the class. Which menus provide the most complete information?

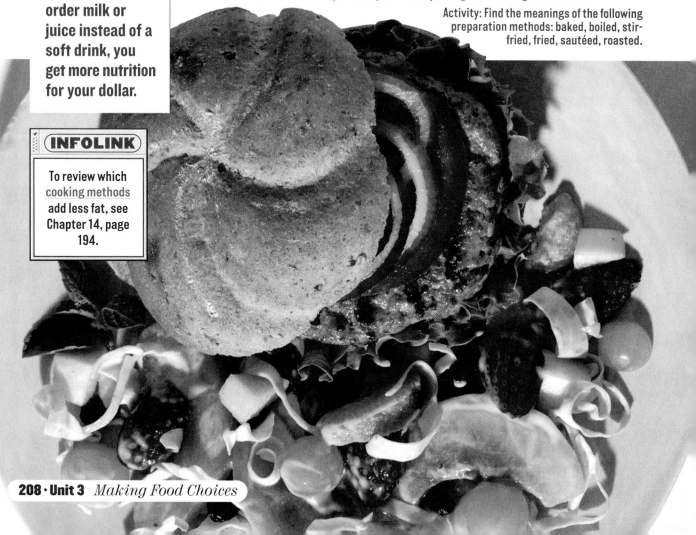

Tip

Want to save money when you eat out? As a bonus, some of the strategies suggested for improving nutrition may also help you use your food dollar wisely. For instance, ordering smaller portions takes a bite out of the restaurant bill. When you order milk or juice instead of a soft drink, you get more nutrition for your dollar.

INFOLINK

To review which cooking methods add less fat, see Chapter 14, page 194.

Ordering on the Lighter Side

Fat and calories really can add up when you eat out regularly. The amount depends on how you order. Pay special attention to:

Preparation methods. Did you know that a sandwich made with breaded, fried chicken could have more than three times as much fat as a broiled chicken sandwich? To reduce fat and calories, choose baked or broiled fish, meat, or poultry, and limit your orders of fried foods. Paying attention can pay off even when making a selection from a vending machine. For example, choose baked pretzels rather than fried potato chips.

Side dishes. In some restaurants, an **entree**, or *main dish*, comes with one or more side dishes. Find out what side dishes are included before you order. If they're high in fat, you can ask for a lower-fat choice, or ask for the entree **a la carte** (*served separately, without side dishes*).

To slightly vary a menu item, you can make a special request. You might ask the server for mustard instead of mayonnaise or fresh fruit instead of french fries. What are some other special requests that you might make for good nutrition?

Activity: Find the meanings of the following preparation methods: baked, boiled, stir-fried, fried, sautéed, roasted.

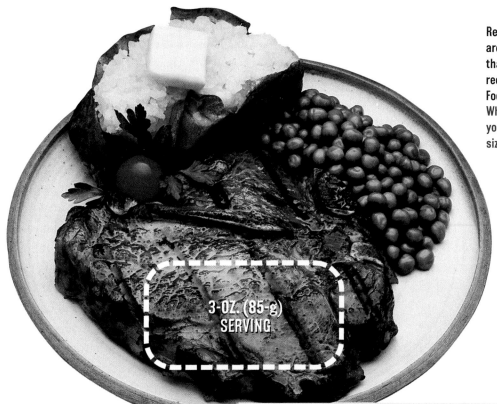

Restaurant portions are often much larger than the serving sizes recommended in the Food Guide Pyramid. What are three ways you could cut portion sizes?

3-OZ. (85-g) SERVING

Toppings. The fat in some foods often comes from toppings such as butter, cream sauce, and gravy. For less fat, you can ask to have the topping served on the side so that you can add only what you want. You can also ask for your food to be served without the topping or with a lighter alternative, such as reduced-fat salad dressing.

Portion size. One order of a restaurant dish may actually count as two, three, or even four servings from the Food Guide Pyramid. You can reduce the fat and calories just by eating a smaller portion.

More About Special Requests: Whether a special request can be honored depends on the restaurant as well as the request. Some foods are prepared in advance and the ingredients or cooking methods can't be changed.

Check This Out!

FIVE WAYS TO CUT PORTION SIZES

Do restaurants fill your plate with more food than you want? Try these tips to cut portions down to size.

- Order the regular-size portion rather than the large or deluxe size.
- Ask whether you can order a half portion.
- Share an order with a companion.
- Eat part of the order and take the rest home. (For food safety, refrigerate the leftovers right away.)
- Make a meal of several healthful appetizers or side dishes. For instance, you might choose hearty soup plus bread, a small tossed salad, and fruit.

It's Your Turn!

Write a courteous letter to a restaurant manager (real or imaginary) expressing your opinion about the portion sizes offered and suggesting changes that would offer more choices.

Passport to Ethnic Restaurants

INFOLINK

To learn about guidelines for dining out with courtesy and confidence, see Chapter 2, page 42.

Have you ever tried foods from Thailand, Brazil, India, or Ethiopia? How about specialties from different parts of the United States? You don't need to travel around the world to learn about foods from other places. For a taste adventure and new flavor combinations, try an ethnic restaurant or one featuring regional American cooking.

You may feel a little unsure about ordering foods that are unfamiliar to you. That's natural, but don't let that stop you from trying something new. Ask the server plenty of questions—such as what the ingredients are, how the dish is prepared, and whether it's spicy or mild. If you still can't decide, ask the server for a recommendation, or consider ordering a sampler plate that includes a variety of items. If you are with family or friends, you could order a variety of dishes and share so that everyone gets a sampling. As for any tongue-twisting names on an ethnic menu, make it a learning experience. There's no need to worry about pronouncing them exactly right. Ask the server how to say the names—or just point to them!

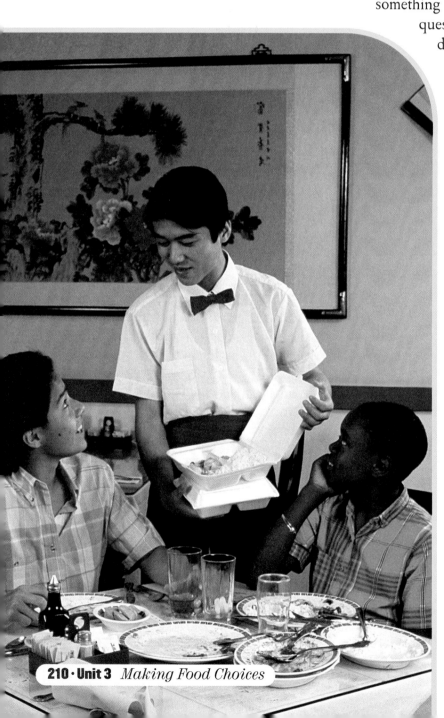

Activity: Find ethnic foods in grocery stores. Report: What types did you find? What countries or regions are they from? What are the ingredients? What are the preparation methods? Are they nutritious? Would you try these foods? Why or why not?

You can take a trip to another country for the price of a meal. Find an ethnic food on a restaurant menu. Look for a recipe for that dish.

HELP WANTED

Food Court Coordinator

The City Zoo is seeking a coordinator to oversee staffing and promotional programs for our new food facility. Must be able to work at a fast pace, be customer service oriented, and have two years of supervisory experience. Flexible schedule including evenings, weekends, and holidays. Hourly wage, bonus, and health insurance. Send resume to Human Resources, City Zoo.

Chef Manager

Experienced chef needed to oversee all banquet and catering functions in college setting. Must be creative, possess excellent business skills, and be knowledgeable in food service management. Degree preferred. Please send resume to Human Resources Manager, University Hospitality Services.

Assistant Food Production Manager

Do you have experience in a fast food restaurant? We are looking for assistant managers to enter our training program. You will assist in supervising staff, purchasing, inventory control, and enforcing health regulations. Ability to handle diverse situations and changing staff a must. Education and training in food service management a plus. Send resume to Recruiting Department, Bagel Shop, Inc.

Catering Specialist

Choice Catering, Inc. is growing rapidly and needs a qualified individual interested in the fast-paced catering environment. The Catering Specialist is responsible for organization of daily events and training and managing staff. Should be self-motivated, creative, and able to work a flexible schedule. Catering experience required. Drug testing and background checks are a part of our hiring process. Contact us today!

Counter Attendants

New theater complex opening soon needs counter attendants to take orders, assemble, and serve food in a fast-paced environment. Basic math skills needed to operate cash register. Minimum wage, flexible work schedules, and movie passes offered. Apply in person at the Theater Complex 24.

Restaurant Cook

Opening for an experienced cook with creative talent and artistic flair! Manage all areas of food preparation for our full service menu. Post-secondary training required with proven abilities as a successful cook. Must work evenings and every other weekend. Excellent salary and benefits package. Send resume to The American Grill.

LINKING *to the* WORKPLACE

❶ **Career Goals:** Many people set a long-term career goal. To get there, they set and reach short-term goals. Describe a career path made up of short-term and long-term career goals, including at least one of the jobs listed above.

❷ **Your Own Restaurant:** Choose a theme for a unique restaurant of your own design. Describe how you would carry out the theme in the menu and decor.

LOOKING BACK

- Where you eat out depends on what you want to eat, where you are, how much time you have, and your budget.
- Your knowledge of the Food Guide Pyramid and Dietary Guidelines can guide your food choices when you eat out or eat in.
- An ethnic restaurant or one featuring regional American cooking gives you a chance to try new tastes and flavors.

UNDERSTANDING KEY IDEAS

1. If you had to choose between eating at a fast-food or full-service restaurant, what factors would influence your decision?

2. How might you find out about foods before you order?

3. Which of the following menu items might you choose if you were following a low-fat eating plan: a baked potato or potatoes au gratin? Asparagus in cream sauce or asparagus sprinkled with lemon and garlic? Why?

4. When ordering a chicken dinner, what requests could you make to cut back on fat and calories? Consider the portion size, preparation methods, and side dishes.

DEVELOPING LIFE SKILLS

1. **Communication:** Your English teacher has assigned the essay topic: "Teens Can Eat Smart on Fast Food." How might you argue in favor of this claim?

2. **Leadership:** You would like to try an Indian restaurant that has just opened in your neighborhood. However, your friend says that she will not join you. She heard that Indian food is very spicy, and she is unfamiliar with the dishes on the menu. How might you encourage her to join you?

Wellness Challenge

Whenever Lamar eats at a local restaurant, he orders the same meal that he knows is low in fat. He wants to try something different, but he is unfamiliar with some of the foods on the menu. He doesn't want to order something that he may not like.

1. How can Lamar get information about menu items?

2. What challenges might Lamar face?

3. How can he meet those challenges?

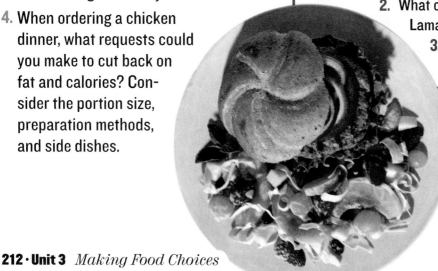

APPLYING YOUR LEARNING

1. **Create a Restaurant Meal:** Imagine that you are opening a restaurant. Write descriptions of foods that will appear on your menu. Base your decisions on nutrition and variety. Create a finished menu to share with the class.

2. **Simulation:** With two of your classmates, act out the most appropriate way to handle the following situations. (a) You are at a fast-food restaurant. After you pick up your order, you discover that there are no clean tables. (b) The bill indicates that each person's meal costs about the same, and you suggest dividing the cost evenly. One friend insists that she will pay only the exact cost of her meal.

EXPLORING FURTHER

1. **Nutrition Claims:** Government laws regulate nutrition claims on restaurant menus. Find out which federal government agency ensures that restaurants follow the regulations. What claims can be made under these laws? What guidelines must the foods meet?

2. **Menu Evaluation:** Obtain menus from two or three local restaurants. Evaluate them for variety, appeal, and nutritional information. Present your findings to the class.

Making CONNECTIONS

1. **Social Studies:** Choose a foreign country and investigate its restaurant industry. What types of restaurants are most common? How often does the average person eat out? How does the cost of eating out compare with such costs in the United States? Report your findings to the class.

2. **Math:** How much money do you spend in an average week on eating out, including school meals and snacks from vending machines? Keep track of what you spend for a typical week. What percentage is it of your budget? Explain ways you could get more for your money.

FOODS LAB

What's your favorite fast food? Tacos, hamburgers, pizza? Find a recipe for your favorite and prepare it. How does it compare in taste to the fast food? How do the calories and fat of each compare? What about the costs? What can you conclude?

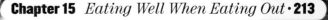

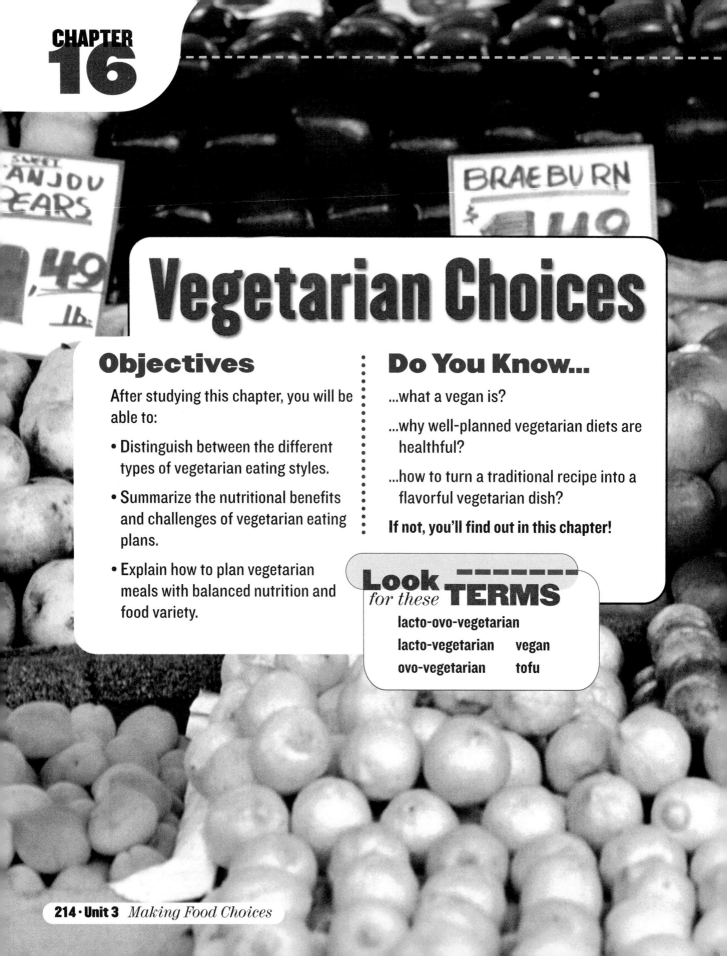

Vegetarian Choices

Objectives

After studying this chapter, you will be able to:

- Distinguish between the different types of vegetarian eating styles.

- Summarize the nutritional benefits and challenges of vegetarian eating plans.

- Explain how to plan vegetarian meals with balanced nutrition and food variety.

Do You Know...

...what a vegan is?

...why well-planned vegetarian diets are healthful?

...how to turn a traditional recipe into a flavorful vegetarian dish?

If not, you'll find out in this chapter!

Look *for these* TERMS

lacto-ovo-vegetarian

lacto-vegetarian   vegan

ovo-vegetarian   tofu

Vegetarian means...

a style of eating! Vegetarians eat foods from plant sources—vegetables, fruits, grains and grain products, dry beans and peas, nuts, and seeds. They don't eat meat, poultry, and fish. They may avoid eggs and dairy products, too. With careful food choices, a vegetarian style can be a healthful—and delicious—way to eat.

The common element among vegetarian eating plans is that they are based mainly or entirely on foods from plant sources. How do vegetarian eating plans differ?

Eating the Vegetarian Way

Vegetarian eating plans—and the people who follow them—are often described by the foods eaten:

- **Lacto-ovo-vegetarians** *eat dairy foods and eggs in addition to foods from plant sources.* This is the most common vegetarian eating style.
- **Lacto-vegetarians** *eat dairy foods in addition to foods from plant sources.*
- **Ovo-vegetarians** *eat eggs in addition to foods from plant sources.*
- **Vegans** (VEE-guns) *eat only foods from plant sources.*

Some people consider themselves "part-time" vegetarians. They may eat vegetarian meals several times each week but enjoy meat, poultry, and fish once in a while. You don't have to be a vegetarian to enjoy the flavors and food variety of this eating style!

Why choose a vegetarian eating style? Some people are vegetarians for religious or cultural reasons. Others choose to be vegetarians because they are concerned about animals or the world food supply. Many people are vegetarians because they want to follow a healthful eating style.

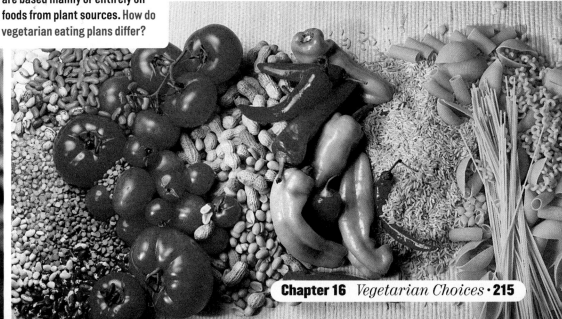

Check This Out!

PROTEIN THAT'S SOY GOOD

Soybeans are a good source of protein and other nutrients. They're versatile, too, because they're made into hundreds of different products. Look for these foods in supermarkets and specialty stores.

- **Tofu,** or *soybean curd,* is a cheeselike food that takes on the flavor of whatever you cook with it. It comes in firm, soft, and creamy textures and can be used in many ways.
- Tempeh (TEM-pay) is a fermented soybean patty with a nutty or smoky flavor. You can marinate and grill tempeh and crumble it into soups, casseroles, or chili.
- Soy milk is made by processing soybeans. It can be used as a beverage and in cooking. Soy milk is also made into other products such as soy cheese, soy yogurt, and frozen desserts.
- Textured soy protein (TSP) is sold as dry granules. When soaked in liquid, TSP has a texture similar to that of ground meat.
- Meat alternatives made from soy protein or tofu are designed to be used just like the foods they replace. Soy burgers are one example.

It's Your Turn!

Find a recipe using tofu and bring it to class. Compare with your classmates and see how many different uses for tofu you found.

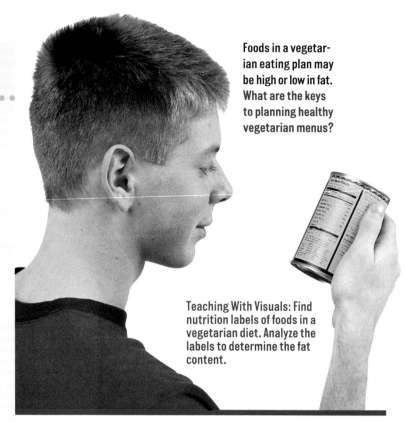

Foods in a vegetarian eating plan may be high or low in fat. What are the keys to planning healthy vegetarian menus?

Teaching With Visuals: Find nutrition labels of foods in a vegetarian diet. Analyze the labels to determine the fat content.

The Health Connection

Of course, the vegetarian style of eating isn't the only one that can be healthful! It's really a matter of your food choices. A well-planned vegetarian diet offers the health benefits of an eating plan that's often low in fat and cholesterol and high in fiber. Vegetarian eating plans aren't automatically more healthful than others, however. Any plan—including a vegetarian plan—is less healthful if it includes too many high-fat foods or sweets. Also, a vegetarian plan that lacks variety may come up short on certain nutrients.

Nutrition for Vegetarians

Eating more foods from plant sources matches the advice of the Dietary Guidelines for Americans: choose a diet with plenty of grain products, vegetables, and fruits. The key is to eat a variety of foods every day in recommended amounts!

The Pyramid for Vegetarians

The Food Guide Pyramid is flexible and can guide vegetarians in their food choices. In the Meat, Poultry, Fish, Dry Beans, Eggs, and Nuts Group, vegetarians can choose from a variety of nonmeat protein sources. Dry beans and peas, soy burgers, tofu, peanut butter, eggs, and sunflower seeds are good choices. In the Milk, Yogurt, and Cheese Group, vegans can substitute calcium-fortified soy milk and soy yogurt for dairy products.

To get enough energy and fill in nutrient gaps, vegetarian teens may need extra servings from the Fruit Group, the Vegetable Group, and the Bread, Cereal, Rice, and Pasta Group. A vegetarian plan is okay for kids, too, as long as they get enough variety and food energy for their growth and health.

Vegetarian Nutrition Challenges

Just as everyone does, vegetarians need to choose foods carefully. That helps ensure they get enough of each nutrient! Since the vegan eating plan excludes more foods, it presents special nutrition challenges.

Energy. Typical vegetarian meals—especially vegan meals—are filling when they're high in fiber. Therefore, children and teens following vegan diets may feel full before they get enough calories. Including some higher-calorie foods such as peanut butter, dried fruits, and nuts helps supply enough food energy for growth and development.

Protein. It's easy to get enough protein from plant foods. Remember, variety is the key! Eating a variety of plant-based foods each day can provide all the essential amino acids you need. Proteins in eggs and dairy foods also fill this need for lacto-ovo-vegetarians.

(**INFOLINK**)

You'll learn more about <u>nonmeat protein sources</u> in Chapter 26.

Discuss: What kinds of soybean products have you tried? Describe each product's taste, texture, and flavor.

Children and teens eating vegan meals may feel full before getting enough calories. Adding peanuts and nuts to dishes is one good way to get additional nutrients and calories. What role can these foods play in a healthful vegetarian eating plan?

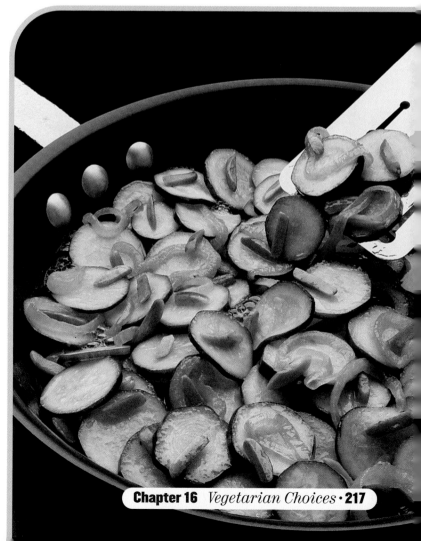

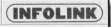

Tip

To see if foods are fortified with certain nutrients, such as vitamin B₁₂, vitamin D, and calcium, read food labels carefully. Added vitamins and minerals are listed on the Nutrition Facts panel.

INFOLINK

To review the functions of these nutrients, see Chapter 6.

Calcium. For lacto-vegetarians, dairy foods provide calcium for healthy bones and teeth. Vegans can get enough calcium from various sources. These include dry beans; seeds; certain vegetables such as broccoli, kale, and mustard greens; calcium-processed tofu; calcium-fortified soy milk; and calcium-fortified orange juice. Vegan teens and children need to pay special attention to getting enough of this nutrient.

Vitamin D. Milk fortified with vitamin D is a source for lacto-vegetarians. Vegans can get vitamin D from many fortified breakfast cereals and some soy beverages.

Vitamin B₁₂. Getting enough of this vitamin is easy for vegetarians who eat eggs and dairy products. Vegans can get vitamin B₁₂ from fortified foods, such as cereal, soy milk, and soy burgers.

Iron. For iron, vegetarians can choose enriched, fortified, and whole-grain cereals and breads, dry beans, seeds, dried fruits, and some dark green leafy vegetables. To help the body absorb iron, vegetarians should eat foods rich in vitamin C along with plant-based sources of iron.

Zinc. Whole-grain breads and cereals, dry beans, nuts, seeds, wheat germ, and tofu provide zinc. Eating a variety of these foods helps vegetarians get enough of this mineral. Dairy products also supply zinc.

Planning Vegetarian Meals

Vegetarian meals can be a feast of colors, flavors, and aromas. They can include many familiar foods and introduce you to new favorites, too. As an added benefit, vegetarian meals can be economical.

Planning and preparing healthful vegetarian meals can be a snap! Take your cues from the Food Guide Pyramid and keep the importance of food variety in mind. The chart on page 219 shows sample menus. Notice how many Pyramid servings are included in each. Which menu would a vegan enjoy?

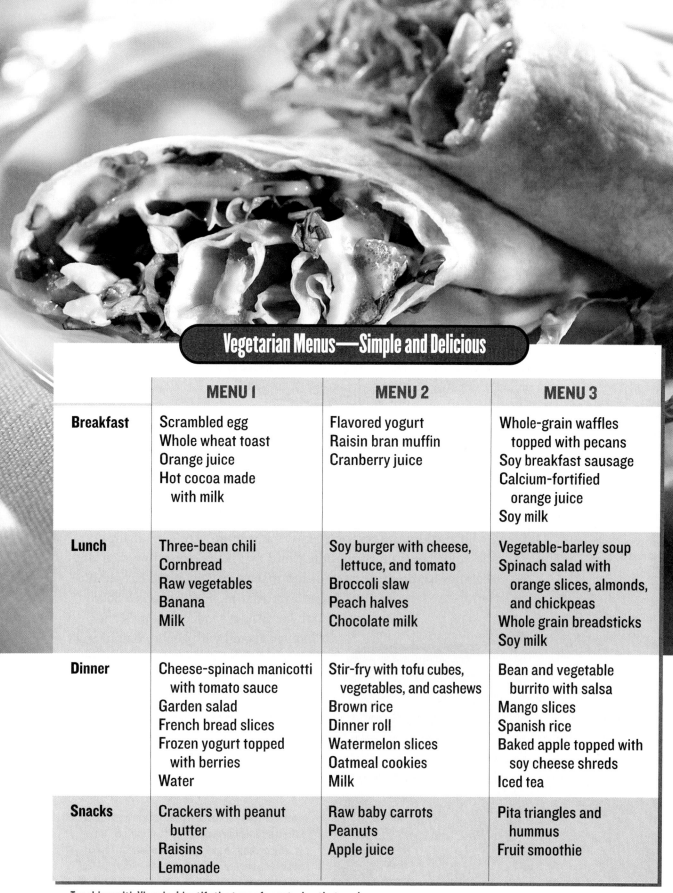

Vegetarian Menus—Simple and Delicious

	MENU 1	MENU 2	MENU 3

Breakfast	Scrambled egg
	Whole wheat toast
	Orange juice
	Hot cocoa made
	  with milk
		Flavored yogurt
		Raisin bran muffin
		Cranberry juice
			Whole-grain waffles
			  topped with pecans
			Soy breakfast sausage
			Calcium-fortified
			  orange juice
			Soy milk

Lunch	Three-bean chili
	Cornbread
	Raw vegetables
	Banana
	Milk
		Soy burger with cheese,
		  lettuce, and tomato
		Broccoli slaw
		Peach halves
		Chocolate milk
			Vegetable-barley soup
			Spinach salad with
			  orange slices, almonds,
			  and chickpeas
			Whole grain breadsticks
			Soy milk

Dinner	Cheese-spinach manicotti
	  with tomato sauce
	Garden salad
	French bread slices
	Frozen yogurt topped
	  with berries
	Water
		Stir-fry with tofu cubes,
		  vegetables, and cashews
		Brown rice
		Dinner roll
		Watermelon slices
		Oatmeal cookies
		Milk
			Bean and vegetable
			  burrito with salsa
			Mango slices
			Spanish rice
			Baked apple topped with
			  soy cheese shreds
			Iced tea

Snacks	Crackers with peanut
	  butter
	Raisins
	Lemonade
		Raw baby carrots
		Peanuts
		Apple juice
			Pita triangles and
			  hummus
			Fruit smoothie

Teaching with Visuals: Identify the type of vegetarian that each
menu is tailored to. (1. lacto-ovo; 2. lacto; 3. vegan)

Adapting Traditional Recipes

It's easy to modify many family favorites to make them vegetarian. Just make nutrient-rich substitutions for meat, poultry, and fish. Here are some ideas to get you started.

- Use extra beans in place of meat in chili.
- Substitute cooked beans or lentils in a casserole. Top with toasted nuts or seeds for added flavor and crunch.
- Add a variety of chopped vegetables to meatless spaghetti sauce.
- Top a pizza with extra vegetables and crumbled soy burgers.

For a vegan meal, replace dairy products, too.

- Use soy cheese in place of mozzarella on pizza.
- Try crumbled tofu in place of ricotta cheese for lasagna.
- Use soy milk or soy yogurt in baked goods.

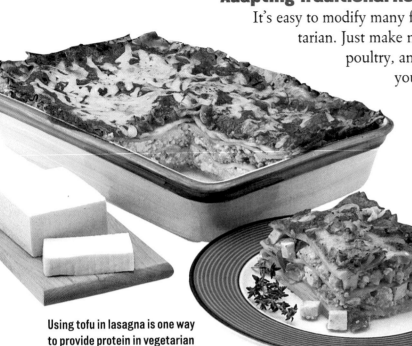

Using tofu in lasagna is one way to provide protein in vegetarian dishes. Think of a main dish with meat, poultry, or fish. How could you adapt it for a vegetarian meal?

Activity: Research and report on the following ethnic foods: *tabbouli, hummus, baba ghanoush, kasha varnishkas, colcannon, succotash,* and *ratatouille.* Which types of vegetarians could eat which foods?

Exploring Vegetarian Foods

Take your taste buds on a flavor adventure! Try some plant-based dishes from around the world that may be new to you. Many cultures feature vegetarian dishes that are delicious and easy to prepare. For instance, *mujudarah* is a Saudi Arabian dish. It's made from rice and lentils flavored with lemon, onion, and cumin. Look in ethnic and vegetarian cookbooks for recipes. Remember to explore the choices at ethnic restaurants, too. They offer many options for vegetarians.

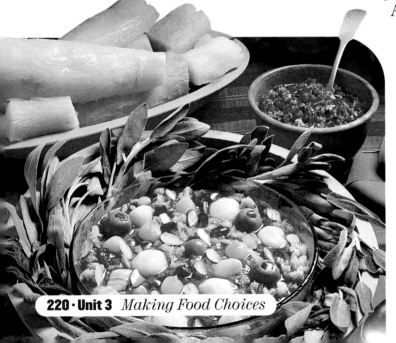

Vegetarian dishes are everyday fare in many parts of the world. Ethnic foods offer food variety, interest, and perhaps a new taste experience. **Find a recipe for a vegetarian dish you have not tried. Tell your classmates about it.**

NOW You're COOKING!

SKILL
Preparing a Vegan Side Dish

*C*ouscous—the name sounds exotic! Actually, it's a tiny pasta you can prepare quickly. In fact, it goes with any meal. Just mix in chopped nuts or cooked beans, and your couscous dish is a good source of protein.

RECIPE

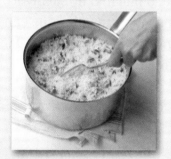

Orange-Thyme Couscous

CUSTOMARY	INGREDIENTS	METRIC
1 cup	Orange juice	250 mL
¾ cup	Couscous	175 mL
¼ cup	Chopped toasted pecans	50 mL
1 tsp.	Dried thyme leaves	5 mL

Yield: 4 servings, ½ cup (125 mL) each

❶ In tightly covered medium saucepan, bring orange juice to a boil. Stir in couscous and thyme.

❷ Remove from heat and cover pan. Let stand 5 minutes. Add pecans and fluff couscous with a fork before serving.

Per serving: 172 calories, 4 g protein, 28 g carbohydrate, 5 g fat, 6 mg sodium, 5 g fiber

Percent Daily Value: vitamin C 35%, thiamin 10%

More Ideas When you cook couscous, rice, oatmeal, and other grain products:

- Use a flavorful cooking liquid, such as juice or broth. What could you use in place of the orange juice?
- Add a spice, such as cinnamon or ginger, or herbs, such as chives.
- For more nutrition, add dried fruit or cooked beans.

Your Ideas Orange juice provides vitamin C, which helps your body use the iron in the nuts. It adds flavor, too. What other vitamin C–rich fruits or vegetables could make good "mix-ins" for this couscous dish?

LOOKING BACK

- Vegetarian eating plans are named after the type of foods eaten and are chosen for many reasons.
- The Food Guide Pyramid can guide vegetarians as they make their own healthful eating plans.
- Vegetarian meals may include familiar foods or introduce you to new plant-based dishes.

UNDERSTANDING KEY IDEAS

1. What type of vegetarian eating plan could include a cheese omelet? Compare a lacto-vegetarian eating plan with a vegan eating plan.
2. How might vegetarians use soy products at lunchtime?
3. What nutritional challenges do many vegans face? How might a vegan avoid potential nutritional gaps?
4. Describe two strategies for vegetarian meals that feature nutrition and variety.

DEVELOPING LIFE SKILLS

1. **Communication:** A vegetarian has been invited to a non-vegetarian's home for dinner. How can both of them use good communication and interpersonal skills to help make sure the dinner goes smoothly?
2. **Critical Thinking:** Rafael has several friends who have recently become vegetarians. They told him that by simply giving up meat, poultry, and fish, he can follow a healthful vegetarian eating plan. Is this information accurate? Explain.

Wellness Challenge

Nina is the only vegetarian in her large family. Her parents usually cook meals that include meat or poultry. They are too busy to make two separate dinners each night. Nina would like to have enjoyable meals with her family and maintain her vegetarian eating style.

1. How might Nina approach her parents with her concerns?
2. What solution might help Nina and her parents?

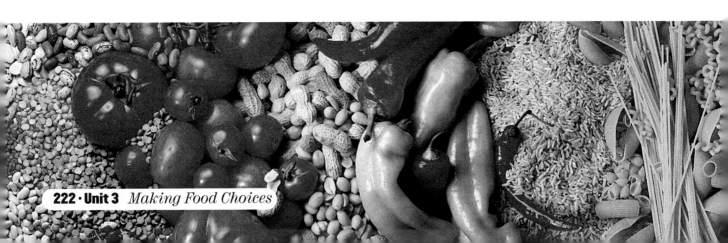

APPLYING YOUR LEARNING

1. **Simulation:** Obtain a take-out menu from a local deli or pizza parlor. In class, divide into groups and role-play the following situation: Several teens are having lunch at a deli or pizza parlor. One isn't a vegetarian, one is a vegan, and the others are lacto-ovo and lacto-vegetarians. Simulate the conversation the teens would have about the menu. Each student can describe what he or she would order and explain the reasons for that choice.

2. **Recipe File:** Vegetarian dishes are enjoyed around the world. Collect six recipes from different countries. Identify the nonmeat protein sources in each one. Add these recipes to your file.

EXPLORING FURTHER

1. **All About Soy:** Learn more about one food product made from soybeans. Choices may include tofu, tempeh, soy milk, or textured soy protein (TSP). What are the product's health benefits?

2. **Other Options:** Soy milk is a substitute for cow's milk. Find out about several other protein-rich, nondairy foods vegans can enjoy by doing research or by doing some food shopping. List the nutrients provided by each. If possible, sample a food or beverage and describe its flavor and texture.

Making CONNECTIONS

1. **Child Development:** Can pregnant women and young children healthfully follow a lacto-ovo-vegetarian eating plan? Find out how these groups can meet their special needs without eating meat, poultry, or fish. Present your findings to the class.

FOODS LAB

Cook and taste a soy burger. Describe its texture, color, and flavor. How does it rate nutritionally? How might you use a soy burger in different types of recipes?

2. **Math:** Would adopting a vegetarian eating plan save money? Compare the cost of a stir-fry dish using meat, poultry, or fish, vegetables, and a grain product to that of the same dish using tofu as a substitute for the meat, poultry, or fish. Share your findings with the class.

BREAD LINES

Next time you bite into a sandwich, you can thank John Montague for being the person credited with inventing it. Montague, a British nobleman, was the Fourth Earl of Sandwich. Legend has it that in the 1700s, he came up with the idea of placing meat or cheese between two thick slices of bread. No one is absolutely certain what gave him the idea, but it caught on. Soon, people all over Britain were eating this newfangled food. What to call it? The sandwich, of course! ■

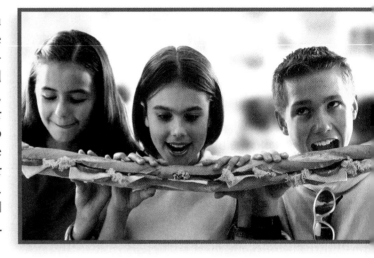

Like other sandwich fans, these kids can thank ▶ John Montague for his idea.

Truffle Snuffles

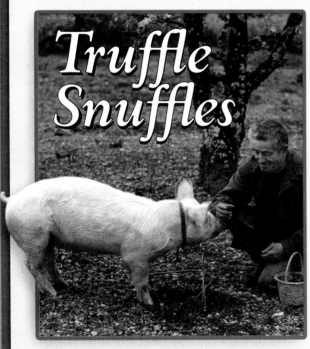

▲ **This little oinker in France has an expert snout for truffles.**

Truffles are one of the most prized delicacies in France and Italy and on the Italian island of Elba. A truffle, which is a type of fungus, can be the size of a small ball. They are used as flavorings and garnishes in dishes from eggs to chicken and beef. Black truffles generally grow in France. White truffles grow in Italy.

Truffles cost several hundred dollars each. Why so expensive? Truffles are rare. They grow in the fall and winter hidden underground near the base of forest trees. In Europe, truffle hunters use specially trained dogs to sniff them out. Female pigs are also used to find truffles, as the sows are naturally attracted to the truffle scent. Truffle seekers need to be careful with pigs, however, as the animals dig up the truffles and eat them. If pigs are used, they are gently muzzled. Dogs don't care for the fungi as much, and so they won't snack on them. ■

Food for thought

The Greeks have been eating ▶ olives since ancient times.

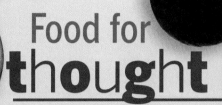

Olé to the doughnut

It seems the Spanish love garlic, rice, olives, and American doughnuts! Two well-known American doughnut chains have opened stores throughout the Mediterranean nation and report their doughnuts are selling like—hotcakes! Jelly and cinnamon flavored doughnuts appear to be favorites among the Spanish, who don't eat them for breakfast but enjoy them much later in the day. "The most doughnut sales in Spain take place after 5 in the afternoon," reports a spokesperson for one of the dough-nut chains. ■

Archaeologists and experts on ancient Greek literature have figured out what Greeks thought about food and what they ate some 4,000 years ago. Good diet was important to the ancient Greeks. They consumed foods that they thought would help keep them in good health and make them strong. Apparently, boiled beef—including large amounts of animal feet and noses—did the trick. Ancient Greeks also ate mutton, goat, wild boar, blackbirds, cuckoos, ducks, owls, and peacocks. Milk was drunk only if a person was sick. Butter was considered a food for people who didn't know better. Acorns were used as seasonings, and figs were a favorite fruit.

Greeks in cities, which were usually built by the sea, most likely ate more fish than meat. Octopus, shark, squid, and anchovies were eaten with gusto.

Some things never change, however. Then, as now, olives and olive oil were widely used. Wheat is still turned into bread, and honey is still a common sweetener. Modern Greeks eat lots of fish. Tomatoes, which were unknown to the ancient Greeks, are extremely popular today, as is creamy, thick yogurt. ■

Europe

From the Baltic Sea to the sunny shores of the Mediterranean, the British Isles, Western Europe, Russia, and Eastern Europe are filled with all kinds of wonderful and interesting foods to eat. Here's a tasty sampling.

Sweden In Swedish, *smörgås* means "open sandwich" and *bord* means "table." A smörgåsbord (SHMORE-gaz-bord) is not a table full of sandwiches, however. It's a buffet made up of many small dishes. There's always something fishy going on in a typical smörgåsbord. You'll find fresh and pickled herring and a dish made of sliced herring, potatoes, and onions baked in cream. You can dine on fresh salmon, roasted salmon, or salmon cured with salt and dill. For meat lovers, Swedish meatballs—made from a combo of meats (veal, pork, and beef) and flavored with spices and mustard—are a staple. Fill it all out with various beet, fish, and egg salads, breads, boiled and fried potatoes, and

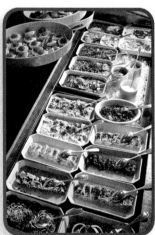

▲ What's to eat? Plenty in this Swedish feast!

Spaghetti with tomato sauce and basil is an Italian staple. ▶

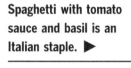

pies. In the 18th century, Swedes served smörgåsbord as an appetizer before the main course. Over the years, however, it has become a meal in itself.

Italy The cuisine in southern Italy includes many of the familiar dishes that Americans think of as Italian food. However, they tend to be simpler and have fewer ingredients than their American counterparts. Pasta is often a small first course followed by a meat, fish, vegetable, or pizza dish. Traditional foods in northern Italy include polenta, made from cornmeal; risotto, a creamy rice dish; and many hearty bean soups.

Russia "No dinner without bread," goes the Russian saying. Loaves made from wheat come in dozens of varieties. As for rye bread, more of it is eaten in Russia than in any other nation in the world. The bread often goes with cabbage and beet soups, as well as pelmeni (pell-m'ye-nee), small meat pies boiled in

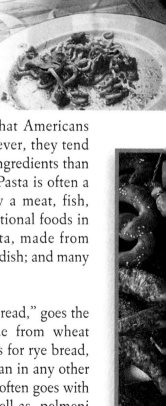

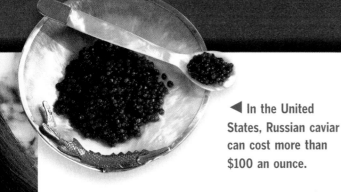

◀ In the United States, Russian caviar can cost more than $100 an ounce.

What's in a Name?

Some foods in the British Isles have unusual names.

Bangers and Mash: Sausages and mashed potatoes

Baps: Little white flour rolls

Cuppa: A cup of tea

Hotch Potch: A meat and vegetable stew

Rumbledethumps: Potatoes, onions, cabbage, and butter mashed together

Toad in the Hole: Link sausages and Yorkshire pudding (a type of popover)

broth. While regional cooking changes from area to area, some dishes are popular everywhere. These popular dishes include caviar (fish eggs from sturgeon), bliny (blee-nee), which are pancakes, and beef stroganoff—a delicious blend of meat and sour cream.

Russians start the day with a hearty breakfast of eggs, sausage, cold cuts, cheese, and bread and butter with tea or coffee. The main meal of the day is served around 1:00 P.M. It starts with appetizers such as caviar, pickles, smoked fish, and various vegetables. Go on to soup, and then the main course of meat or fish. The main dish is usually accompanied by a starch, such as potatoes, rice, or noodles, and fresh or marinated vegetables. Finally, there is dessert, which might be cake, stewed fruit such as apples and pears, or chocolates.

The evening meal is served around 7:00 P.M. or later. It's similar to the afternoon meal but without the soup and, often, dessert. All day long, Russians sip tea, and children often drink the sweet liquid from stewed fruit.

Germany Germans love sausages called "wursts" (verstz), and Germany has over 1,500 different

kinds. In fact, sausages are German snack food and can be purchased from street vendors. The meat is served on a roll with mustard, similar to the American hot dog.

All sorts of spicy sausages, salamis, and cold hams are served at a typical evening meal. Germany is famous for its sauerkraut (pickled cabbage) and spaetzle (SHPEHT-slee)—dumpling-like pieces of dough that are boiled and then served with meat dishes such as veal. Rabbits are a traditional food and are often served with juniper berries and the wild mushrooms that grow within Germany's many forests. Mustard and horseradish are two of the country's most popular condiments.

Germany's most famous dessert is probably strudel. It's made with a paper-thin dough that is rolled by hand. Fillings are usually cherry, apple, or cheese. ■

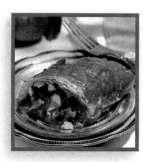

▲ Strudel is one of Germany's best-known desserts.

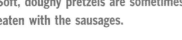

◀ Sausages are a German staple. Soft, doughy pretzels are sometimes eaten with the sausages.

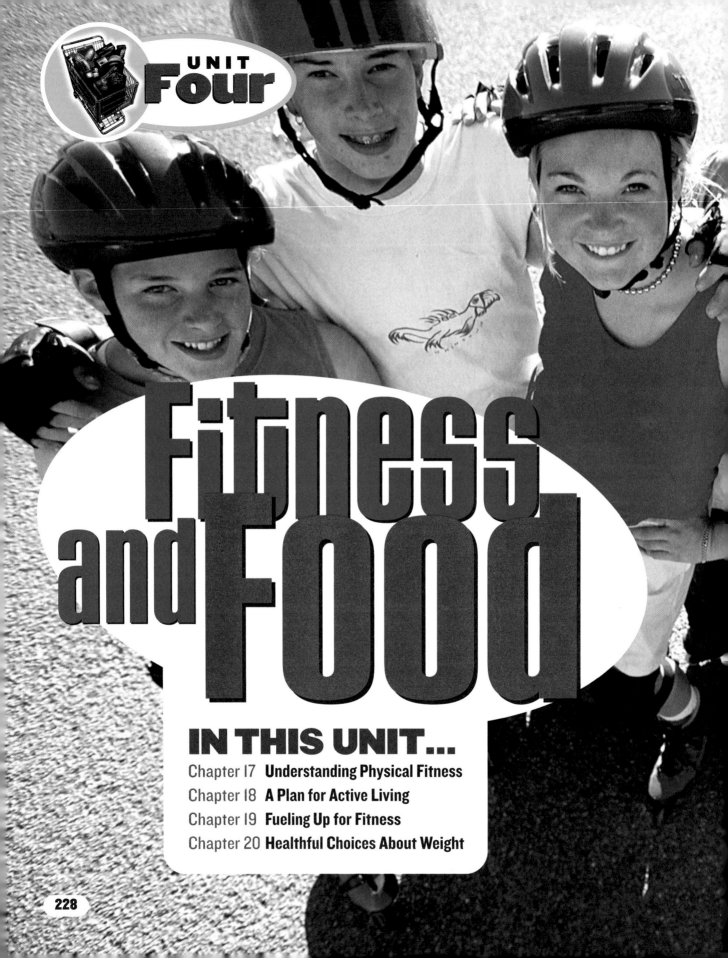

Fitness and Food

IN THIS UNIT...

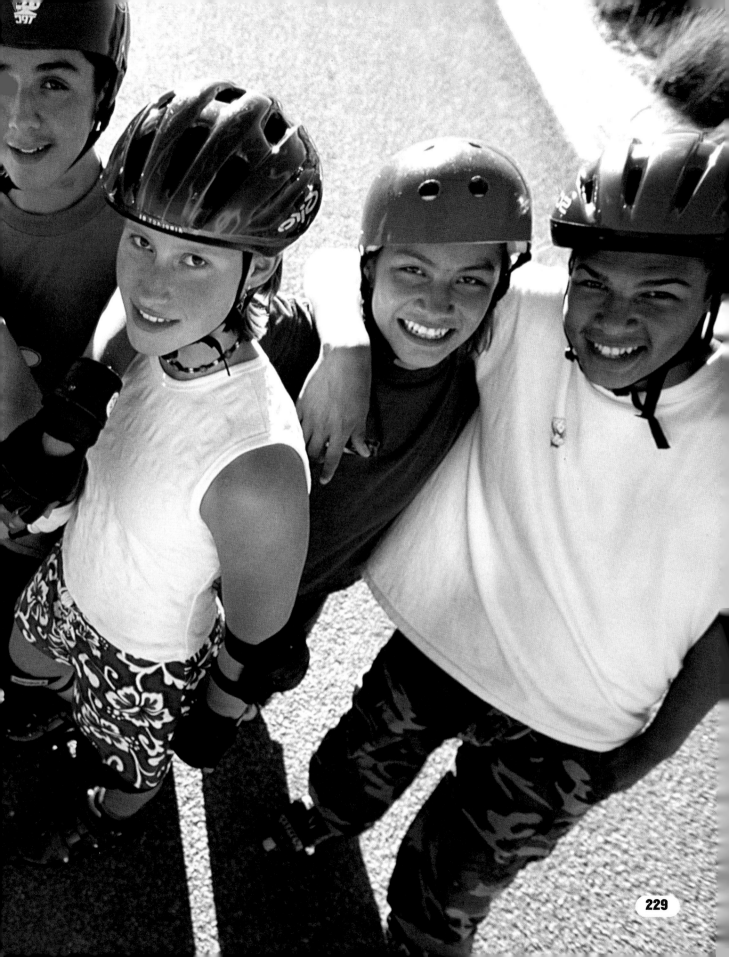

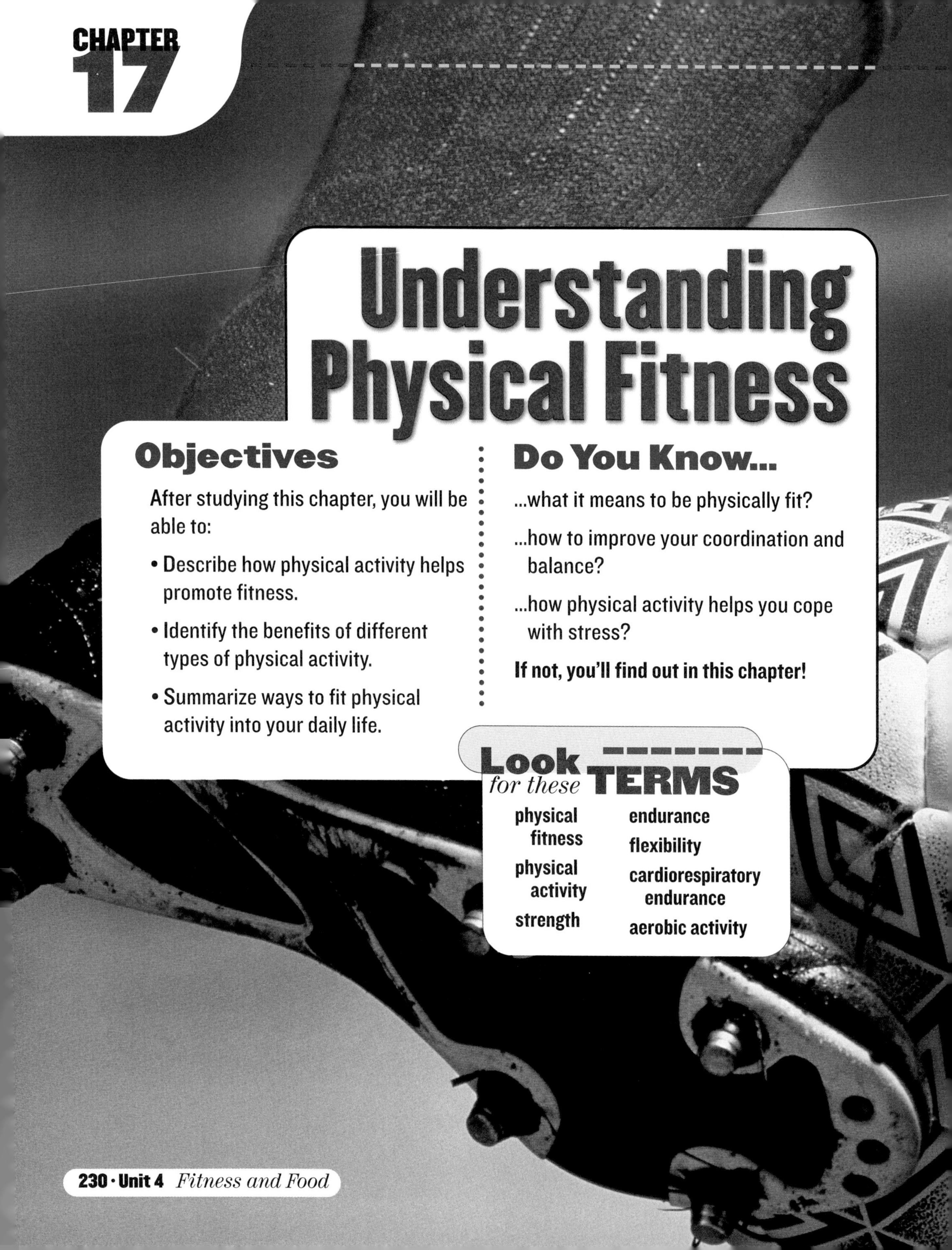

Understanding Physical Fitness

Objectives

After studying this chapter, you will be able to:

- Describe how physical activity helps promote fitness.

- Identify the benefits of different types of physical activity.

- Summarize ways to fit physical activity into your daily life.

Do You Know...

...what it means to be physically fit?

...how to improve your coordination and balance?

...how physical activity helps you cope with stress?

If not, you'll find out in this chapter!

Look *for these* TERMS

physical fitness

physical activity

strength

endurance

flexibility

cardiorespiratory endurance

aerobic activity

Would you like to

know how you can be stronger, feel more energetic, and look your best? The answer is quite simple—active living! These are just some of the rewards that come with being active. If you're not already active, challenge yourself to get up and get moving!

What Is Physical Fitness?

Being physically fit is more than the ability to lift heavy weights, run for long distances, or touch your toes. **Physical fitness** is *having the energy and ability to do everything you want and need to do in your daily life*. You're fit if you can meet the physical demands that come your way. **Physical activity**—*using your muscles to move your body*—helps you develop fitness. The more physically active you are, the more fit you're likely to be. You don't need to be an athlete to be active and physically fit!

There are several components of physical fitness.

Muscular strength and endurance. **Strength** is the *power to work your muscles against resistance*. When you have strength, you can lift heavy objects, such as bags of groceries or sports equipment, without strain. **Endurance** is *the ability to keep working your muscles without becoming overly tired*. Carrying a book-filled backpack for several blocks is a sign of muscular endurance.

Flexibility. Having *the ability to move your muscles and joints through their full range of motion* is a sign of **flexibility.** When you're flexible, you can more easily do everyday activities that require bending, reaching, and stretching.

Physical activity helps you develop fitness. What do you do to stay fit?

Coordination and balance. Having coordination and balance allows you to do things like hit a tennis ball and ride a bike. You're able to control your muscles and stay upright as you move your body.

Body composition. This is a measure of the proportions of fat, muscle, bones, and fluid that make up your weight. Chances are the more active you are, the greater the amount of your body that's made up of muscle. When you have more muscle, you're better able to be active!

Cardiorespiratory endurance. Can you walk up three flights of stairs without breathing heavily? **Cardiorespiratory endurance** is *how well your heart and lungs can keep up with your activity.* Doing aerobic activities increases your cardiorespiratory endurance. **Aerobic activities** are *activities that work your heart and lungs.* They rely on your ability to take in oxygen so that you can keep your muscles moving. The better your body uses oxygen, the more active you can be without tiring.

Varying the types of activities you do helps to develop each of the components of physical fitness. The chart that follows shows you how.

Different Activities, Different Benefits

Activity	Muscular Strength and Endurance	Flexibility	Coordination and Balance	Cardiorespiratory Endurance
Brisk walking	✔ (lower body)		✔	✔
Vigorous biking	✔ (lower body)		✔	✔
In-line skating	✔ (lower body)		✔	✔
Jumping rope	✔ (lower body)		✔	✔
Aerobic dancing	✔ (upper and lower body)	✔	✔	✔
Swimming	✔ (upper body)	✔		✔

Benefits of Physical Fitness

Being fit gives you a chance to look and feel your best. You can feel the benefits of active living today—and for a lifetime!

Looking Good

Smart eating and active living can have a positive effect on how you look! Physical activity helps you manage your weight by burning calories so that the extra you consume won't get stored as body fat. You may use up some energy reserves stored as body fat, too. By building muscle, physical activity also helps your body become more firm and toned.

Moving with Ease and Speed

Your muscles help you control your movements and posture. As you work your muscles and joints through regular physical activity, you become stronger, more coordinated, and more flexible. You have better balance and you move with more steadiness. Strong muscles and joints allow you to move with agility—and with speed.

Managing Stress

Physical activity is a healthful way to cope with stress. It gives you stamina so that you feel energetic and ready to handle whatever comes your way. It helps improve your mood, making it easier to concentrate and think positively. You'll sleep more soundly and feel more refreshed when you wake up. Being physically active helps you feel good about yourself, and that's bound to be reflected in everything you do!

Activity: What are your favorite activtities? How many calories are burned in a **30** minute period of each physical activity? Record your findings in a graph.

Physical activity can have psychological as well as physical benefits. It may help improve your mood and help you deal with stress. How does physical activity help you cope with stress?

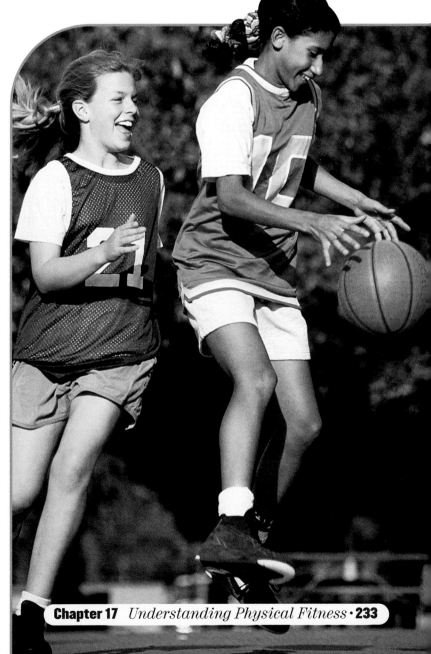

Activity: Compile a list of exercise classes or sports available in your community. Check out places such as local schools, the YMCA, and local park districts.

Activity: Work in small groups to brainstorm ways of getting more physical exercise in everyday activities. Share your group's ideas with the class.

Staying Physically Healthy

A physically fit body is often better able to fight disease and illness. Make physical activity a habit now—you'll reduce your chances of health problems as you get older! For instance, you can strengthen your bones with weight-bearing activities such as walking, soccer, or dancing. Combine this with getting enough calcium from your food choices, and your strong, dense bones will be less likely to break.

Having Fun

Physical activity should be fun! Try different activities until you find some you enjoy doing. If it seems like a chore, you won't stick with it. Being physically active with friends and family is a great way to spend quality time together. Team activities offer more than fitness, too. You build friendships and learn how to interact with others.

Getting and Staying Fit

Everyone has his or her own fitness potential. You can be as fit as your personal potential allows, whatever your shape or size. Your level of physical fitness depends on what you do and how often you do it. Even if you're busy, you can fit physical activity into your daily routine. It may just take a little thought and planning. Remember, eating smart and getting enough rest are important, too.

How Much Physical Activity?

You know it's smart to be physically active, but just how much activity is enough? Each day, try for about 60 minutes of moderately intense physical activity. Whatever you do, choose activities that you enjoy!

Activity doesn't need to be strenuous to have benefits. You might walk the dog, ride your bike, shoot baskets, dance fast to your favorite music—or help out with chores that keep you moving. If you can't carve out an hour at one time, do several shorter sessions during the day.

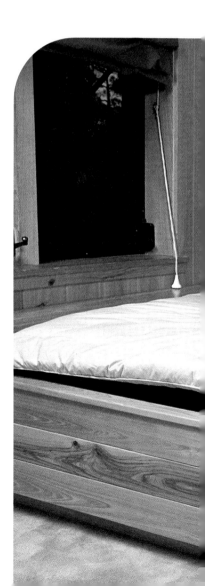

Another option is doing 20 to 30 minutes of more intense activities at least four days a week. Activities you might do include swimming, running, or playing basketball.

Can You Be Too Active?

Even for physical activity there are limits. Too much activity may cause injury and make you feel too tired to do other things. In females, it may cause problems with the reproductive cycle. Whenever you increase your activity level, do so gradually. Get plenty of rest and eat enough to fuel your active lifestyle. Talk to your doctor or a qualified expert to find out how much physical activity is too much for you.

Activity: Make a fitness contract with a friend or family member. Include fitness goals, benefits, and rewards.

Check This Out!

CHECKING YOUR FITNESS LEVEL

Perhaps you'd like to raise your current level of fitness. You can start by determining how well you perform on standard fitness tests, such as the President's Challenge. Fitness tests usually measure your abdominal strength and endurance, speed, heart and lung endurance, upper body strength, and flexibility.

Knowing your fitness level can motivate you to achieve more physically. It also can help you set realistic goals. Then as you continue your fitness program, you can compare your progress with your original test results. Your teacher or coach can help you learn more about fitness tests.

It's Your Turn!

Find out what activities are included in the President's Challenge. What does each activity measure?

INFOLINK

You can learn more about fitting physical activity into your life by reading Chapter 18.

How much time do you spend in front of a computer? Perhaps it's time to turn it off and enjoy some outdoor activities. What are other behaviors that cause you to be sitting instead of being active?

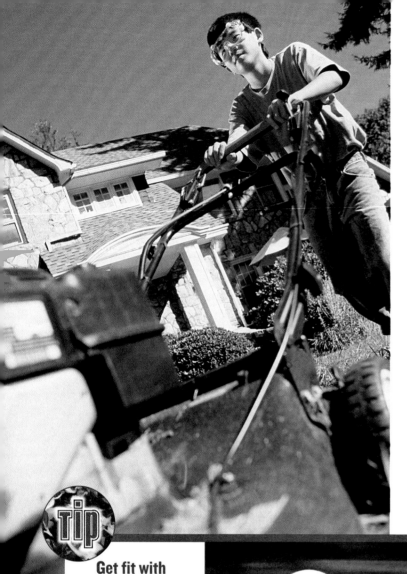

Physical activity doesn't have to be strenuous to be beneficial. Even everyday activities and chores, such as raking leaves or mowing the lawn, can count toward your 60 minutes. What chores contribute to your being physically active?

Physical Fitness— For Your Life!

Make physical fitness a lifelong goal! Being physically active when you're young gets you off to a healthy start. When you enjoy physical activity—and you do it regularly—it becomes a habit you'll want to continue for a lifetime! The activities you choose may change, but as long as you stay active, you'll continue to enjoy the benefits.

Activity: Create a life-cycle mural showing ways that people of different ages can keep active.

Tip

Get fit with friends. For instance, instead of sitting around talking, go skating or take a bike ride. Walk as you talk. Do laps around the mall as you window shop. What other fitness activities can you do with friends?

WELLNESS *in* ACTION

TEENS COMBAT "Too-Thin" Image

Physical fitness helps you look good—but is there too much pressure on teen girls to be thin? Too-thin models and very small clothes at stores make many girls feel fat when they aren't.

Students from Redmond High School in Washington decided to do something about it. "Rather than trying to conform," said Allie Kingsley, "we need to respect ourselves and our different body sizes. That's healthier than putting ourselves down!"

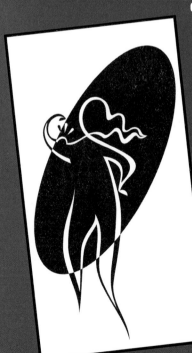

The teens took action as part of GO GIRLS, a program created by the National Eating Disorders Association. They talked and wrote to advertisers and store managers. As a result, a Seattle department store agreed to show some trendy teen clothes on larger mannequins and display size 13 jeans, not just size 3.

The students' Great Jeans Exchange told growing teens: "Don't fight your genes. Change your jeans!" In other words, get the size that fits you now. Students turned in 200 pairs of jeans for a fundraiser.

"We need to get the message to younger kids—before their attitudes are formed," said Brandy Gove, who talked to fourth-grade girls about body image. Bri Odle was so committed that she created a public relations campaign to share the program.

Take Action

What teen-targeted marketing messages about body size and shape do you see? How do they compare with what you're learning about fitness, growth, and being the size that's right for you? Do something to help promote a healthy body size for teens.

LOOKING BACK

- Physical fitness involves muscular strength and endurance, flexibility, coordination and balance, body composition, and cardiorespiratory endurance.
- Physical fitness can help you look good, move with ease and speed, manage stress, stay physically healthy, and have fun.
- Your level of physical fitness depends on what you do and how often you do it. You can fit physical activity into your daily routine even if you're busy.
- Make physical fitness a lifetime goal.

UNDERSTANDING KEY IDEAS

1. What is cardiorespiratory endurance? How might improving it enable you to reach new fitness goals?
2. Why might aerobic dancing be a wise choice for all-around fitness?
3. How might physical activity improve your mental and emotional health?
4. Describe several ways you might fit physical activity into your daily life if you have a busy schedule.
5. Why are there limits to the amount of physical activity a person should do?

DEVELOPING LIFE SKILLS

1. **Critical Thinking:** Jamal recently decided to fit physical activity into his daily routine. He invited his friend Derek to join him three mornings a week before school for a brisk 30-minute walk. Derek says that if he has to get up early to perform physical activity, he will be tired for the rest of the day. What is the flaw in Derek's logic?
2. **Leadership:** How might teens encourage older adults in their family to be physically active? Why is this important?

Wellness Challenge

Through this past summer and the early months of autumn, Mieko and her friends went in-line skating and played tennis and volleyball outside at least three or four times a week. Now that the winter months and snow have arrived, they haven't been doing much physical activity. Mieko would like to stay fit even if she can't be active outdoors, and she'd like to encourage her friends to do the same.

1. What options might help Mieko and her friends stay active?
2. How might Mieko encourage her friends to join her in staying fit?

APPLYING YOUR LEARNING

1. **Personal Fitness Record:** Keep track of your schedule for three typical days. Count physical activity sessions that last at least ten minutes. Be sure to include team practices, helping out with chores, and other activities that keep you moving. Do you need to be more active? Look at your schedule to see how you can fit in more activity.

2. **Job Application:** Write a letter of application for a job at a local physical fitness center. In your letter, describe how you would use your knowledge of physical fitness and its benefits to motivate people.

EXPLORING FURTHER

1. **All-around Sports:** Athletes who compete in triathlons must be in top condition. Using library or Internet research, find out what a triathlon is, what events it includes, and how athletes train for this competition.

2. **Safe Stretches:** Investigate recommended stretches to improve flexibility. What muscle(s) does each stretch? What are correct and incorrect ways to perform the stretch? Prepare a visual report or video for the class.

Making CONNECTIONS

1. **Health:** Find out more about the Presidential Physical Fitness Award program. When did it start? What is its purpose? How do you participate? Create a poster promoting this program.

2. **Science:** During physical activity the brain releases endorphins, a type of chemical, into the body. Learn more about this chemical. What role does it play in the relationship between physical activity and reduced stress? Share your findings with the class.

FOODS LAB

Weight-bearing exercises and calcium are great ways to strengthen your bones during your teen years. Yogurt is a good source of calcium and a convenient, healthful snack. Compare yogurt that has fruit already mixed in with plain yogurt to which you add your own choice of fruit. How does the flavor compare? The costs?

A Plan for Active Living

Objectives

After studying this chapter, you will be able to:

- Propose solutions to common obstacles to active living.

- Explain how to develop and carry out a plan for physical activity.

- Describe factors to consider when choosing physical activities.

- Identify ways to keep physical activity safe and healthy.

Do You Know...

...how to make a fitness plan and stick with it?

...why you need to warm up and cool down in your workout?

...how to make physical activity fun?

If not, you'll find out in this chapter!

Look *for these* **TERMS**

sedentary   intensity

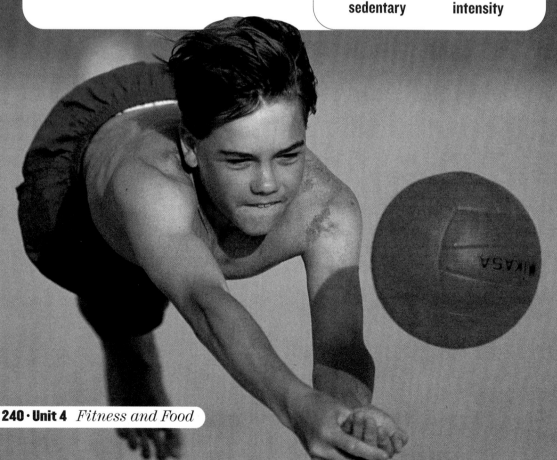

What's the right

path to fitness for you? The answer depends on you and your interests and goals. In Chapter 1, you learned about making an action plan for wellness. That step-by-step approach works just as well for increasing your level of activity as it does for reaching any other wellness goal. This chapter will show you how!

How Active Are You?

How would you give someone directions to your home or your school? Wouldn't you need to know where the person is starting from? The same is true of setting fitness goals. Start by taking a look at how active you are now. Knowing your starting point will help you decide what goals to set and how to reach them!

Over the past week, how much did you get up and move? Remember the guidelines you learned in Chapter 17—about 60 minutes of moderately intense physical activity each day, or 20 to 30 minutes of more intense activities at least four days a week. Did you get that much physical activity? If so, great! If not, what gets in your way? Some common reasons that people give for not being active are listed here. As you'll see, there's usually a simple solution.

• *"I don't have time."* Just as you do for other priorities in your life, you can find the time to be active. It's up to you! Remember, you can break up physical activity into short sessions that fit easily into your day. It can be as simple as taking the stairs instead of the elevator.

• *"It isn't fun."* Just choose a variety of activities you enjoy! You'll find ideas throughout this chapter.

• *"I don't like to sweat."* Physical activity doesn't have to be strenuous. Anything you do to get moving helps. There's nothing wrong with sweating, though—it cools you off.

Remember playing tag as a kid? Now that you're a teen, you may have outgrown tag—but not the fun of physical activity. How can you make physical activity part of your everyday routine?

• *"None of my friends do it."* You're being active for you—not your friends. If friends won't join you, you might let them know how good you feel from being active. Before long, they'll want to experience the same benefits!

• *"I'm too uncoordinated."* Becoming more coordinated is one of the benefits of becoming more physically fit. Start with an activity that suits your abilities. As you gain confidence, add different activities.

Setting Your Goals

Spending more time being active, if you need to, is a great goal for a fitness plan. Perhaps you have other goals, too. What would you like to gain from being physically active—feeling good, looking your best, improving your health? Perhaps you want to be able to run a distance without getting too breathless or to qualify for a sports team.

Setting goals helps you design and stick with a fitness program. You can check your progress with your goals in mind. The best goals are challenging but realistic for you.

Choosing Physical Activities

For your action plan to succeed, you need to decide how to work toward your goal. When it comes to physical activity, you have plenty of options! Here are just a few ideas to get you started.

Outdoor recreation: biking, in-line skating, running, walking, hiking, downhill or cross-country skiing, canoeing.

Indoor recreation: stationary cycling, all kinds of dancing, stair climbing, aerobics, jumping rope, exercise videos and classes.

Team sports: basketball, field hockey, soccer, volleyball, softball, football, baseball, track, cross-country running, water polo.

Activity: Make a "Top 5" list of favorite activities. What are the benefits of each? Review the chart on page 232. Are your activities meeting all your needs?

Individual and partner sports: tennis, racquetball, handball, squash, swimming, rowing.

Lifestyle activities: walking to school, mowing the lawn, washing the car, shoveling snow, vacuuming, raking leaves.

How can you choose? Start by thinking about what you might enjoy most. Remember, too, that different activities have different benefits. Some work your heart and lungs; some help strengthen your upper or lower body; some help you stay flexible. Choose activities with benefits that match your goals.

The activities you choose can be recreational—just for fun—or part of an organized sport. They can be individual, partner, or team activities. It's up to you! Survey the members of your school sports teams. Why do the students participate? What do they feel are the benefits?

Activity: Make a "wish list" of activities you would enjoy doing. How can you get started?

INFOLINK

To review the benefits of different activities, see Chapter 17, page 232.

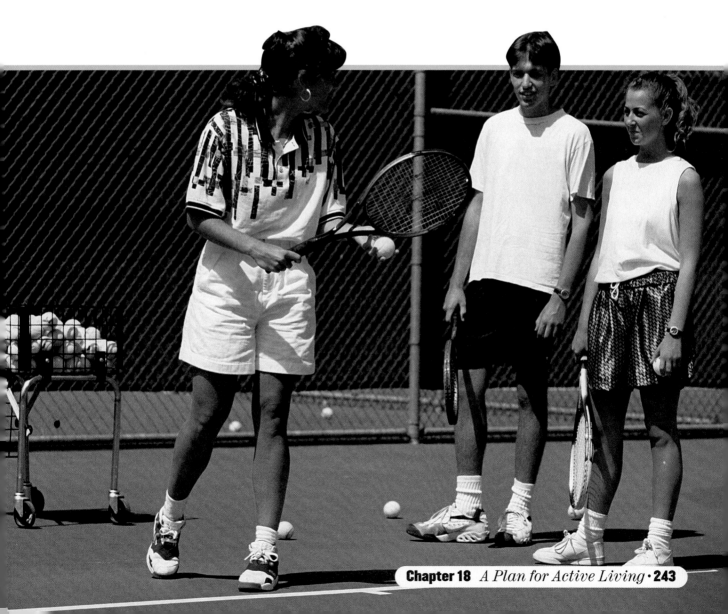

Chapter 18 *A Plan for Active Living* · **243**

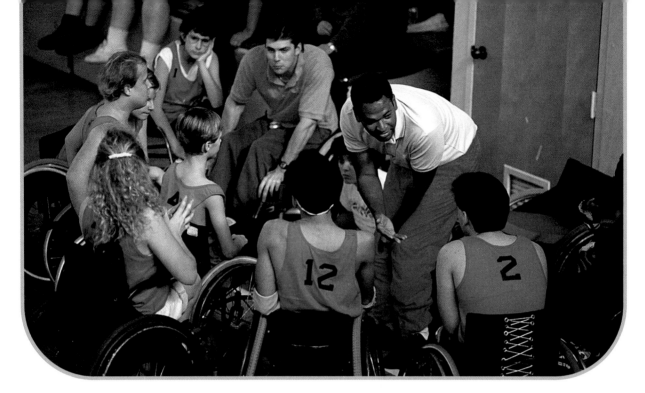

Everyone can benefit from physical activity. Find out what opportunities for physical activities exist for physically challenged teens in your area.

Tip

Lifting heavy weights isn't recommended for younger teens because you can damage your growing bones easily. To build muscle strength and endurance, work your muscles using your own weight as resistance. For instance, you can do push-ups or leg lifts.

Also consider whether the activity is convenient and affordable for you. Some activities require special equipment or clothing or access to a specific place, such as a swimming pool. Other activities, such as walking, have few special requirements.

You don't have to settle on one activity. For all-around fitness—and fun—it's a good idea to vary your fitness routine. That way you can combine the benefits of different activities, and you won't get bored.

Ready, Set, Go!

You've set your goals and picked your activities. Now it's time to put some action into your plan!

Remember to break your goals into small, achievable steps. Take one step at a time. If one of your overall goals is to build strength, you might set a mini-goal of doing a certain number of push-ups. Work up to it gradually by trying to do just a few more each time you work out. When you achieve a mini-goal, challenge yourself with another target.

Starting slowly is especially important if you've been **sedentary**, or *physically inactive*. Work up to your goal gradually while you get used to the increased activity.

Discuss: What kinds of safety gear are needed for your favorite physical activity?

GET FIT WITH F.I.T.

*P*ay attention to the **F.I.T.**—*F*requency, *I*ntensity, and *T*ime (duration)—of your workouts. To improve your level of physical fitness, gradually increase all three factors over time.

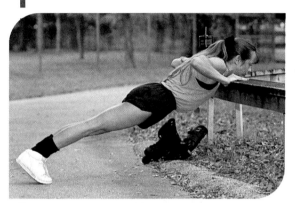

FREQUENCY—*how often you work out.* You might begin with two or three days a week and gradually increase to five days.

INTENSITY—*the speed and power of your movements.* This might mean how much you hustle on the basketball court or the height of the step in step aerobics. Over time, the same level of intensity will begin to seem easier as you build strength and endurance. Gradually turn up the intensity to give your body a new challenge.

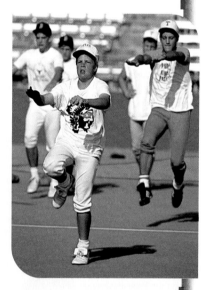

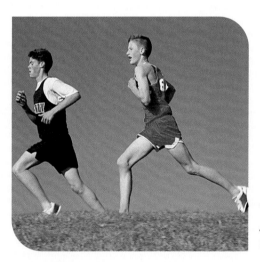

TIME (duration)—*how long you work out at each session.* Begin with just a few minutes at a time. Gradually work up to longer sessions.

Investigate Further

Talk to a school coach to find out how he or she increases the frequency, intensity, and time of workouts to get the players into shape for the sports season.

The Talk/Sing Test

Check your intensity level by talking and singing. If you can talk while working out, you're probably moving at a pace that's right for you. Slow down if you're too breathless to talk. If you can sing, you may not be working hard enough.

Chapter 18 *A Plan for Active Living* • **245**

Playing It Safe

Emphasize: Never run alone. Make sure you wear clothing that allows you to be seen easily by others.

Whether your physical activity is for fun, fitness, or competition, make health and safety a priority. You can prevent injuries and discomfort that may occur with physical activity.

Get in Gear!

Always wear protective gear, such as a helmet and knee pads, for activities that require them. These include in-line skating, biking, and snow skiing. Before outdoor physical activity, consider the weather and choose appropriate clothing. Use sunscreen when you're in the sun.

Warming Up and Cooling Down

Discuss: What can you do to warm up and cool down for your favorite physical activity?

With more intense activity, it's important to warm up before your workout, then cool down afterward. You'll experience less soreness and lower your chance for injury.

Warming up prepares your muscles for a workout and increases your heart rate gradually. Do 5 to 10 minutes of a slower, gentler version of your activity. For instance, you might walk before jogging, do some light marching in place before aerobics, or bike slowly before going all out.

People who stay active throughout their lives can delay the loss of strength, flexibility, and endurance that's associated with aging. Survey older adults to find out which physical activities they enjoy. How do they stick with their physical fitness plan?

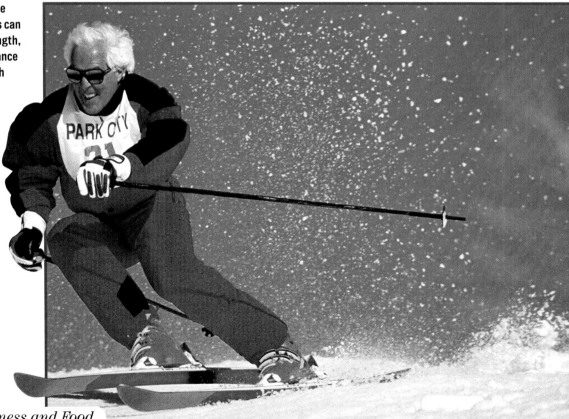

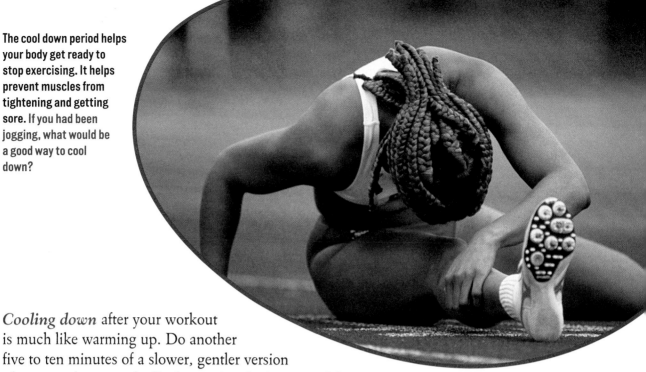

The cool down period helps your body get ready to stop exercising. It helps prevent muscles from tightening and getting sore. If you had been jogging, what would be a good way to cool down?

Cooling down after your workout is much like warming up. Do another five to ten minutes of a slower, gentler version of your workout, gradually decreasing the intensity. Now is a good time for some gentle stretching exercises, too. Your muscles are more elastic after working out, which means they stretch more easily and safely. Stretching can improve your flexibility and may help prevent stiffness and soreness.

Fluids and Fuel to Go On

To help performance and prevent dehydration, drink plenty of fluids before, during, and after your activity. Be sure to eat enough to fuel your active lifestyle, too.

Keep It Up!

If something keeps you from being physically active for a day or more, figure out what the obstacle is. Look at your fitness plan. Do you need to revise it a little to overcome the obstacle? For example, if you're too tired, try working out at a different time of day. If you're not enthusiastic, consider a different type of activity. Do you just "forget" to make time for physical activity? Try scheduling it for a specific time and writing it on your calendar.

Let the people around you—family, friends, coaches—know about your fitness plan and your goals. Their support can encourage you to succeed. Invite others to join you in your routine. Being active with a friend can make it more enjoyable—and you can motivate each other. It's also a great way to spend quality time with others. Everyone benefits!

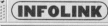

You'll learn more about fueling up for physical activity in Chapter 19.

Discuss: Why do people who exercise with a partner tend to stick with it longer than if they were exercising alone?

Emphasize: You can exercise while watching your favorite television program. You could bicycle on a stationary bike, jog in place, or do sit-ups and push-ups.

Checking Your Progress

Keeping a fitness log will help you keep track of your activities. Write down all your daily physical activities, including their intensity and duration. Are you achieving your goals and following your strategies?

Progress can also be measured in other ways: Do you feel more energetic? Can you run for the bus without feeling out of breath? Are you swimming more laps in a shorter amount of time? How you measure your progress depends on your goals and your personal action plan.

If you're not making progress, use your log to see how you've been following your fitness plan. You may need to change your strategies or overcome some challenges. Perhaps your original goal was too ambitious. Maybe you need to allow yourself more time. Don't let slower progress or obstacles keep you from your goal.

If you've achieved your goal, congratulations! Give yourself a pat on the back. Now you're ready to set a new, more challenging goal. It's another step on your path to fitness!

More About Your Fitness Plan: Review your fitness log. If needed, substitute activity for inactivity. For example, instead of talking on the phone with your best friend, go for a walk together and talk.

Try to be patient. Achieving fitness takes time. Keep a physical activity log for the next four weeks. Record your progress. In what areas have you improved?

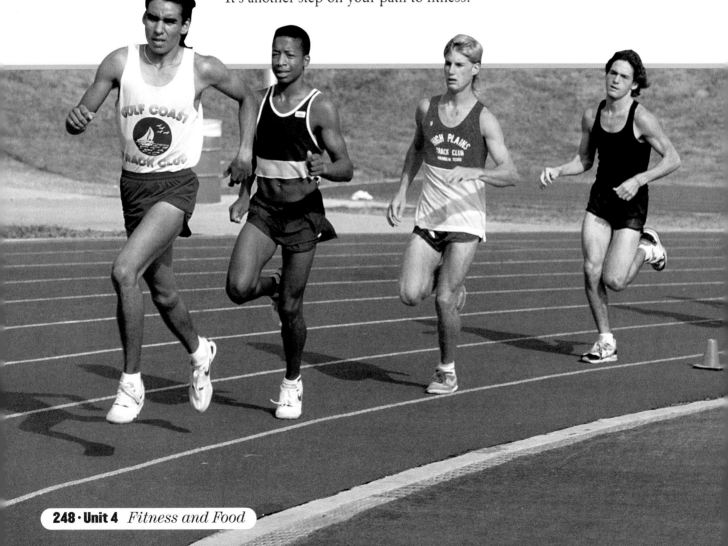

CAREERS *in*

HELP WANTED

Nutrition/Health Educator

Large food company has business opportunity for a dynamic, motivational educator to inform and inspire our distributors. Represent our nutrition and health products at large public speaking engagements and small group workshops. Ideal candidate must be a registered dietitian and have at least two years of experience as an educator. Must be able to work evenings and weekends. Send resume to Human Resources, New Way Foods, Inc.

Merchandise Displayer

Retail supermarket has an entry level opening for a merchandise displayer. Design and create settings to show off merchandise and attract customers' attention. On-the-job training. High school diploma required. Must be creative and have good mechanical aptitude. Apply at the National Stores.

Business Dietitian

New opportunity for a Registered Dietitian to assist in developing sales and promotional ideas for our new line of low-fat products. Work in our corporate headquarters using your background and knowledge in nutrition. Excellent oral and written communication skills required. Competitive salary and benefits. Send resume to Executive Director, Nutrition Resources.

Account Manager

Advertising and public relations firm seeks an Account Manager for restaurant accounts. Oversee development of high quality ads for print and electronic media. Must be able to motivate and manage creative teams. Bachelor's degree required with advertising related internship preferred. Apply in person at Chavez & Associates.

Assistant Art Director

Advertising firm has an immediate opening for an Assistant Art Director specializing in food. Develop visual concepts and designs for weekly print advertisements for supermarket chain. Must be creative, have excellent computer skills, and be willing to keep pace with advancing technology. Two-year degree from art or design school preferred. Send resume to Washington Design, Inc.

Food Writer

The Community Journal has position open for a Food Writer. Develop weekly section on food including recipes, health issues, fitness trends, and nutrition. Registered dietitian preferred with good writing skills. Must express ideas clearly and be able to meet deadlines. Send resume and writing sample to Editor, *The Community Journal*.

LINKING *to the* WORKPLACE

❶ Ad Campaign: Develop a print ad campaign for a new brand of canned soup.

❷ Entrepreneurship: Someone who owns his or her own business is an entrepreneur. List ideas for starting businesses in the nutrition and food industries.

LOOKING BACK

- Set realistic fitness goals by determining how active you are now and deciding what you want to accomplish.

- Break your goals into achievable steps. Check your progress with a fitness log.

- Play it safe. Wear protective gear, warm up before a workout and cool down afterward, and get adequate amounts of fluids and food.

- If you aren't physically active for a day or more, figure out what the obstacle is and adjust your fitness plan if necessary.

UNDERSTANDING KEY IDEAS

1. How could a busy teen involved in several after-school activities overcome the obstacle of not having time for physical activity?

2. Describe the steps you'd take to create and carry out a physical activity plan.

3. If you lived in a warm climate and didn't have any special fitness equipment, what physical activities might you choose?

4. What does F.I.T. mean? How can increasing your F.I.T. help you carry out a fitness plan?

5. How do warming up before and cooling down after activity lessen the risk of injury?

6. What might you do if you're not achieving your fitness goals?

DEVELOPING LIFE SKILLS

1. **Critical Thinking:** Elena feels awkward with activities that require a lot of coordination such as gymnastics and dance. She'd like to try out for the field hockey team, but she doubts her athletic ability. What assumptions might Elena be making? What might she consider to help her give field hockey a try?

2. **Management:** What might happen if someone set fitness goals that are too high? Too low? How can you tell whether you're setting goals that are right for you?

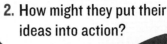

Wellness Challenge

Rahim and Josh realize that they aren't as physically active as they need to be and that many of their friends aren't either. They'd like to find ways to be more active after school and on weekends. As an added benefit, they hope to encourage physical activity among their peers and younger children in their community.

1. What are several alternatives that Rahim and Josh could suggest?

2. How might they put their ideas into action?

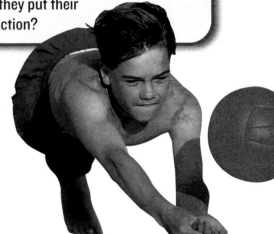

APPLYING YOUR LEARNING

1. **Fitness Survey:** Take a survey of family members, friends, and classmates to find out what reasons people give for not being active. Also ask them to suggest solutions for overcoming fitness obstacles. Create a chart that shows the results of your survey and compare them to the obstacles and solutions identified in this chapter. Are they the same or different?

2. **In the News:** Imagine it is two years from now. Write a news article about yourself and how you achieved a fitness goal. Describe what your fitness level was when you began and the steps you took to reach your goal.

EXPLORING FURTHER

1. **Preventing Injury:** Many sports-related injuries occur when inactive people suddenly begin vigorous activity or when people don't warm up and cool down. One common activity-related injury is shin splints. Learn more about shin splints, including the symptoms, causes, and methods of prevention.

2. **Expert Advice:** Using library or Internet research, choose an athlete whom you admire. What activities are part of the athlete's training program during a typical week? What does he or she do to stay motivated?

Making CONNECTIONS

1. **Language Arts:** Protective gear such as knee, wrist, and elbow pads; helmets; and mouthpieces can prevent serious injuries, but not all teens use them. Find out how many sports-related injuries occur among teens each year. Write an article for the school or community newspaper encouraging teens to use protective gear.

2. **Math:** Survey friends, family, students, and directors of community centers to find out which activities people are enjoying. Divide them into the categories shown on page 243 and create a bar graph to show the percentages. Compare your findings in class.

FOODS LAB

Imagine that you are planning a day-long hike or canoe trip. Find recipes for some snacks you could take along. Prepare one of the snacks. Rate its flavor, texture, and appeal. How does it rate nutritionally? Why would the snack be easy to take along on a hike?

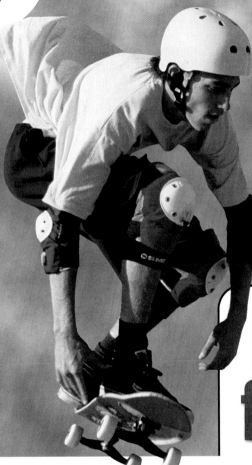

Fueling Up for Fitness

Objectives

After studying this chapter, you will be able to:

- Describe how physical activity affects your nutrient needs.

- Explain why fluids are important before, during, and after physical activity.

- Discuss smart food and beverage strategies for peak performance.

- Distinguish between facts and myths about sports nutrition.

Do You Know...

...why you need to drink fluids even if you're not thirsty?

...what helps build bigger muscles?

...what's best to eat and drink before, during, and after a workout or competition?

If not, you'll find out in this chapter!

Look *for these* TERMS

electrolytes

carbohydrate loading

Nutrition fuels

fitness! An eating plan with the right amount of nutrients and energy for you is a smart strategy for peak performance. Whether you're preparing for tryouts, competing in a sports event, or being active for fun and fitness, smart eating can help you do your very best.

Nutrients for Active Living

The best eating plan for active living follows the advice of the Food Guide Pyramid. Whether you're an athlete or not, the Pyramid plan supplies all the nutrients you need. With increased energy needs, you'll need to consume more than the minimum number of servings.

Plenty of carbohydrates. Active teens need extra calories for energy. Get most of them from nutrient-dense foods high in complex carbohydrates—bread, cereal, rice, pasta, dry beans and peas, vegetables, and fruits. Remember, "carbs" are your body's main energy source!

Enough, but not too much, protein. Getting enough protein is easy when you eat two to three servings each day from the Meat, Poultry, Fish, Dry Beans, Eggs, and Nuts Group. Beyond that, extra protein won't help you build bigger muscles. Physical activity—along with just enough protein—does that. Your body uses extra protein for energy or stores it as fat.

Enough vitamins and minerals. Following Pyramid guidelines—with a variety of foods—provides vitamins and minerals in the amounts you need. Eat calcium-rich foods for healthy bones and iron-rich foods for healthy blood.

Enough water. During intense activity, your body sweats to help reduce the heat generated by muscles and to cool you down. By drinking plenty of fluids, you will help replace what you lose by perspiring. Each pound of weight loss from sweating requires 2 cups (500 mL) of water to replace it!

Activity: Study the school lunch menu and decide what foods need to be eaten in other meals for a balanced diet for a physically active teen.

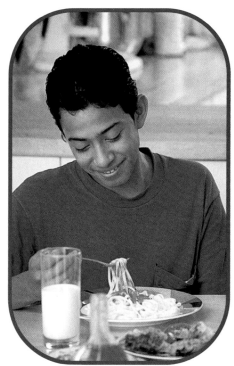

Smart eating should be part of your body's ongoing fitness program. What are some of the nutrients these foods supply?

Check This Out!

HIGH-PERFORMANCE MEALS

These examples of high-carbohydrate meals can help fuel your body for a heavy workout or competition. Although you can eat them at any time of the day, they're good a few hours before physical activity.

- Orange juice
- Bagel
- Peanut butter
- Apple slices

- Apple juice
- Pancakes and syrup
- Low-fat yogurt
- Strawberries

- Grapefruit juice
- Cornflakes with low-fat milk
- Banana
- Wheat toast with jelly

- Baked potato with broccoli and shredded low-fat cheese
- Low-fat pudding
- Apple juice

- Spaghetti and tomato sauce with mushrooms
- French bread
- Low-fat milk

- Tomato soup
- Grilled cheese sandwich
- Fruit salad
- Low-fat milk

It's Your Turn!

Plan three other meals an athlete could eat before a workout or competition. Trade with a classmate and evaluate each other's plans.

Tip

Energy bars that contain carbohydrates, protein, and fat can be convenient— but expensive— ways to get energy before or during physical activity. The food suggestions in this chapter work just as well.

Choices for Peak Performance

When you're involved in strenuous or prolonged physical activity, eat smart. Choosing foods carefully can help you perform your best. What you eat and drink before, during, and after physical activity takes thought and planning.

Before You're Active

About three to four hours before a vigorous workout or competition, enjoy a meal that's high in starches and low in fat and protein. This nutrient combination is easy to digest, a plus before physical activity. Also, it provides your body with energy to power your working muscles. Eat enough so that you are satisfied but not too full. Drink plenty of fluids as well. If necessary, you can eat a light snack, such as fruit, about a half hour before you're active. Eating sugary foods such as candy before a workout or event does not provide quick energy. Instead, it may leave you feeling shaky or cause you to tire more quickly.

While You're Active

Unless your workout or competition lasts more than one hour, you probably don't need to eat during physical activity. If you feel you need extra energy, enjoy carbohydrate-rich foods that are easy to eat and digest, such as a banana, rice cakes, or cereal bars.

Fluids are your top priority during physical activity. Drink plenty of them. If you don't replace the fluids you lose by sweating, your strength, endurance, and coordination may be affected. You may also risk dehydration. That can lead to serious problems such as muscle cramps and heat exhaustion.

Teaching With Visuals: Measure and pour 2 cups of water into a water bottle. Mark the 2-cup water line as a reminder of the least amount of water to drink before physical activity and after physical activity (for every pound of weight lost during activity).

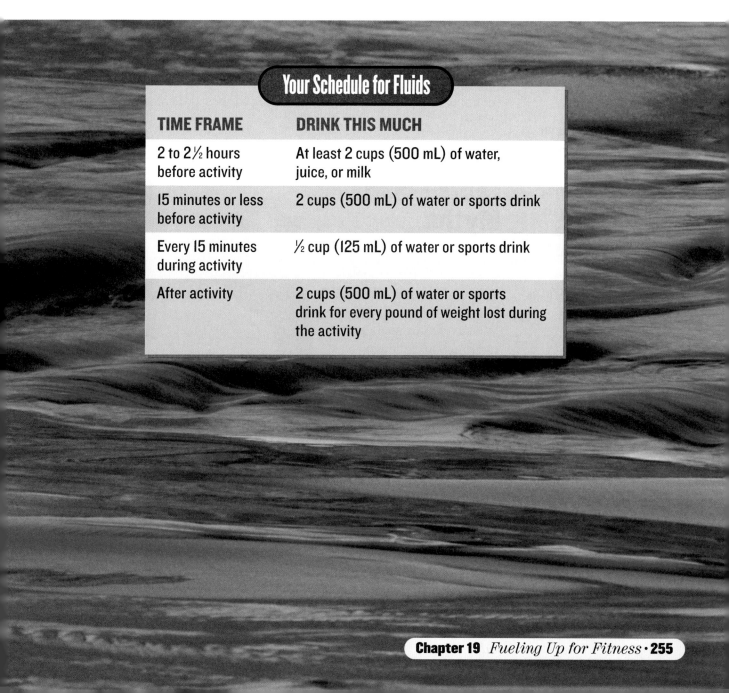

Your Schedule for Fluids

TIME FRAME	DRINK THIS MUCH
2 to 2½ hours before activity	At least 2 cups (500 mL) of water, juice, or milk
15 minutes or less before activity	2 cups (500 mL) of water or sports drink
Every 15 minutes during activity	½ cup (125 mL) of water or sports drink
After activity	2 cups (500 mL) of water or sports drink for every pound of weight lost during the activity

Emphasize: Your body absorbs cool drinks more quickly than warmer ones.

Fluid Choices

Cool water is one of the best ways to replace fluids. Besides water, you might drink juice and milk, which supply carbohydrates to fuel your working muscles. Sports drinks, with their easily absorbed glucose (a form of sugar), are a good idea for activities that last over one hour.

Sports drinks also supply **electrolytes**—*sodium, chloride, and potassium, which work together to help maintain your body's fluid balance.* Your body loses some electrolytes as you perspire. Caffeine drinks such as cola aren't the best choice because they can make your body lose fluids. Carbonated drinks may upset your stomach.

After You're Active

After an intense workout or competition, refuel your body with food and fluids. Immediately after, drink enough water, sports drink, or fruit juice to replace lost fluids. Within one to four hours, eat a meal that includes plenty of carbohydrates and some protein and fat.

Sports Nutrition Facts—and Myths

Are you looking for a way to gain a competitive edge? Perhaps you hope for faster results from your workouts. Whatever your goal, be careful about following eating regimens or using nutrition supplements and other sports products with promises of top performance. Use caution!

TIP

Some people believe that after a workout or competition, electrolytes need to be replaced by taking salt tablets or getting extra sodium. The best way is the familiar sound advice—eat a variety of foods.

Some athletes and active people choose sports drinks over water because they like the taste. Just remember that these drinks have calories, which can add up if you select sports drinks often. Name two endurance events or sports for which an athlete might choose a sports drink instead of water.

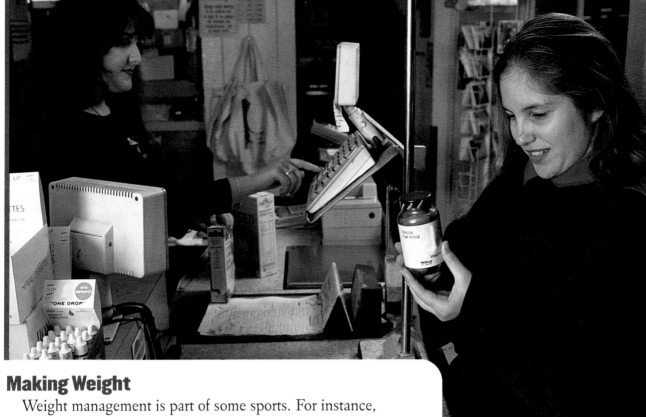

Making Weight

Weight management is part of some sports. For instance, wrestlers compete in weight classes. In other sports, such as gymnastics, athletes may think they need to compete at a low weight—even if they don't. You need to take growth into account when you choose a weight class for competition. Managing weight for competition should be part of everyday training, not something you do just before an event. Fasting, crash dieting, or trying to sweat off weight may cause dehydration and fatigue—and keep you from doing your best. Over time, these practices can affect your growth and development, too.

Bulking Up

Some athletes, such as hockey and football players, may improve their performance with more muscle weight. Trying to bulk up too fast and without physical activity may put on extra fat instead of more muscle. Slow, steady weight gain of no more than two pounds a week is best. To build muscle while gaining weight, work out more, especially with strength-building activities. Extra calories should come from nutrient-dense, high-carbohydrate foods. Remember, too, that teens' bodies will start to bulk up according to their own genetic time clock.

Stay away from steroids! Using steroids as muscle builders can have dangerous and permanent side effects. Steroids are drugs that act like male hormones. Among other problems, they can damage the reproductive system.

Products such as bee pollen, caffeine, glycine, carnitine, lecithin, brewer's yeast, and gelatin are sometimes promoted as substances that will improve strength or endurance. Science does not support these claims. Name several other products that are inappropriately promoted as substances that will improve strength or endurance. How would you evaluate the claims?

Emphasize: Steroids are prescription drugs. Using them without a prescription is illegal.

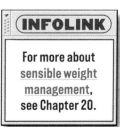

INFOLINK

For more about sensible weight management, see Chapter 20.

Activity: Read the labels of protein powders and amino acid supplements to find out what the ingredients include.

Tip

Eating a steak dinner before competing won't give you an athletic edge. In fact, a high-fat, high-protein meal may hinder your performance. Instead, choose a low-fat, high-carbohydrate meal. It's easier to digest, too.

High-Protein Diets

Contrary to a common sports myth, a high-protein, low-carbohydrate eating plan won't improve your performance. This kind of eating plan may not provide the variety and balance of foods your body needs for good nutrition. Extra protein from protein powders and amino acid supplements won't build muscle either. Remember, your body uses extra protein for energy or stores it as fat. Supplements are expensive and often have no more protein than a serving of meat or glass of milk.

Carbohydrate Loading

Carbohydrate loading is *a way of training and eating several days before an athletic event.* Athletes gradually decrease their training as they increase their carbohydrate intake. For trained endurance athletes, it helps build the amount of carbohydrates stored in the body. Most people, though, will not benefit from carbohydrate loading. Because this practice may affect growth if used repeatedly, it's not advised for teen athletes.

Protein-rich foods supply other important nutrients, such as iron and calcium, whereas amino acid supplements supply only amino acids. What are some protein-rich foods that supply iron and some that provide calcium?

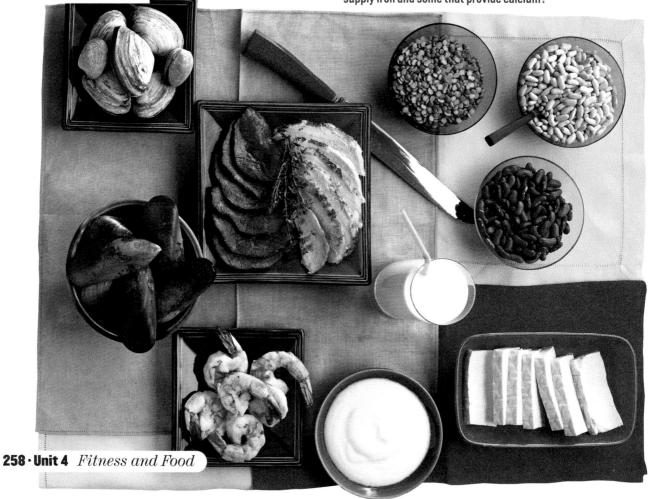

NOW *You're* COOKING!

(SKILL) Microwaving a Portable Snack

*C*reate an easy snack to enjoy now or to take in your backpack to eat after sports practice or a workout. Share it with your friends when you're out having active fun.

RECIPE

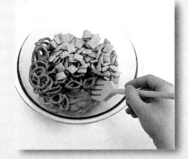

Cereal Crunch

CUSTOMARY	INGREDIENTS	METRIC
2 Tbsp.	Honey	30 mL
2 tsp.	Margarine or butter	10 mL
½ tsp.	Ground cinnamon	2 mL
2 cups	Rice flakes cereal	500 mL
2 cups	Small twist pretzels	500 mL

Yield: 4 servings, 1 cup (250 mL) each

1. In large microwave-safe bowl, place honey, margarine, and cinnamon. Microwave on high power for 1 to 1½ minutes or until margarine is melted. Stir until blended.

2. Add cereal and pretzels; toss to combine. Microwave on high power for 3 minutes, stirring after every minute.

3. Pour onto baking sheet. Let cool and store in airtight container.

Per Serving: 278 calories, 5 g protein, 56 g carbohydrate, 4 g fat, 856 mg sodium, 0 g fiber

Percent Daily Value: iron 10%, vitamin C 11%, thiamin 20%, niacin 21%, vitamin B_6 11%, folate 12%, vitamin B_{12} 11%

More Ideas For more mix-and-match nutrition:

- For a flavor twist, stir in your favorite dried fruits, popcorn, or nuts after microwaving. Let cool on the baking sheet.

- Use your favorite breakfast cereal. This snack even makes a great grab-and-go breakfast!

Your Ideas Check out the variety of dried fruits in the grocery store. List the ones you think would taste good in a snack mix.

LOOKING BACK

- Follow the advice of the Food Guide Pyramid to get enough nutrients for peak performance. Get most of your food energy from complex carbohydrates.

- For peak performance, plan carefully what you eat and drink before, during, and after physical activity.

- Use caution before following an eating regimen or using nutrition supplements that promise top performance.

UNDERSTANDING KEY IDEAS

1. How does physical activity affect your nutrient needs?

2. Why is it important to drink fluids before, during, and after physical activity? Which fluids are the best choices?

3. Which would be a better main dish for lunch on the day of a late afternoon gymnastics meet—a steak sandwich or spaghetti? Why?

4. What problems might you experience if you fasted to lose weight quickly? What problems might you experience from trying to bulk up too quickly?

5. What advice would you give to a friend who decided to try a high-protein eating plan?

6. Define carbohydrate loading. Why isn't it recommended for teens?

DEVELOPING LIFE SKILLS

1. **Management:** Making a plan and putting it into action are important management skills. If you were a long-distance runner on the track team, how could you use management skills to make sure you get enough fluids?

2. **Leadership:** Imagine that you are on the wrestling team. You notice that some team members are following unsafe practices in trying to compete in a weight class lower than their appropriate weight. How could you show leadership and help them understand the potential dangers?

Wellness Challenge

Lauren and several of her friends have signed up to participate in a jump-rope-a-thon to raise funds to combat heart disease. The event is scheduled to last late into the night, and Lauren's friends have planned a breakfast to take place immediately afterward. Lauren is concerned about what they will eat before and during the event. She wants to make sure that she and her friends have enough energy to last the night and raise money for the charity.

1. How might Lauren convey her concerns to her friends?
2. What solutions might help her and her friends?

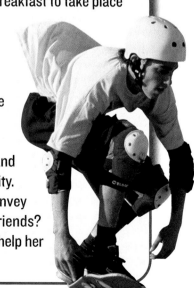

APPLYING YOUR LEARNING

1. **Promote Nutrition:** Create your own ad for a nutrient-dense food that is high in complex carbohydrates. Also promote the other nutrients provided by this food.

2. **Menu Planning:** Plan five original menus that include foods you like and that would help fuel your body before a big competition. If possible, make one of the meals at home.

EXPLORING FURTHER

1. **Dangers of Steriods:** Steroids can have hazardous and permanent side effects. Research the damage steroids can do to the body. Create a public service announcement warning teens of the danger.

2. **Protein Powders:** Some athletes believe that protein powders and amino acid supplements help build muscle. Visit a store and read the labels of such products to find out what they contain and their costs. Compare those costs to the same amount of protein in a serving of meat or glass of milk. What can you conclude?

Making CONNECTIONS

1. **Science:** Your body loses electrolytes as you perspire. Learn more about how electrolytes maintain your body's fluid balance. What are some ways to replace lost electrolytes? Share your findings with the class.

2. **Language Arts:** In teams of three or four students, write a poem or rap dispelling sports myths and promoting good food choices for peak performance. Present your finished piece to the class.

FOODS LAB

Create a juice beverage you would enjoy after a workout. You might try a mixture of half water and half fruit juice or vegetable juice. Consider using more than one juice for your own personal blend. Compare your drink with those of your classmates.

Healthful Choices About Weight

Objectives

After studying this chapter, you will be able to:

- Explain why appropriate weight is not the same for everyone.
- Describe smart ways to achieve and maintain appropriate body weight.
- Distinguish between fad diets and sensible weight management plans.

Do You Know ...

...why there's no perfect weight, size, or shape for teens or anyone else?

...why "dieting" isn't right for most teens?

...how to judge popular diets from magazines?

If not, you'll find out in this chapter!

Look for these TERMS

Body Mass Index
energy balance
fad diets

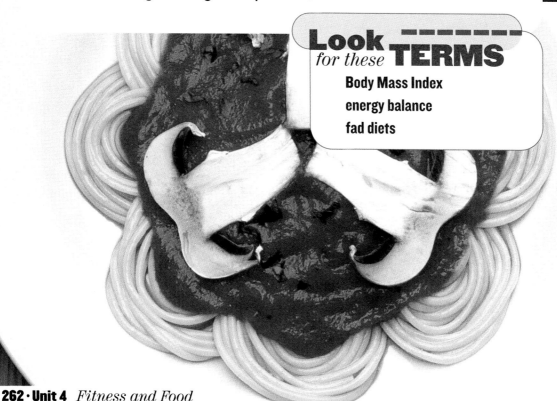

Look around you

...it's easy to see that people come in many sizes and shapes. Some are tall and slender. Others are short and stocky. Like differences in hair color, your body structure is a trait that helps make you unique. No one is just like you!

Your Appropriate Weight

There's a wide range of normal body weights for teens. Your appropriate weight fits somewhere within that range. It's not too high or too low for your age and height. It doesn't mean "the lowest weight you think you can be"!

Remember, you need some body fat. Body fat acts as insulation to protect you from cold and heat. It cushions your bones and your heart, lungs, and other organs. A small amount also serves as an energy reserve.

Being at your appropriate weight increases your chances for good health. Later in life, you'll be less likely to develop health problems related to being too heavy or too thin. You'll probably feel best at your right weight, too.

The weight that's right for you depends on your growth pattern and body type, which are both determined by your genes and gender. Trying to weigh the same as a friend, a celebrity, or a fashion model makes no sense. No single body weight is ideal at any age!

You're Still Growing!

Do your school clothes from last year or the year before still fit? Probably not—at least not like they did. When your teen growth spurt ends, you'll probably be 20 percent taller and weigh 50 percent more than before it began. Almost half of your adult skeleton is forming now. That's the fastest growth rate since you were an infant!

Being different is absolutely normal! What qualities make you unique and special?

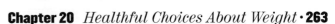

Weight gain is a normal part of the teen years. Your body shape is developing, not getting fat. Males develop broader shoulders. In females, the hips widen and body fat increases as a womanly shape develops.

Your body grows according to your own inborn "growth clock." Females usually start their teen growth spurt before males do. Some teens put on extra body fat before they grow taller. Others grow tall first and put on weight later. If they are physically active and eat smart, they'll probably grow into their appropriate body weight.

Many teens keep on growing into their adult shape until their early 20s. Your body will continue to change all through your life, even after you stop growing. It's normal and part of a lifelong process.

Every Body's Different!

Some people have a small body frame; others have a large one. Some are more muscular. There is no ideal body shape and size because everyone is an individual.

As you grow into your adult size, remember that body structure is inherited. Your body type and growth pattern may mirror those of a parent or a relative. Smart eating and active living are choices for keeping an appropriate weight for you. That's what counts for wellness!

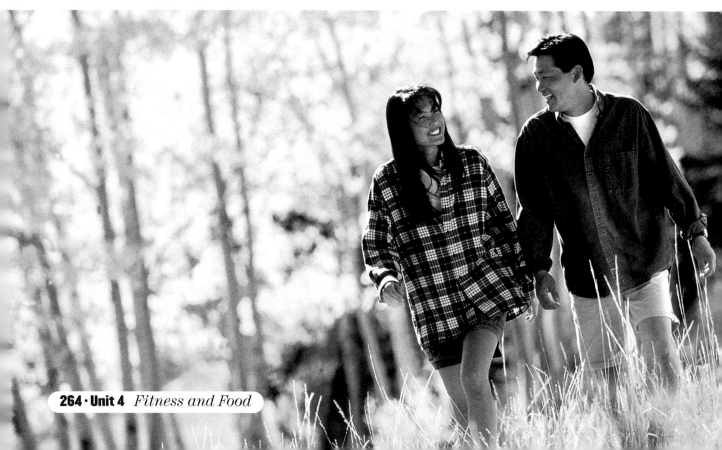

Finding Your Appropriate Weight

Two charts help you look at your height and weight patterns in a realistic way. The first is a height chart, which shows height in relation to age. The second is a **Body Mass Index** (BMI) chart, *a tool that looks at weight in relation to height.* The BMI charts for teens on page 266 show the wide range of appropriate weights. The pattern you plot on the chart takes your height, weight, and age into account. However, it doesn't measure body composition. Also, it's only a guide, since teens' bodies are changing.

Tip

If you're concerned about your weight or place on the BMI chart, talk to an adult you can trust. The school nurse or your physician can offer sound advice.

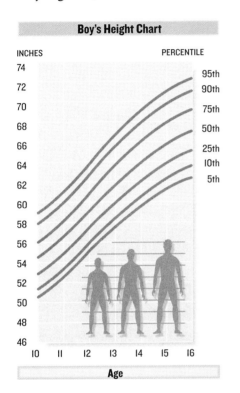

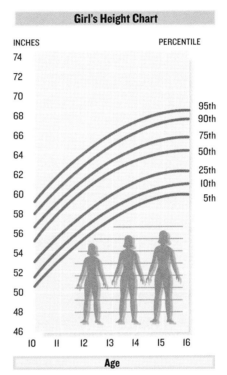

INFOLINK

For more about appropriate weight, underweight, and overweight, see Chapter 7.

Read about body composition in Chapter 17.

Track Your Height

I. Measure your height in inches.

2. Find your height along the left side of the chart.

3. Find your age along the bottom of the chart.

4. Note where your age and height cross on the chart.

5. What percentile line comes closest to your spot? The percentile shows how you compare with an average group of males or females your age. These charts are estimates and not the only way to judge growth.

Teaching With Visuals: Write down the height and weight of a fictitious friend. Trade with a classmate and calculate the BMI of the "person" you are given.

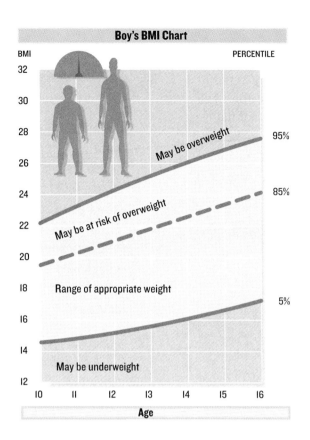

Boy's BMI Chart

BMI

PERCENTILE

32
30
28 — May be overweight — 95%
26
24 — 85%
22 — May be at risk of overweight
20
18 — Range of appropriate weight
16 — 5%
14
12 — May be underweight

10 11 12 13 14 15 16
Age

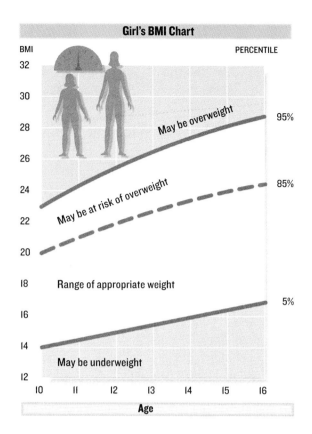

Girl's BMI Chart

BMI

PERCENTILE

32
30
28 — May be overweight — 95%
26
24 — 85%
22 — May be at risk of overweight
20
18 — Range of appropriate weight
16 — 5%
14
12 — May be underweight

10 11 12 13 14 15 16
Age

Tip

During the growth spurt of your teen years, certain nutrients need special attention. Getting enough zinc is essential for growth. Iron is needed to support increasing muscle mass, and females need it to avoid anemia. Calcium helps you grow bones that will be strong for a lifetime. How can you get all those nutrients? You're right if you said, "By eating enough of a variety of foods!"

Discuss: What foods do you eat that contain the nutrients needed for growth?

What's Your BMI?

To figure your **BMI**, you need to know your height and weight. A calculator may help you with the math.

1. Divide your weight in pounds by your height in inches.
   $weight \div height = x$

2. Divide again by your height in inches.
   $x \div height = y$

3. Multiply by 703.
   $y \times 703 = BMI$

4. Find your age along the bottom of the chart.

5. Find your BMI along the left side of the chart.

Remember, these charts are estimates. Every person has her or his own pattern of growth.

Source: yourSELF, USDA, Food and Nutrition Service, 1999

More about the BMI: The BMI does not measure bone, fat, or muscle. Since teen's bodies are changing, it is not clear whether some teens may be at risk of being overweight or are at an appropriate weight.

Activity: Identify the kinds of foods that contain the nutrients essential for growth: zinc, iron, and calcium. Make a poster of each nutrient showing pictures of the foods that contain them.

Smart Choices for You

No matter what your size or shape, or where you fit on the BMI chart, the advice for health is the same. Follow a healthful eating plan and stay physically active! To keep weight within an appropriate range:

- Follow guidelines from the Food Guide Pyramid. Be sure your choices provide enough food energy for growth—many teens need 2,400 to 3,000 calories a day. Remember, teens need three servings from the Milk, Yogurt, and Cheese Group.
- Stay physically active. Besides other health benefits, you'll burn calories, which gives you more "room" to enjoy a variety of food.
- Accept the weight that's right for you as your body grows.
- Forget the notion of "dieting." Following unhealthy diets or skipping meals isn't a smart way to keep your weight on track. You may not get all the nutrients and food energy you need for growth and health.

INFOLINK

Review the discussion of energy and calories in Chapter 5.

INFOLINK

Read about the benefits of physical activity in Chapter 17.

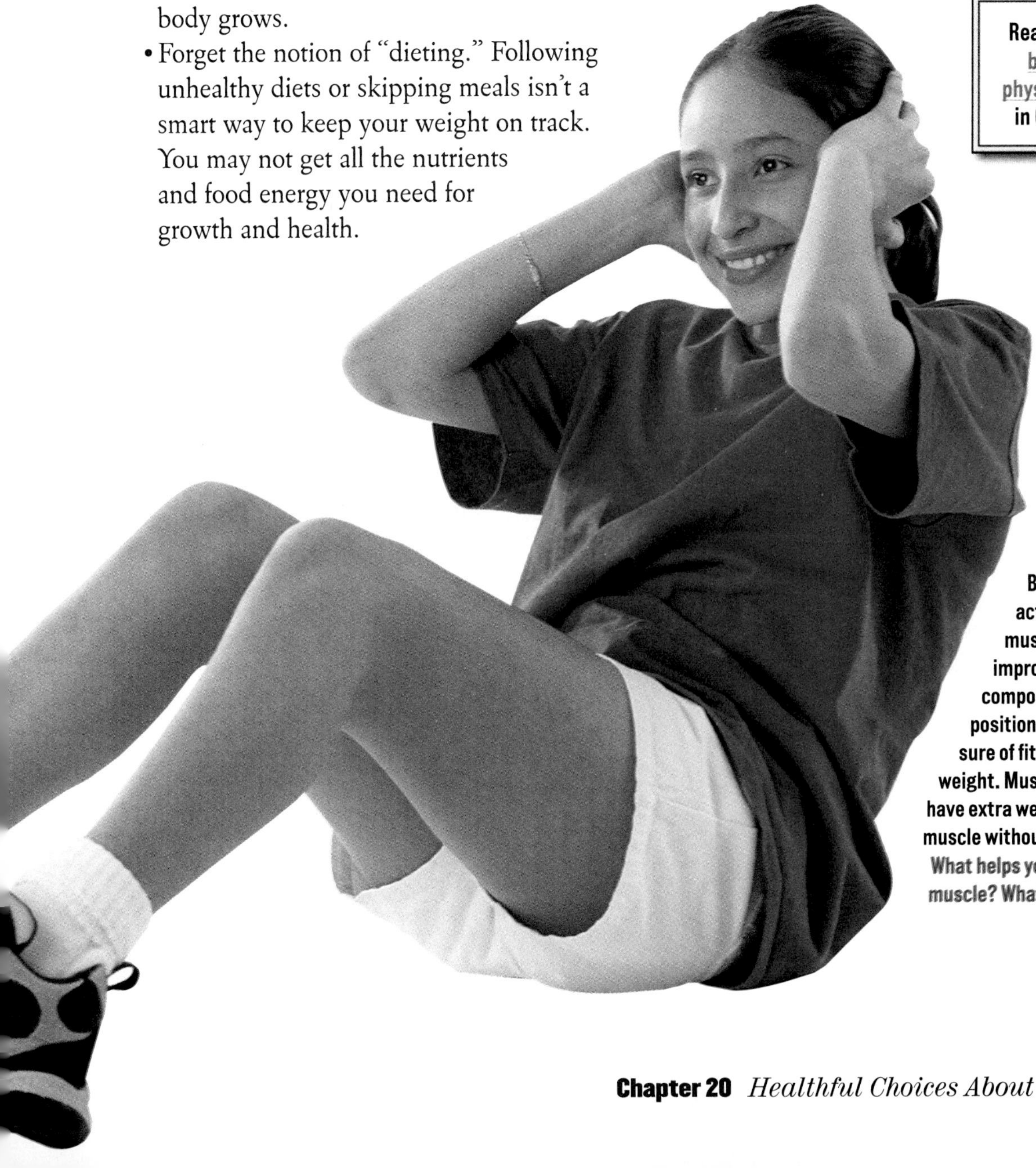

Being physically active can build muscles and improve your body composition. Body composition is a better measure of fitness than body weight. Muscular people may have extra weight from muscle without being overfat. What helps you build and keep muscle? What doesn't?

INFOLINK

Review how to set goals and make an action plan in Chapters 1 and 18.

Tip

Eating to relieve boredom or anxiety may lead to overeating. Learn to handle stress and boredom by doing something active.

Reaching Weight Goals— Slowly and Sensibly

At some point in life, you may need to lose or gain weight. Talk to your doctor first. Then set smart goals that are right for your body size, shape, and age. Losing or gaining ½ to 1 pound (0.25 to 0.5 kg) a week may be realistic and safe. Next, make a healthwise action plan to reach your goals. To check your progress, weigh yourself just once a week, not every day. It's normal to hit a weight plateau now and then.

Strategies for Losing Weight

- Fit more physical activity into your lifestyle whenever you can. That may be all you need to do to reach your weight goal!
- Eat at least the minimum number of Pyramid servings from the five food groups. That's about 1,700 calories if you make low-fat and low-sugar choices. Getting fewer calories can be dangerous to your health.
- Eat plenty of fruits and vegetables to avoid being too hungry. They're usually low in fat and calories.
- Don't go for long periods of time without eating. Eat nutrient-dense snacks. Cut back on foods high in fat and sugar.
- Use Nutrition Facts on food labels to find foods with fewer calories.
- Don't give up higher-calorie favorites; just eat smaller amounts.
- Compare your portions to Pyramid servings. Eat from a plate, not the package, so that you know how much you've eaten.

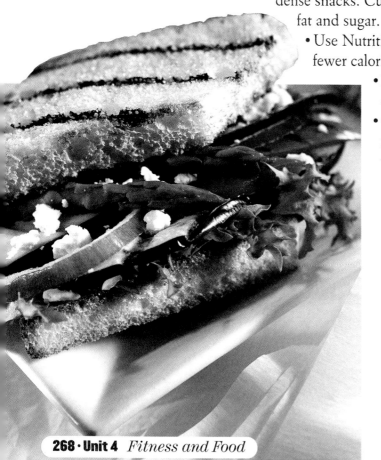

You can control your calorie intake and still enjoy great-tasting foods. Look for a tasty, low-fat recipe you would like to prepare.

Critical Thinking: Ask: If you are trying to lose weight, why is it recommended that you not go for long periods of time without eating?

Emphasize: It takes twenty minutes for your body to feel full after eating a snack or meal. Eat slowly so you eat less in the amount of time it takes to relieve hunger pains.

Strategies for Gaining Weight

- Stay physically active. That way, the weight you gain will be muscle.
- Eat a moderate amount of foods that contain some fat and sugar. Go easy on fats and sweets from the Pyramid tip.
- Eat nutrient-dense snacks often. Don't go for long periods of time without eating. Time your snacks two to three hours before meals so that you're hungry for lunch or dinner.
- Choose more than the minimum number of servings from the five food groups, especially foods high in complex carbohydrates, such as pasta, rice, bread, and starchy vegetables. Take bigger portions or second helpings.
- Use Nutrition Facts on food labels to find nutrient-dense foods with more calories.
- Eat several small meals if your appetite is small. Avoid meal skipping.
- Give it time. Don't try to gain weight too fast, or you may add a layer of fat. Building muscle takes time.

Choosing nutrient-dense foods from the five food groups is a good strategy for gaining weight. What food group snack are these teens enjoying?

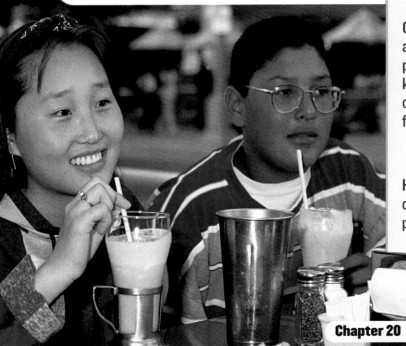

Check This Out!

BALANCING THE ENERGY EQUATION

You don't need to count calories when you're being careful about weight. However, learning about **energy balance**—*balancing energy from food with energy your body uses*—helps you understand how your body uses food energy. Remember, your body uses energy—measured in calories—for physical activities. You also use energy for body processes, including growth. The rate at which energy is used for body processes varies from person to person.

- If over time the food energy from your meals and snacks equals the amount of energy your body uses, you stay the same weight.
- If over time you take in *less* food energy than the amount of energy your body uses, you will lose weight.
- If over time you take in *more* food energy than the amount of energy your body uses, you will gain weight.

One pound (0.5 kg) of body fat is worth about 3,500 calories. For example, a person who wants to gain I pound (0.5 kg) per week could do so by adding 500 calories, with mostly nutrient-dense foods, to each day's food plan.

It's Your Turn!

How would a person need to change his or her energy balance in order to lose ½ pound (0.25 kg) of body fat per week?

Check This Out!

RATE THE PLAN

A sound eating and lifestyle plan:
- Follows the Food Guide Pyramid.
- Lets you eat foods you enjoy.
- Matches your food budget.
- Fits your lifestyle.
- Includes regular physical activity.
- Is a plan you can follow for life.

It's Your Turn!

Explain why each of these points is important for the success of an eating and lifestyle plan.

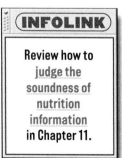

Tip

Smoking, as a substitute for eating, is a poor way to lose weight or maintain a low weight. It robs the body of nutrient-rich food. Besides, smoking is linked to many health problems, including cancer and heart disease. It's not smart to start!

Why Fad Diets Aren't Smart!

Have you heard about so-called magical or effortless ways to melt away body fat? Many fad diets make that promise but can't deliver. **Fad diets** are *weight-loss plans, often based on misinformation, that are popular for a short time.* Most won't effectively help people reach or stick to a weight goal for long. Fad diets don't help people develop healthful patterns of eating and enjoying physical activity, which are the long-term way to maintain weight.

Some fad diets restrict the amount and type of foods too much, so they don't provide the nutrients and food energy needed for growth and health. When people follow one fad diet after another, their weight may "seesaw" up and down, which isn't healthful. The weight they lose may be muscle. Without exercise, it may be replaced with body fat.

If at some time you need a weight-loss diet, look for one with sensible advice for a long-term way of eating. Avoid these risky ones.

Liquid diets. A very low-calorie liquid diet won't provide enough food energy. You may feel tired, and the diet may have other harmful side effects. You won't get all the nutrients and fiber you get from food.

Fasting. Denying your body food, even for a short time, means you miss out on nutrients and energy. Your body uses up some protein, which is stored in muscle, for fuel. You may become dehydrated without fluids.

Diet pills. Diet pills may suppress appetite. However, they can have harmful side effects, such as making you drowsy or anxious or giving you a rapid heart rate. Some diet pills increase water loss, promoting dehydration. Some may be addictive.

Emphasize: One of the keys to losing weight is getting support from family members, friends, a doctor, or a support group.

INFOLINK

Review how to judge the soundness of nutrition information in Chapter 11.

HELP WANTED

Consumer Services Consultant

Opening for Consumer Services Consultant to organize and provide consumer education services for local schools and community organizations. Also advise individuals and families on home management practices. Must have excellent organizational and presentation skills. Experience and masters degree required. Apply at University Extension Services Office.

Home Health Aide

Caring individuals needed to assist patients in their homes. Provide personal care services, plan nutritional meals, shop for food, and cook. High school diploma, driver's license, and reliable transportation required. Attractive benefit program. Complete application in person at Home Health Services.

Health Commissioner

The Hamilton County Board of Health is accepting applications for a full-time Health Commissioner. Must have experience in a public health department, hold a master's degree in a related field, and be a licensed physician. Strong leadership skills and knowledge of public health practices required. Submit resume to the Hamilton County Board of Health.

Dietetic Technician

Dietetic Technician needed for government-funded WIC (Women, Infants, and Children) nutrition program. Work under the direction of a registered dietitian instructing clients on menu planning, shopping, and meal preparation. Provide referrals for other health-related needs. Associate degree required. Apply to Director, Newark County WIC Program.

Community Dietitian

Community health organization needs a registered dietitian to manage nutritional health care services that promote healthy eating habits. Plan, conduct, and evaluate dietary studies. Direct and train professional staff. Competitive salary and benefits. Submit resume to Carmel Health Services.

Food Bank Coordinator

Social service agency seeks a coordinator for food bank program. Caring individual will direct daily preparation and service of meals. Must have excellent people skills to recruit and work with volunteers. Two-year degree preferred. Experience in food preparation a plus. Contact St. Johns Outreach.

LINKING *to the* WORKPLACE

❶ **Personal Characteristics:** Select one of the jobs listed above. What personal characteristics, in addition to any listed in the ad, would be an asset for a person in that occupation? Do you think the job would be a good fit for you? Why or why not?

❷ **Terminating Employment:** An employee who decides to leave a job should give ample notice, preferably in writing. Find out what a letter of resignation should include. Then write one in proper business letter format.

CHAPTER 20

Review & Activities

LOOKING BACK

- There's a wide range of appropriate body weights for teens.
- For an appropriate weight, follow a healthful eating plan and stay physically active.
- If at some point in life you need to lose or gain weight, follow a health-wise action plan to reach your goals.
- Fad diets may not follow guidelines of healthful eating or promote a long-term way to maintain your appropriate weight.

UNDERSTANDING KEY IDEAS

1. If you were 2 inches shorter and weighed 10 pounds more than your best friend, would it be appropriate for you to go on a weight-loss diet? Explain your answer.
2. What are some specific ways teens can keep their weight within an appropriate range?
3. How might you gain weight sensibly?
4. If a friend were considering taking diet pills, what advice would you give to him or her?
5. Explain how the relationship between the energy you take in from food and the energy your body uses affects your weight.
6. What are fad diets? Why should they be avoided?

DEVELOPING LIFE SKILLS

1. **Communication:** In what ways do you think society communicates a "thin is in" message to young people today? What effects does this message have? What could be done to counter this message with more healthful, positive ones?
2. **Critical Thinking:** If you read about a new diet in a magazine, what clues would help you judge whether it was a legitimate weight-loss plan or a fad diet?

Wellness Challenge

Tyrone's friend Paul wants to lose 5 pounds before the school dance next week. Paul plans to try a diet that claims you can lose a pound each day by drinking only grapefruit juice. Tyrone, however, is concerned that this diet is not healthful and may even harm his friend. Tyrone would like to encourage Paul to follow a sensible eating and lifestyle plan instead of relying on fad diets.

1. What challenges does Tyrone face?
2. What can Tyrone do to encourage Paul to follow a healthful eating plan?

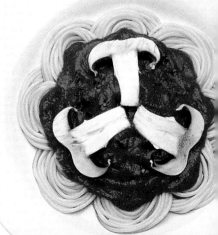

APPLYING YOUR LEARNING

1. **Web Page Design:** Create a web page design or make a poster that promotes the beauty of the individual, no matter what shape or size.

2. **Menu Planning:** Plan a menu for a day that includes at least 1,700 calories and fits Food Guide Pyramid guidelines for teens. Using Nutrition Facts panels or other sources of nutrient information, calculate whether the menu provides 100% of the RDA for zinc, iron, and calcium for teens your age. (Find the RDAs in the Appendix.)

EXPLORING FURTHER

1. **Smart Strategies:** Using the Internet or library resources, find out how many calories you can burn from 30 minutes of swimming, running, brisk walking, biking, aerobic dancing, in-line skating, and jumping rope. Which of these activities might you fit into your weekly schedule?

2. **Expert Opinion:** Investigate a currently popular weight-loss plan. Is it safe and effective? What are its drawbacks, if any? To find out, interview a qualified nutrition expert or find an article written by one. Present your findings to the class.

Making CONNECTIONS

1. **Language Arts:** Write a short story in which a fictitious teen is growing and developing at a different rate from that of friends and classmates. Tell how the teen overcomes feelings of being "different" and learns to celebrate his or her uniqueness.

2. **Social Studies:** Labor-saving devices have enhanced the lives of Americans and impacted public health. Choose a historical period before the Industrial Revolution and find out a typical person's amount of physical activity. Was overweight a concern then? Why or why not?

FOODS LAB

Find a recipe for a nutritious food-group snack. Adapt the recipe to meet the needs of two people: an active teen who wants to gain weight and an adult who wants to lose weight. Prepare both versions of your snack. Rate them for flavor and nutrition.

Tandoors Heat Up Indian Cooking

You can't use just any old oven to bake Indian bread (naan) or many other delicious traditional Indian dishes. If you want to prepare these dishes the authentic way, you need a tandoor oven. It looks like a tall, cylindrical clay pot. Burning charcoal provides the heat from the bottom of the oven.

The clay helps distribute the heat evenly. Temperatures in the oven reach about 500 degrees. Foods such as tandoori chicken, lamb, spiced ground lamb sausages, or prawns can be prepared by skewering the meat on a long rod and placing it in the oven. Food cooks quickly due to the high temperatures and the structure of the oven. To make naan, thin disks of dough are slapped onto the inside wall of the tandoor, where they stick and cook until slightly browned and puffed. ∎

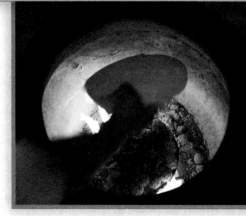

▲ Indian bread (naan) is prepared in a tandoor oven.

tidbits

Wedding guests in Pakistan usually are not served wedding cake. Instead, they enjoy **firini**, a sweet, soupy dessert made from cream of rice and milk.

In Nepal, the herb **turmeric** has two purposes. Besides making food tastier, it's also rubbed on the skin of butchered goats to keep the flies away until the meat can be cooked.

One of the most popular fruits in Sri Lanka is the **mangosteen**.

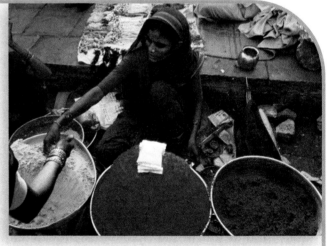

▲ A woman sells turmeric in Nepal.

These juicy sweet-tart fruits are in high demand by natives and visitors alike, but they are extremely hard to come by. The mangosteen season lasts just one month (around July or August), and the purplish ripe fruit is only good for a few days.

Citizens of Bangladesh like to eat **cheese straws** before their meals. They're similar to fried cheese, the popular American appetizer. The main difference is that cheese straws contain a large dose of spicy ground cumin. ∎

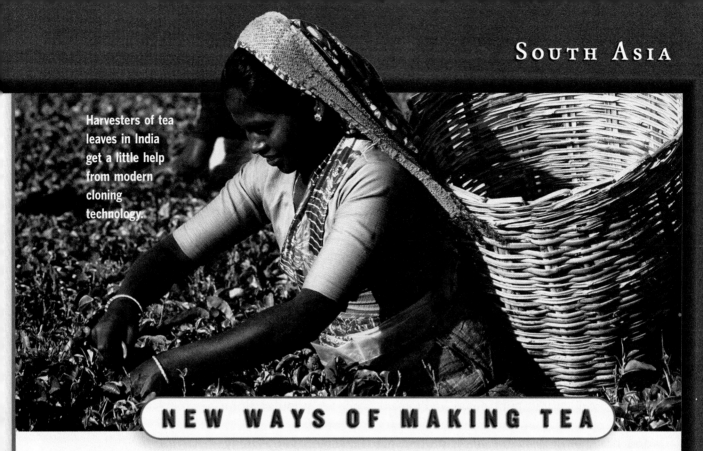

Harvesters of tea leaves in India get a little help from modern cloning technology.

NEW WAYS OF MAKING TEA

Conditions in India are perfect for growing tea leaves. The foothills of the Himalayas have the fertile soil and moist air needed for the tea plant. But in the modern world, Mother Nature isn't always enough. Indian tea growers are using the latest technology to produce the best tea leaves, and to share them with the rest of the world. Companies in India are using modern cloning techniques to increase the amount of tea leaves they can produce. They also use newly developed pesticides to keep unwanted bugs away without harming the environment.

When it comes to processing the tea leaves, the companies use state-of-the-art equipment that helps the teas keep their distinct flavors. Although the technology has changed greatly, the bottom line—tea that tastes good—remains the same. ■

mashed **potatoes** for **dessert**?

One of the most popular desserts in Sri Lanka is made from something you might not normally think of having for dessert. Aluwa (a-LUH-wah), which is similar to toffee, is often made from mashed potatoes, sugar, sweet milk, and the spice cardamom. After being baked and flattened, it is often cut into cookies of various shapes and sizes.

Another kind of aluwa is called rulang (rou-lahng) aluwa. Instead of using potatoes, it calls for roasted semolina, a flour that is often used to make pasta. The semolina is mixed with cashews to form a nuttier version of the sweet dessert. ■

South Asia

The region of South Asia has many differences in landscape, customs, languages, and climate. It makes sense that you'd find a wide variety of foods there. In fact, there's something for everyone!

India Indian food changes in flavor as you travel around the country. In the north, major flavors include garlic, mint, onion, and tomato. Lamb, goat, and chicken are popular meats, and bread is eaten with almost everything. Rice is also very popular. Darjeeling tea leaves, famous for their strong flavor, grow on the hillsides of northeastern India.

In western India, deer and wild boar are part of the regular diet. The meats are often served with vegetables that have been marinated in creamy yogurt and spiced with garlic. Breads made from chickpeas, lentils, and wheat are also popular.

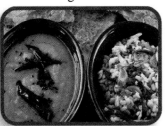

▲ Rice, bread, and lentils make an Indian dinner.

South India, on the other hand, is known for its fiery, spicy foods and savory filled pancakes, called dosa (doe-suh). Spices make people sweat, which helps keep them cool in hot tropical climates. Southern Indians eat rice with many of their meals. The grain is also used to make pancakes, noodles, dumplings, and many kinds of breads. Since many Indians are vegetarian, lentils are the protein source in many meals. Seafood or vegetarian dishes served with coconut, banana, and ginger are popular along the coast.

Indian food is traditionally eaten from small bowls that are arranged on a large plate. Each bowl contains a different kind of food. Main dishes include grilled meats and curries. They are usually served with flatbread, rice, or noodles. Side dishes include a simple stir-fried vegetable and a chutney, which is a mixture of fruit and vegetables, vinegar, sugar, and spices. To add moisture and protein to the meal, creamed lentils or cool yogurt salad is also served.

Pakistan Wheat and other flour products make up much of a Pakistani's diet. An abundance of spices and herbs are used to flavor these basic ingredients. A variety of sauces also give food a unique flavor. Popular spices include chili powder, garlic, paprika, black pepper, red pepper, cloves, ginger, cinnamon,

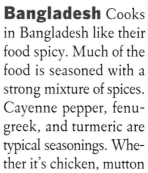

nutmeg, and poppy seeds.

The Islamic religion has influenced the food of Pakistan. Muslim feasts call for special dishes. Goat, lamb, or beef may be eaten as part of a religious gathering. The animals are killed according to strict dietary laws. Many people enjoy shahi tukra (SHAH-he TOO-krah). The dessert is made from slices of bread, milk, cream, sugar, and a spice called saffron.

Nepal

Nepal is a small nation along India's northeast border. The country has an unusual climate that goes from warm to cool. The most common food is dal bhaat (d'hahl-baht), a dish of boiled rice served under a thin sauce made with lentils, garlic, and spices. This dish is prepared in different combinations—some with assorted vegetables, some with chicken, lamb, goat, or fish. It is often served with vegetables and pickled mango.

Most people in Nepal eat dal bhaat twice a day, once around 10:30 A.M. and once just after sunset. Between meals, locals like to drink sweet tea with some milk and eat snacks such as rice, bread, and potatoes.

◀ In Sri Lanka, coconuts and coconut milk are important foods.

Bangladesh

Cooks in Bangladesh like their food spicy. Much of the food is seasoned with a strong mixture of spices. Cayenne pepper, fenugreek, and turmeric are typical seasonings. Whether it's chicken, mutton (sheep), beef, fish, or prawns, the food in Bangladesh is bound to have plenty of kick. As in other nations in the region, rice is a big part of mealtime.

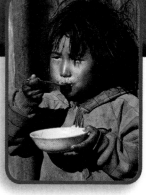

▲ A child in Nepal eats dal bhaat.

Mangos, bananas, papayas, jackfruits, watermelons, pineapples, and coconuts are grown in Bangladesh and are traditionally served as side dishes. Dessert might be a sweet and creamy yogurt pudding.

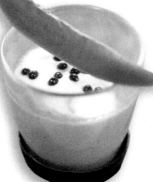

▲ A yogurt drink from Bangladesh

Sri Lanka

In Sri Lanka, an island nation off the coast of India, rice is prepared in a variety of ways and flavored with spices and sauces. Cooked rice can be laden with curry and served with pickled vegetables or with chutney. Instead of being boiled in water, the rice might be cooked in coconut milk. On occasion, meats, seafood, and vegetables are cooked with rice.

Many Sri Lankans love dessert. Juggery is like a fried donut hole with a thick sweet syrup poured over it. Other desserts combine juggery with coconut milk, nuts, and various dried fruits. ■

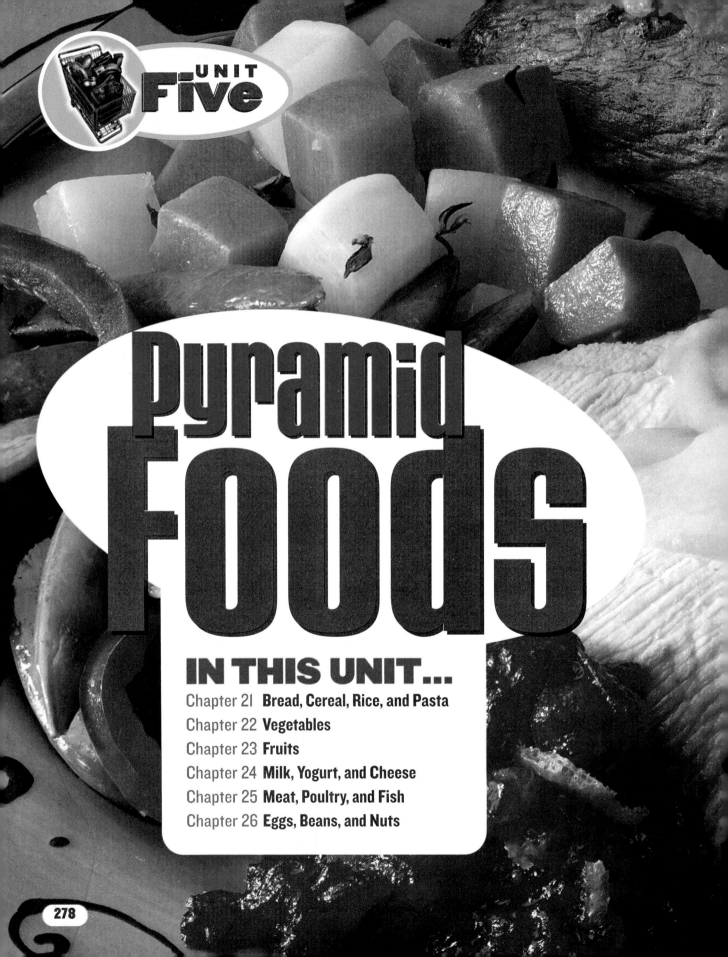

Pyramid FOODS

IN THIS UNIT...

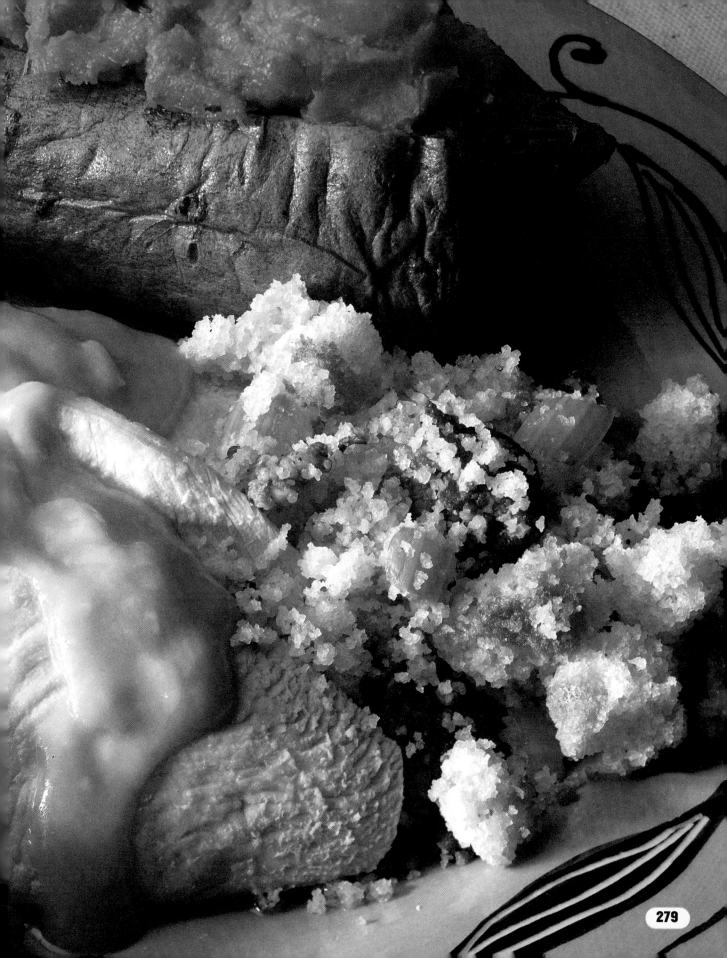

Bread, Cereal, Rice, and Pasta

Objectives

After studying this chapter, you will be able to:

- Explain why grain foods are the foundation of healthful eating.

- Identify various types of grain foods and ways to include them in meals and snacks.

- Summarize smart tips for selecting grain products.

- Describe how to store and prepare grain foods for quality, nutritional value, and appeal.

Do You Know...

...what couscous, triticale, and quinoa are?

...how to tell which loaf is really whole grain bread?

...how to cook pasta so that it won't stick together?

If not, you'll find out in this chapter!

Look for these TERMS

whole grain   germ
bran   al dente
endosperm

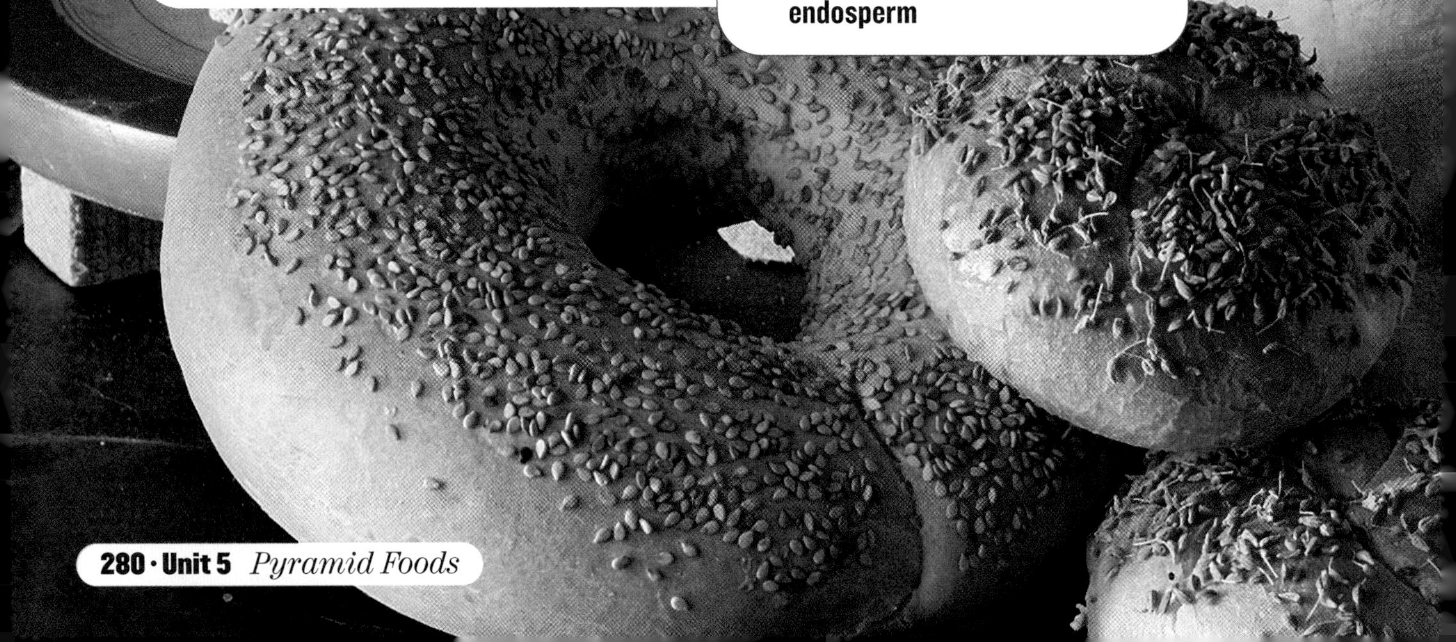

What do bread,

cereal, rice, and pasta have in common? That's right— grains! Grain foods have so much to offer—satisfying flavors, appealing aromas, and hearty textures. Their nutrients help keep you active and healthy. Grains appear at every meal and are served in many different ways. Think about all the foods you'd miss if there were no grains!

Grains... For Energy and More

Grain foods are probably the basis of many of your meals and snacks. They supply key nutrients that fuel your body and contribute to good health.

High in "carbs." The complex carbohydrates in grain products make these foods great sources of food energy. Some grain products also provide simple carbohydrates in the form of added sugar.

Fiber-rich. Foods made with whole grains have an added benefit—fiber! Page 282 shows the parts of a whole grain, including the part that supplies fiber. Remember, fiber helps your digestive tract work properly and may offer protection against heart disease and cancer.

Often low in fat. In their natural state, grains have very little fat and no cholesterol. When grains are processed and prepared, added ingredients sometimes add fat, calories, and cholesterol. This is true of biscuits, croissants, doughnuts, and hush puppies, for example. On the other hand, many grain products— including rice, pasta, and most breads—are low in fat and calories. To keep them this way, go easy on high-fat sauces and spreads.

There is a wide variety of breads, and most are naturally low in fat and cholesterol-free. What spreads are low-fat?

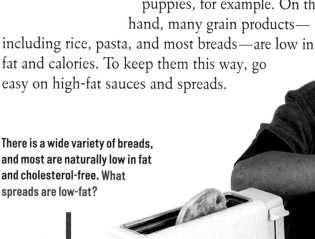

WHAT'S IN A Grain Kernel?

Whatever the type of grain—wheat, oats, barley, or any other—the part of the plant that is eaten is the kernel, or seed. A **whole grain** product *is made from the entire grain kernel,* including the three parts shown below. These parts may also be separated during processing, or refining, and used individually.

Parts of a Grain Kernel

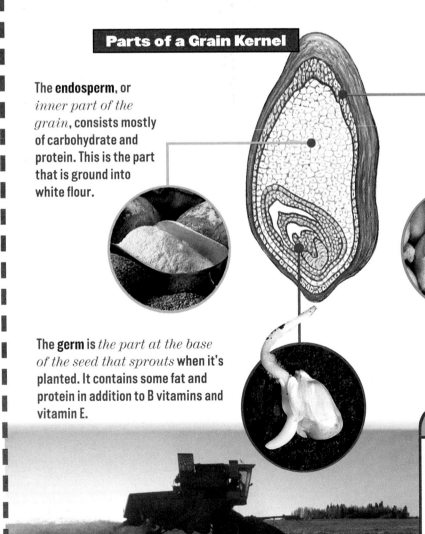

The **endosperm**, or *inner part of the grain*, consists mostly of carbohydrate and protein. This is the part that is ground into white flour.

The **bran** is *the coarse, outer layer of the grain*. It supplies fiber and is a good source of B vitamins and minerals.

The **germ** is *the part at the base of the seed that sprouts* when it's planted. It contains some fat and protein in addition to B vitamins and vitamin E.

Investigate Further

Nutritionally, what do whole grain foods have that foods made with refined grains may not have? Name four whole grain foods you could add to your menu plan.

Packed with vitamins and minerals.
Whole grains are good sources of B vitamins and iron. Refined grains have the bran and germ removed, which takes many nutrients and fiber with them. B vitamins and iron are added back to refined grain products labeled "enriched." Most grain products are fortified with extra folic acid, and some are fortified with additional vitamins and minerals.

Grains in the Pyramid

Foods made from grains form the base of the Food Guide Pyramid. To fuel your body, you need 6 to 11 servings from the Bread, Cereal, Rice, and Pasta Group each day. Foods that equal one serving include:
- 1 slice of enriched or whole grain bread.
- ½ hamburger bun, bagel, pita, or English muffin.
- 1 6-inch (15 cm) tortilla.
- 1 ounce (28g) of ready-to-eat cereal.
- ½ cup (125 mL) of cooked cereal, pasta, rice, or other cooked grain.

You may think that 6 to 11 servings sounds like a lot, but take a look at how quickly servings add up.

Breakfast: ½ cup (125 mL) oatmeal +
   1 English muffin = 3 servings

Lunch: 1 whole wheat hamburger bun =
   2 servings

Snack: 6 crackers = 2 servings

Dinner: 1 cup (250 mL) pasta + 1 slice
   French bread = 3 servings

Total: 10 servings

Check This Out!

HAVE YOU TRIED THESE GRAIN FOODS?

When you're in the mood for a taste adventure, and you want something other than plain white rice, look in your grocery store for one of the following grain foods. Just be sure to check the package for cooking directions.

- *Bulgur.* Whole wheat kernels that have been cooked, dried, and cracked. Gives a nutty flavor and a chewy texture to ground meat dishes, salads, and stuffed vegetables.
- *Couscous.* A type of pasta shaped like tiny beads. Has a nutty flavor. Can be eaten as a cereal, side dish, or sweetened for dessert.
- *Hominy.* Dried and hulled corn. Use in stews, casseroles, and other mixed dishes. Often ground and eaten as grits.
- *Kasha.* Hulled, crushed, and roasted buckwheat. Has a nutty flavor. Use as a cereal or side dish.
- *Millet.* Mild-flavored grain with chewy texture. Use as a cereal or as a substitute for rice.
- *Pearl barley.* Mild-flavored, polished grain. Use in soups and stews for added flavor and a slightly thickened consistency.
- *Quinoa* (KEEN-wah). Small, bead-shaped grain with a sweet, nutty flavor. Can be used as a substitute for rice. Good in salads.
- *Triticale* (trih-tih-KAY-lee). Cross between rye and wheat. Use in main dishes, cereals, or combined with other cooked grains.

It's Your Turn!

How might you substitute one or more of the grain products listed above for rice in a favorite family dish?

Pearl barley with scallions is a nutritious side dish. Find out what quick-cooking forms of barley are available.

All Kinds of Grains

Explore and enjoy the many ways to eat grain foods. Make them the foundation of a healthful eating plan!

- Bite into breads of all sorts—bagels, breadsticks, pita pockets, tortillas, muffins, and more.
- Be adventurous! Try tasty and nutritious grain foods such as the ones listed on page 283.
- Enjoy grain dishes from around the globe. Have some Italian polenta made with cornmeal or Indian basmati rice mixed with onions, chickpeas, and spices. How about the all-American favorite, macaroni and cheese?
- Aim for at least three daily servings of foods made with whole grains.
- For snacking, pair grain products with other foods. Pita bread triangles go great with hummus (chickpea dip), or wash down some light microwave popcorn with fruit juice.

Shopping for Grain Products

You'll find many grain products throughout the supermarket—for example, dry pasta in the grocery aisles and fresh pasta in the refrigerated case. Use the information on food labels and shelf tags to get the most nutrition for your dollar. If products are similar in content, use the unit price to determine the best value.

- Compare products for their fiber and vitamin and mineral content. Remember that you don't need to get 100 percent of your day's vitamin and mineral needs from a single serving of any food.
  - When buying bread, check the ingredient list for whole grain flour for more fiber.

Choosing Pasta and Rice

Pasta, rice, and other grains add variety, texture, and flavor to many dishes. Choose different pasta shapes for different purposes—perhaps noodles or bow ties for soup, shells to stuff with ricotta cheese, spaghetti or vermicelli to have with a tomato-based sauce.

Like pasta, rice gives you many choices.

- Long-grain rice is dry and fluffy, whereas short-grain rice is moist and sticks together. Medium-grain rice is in between.

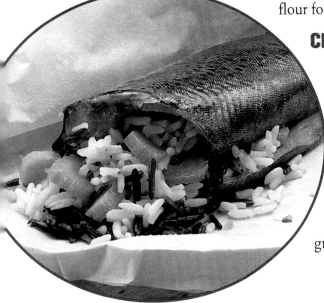

- Brown rice is whole grain rice. It's chewier than white rice, with a nutty flavor. White rice has had the bran and germ removed.
- Converted rice also has no bran or germ, but it has been processed to retain more nutrients.
- Instant rice cooks faster than regular rice, so it's quick and convenient.
- Try flavorful varieties of rice, such as Arborio or jasmine rice.
- Wild rice is not really rice, but it's eaten the same way!

Buying Breakfast Cereal

You have many choices when it comes to breakfast cereal—hot, cold, crunchy, nutty, fruity, and chewy. Dry cereals are ready to pour and eat. To save money, buy plain wheat flakes or cornflakes and add your own extras, such as dried fruits or nuts. To save time with cereals that need cooking—such as oatmeal, grits, farina, and cream of wheat—buy the instant or quick-cooking varieties.

Convenience Options

Take advantage of the many convenient grain food choices. For instance, you can heat frozen waffles or pancakes in the microwave oven or toaster for a quick, easy meal. Other options—such as cornbread mix, refrigerated breadstick dough, and premade pizza shells—are ready to enjoy with just a few quick preparation steps.

More About Wild Rice: Wild rice of northern U.S. and southern Canada, *Zizania aquatica*, is a type of grass with broad blades and long, reedy stems. The Chippewa prepared wild rice with dried blueberries.

Breakfast cereals can be expensive. To save money, avoid expensive packaging and add your own fruit or nuts. At the grocery store, compare prices of cereals packaged in boxes, bags, and bulk.

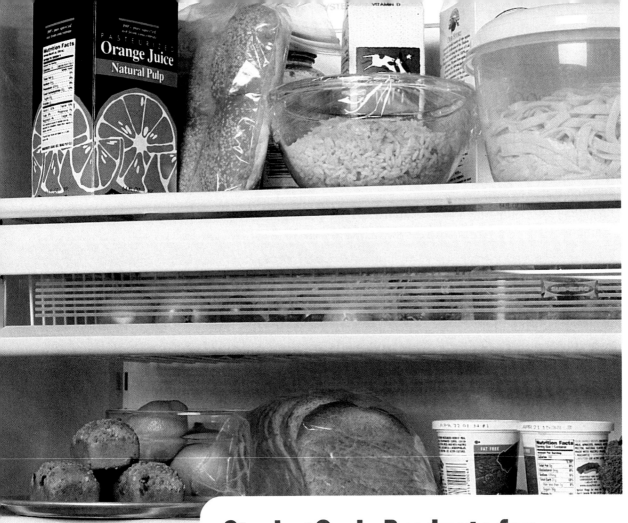

Storing Grain Products for Freshness

To store grain products for maximum freshness, consider their form and ingredients.

- Store breads and rolls in an airtight plastic bag. Refrigerate them in warm, humid weather. If they are whole grain products, refrigeration will keep them fresh longer. Otherwise, keep them at room temperature. If you need to store them longer than a few days, wrap them well and freeze.
- Store dry grain products in a covered container in a cool, dry place. Foods in this category include uncooked rice, pasta, oatmeal, cornmeal, and dry mixes. Most will keep for about a year.
- Store prepared grain products, such as fresh pasta or leftover cooked grains, in the refrigerator if you plan to use them soon. For later use, store them in the freezer.

Whole grain products stay fresh longer when you store them in the refrigerator. Fat in the germ of grains becomes rancid (spoils) when stored too long at room temperature. Not every bread that is brown is whole wheat. Name at least two other types of brown bread.

Discuss: Why keep frozen grain products (waffles, bread dough, and prepared pastas) in the freezer until you're ready to prepare them?

Preparing Grain Products for Healthful Eating

Many grain foods are ready to eat when you buy them. A number of others—including pasta, rice, some cereals, and grains such as bulgur—need to be cooked in liquid. It's really quite simple to cook these grains. To ensure a tasty, tender product, follow package instructions for the amounts of liquid and grain, the method, and the cooking time.

Cooking Pasta

Have you ever eaten pasta that stuck to itself? To make your pasta slippery, not sticky, remember these keys to success.

- Use plenty of water—about 4 quarts (4 L) of water per pound of pasta.
- Heat the water to a vigorous boil before adding the pasta. Keep it boiling during the cooking time. Do not cover.
- Stir occasionally to prevent clumping.

Cook just long enough so that the pasta is **al dente**—*tender but slightly firm.* Use the instructions on the package as a guide to cooking time. The cooking time for fresh or frozen pasta will be shorter than for dried pasta. Drain by carefully pouring the water and pasta into a colander placed in the sink.

Pasta is a type of noodle made from wheat flour, water, and sometimes eggs and other flavorings. It comes in many shapes and sizes—from long strands to corkscrews to shells. Some Asian cultures make noodles from other grains, like rice or buckwheat. What are your favorite kinds of pasta?

Activity: Read and compare the cooking instructions on a variety of dried, fresh, and frozen pasta packages. If possible, demonstrate the cooking procedures for one variety of each type of pasta.

INFOLINK

To learn about baking breads, see Chapter 30. To learn about using grains as thickeners, see Section 4-9 of the Food Preparation Handbook.

INFOLINK

To learn more about cooking pasta, see Section 4-3 of the Food Preparation Handbook.

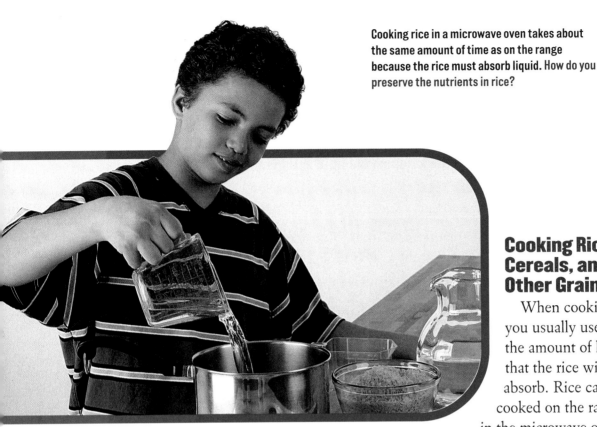

Cooking rice in a microwave oven takes about the same amount of time as on the range because the rice must absorb liquid. How do you preserve the nutrients in rice?

Cooking Rice, Cereals, and Other Grains

When cooking rice, you usually use only the amount of liquid that the rice will absorb. Rice can be cooked on the range or in the microwave oven. Both take about the same amount of time. Cooking methods may vary depending on the type of rice, so check the package directions.

Rice is done when all of the liquid is absorbed and the rice is tender. Brown rice and wild rice typically take longer to cook than white rice. To preserve nutrients, do not rinse rice before or after cooking.

Products such as oatmeal, farina, grits, and whole grains are cooked in much the same way as rice.

Discuss: Suggest combinations of add-ins you would enjoy in rice or grain side dishes and in cooked cereal. Try several of your ideas and report back on the results.

Add-ins for Flavor and Nutrients

For a flavor and nutrition boost, try some of these ideas.
- When cooking rice or other grains for a side dish, use broth or fruit juice as the liquid. Experiment with herbs and spices to enhance flavors without adding salt or fat.
- When cooking cereals, try using milk as the liquid. You can also mix in extras such as dried fruits, nuts, cinnamon, or honey.

NOW *You're* COOKING!

Boiling Pasta

*G*reat-tasting pasta is available in a variety of flavors—such as spinach, whole wheat, tomato, beet, and herb. Pasta can be cooked ahead of time, stored in a covered container in the refrigerator, and then dipped in boiling water to reheat it.

RECIPE

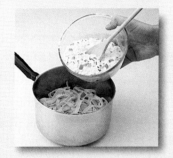

Italian Cheese Noodles

CUSTOMARY	INGREDIENTS	METRIC
2 cups	Bow-tie pasta	500 mL
½ cup	Small curd cottage cheese	125 mL
½ tsp.	Italian seasoning	2 mL
¼ cup	Chopped green bell pepper	50 mL

Yield: 4 servings, ½ cup (125 mL) each

❶ Bring 2 quarts (2 L) of water to a vigorous boil. Add pasta and boil, uncovered, for 8 to 10 minutes or until pasta is al dente, stirring occasionally. Drain.

❷ While pasta is cooking, combine cottage cheese and Italian seasoning. Stir in the bell pepper.

❸ Drain the pasta and return to the pan. Add cottage cheese mixture. Over low heat, warm pasta mixture, stirring constantly. Serve immediately.

Per Serving: 123 calories, 7 g protein, 20 g carbohydrate, 1 g fat, 116 mg sodium, 2 g fiber

Percent Daily Value: vitamin C 13%

More Ideas For more variety:

• Add yesterday's leftover dinner vegetables, meat, poultry, or fish to this pasta dish.

• Try different herbs or herb blends or grated cheeses for an entirely different flavor.

• Pick a different shaped pasta—or perhaps a flavored pasta.

Your Ideas Noodles are eaten around the world. Look for recipes from several countries that use different kinds of noodles such as soba (buckwheat), cellophane (mung bean), soy, and rice noodles. Find out where you can buy these noodles.

Review & Activities

LOOKING BACK

- Grain foods supply key nutrients that fuel your body and contribute to good health.
- When shopping for grain products, check food labels and shelf tags to get the most nutrition for your food dollar.
- To store grain products for freshness, consider their form, ingredients, and when you plan to use them.
- When cooking grain products, follow package directions for the amounts of liquid and grain, the method, and the cooking time.

UNDERSTANDING KEY IDEAS

1. What nutrients are provided by grain foods?
2. Name three different grain foods you could eat at each meal and as snacks.
3. How many Pyramid servings is 1 ounce (28 g) of cornflakes and a whole bagel? How many more servings would you need during the day?
4. How might you save money when buying dry breakfast cereal? What is a time-saving tip for breakfast cereal that needs cooking?
5. What is the best way to store fresh pasta? Uncooked rice?
6. When cooking rice, how can you preserve nutrients? How do you know when the rice is done?

DEVELOPING LIFE SKILLS

1. **Critical Thinking:** What might be the consequences of following an eating plan that limits foods from the Bread, Cereal, Rice, and Pasta Group?
2. **Leadership:** What actions could you take to encourage family members to get the recommended 6 to 11 servings of grain products each day?

Wellness Challenge

Every summer twin brothers Alberto and Emilio spend one month with their cousins. The brothers look forward to their visits but would like more variety in the family meals. Their aunt usually provides doughnuts for breakfast, sandwiches on white bread for lunch, and burgers or hot dogs for dinner along with vegetable and fruit side dishes, milk, and juice. Alberto and Emilio appreciate all their aunt does for them, but they are getting tired of doughnuts and white bread. They miss the greater variety of bread, cereal, rice, and pasta they're used to having at home.

1. What substitutions might help Alberto and Emilio achieve more variety in their meals?
2. How might they suggest these changes while showing thoughtfulness to their aunt and cousins?

APPLYING YOUR LEARNING

1. **Parts of the Grain:** Make a collage of pictures or empty food packages to show grain products that come from the endosperm, bran, germ, or a combination. How do they compare in nutrients and fiber? Why?

2. **Recipe File:** Find recipes for at least five of the grain products listed in "Have You Tried These Grain Foods?" on page 283. Add them to your personal recipe file.

3. **Reading Food Labels:** Compare the labels of several multigrain breads (for example, 5-grain, 7-grain, 12-grain). Which grains are used in the different kinds of bread? How do the breads compare nutritionally? Combine your findings with those of your classmates to make a chart consumers can use to make wise choices.

EXPLORING FURTHER

1. **Processing Grains:** Choose a grain product and learn more about how it's processed. For example, how is enriched flour made? How is converted rice processed? Present your findings to the class.

2. **Fortified Facts:** By law, enriched grain products sold in the U.S. are fortified with folic acid. Find out why and report to the class.

Making CONNECTIONS

1. **Foreign Languages:** How did different pasta shapes get their names? Learn the original meaning of names such as *linguini*, *vermicelli*, *radiatore*, and others. Present your findings using visual aids.

2. **Language Arts:** Write a print or radio ad highlighting the benefits of a specific grain product. Include a brief report describing your target audience, where you would run the ad (for example, what magazines or radio stations), and why you chose that particular product.

FOODS LAB

Prepare two samples of spaghetti. Cook one sample according to the package directions. Cook the other for 7 minutes longer. Compare the appearance and texture of each. What are the differences? What can you conclude from your results?

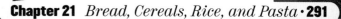

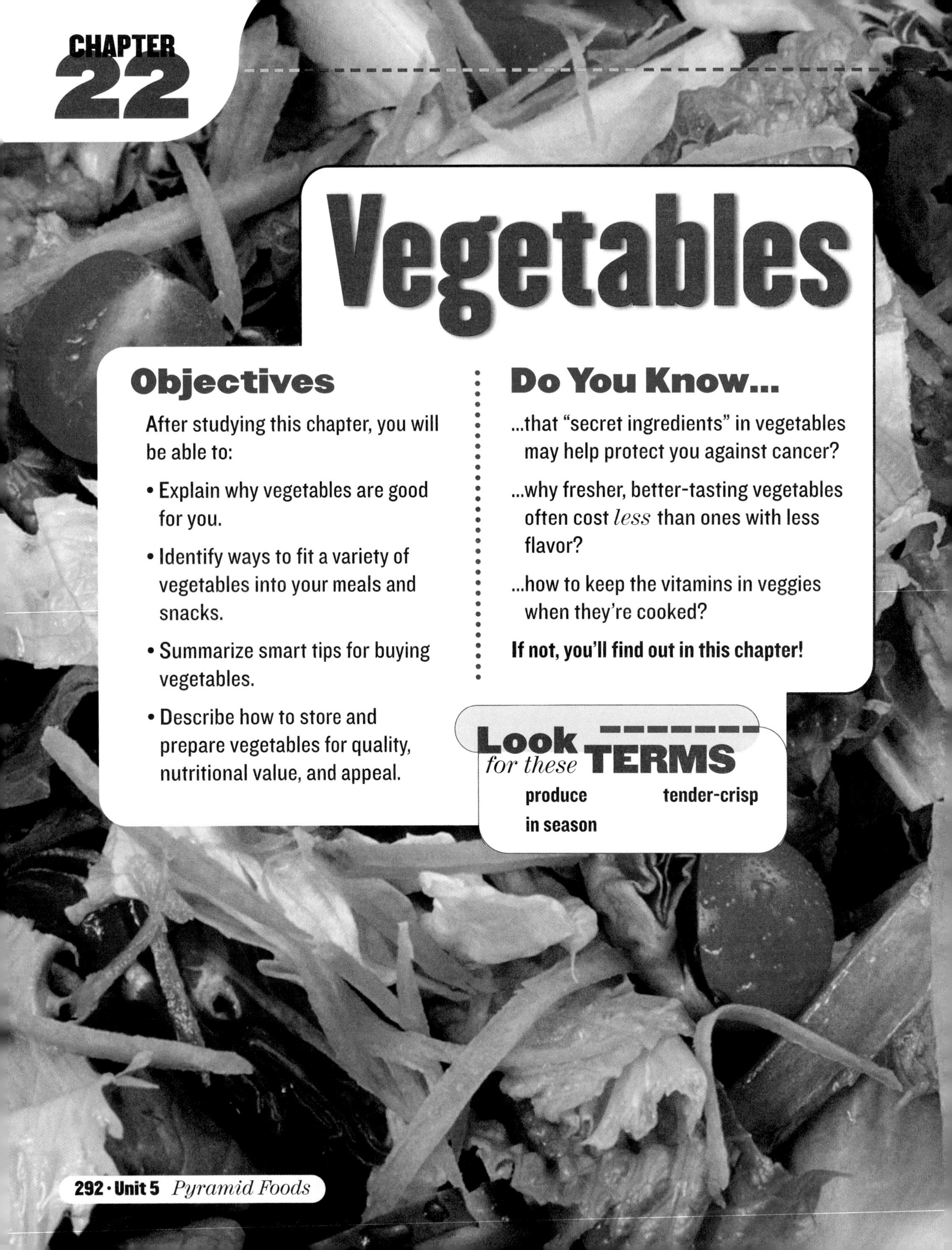

CHAPTER 22

Vegetables

Objectives

After studying this chapter, you will be able to:

- Explain why vegetables are good for you.
- Identify ways to fit a variety of vegetables into your meals and snacks.
- Summarize smart tips for buying vegetables.
- Describe how to store and prepare vegetables for quality, nutritional value, and appeal.

Do You Know...

...that "secret ingredients" in vegetables may help protect you against cancer?

...why fresher, better-tasting vegetables often cost *less* than ones with less flavor?

...how to keep the vitamins in veggies when they're cooked?

If not, you'll find out in this chapter!

Look for these TERMS

produce

in season

tender-crisp

Vegetables are great!

They're packed with nutrition and flavor, they're colorful, and they can be enjoyed in so many different ways. You can eat them as appetizers, salads, side dishes, garnishes, and snacks. They're flavorful ingredients in many main dishes. They even make great additions to baked foods and desserts.

Vegetables— For Your Health

Why is "Eat your vegetables" good advice? For one thing, vegetables taste good—especially if they're prepared properly. Vegetables are also chock-full of nutrients and other health-promoting benefits. No matter what their form—fresh, frozen, or canned—if they're handled properly, they provide these nutritional advantages.

"Carbs" for energy. Most of your food energy should come from carbohydrates: starches and sugars. Vegetables are great sources. Sweet corn, green peas, potatoes, squash, and turnips are high in natural sugars and starches.

Fiber. Fiber gives shape to vegetables. It's part of the celery stalk, the skin of a potato, and the stem in lettuce leaves, for instance. Remember, fiber helps your digestive system work properly.

Low in fat, no cholesterol. Almost all vegetables contain little or no fat naturally. Unless excess fat is added in processing, cooking, or serving, vegetables stay low-fat—and low in calories, too. Another plus: all vegetables are cholesterol-free.

Packed with vitamins and minerals. Different vegetables provide different vitamins and minerals. That's one reason why variety is such a great thing. For a few examples, see "Vegetables for Vitamins and Minerals" on page 294.

Activity: Imagine that you write a nutrition advice column. Answer this reader's question: Which are most nutritious— fresh, frozen, or canned vegetables? Will eating vegetables help my energy level?

Many vegetables contain fiber, which helps your digestive system work properly. Keep the edible skin on vegetables for nutrition. Find out what other vegetables are high in fiber.

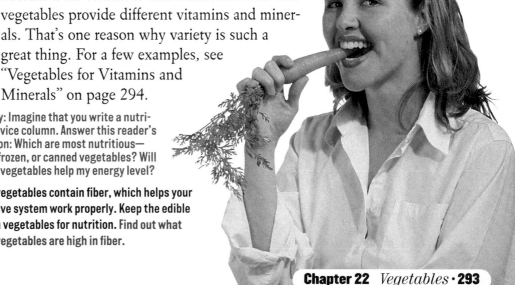

INFOLINK

To read more about phytochemicals, see Chapter 5, page 85.

The latest news—phytochemicals! There's more to vegetables than nutrients. Scientists are starting to learn about phytochemicals—natural chemicals found in plants. Throughout your life, they may help protect you from cancer, heart disease, and other health problems. That's another reason to eat plenty of veggies!

Teaching with Visuals: Work in small groups to create an infomercial about vegetables. Use information from the chart.

Vegetables for Vitamins and Minerals

VEGETABLE	VITAMIN A	VITAMIN C	FOLATE	CALCIUM	MAGNESIUM	POTASSIUM
Bok choy	✔	✔				
Broccoli	✔	✔	✔			
Cabbage		✔				
Carrots	✔					
Green peppers		✔				
Lentils			✔			✔
Okra		✔			✔	
Peas, green		✔	✔			✔
Potato		✔				✔
Spinach	✔	✔	✔	✔	✔	✔
Sweet potato	✔	✔				✔
Tomato	✔	✔				✔
Turnip greens	✔	✔	✔			
Winter squash	✔	✔				✔

✔ = One serving contains at least 10 percent of the Daily Value (DV) of that vitamin or mineral. Calculations based on ½ cup (125 mL) serving, except for potato, sweet potato, and tomato, which are one medium-sized vegetable.

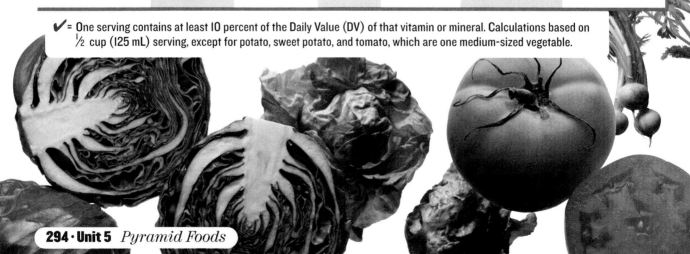

Critical Thinking: Why do legumes belong in both the Vegetable Group and the Meat, Poultry, Fish, Dry Beans, and Nuts Group?

Activity: Survey friends and family members for other veggie snack ideas. Share your survey results in class.

The Food Guide Pyramid's Advice

For the balanced nutrition you need for energy, growth, and health, eat three to five vegetable servings each day. Remember, one serving from the Vegetable Group is:

- ½ cup (125 mL) of nonleafy vegetables (cooked or raw).
- 1 cup (250 mL) of leafy greens.
- 1 small potato.
- ¾ cup (175 mL) of vegetable juice.
- ½ cup (125 mL) of cooked dry beans or peas.

Legumes belong in two food groups: the Vegetable Group and the Meat, Poultry, Fish, Dry Beans, Eggs, and Nuts Group. In a healthful eating plan, you count a serving in one group or the other, not both. You decide.

Veggie Variety

The Vegetable Group has everything from A (for asparagus) to Z (for zucchini). Variety brings you a mixture of nutritional benefits. It also makes meals look and taste more interesting.

When you choose vegetables, go beyond french fries!

- Choose mostly vegetables prepared and served with little or no fat.
- Enjoy different vegetables—and different varieties of the same vegetable (such as green, red, and yellow bell peppers).
- Eat a vitamin A–rich vegetable at least every other day.

Check This Out!

VEGGIES FOR YOUR SNACK ATTACK

When you get the hungries, think veggies! Snacks are a great way to tuck vegetable servings into your eating plan.

- Cut raw veggies into easy-to-eat slices or sticks.
- Dip crisp, raw veggies or chips into spicy salsa.
- Pour a tall glass of tomato or vegetable juice over ice.
- Load a home-baked pizza with chopped tomatoes, broccoli, or bell peppers.
- Cut broccoli or cauliflower into bite-size florets. Serve with a light dip.
- Just wash and eat baby carrots or cherry tomatoes.

It's Your Turn!

Challenge yourself to add one vegetable serving a day through your snack choices. Keep track for a week. How did you do?

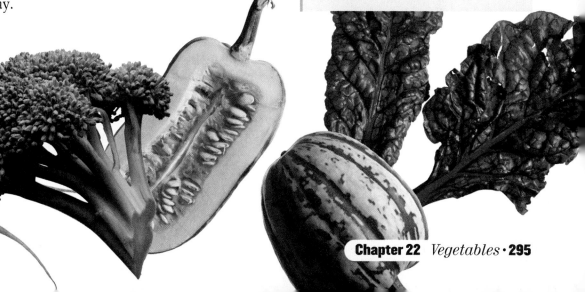

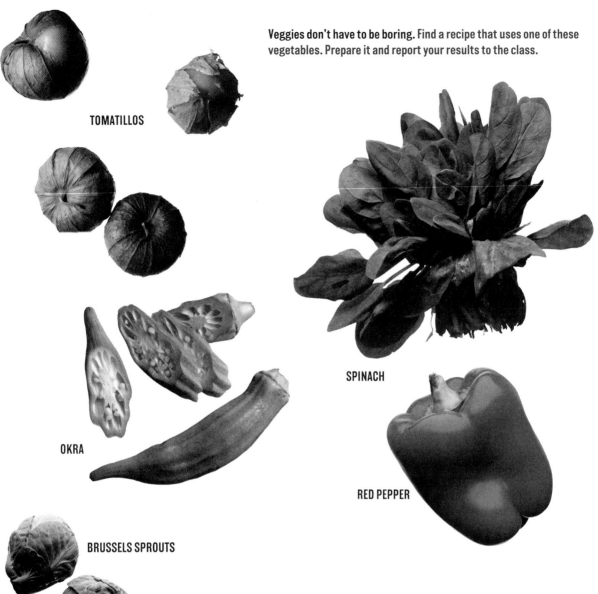

Veggies don't have to be boring. Find a recipe that uses one of these vegetables. Prepare it and report your results to the class.

TOMATILLOS

SPINACH

OKRA

RED PEPPER

BRUSSELS SPROUTS

How Are You Doing?

Are you following the Pyramid's advice when it comes to vegetables? If not, think about the possible reasons.

- *Not handy?* Then ask your family to keep more vegetables on hand.
- *Boring?* Try new varieties—a new vegetable each week. Have you ever eaten brussels sprouts or bok choy? What about jicama (HE-kuh-muh) or okra?
- *Don't like them?* Learn to prepare vegetables properly or in a new way. Maybe you'd like them as raw, crispy finger foods.
- *Not in the habit?* Make a point to have an additional vegetable serving each day for the next month. It can become a new habit!

Shopping for Vegetables

Do you pick the vegetables on the family shopping trip? Knowing your options and the qualities to look for helps you make smart choices.

Selecting Fresh Vegetables

Today's supermarkets sell more fresh vegetables than ever. You can find them in the produce department. **Produce** includes *fresh vegetables, fruits, and herbs.* In some areas, vegetables are also sold at farmers' markets and roadside stands.

As you choose from the colorful array, try to get the most vegetable nutrition for your food dollar.

• Choose vegetables at their peak. See "Fresh Vegetables—What to Look For" below.

• Look for Nutrition Facts—perhaps on a sign or in a brochure.

• Buy only the amount you need. Since fresh vegetables are perishable, they will keep their peak quality for a short time and may spoil quickly.

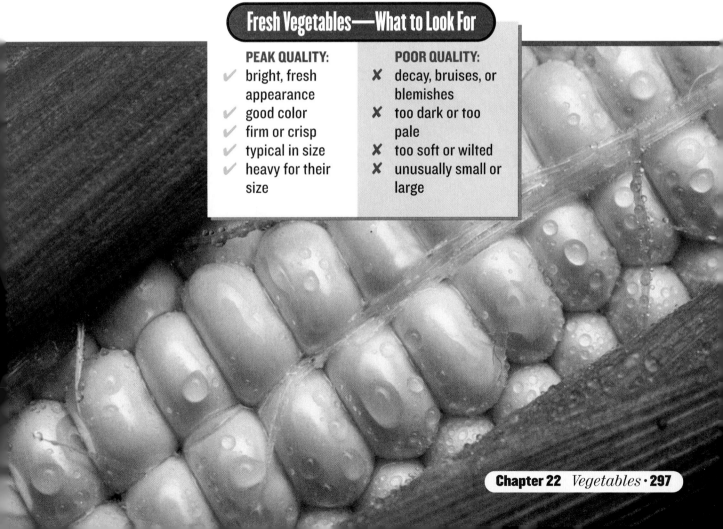

Fresh Vegetables—What to Look For

PEAK QUALITY:	POOR QUALITY:
✔ bright, fresh appearance	✘ decay, bruises, or blemishes
✔ good color	✘ too dark or too pale
✔ firm or crisp	✘ too soft or wilted
✔ typical in size	✘ unusually small or large
✔ heavy for their size	

Activity: Research when certain vegetables are in season. Make charts showing the vegetables in season during each month. **Vegetables purchased in season generally cost less than at other times of the year.** Ask the produce manager at your local supermarket which vegetables are currently in season and how their prices compare with the prices when they are not in season.

Buying in Season

Produce is shipped from all over the world, wherever it grows. That's why you can buy so many varieties of fresh vegetables all year.

However, many vegetables have a certain time of year when they are **in season**. That's when they are *highest in quality, most plentiful, and lowest in cost.* In the summer, for instance, you may find vine-ripened tomatoes fresh from local growers. These usually have better flavor than tomatoes purchased at other times of the year. They generally cost less, too, because they are plentiful and don't have to be shipped far. Vegetables purchased in season are a great value.

Convenience Options

Partly or fully prepared vegetables often cost more than fresh vegetables. You spend more to save time. It's a trade-off.

For vegetables in convenience forms, check throughout your store.

Grocery aisles. Canned vegetables are great to keep on hand and may cost less than fresh or frozen. Also look for dried vegetables, such as onion flakes and vegetable soup mixes.

Freezer case. Frozen vegetables range from simple bags of corn and peas to creative mixtures in microwave-safe containers.

Produce department. Look for salad mixes, stir-fry vegetable mixes, washed veggie snacks, and ready-made salsa.

Deli. Delis may sell premade salads or heat-and-eat vegetables.

Salad bar. You can mix all kinds of vegetables from the salad bar to match your appetite and budget.

More About Buying in Season: Freeze or can in-season vegetables to use when they're out of season and expensive.

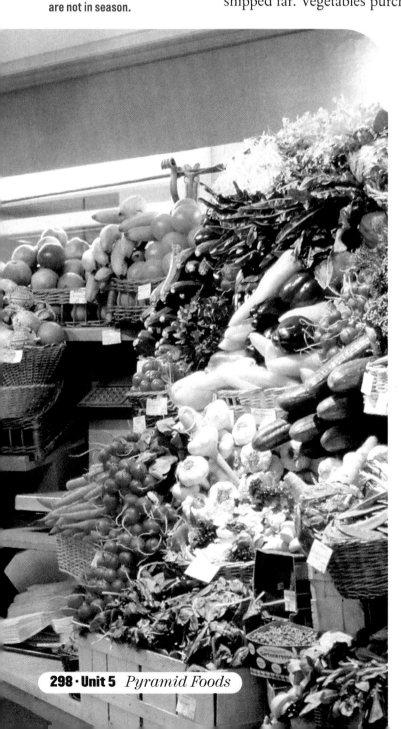

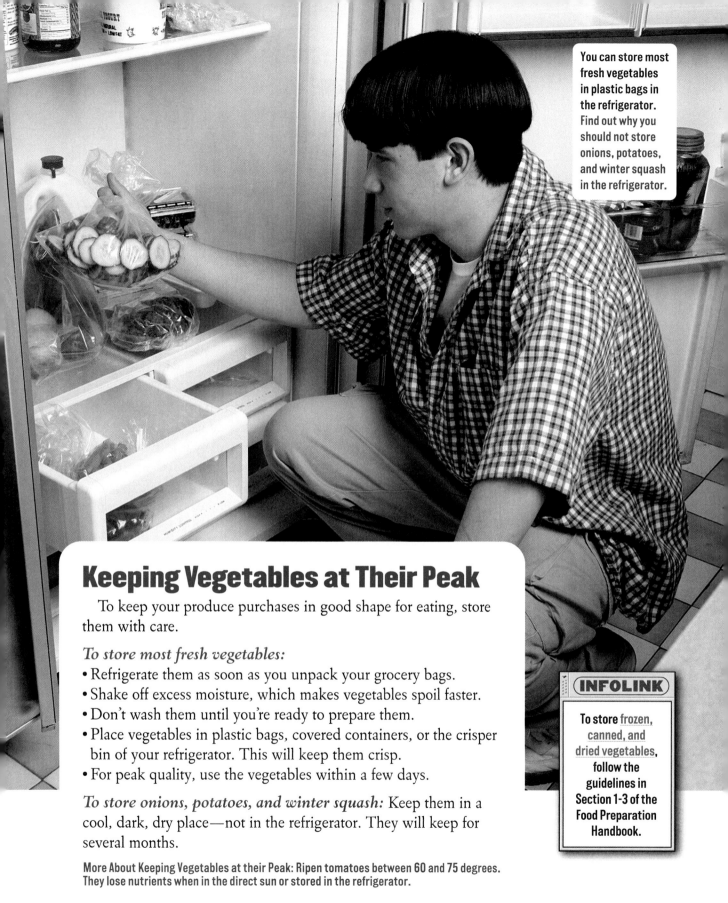

You can store most fresh vegetables in plastic bags in the refrigerator. Find out why you should not store onions, potatoes, and winter squash in the refrigerator.

Keeping Vegetables at Their Peak

To keep your produce purchases in good shape for eating, store them with care.

To store most fresh vegetables:
• Refrigerate them as soon as you unpack your grocery bags.
• Shake off excess moisture, which makes vegetables spoil faster.
• Don't wash them until you're ready to prepare them.
• Place vegetables in plastic bags, covered containers, or the crisper bin of your refrigerator. This will keep them crisp.
• For peak quality, use the vegetables within a few days.

To store onions, potatoes, and winter squash: Keep them in a cool, dark, dry place—not in the refrigerator. They will keep for several months.

More About Keeping Vegetables at their Peak: Ripen tomatoes between 60 and 75 degrees. They lose nutrients when in the direct sun or stored in the refrigerator.

INFOLINK

To store frozen, canned, and dried vegetables, follow the guidelines in Section 1-3 of the Food Preparation Handbook.

Preparing Vegetables for Healthful Eating

No matter where vegetables belong in your day's food choices, prepare them with these goals in mind.

- Make sure they're clean.
- Keep in nutrients.
- Maintain their flavor, texture, and color.
- Add flavor with little or no fat.
- Enjoy preparing and eating them!

Cleaning Fresh Vegetables

Fresh and firm, crisp and colorful—how do you make fresh vegetables ready to eat? Start by cleaning them well. Cleaning removes dirt, bacteria, and residues.

- Wash vegetables under cold running water. Skip soap unless it's sold especially for cleaning produce. To retain nutrients, don't soak.
- Use a brush on firm vegetables, such as potatoes and squash.
- Trim parts you can't eat, such as tough stems. Cut out rough spots or soft spots.
- Remove outer leaves of lettuce, cabbage, and other leafy vegetables.

Raw Veggies as Finger Foods

Salads and sandwiches are made with all kinds of raw vegetables. Once cleaned, many vegetables make great finger foods, too. Cut them into slices, sticks, or chunks for easy eating. Then refrigerate them in an airtight container so that they're ready to eat when you want them.

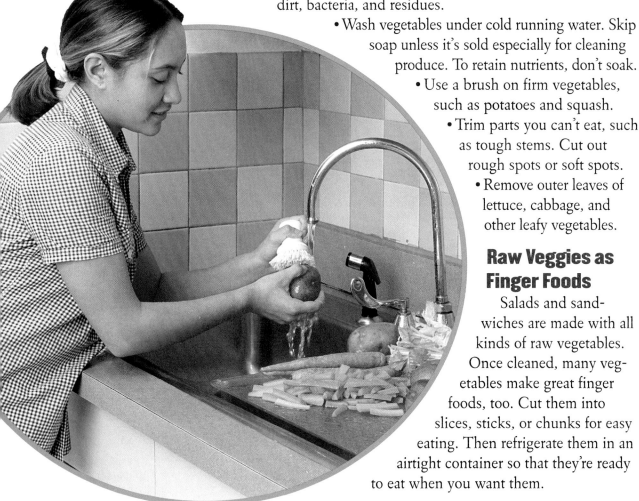

Emphasize: Wash vegetables before eating (skin may contain pesticides or bacteria). Scrub carrots, sweet potatoes, white potatoes, and celery with a vegetable brush to remove dirt. Rinse lettuce and cabbage under cold running water.

Clean fresh vegetables well to remove dirt. What are other ways you can make fresh vegetables ready to eat?

Many vegetables are crunchy and tasty when raw—carrots, broccoli, snow peas, jicama, cucumber, zucchini, and bell peppers, to name a few. What raw vegetables would taste good to you?

Cooking Vegetables

Cooking softens vegetables, making them easier for you to chew. It also changes their flavor, offering another taste experience. Some vegetables, such as potatoes, winter squash, and artichokes, must be cooked before you can eat them.

Choosing a Cooking Method

Vegetables can be cooked in many ways. To preserve nutrients without adding fat, you might choose to bake, simmer, steam, or microwave them. Grilling, another low-fat cooking method, can give vegetables a char-broiled flavor. Stir-frying adds only a little fat. With other forms of frying, vegetables soak up fat and calories.

When you're in a hurry, stir-frying and microwaving may be the quickest. For convenience, bake potatoes, sweet potatoes, and winter squash in their own skins. If you have more time, a baked vegetable casserole might match the occasion. It's also a convenient way to cook for and serve a crowd.

Keeping in Nutrients

Vegetables need to be prepared properly to lock in nutrients and fiber.

- Leave edible skins on vegetables such as carrots, potatoes, or zucchini. The skin provides fiber. Together the skin and the area just below it supply most of the nutrients.
- If you need to cut up vegetables for cooking, leave the pieces as large as you can. With greater surface area, they'll lose fewer vitamins when they're cooked in water.

Emphasize: Potatoes boiled or baked in the skin retain almost all their vitamins. A whole cooked sweet potato keeps 90% of its vitamin C, but if cut in half, only about 30%. Vegetables, cooked ahead, stored, and reheated, lose large amounts of vitamins.

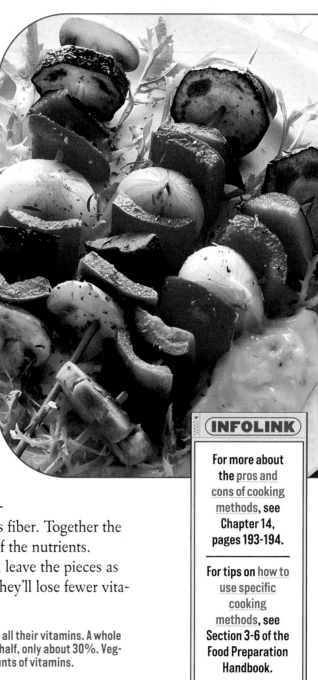

Grilling is a low-fat cooking method that gives vegetables a distinct flavor. Compare the taste of a vegetable made several different ways. You might bake it, steam it, or fry it. Report your findings to the class.

INFOLINK

For more about the pros and cons of cooking methods, see Chapter 14, pages 193-194.

For tips on how to use specific cooking methods, see Section 3-6 of the Food Preparation Handbook.

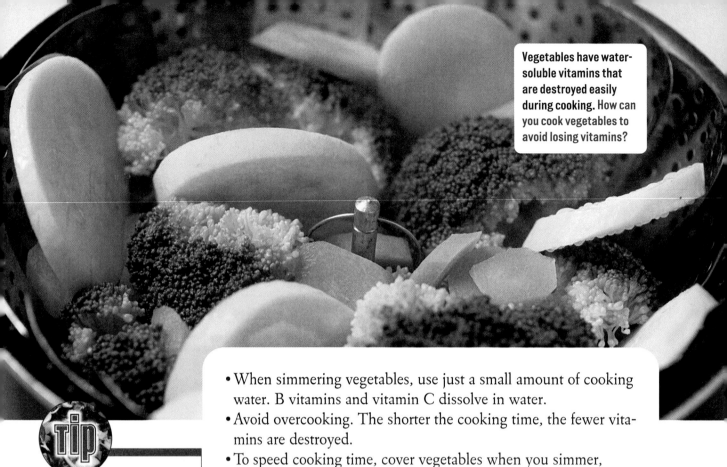

Vegetables have water-soluble vitamins that are destroyed easily during cooking. How can you cook vegetables to avoid losing vitamins?

- When simmering vegetables, use just a small amount of cooking water. B vitamins and vitamin C dissolve in water.
- Avoid overcooking. The shorter the cooking time, the fewer vitamins are destroyed.
- To speed cooking time, cover vegetables when you simmer, steam, or microwave them.

Preserving Flavor, Texture, and Color

Paint your plate with veggies! They add color, flavor, and texture to your meals. Cooked properly, they keep these great qualities.

Remember to keep the cooking time short. Besides helping nutrients stay in, this will:

- Keep the naturally fresh taste. Broccoli and cauliflower, for instance, develop stronger flavors as they're cooked.
- Prevent vegetables from getting too soft or mushy. For most cooked vegetables, your goal is **tender-crisp**. That means they're *tender, but still firm and slightly crisp.*
- Help green vegetables stay bright green instead of turning brownish-green or yellow-green.

Adding Flavor Without Fat and Salt

To enhance the flavor of vegetables, you might add herbs or lemon juice. Go easy on salt, or skip it altogether. Salt can mask a vegetable's natural flavor.

For a buttery flavor, toss vegetables with just a touch of butter or margarine. The flavor is more intense if it's added just before serving.

Tip

Save leftover cooking liquid for its vitamin value. Add it to soup, stews, or gravy, or use it to moisten mashed potatoes.

INFOLINK

For more about the food science behind the colors of vegetables, see Section 4-4 of the Food Preparation Handbook.

Activity: Cook green vegetables at home using different cooking methods and times. Log the flavor, texture, and color. Discuss which methods and times were best for each vegetable.

NOW *You're* COOKING!

SKILL
Stir-Frying

*S*tir-frying is an easy way to prepare vegetables. Because it's quick, the vegetables can keep their bright color and tender-crisp texture.

RECIPE

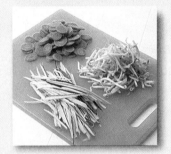

Colorful Vegetables

CUSTOMARY	INGREDIENTS	METRIC
1½ tsp.	Vegetable oil	7 mL
1 cup	Thin, diagonally sliced carrots	250 mL
1 cup	Julienned zucchini	250 mL
1 cup	Bean sprouts	250 mL

Yield: 4 servings, ½ cup (125 mL) each

1. Heat a wok or heavy skillet over high heat. Add oil and then carrots. Stir-fry for 2 minutes.
2. Add zucchini and continue stir-frying for 1 minute.
3. Add bean sprouts; stir-fry for 45 to 60 seconds or until hot. Serve immediately.

Per Serving: 39 calories, 1 g protein, 5 g carbohydrate, 2 g fat, 12 mg sodium, 2 g fiber
Percent Daily Value: vitamin A 78%, vitamin E 10%, vitamin C 14%

More Ideas Try these additions to create a stir-fry dish with more flavor, color, or nutrients:

- Sprinkle with lemon pepper, fresh or dried herbs, or a splash of low-sodium soy sauce.
- Stir-fry thin strips of chicken or beef first, and then frozen stir-fry vegetables (thawed). When they're cooked, toss with cooked noodles for a meal in one.

Your Ideas

- Check cookbooks for stir-fry recipes from three Asian countries. Prepare one of the dishes for your family.
- Suggest vegetable combinations that appeal to you and write your own recipe. Consider colors, flavors, and cooking times as you create your recipe.

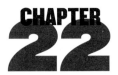
LOOKING BACK

- Vegetables are valuable for their nutrients and other health benefits.

- Eating a wide variety of vegetables, instead of just a few, boosts the nutrition and appeal of your eating plan.

- When buying vegetables, try to get the most nutrition for your money.

- Vegetables will keep their quality and nutrition longer if stored properly.

- Smart preparation helps vegetables keep their nutrients, color, flavor, and texture.

UNDERSTANDING KEY IDEAS

1. What are the nutritional advantages of vegetables?

2. What might encourage you to include a greater variety of vegetables in your eating plan?

3. If you were buying fresh carrots, how could you tell which bunch to buy and which to pass up?

4. How should you store fresh broccoli? Potatoes?

5. When simmering fresh zucchini, what can you do to retain as many nutrients as possible? Give at least three strategies.

DEVELOPING LIFE SKILLS

1. **Critical Thinking:** Jorge eats about one or two servings of vegetables a day. Predict what might happen as a result of his vegetable eating habits.

2. **Leadership:** How could parents, teachers, and caregivers help young children learn to like a variety of vegetables? Why is this important?

3. **Communication:** If you managed the produce department of a supermarket, what would you want your customers to know about vegetables? How could you communicate it in an interesting way?

Wellness Challenge

Two friends, Tonya and Garrett, have an idea for a new teen community group. They want to clean up an empty lot near the school and plant a vegetable garden. By allowing volunteer gardeners to take home a portion of the produce, Tonya and Garrett hope to promote good eating habits. They plan to sell the remainder of the vegetables at a local farmers' market and donate the profits to a center that helps needy members of the community.

1. What challenges might Tonya and Garrett face in starting their project and keeping it going?

2. How could they go about finding solutions?

APPLYING YOUR LEARNING

1. **Menu Planning:** Imagine you are planning to serve a fresh vegetable tray at a party. What six kinds of vegetables would you include? Aim for a variety of nutrients, colors, textures, and flavors. Identify the major nutrients provided and their sources.

2. **Recipe File:** Collect at least ten vegetable recipes or preparation ideas. Each should use a different type of vegetable and be practical for use at home. Try to find low-fat recipes. Add these to your recipe file.

EXPLORING FURTHER

1. **New-to-You Vegetable:** Learn about a vegetable you have never eaten before. Where and how is it grown? What nutrients does it provide? What are some ways to prepare it? If possible, sample the vegetable and describe its flavor and texture.

2. **Local Produce:** Find out what locally grown vegetables are available in your area at different times of the year. (Hint: You might use resources such as the Cooperative Extension Service or the produce manager at a local supermarket.)

Making CONNECTIONS

1. **Math:** Compare the prices and nutrition labels of several different forms of a vegetable, such as fresh whole, prewashed and cut, canned, and frozen. How does the cost per serving compare? How does the nutrient content compare? Show your findings in chart form.

2. **Science:** How much longer do fresh vegetables keep their quality when stored according to the advice in this chapter? Plan and carry out an experiment to find out. Choose one specific storage guideline to test. Write a report that includes your hypothesis, procedure, observations, and conclusions.

FOODS LAB

Prepare two samples of fresh or frozen broccoli: one cooked just until tender-crisp, the other cooked until very soft. Compare the texture, color, and flavor of each. Which one is more appealing to you? Why? How do you think they compare nutritionally? Why?

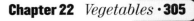

Fruits

Objectives

After studying this chapter, you will be able to:

• Explain how fruits contribute to good health.

• Identify ways to include a variety of fruits in meals and snacks.

• Summarize smart tips for selecting fruits and juices.

• Describe how to store and prepare fruits for quality, nutritional value, and appeal.

Do You Know....

...why it's wise to eat the edible skins and seeds of some fruits?

...what happens during ripening that makes fruits more flavorful?

...how to tell if fruits are at their prime?

If not, you'll find out in this chapter!

Look *for these* TERMS

citrus fruit   fruit concentrate

ripe   fruit nectar

Think of fruits

as nature's gems! Their bright colors, natural sweetness, and refreshing juiciness make them appealing to eat alone or with other foods. They add nutrients and flavor to appetizers, salads, side dishes, snacks, and desserts. Fruits can also enhance the flavors of many main dishes. With so many varieties of fruits available, the possibilities seem endless!

Fruit—Good for You

Chances are you've heard the saying, "An apple a day keeps the doctor away." The saying may not be literally true, but eat a variety of fruits and you'll get many health benefits!

Energy. Fresh fruits are a source of the carbohydrates needed to supply your body with energy. Much of these carbohydrates are natural sugars. They give fruits their sweet flavor. Some canned, frozen, and dried fruits contain added sugar, too, which adds calories.

Fiber. The fiber in fruit helps your digestive tract work properly. It may also help protect against cancer and heart disease. Fiber is part of the edible skins of fruits such as apples, pears, and grapes. It's also part of the pulp, for example, in **citrus fruits** (*oranges, tangerines, and grapefruits*). Edible seeds in strawberries and kiwi fruit offer fiber, too.

Low-fat, cholesterol-free. Most fruits contain no fat. Avocados do contain fat, so eat them less frequently than other fruits. Like vegetables, all fruits are cholesterol-free.

Nutrition bargains. Fruits are brimming with vitamins and minerals. Choose a variety of fruits and juices to get the benefits of their different vitamins and minerals. The chart on page 308 shows some of the nutrients in different fruits. One serving of the fruits listed provides at least 10 percent of the Daily Value for the nutrients shown. Which fruits are good sources of two or more of these nutrients?

Fresh fruits make a great snack because they are naturally sweet. Name several fruits you might choose to eat for dessert or as a snack.

(INFOLINK)

For more about
<u>phytochemicals</u>,
see Chapter 5,
page 85.

More benefits. Phytochemicals in foods from plants may help protect you from cancer, heart disease, and other health problems. These potential benefits are just another reason to eat plenty of fruits!

Teaching with Visuals: Prepare posters to instruct children on the health benefits of eating fruit. Include information from the chart.

Fruits for Vitamins and Minerals

FRUIT	VITAMIN A	VITAMIN C	FOLATE	POTASSIUM
Apple*		✔		
Apricot	✔	✔		✔
Avocado			✔	✔
Banana*		✔		✔
Cantaloupe	✔	✔		✔
Grapefruit		✔		
Guava	✔	✔		
Kiwifruit		✔		
Mango	✔	✔		
Orange*		✔	✔	
Papaya		✔		
Peach*	✔	✔		
Pear*		✔		
Pineapple		✔		
Pomegranate*		✔		✔
Raspberries		✔		
Starfruit		✔		
Strawberries		✔		
Watermelon		✔		

✔ = One serving of the fruit contains at least 10 percent of the Daily Value (DV) of that vitamin or mineral. Calculations are based on a ½ cup (125 mL) serving, except where noted by an asterisk (*), which denotes a medium piece of fruit.

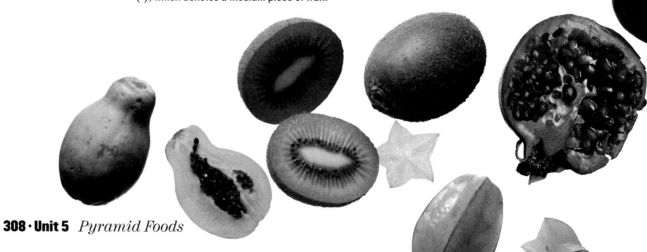

The Food Guide Pyramid's Advice

To obtain the nutrients you need for energy, growth, and health, eat two to four servings of fruit each day. One serving is:

• 1 medium whole fruit, such as an apple, pear, orange, or banana.
• ½ of a grapefruit, mango, or papaya.
• ½ cup (125 mL) berries or cut-up fruit.
• ½ cup (125 mL) canned, frozen, or cooked fruit.
• ¾ cup (175 mL) of fruit juice.
• ¼ cup (50 mL) of dried fruit.

Products such as jelly, jam, and fruit-flavored drinks don't count as servings from the Fruit Group. They contain mostly added sugar and flavorings and only a small amount of fruit juice. Instead, these foods belong in the tip of the Food Guide Pyramid.

Fruit Variety

Take advantage of the array of colors, shapes, and textures of fruits. They add interest as well as nutritional benefits to your meals and snacks. Enjoy the refreshing flavors of fruits and juices anytime—at the start of a meal, with a meal, as a naturally sweet dessert, or as a snack.

Follow these tips to get the most from your fruit choices.

• Eat a vitamin C-rich fruit or juice every day. Breakfast is a good time to enjoy choices such as citrus juice, melon, or strawberries.
• Choose mostly fruits and juices without added sugar.
• Be adventurous! Try a fruit you've never tasted. Do you know what mangoes, kumquats, persimmons, and pomegranates taste like?
• Use dried, canned, and frozen fruit when fresh fruits aren't available.
• Choose fresh fruits with edible skins for extra fiber.

Discuss: How can you include a variety of fruits in your meals?

Activity: Keep a log of the number of servings and kinds of fruits you eat over a period of three days. Plan how to increase, if necessary, the number of servings or the variety.

HOW DO YOUR CHOICES STACK UP?

During a typical week:

✔ Do your daily food choices include two or more servings from the Fruit Group?

✔ Do you regularly eat fruits with edible skins or seeds?

✔ Do you choose canned fruits and fruit juices without added sugar?

✔ Do you eat a vitamin C-rich fruit or drink a vitamin C-rich fruit juice each day?

If you can answer "yes" to these questions, you're getting plenty of nutrition from your fruit choices!

Shopping for Fruits

Do you know what to look for when shopping for fruits and fruit juices? Getting the best quality and nutrition from your fruit choices should be your goal. Read on to learn how!

Tip

For Nutrition Facts for your choices, look for signs or brochures placed nearby in the produce department of a supermarket.

Ripe or Unripe?

You can find many varieties of fresh fruits in today's supermarkets and at local farmers' markets and roadside stands. Use these tips to make tasty selections.

Ripe fruit is generally *full of flavor and color and ready to be eaten*. Unripe fruit is usually hard to the touch and less flavorful. Ripe fruits taste sweeter because the carbohydrate has turned from starch to sugar.

- Cherries, grapes, citrus fruits, and pineapples should be ripe when you buy them. They don't ripen further once they're harvested. Buy only the amount you plan to use within a day or two.
- Apricots, avocados, bananas, and peaches continue to ripen after they're harvested. If you want to use them within a day or two, buy ripe ones. For later use, buy unripe ones and let them ripen at home.

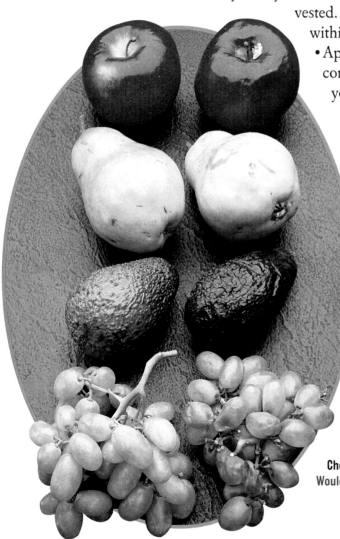

Fresh Fruit—What to Look For

Use your senses when selecting fresh fruit.

Sight. The color should be bright and fresh-looking, without dark spots.

Touch. The fruit should be free of dents or bruises. Some ripe fruit will be slightly soft when pressed gently.

Smell. Some ripe fruit such as peaches, nectarines, and melons will have a sweet aroma.

Choose fresh fruits that are not bruised or too soft. Would you pass up any of these fruits? Which ones and why?

Calendar for Buying Fruit in Season

	JAN.	FEB.	MAR.	APR.	MAY	JUNE	JULY	AUG.	SEPT.	OCT.	NOV.	DEC.
Apple									✓	✓	✓	
Apricot						✓	✓					
Avocado	✓	✓	✓	✓	✓	✓	✓	✓	✓	✓	✓	✓
Cherry					✓	✓	✓	✓				
Grapefruit	✓	✓	✓	✓	✓	✓	✓	✓	✓	✓	✓	✓
Mango					✓	✓	✓	✓	✓			
Melon								✓	✓	✓		
Orange (navel)	✓	✓	✓	✓	✓						✓	✓
Peach					✓	✓	✓	✓	✓	✓		
Pear	✓	✓	✓				✓	✓	✓	✓	✓	✓
Plum					✓	✓	✓	✓	✓	✓		
Strawberry				✓	✓	✓						

Teaching with Visuals: Choose a month and plan a snack using the fruit in season for that month.

Buying Fruit in Season

As with vegetables, some fruits are "in season" at a specific time of the year. That's when they are most plentiful, highest in quality, and lower in price. Look for these bargains when you shop.

Buying Fruit for Convenience

Browse in your supermarket and you'll discover many convenient options for buying fruits. These options may cost more but can save time and allow you to enjoy the flavors and nutrients from fruit all year.

Produce department and salad bar. Look for precut fruits, such as melon and pineapple, and premade fruit salads. You'll also find dried fruits, such as raisins, prunes, cherries, cranberries, apricots, and bananas.

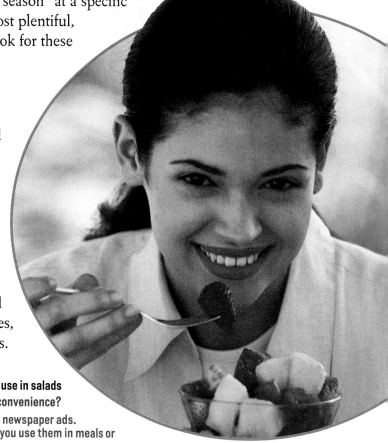

You could save time by buying precut or canned fruit to use in salads and other recipes. What is the trade-off of buying this convenience?

Activity: Find out what fruits are featured as specials in newspaper ads. Which fruits would be a good buy this week? How could you use them in meals or snacks?

Grocery aisles. Many fruits are available in cans or jars. Canned fruits may be whole, sliced, halved, or crushed and may be packed in water, juice, or a sugary syrup. Canned fruits are great to keep on hand and may cost less per serving than fresh or frozen. Look for bottled and boxed juices, too.

Dairy case. You'll find cartons of chilled, ready-to-serve fruit juices in the dairy case. These perishable fruit juices may be made from oncentrated juices.

Freezer case. Fruits in the freezer case include sliced peaches and whole or crushed berries, such as strawberries, raspberries, and blueberries. Some berries are frozen in a sugar syrup. You'll also find frozen **fruit concentrates** (*juice with most of the water removed*) for making juice.

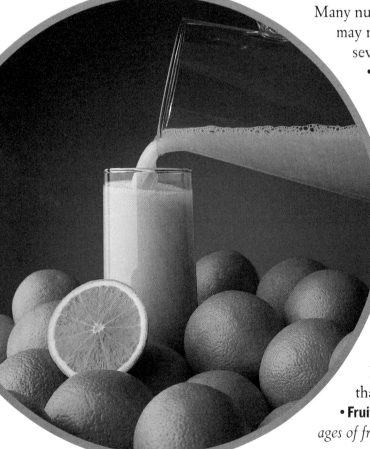

Fruit juices allow you to enjoy the flavor of fresh fruit all year. What is the difference between a product labeled "juice" and one labeled "fruit drink"?

Buying Fruit Juice

The next best thing to whole fruits is their juice. Many nutrients of fruits stay in the juice, but juice may not contain fiber. Look for fruit juices in several different forms.

- Beverages labeled "juice" must be 100 percent juice. They may be bottled, concentrated, or sold chilled and ready-to-serve. Some may contain added vitamins and minerals. Sometimes sweeteners are added to tart juices, such as cranberry juice.

- Products labeled "fruit punch," "fruit drink," "juice blend," or "juice cocktail" contain only a portion of juice. The label tells how much, such as 10 percent. The rest is water, added flavorings, and added sugar. Vitamin C or other nutrients may be added. These beverages often have fewer nutrients, but more calories, than 100 percent juice.

- **Fruit nectars** are *thick, sugar-sweetened beverages of fruit juice and pulp,* which contains fiber.

Activity: Chart the comparison of the amount of fruit juice, nutrients, and other ingredients in various forms of fruit juices and fruit drinks. Which is the most nutritious?

Calcium, a bone-building mineral, is added to some fruit juices and juice drinks. These fortified products aren't meant to replace calcium-rich choices from the Milk, Yogurt, and Cheese Group. However, they do offer an extra way to get calcium.

Storing Fruit for Top Quality

Handle your fresh fruit purchases properly to preserve their quality and freshness. How you store fresh fruits depends on their ripeness.

To store unripe fruits:
- Less ripe fruits can be allowed to ripen slowly on a counter or in a basket. You can speed up the ripening of some fruits, such as peaches, plums, bananas, nectarines, and apricots, by placing them in a loosely closed paper bag at room temperature for a day or two.
- Once they're ripe, eat and enjoy.

To store ripe fruits:
- Refrigerate ripe fruits to prevent further ripening and spoilage.
- Wait to wash fruits until you're ready to eat or prepare them. The added moisture speeds up spoiling.
- Use ripe fruits within a few days to enjoy them at their peak quality.

Activity: Make an illustrated checklist as a reference for storing ripe and unripe fruits. Place it on the refrigerator at home.

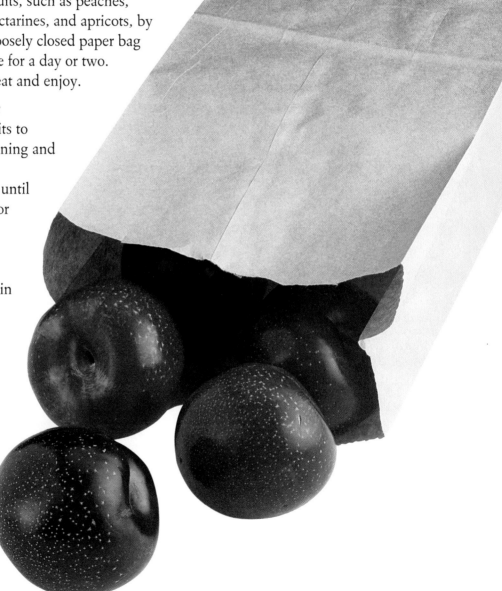

You can ripen some fruits, such as these plums, by placing them in a paper bag at room temperature for a day or two. Find out why this speeds up the ripening process.

Teens Teach Preschoolers to

Eat Smart

Green apples, kiwifruit, broccoli, snow peas—it's a "tasting of the green" for St. Patrick's Day! Through the school year, teens in the child care program at Lawrence Central High School in Indianapolis made nutrition come alive for preschoolers. Together they explored foods—their colors, textures, flavors, shapes, and smells. Teens tasted foods with the children, setting a good example.

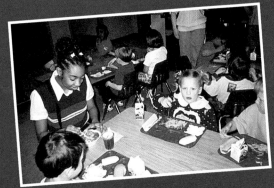

"We help kids become food 'tryers,'" said Andrea Strossner. "Once kids talk about a food, they'll try it." Megan Evers agreed, "From us, they learn that fruits and vegetables are good for you and help your body as you grow."

The teens helped children learn in other ways, too. They taught about the alphabet as they spelled food names and about math as they charted foods that kids tried. Andrea Thomas shared a science lesson, showing that celery is a stalk, carrots are roots, and lettuce is a leaf. Another time, each preschooler "became" a food as they built a human Food Guide Pyramid!

What's the best part of teaching kids about nutrition? Andrea Strossner summed it up: "We know we've made a difference!"

Take Action

Think of an opportunity you have to teach children about food and healthful eating—perhaps when you baby-sit, spend time with a younger sibling, or visit relatives with children. Plan and carry out a fun learning activity. Be creative! Tell your class about your activity and what you learned together.

Preparing Fruit for Your Health

Fresh fruits are one of "nature's fast foods"—ready to eat and enjoy with little effort. Preparing fresh fruits properly helps keep their nutrients, flavor, and quality. Before eating, slicing, peeling, or cooking fruits, wash them thoroughly to remove dirt, bacteria, and pesticides.

To clean fresh fruit:
- Rinse fruits under cold running water. Use a small knife to remove any bruised spots.
- Rinse small fruits, such as berries and grapes, in a colander. Gently turn them to clean all surfaces. Remove any brown or mushy pieces.

To keep cut-up fresh fruits at their best:

For best flavor and appearance, cut fruit just before eating.
- Sprinkle lemon juice or orange juice on cut apples, pears, and peaches. The citrus juice prevents them from turning brown.
- Store cut fruit in an airtight container in the refrigerator.

Emphasize: Wash fruit thoroughly before eating to remove pesticides or bacteria on the skins.

Activity: Prepare one of the snacks described. Share with the class and vote on your favorite.

Check This Out!

FRUIT FOR SWEET, EASY SNACKING!

When you have a taste for a sweet snack, try one of these nutrient-packed snack ideas that feature fruit.
- Mix fresh or canned fruit pieces with plain low-fat yogurt. Top with granola or cereal flakes.
- Spread a dab of peanut butter on apple or pear slices.
- Freeze grapes, banana slices, watermelon cubes, or berries. Pop them into your mouth for a cold, crunchy treat.
- Make a fruit smoothie. Blend pieces of your favorite fruit, plain low-fat yogurt, ice cubes, and fruit juice.
- Make your own trail mix. Combine dried fruits such as cherries, raisins, or apricots with pretzels, dry cereal, and nuts.

It's Your Turn!

If you were making a fruit smoothie, which fruit and fruit juice would you use? What kind of fruit would you add to yogurt? What nutrients are supplied by your choices?

INFOLINK

To learn why some cut fruit turns brown when exposed to air and how to avoid this reaction, see Section 4-4 of the Food Preparation Handbook.

Cooking with Fruit

Cooked fruit is easy to prepare and delicious. You can simmer, steam, bake, sauté, or broil many fruits. When fruits are cooked, their sweet flavor often becomes more intense. To minimize nutrient loss, keep cooking times short.

- *To make a fruit sauce,* add a small amount of liquid, such as water or juice, to fruit or fruit pieces and cook over low heat. If the fruit is too tart, add a small amount of sugar after cooking. Fruit sauces are terrific served alone or as a topping for pancakes, ice cream, or meat.
- *To cook whole fruits* such as apples, pears, peaches, or nectarines, remove the core or pit. Stuff with nuts, oats, or dried fruits, and sprinkle with cinnamon or nutmeg. Bake or microwave in a small amount of liquid.
- *Mix dried fruits* into cookie or muffin batter, cooked cereals, or casseroles for extra flavor and nutrients.

You can make a fruit sauce by cooking fruit pieces and a liquid over low heat. How might you use a fruit sauce to add natural flavor to a breakfast food?

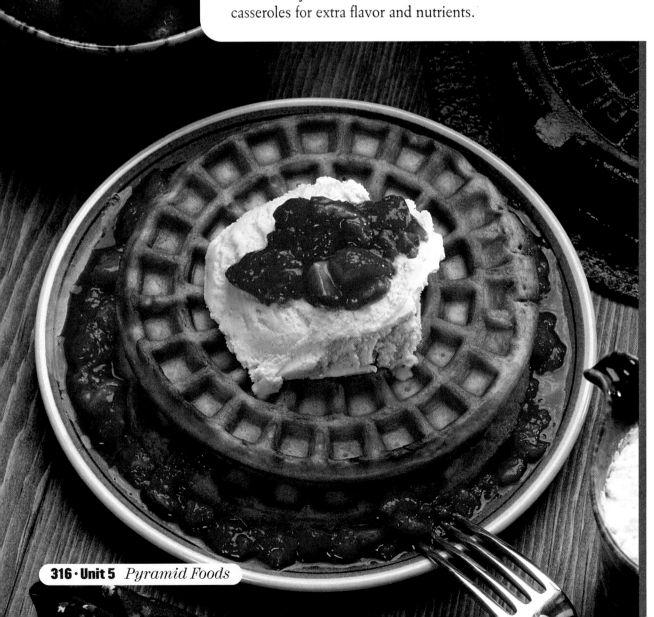

NOW You're COOKING!

SKILL
Simmering Fruits

*C*ooking fruits to make a sauce gives you another flavor experience. Try doubling this recipe for homemade applesauce. Use half today as a side dish and the rest tomorrow over a toasted waffle, on top of your cereal, or even in a fruit smoothie.

RECIPE

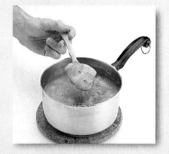

Chunky Cinnamon Applesauce

CUSTOMARY	INGREDIENTS	METRIC
4	Medium cooking apples	4
½ cup	Water	125 mL
3 to 4 Tbsp.	Sugar	45 to 60 mL
½ tsp.	Ground cinnamon	2 mL

Yield: 4 servings, ½ cup (125 mL) each

1. Peel, quarter, and core apples.
2. Place apples in saucepan and add water. Simmer over medium heat, covered, for 12 to 15 minutes or until apples are tender when pierced with a fork.
3. Add 3 tablespoons sugar and the cinnamon; stir until sugar is dissolved and apples are broken apart to make a chunky sauce. Taste; add additional sugar if apples are not sweet enough. Serve warm or cold.

Per Serving: 108 calories, 0 g protein, 28 g carbohydrate, trace fat, 1 mg sodium, 2 g fiber

More Ideas For a different flavor and texture:

- Add a dash of vanilla extract, raisins, or other dried fruit.
- Keep the apple peels on for more fiber. Just coarsely chop them before cooking.
- Try different varieties of apples and compare the flavors.

Your Ideas Make a list of other fruits that might make a good sauce. Look through cookbooks for tips on preparing them. How could you use these sauces?

LOOKING BACK

- Fruits are appealing sources of nutrients and offer important health benefits.
- Eating a variety of fruits and juices provides different nutrients and flavors.
- When buying fresh fruit, look for signs of ripeness and quality to ensure good flavor.
- Fresh fruits keep their nutrients, flavor, and quality when stored and prepared properly.

UNDERSTANDING KEY IDEAS

1. What are the nutritional contributions of fruits?
2. When might you buy fruit that is less ripe? Which fruits could you buy unripe and allow to ripen at home? How can you help speed up the ripening process?
3. What should you look for when buying fruit juices?
4. How can you preserve nutrients, quality, and appeal in fresh fruits? Name at least three strategies.
5. When making fruit sauce, when might sugar be added?

DEVELOPING LIFE SKILLS

1. **Creative Thinking:** What are some creative ways you might serve fruit at a party?
2. **Critical Thinking:** Some teens may not choose fruits for a snack because they think they are too expensive or that they don't fit into an on-the-go lifestyle. What might be the basis for these opinions? What could you say to offer these teens another point of view on the subject?

Wellness Challenge

LaDonna and Alison volunteer once a week at a retirement center. They would like to provide further encouragement to the residents and get others involved in this service. The teens have decided to sell fruit baskets to students and parents. Each basket will have the name of a retirement center resident attached. Once baskets have been sold for all the residents, LaDonna and Alison will hold a party where the purchasers and residents will meet each other.

1. What challenges might the teens face in carrying out their idea?
2. What steps might they take to get started?

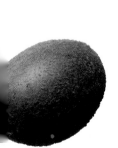
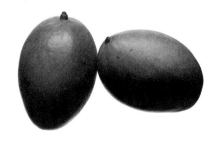
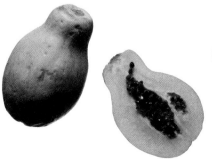
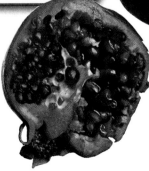

APPLYING YOUR LEARNING

1. **Meal Planning:** How might you fit more fruit in your eating plan? Create a two-day menu with the fruit servings highlighted. Try not to repeat a fruit.

2. **Reading Food Labels:** Compare canned peaches packed in heavy syrup with canned peaches packed in water or juice. What are the differences in ingredients, nutrients, and calories? Which would you choose and why?

3. **Storage Test:** Obtain four pears or other whole fresh fruits at the same stage of ripeness. Put one in a loosely closed paper bag on a kitchen shelf, one in an airtight container in the refrigerator, one uncovered on a refrigerator shelf, and one uncovered at room temperature. After three days, compare the texture, color, and flavor.

EXPLORING FURTHER

1. **Local Fruit:** Find out what types of fruit are grown in your state or province. Where is the produce sold? What conditions are necessary for each type of fruit to grow?

2. **Pectin Power:** Find out about pectin, a natural substance in some fruits. Which fruits are high in pectin? What special power does pectin have? How is this information useful?

Making CONNECTIONS

1. **Social Studies:** Many fruits we eat are imported from countries around the world. Find out where the fruits in the produce departments of your local stores come from. Use a map of the world to locate each country.

2. **Math:** Compare the cost of four types of fresh fruits when they are in season and when they are out of season. (Check with the produce manager at your local supermarket for information about costs.) Display your results in a chart. How do the costs compare? What can you conclude?

FOODS LAB

Bake or microwave an apple, pear, or peach in a small amount of liquid. Add a little cinnamon or nutmeg for additional flavoring if you prefer. Compare the texture, color, and flavor of the cooked fruit with that of uncooked fresh fruit.

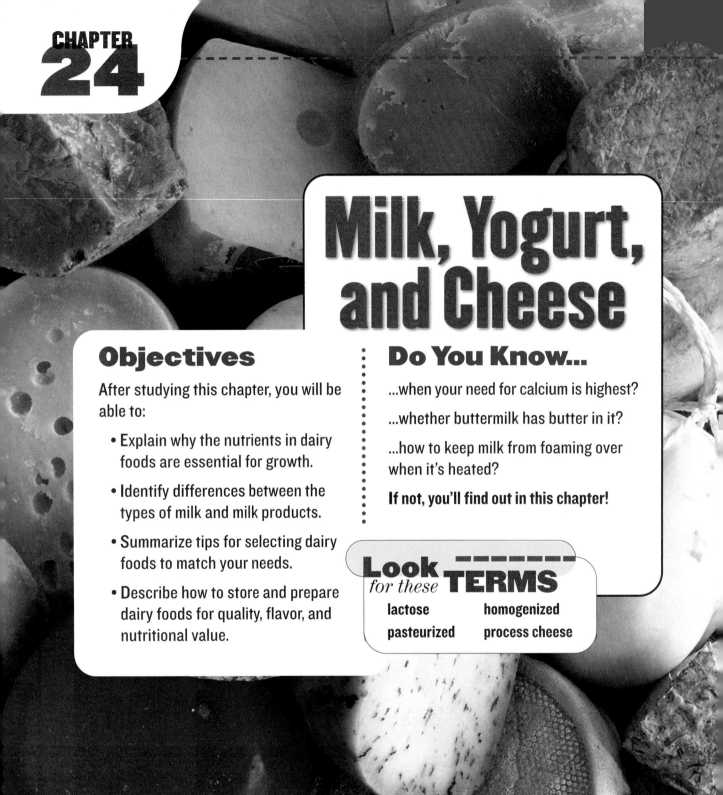

Milk, Yogurt, and Cheese

Objectives

After studying this chapter, you will be able to:

- Explain why the nutrients in dairy foods are essential for growth.

- Identify differences between the types of milk and milk products.

- Summarize tips for selecting dairy foods to match your needs.

- Describe how to store and prepare dairy foods for quality, flavor, and nutritional value.

Do You Know...

...when your need for calcium is highest?

...whether buttermilk has butter in it?

...how to keep milk from foaming over when it's heated?

If not, you'll find out in this chapter!

Look for these TERMS

lactose	homogenized
pasteurized	process cheese

Dairy foods

include milk and foods made from milk—buttermilk, cheese, yogurt, pudding, frozen yogurt, and more. They're great-tasting, versatile, and nutrient-packed. You can enjoy them anytime, anywhere—as part of any meal or snack. How do you like *your* milk?

Dairy Foods—Good for You and Your Bones

Drink your milk—that's smart advice, especially for teens! Dairy foods make many important contributions to your health.

Bone-building nutrients. Dairy foods give you calcium and phosphorus. Most milk is fortified with vitamin D to help your body absorb the calcium. Your need for calcium will never be greater than during the teen years—your body is growing rapidly, and your bones are growing longer and stronger.

Other vitamins and minerals. Dairy foods also provide riboflavin (a B vitamin), vitamins A and D, potassium, and other vitamins and minerals you need for good health.

Protein power. The complete protein in dairy foods helps to build, repair, and maintain your body's tissues. Just 1 cup (250 mL) of milk provides about 16 percent of the protein you need for the day!

Carbohydrates for energy. **Lactose** is a *natural sugar found in milk and milk products*. It contributes food energy and a unique, pleasing flavor to dairy foods.

What about fat? Today you can find many dairy foods in low-fat, reduced-fat, or fat-free versions. That makes it easier than ever to fit plenty of dairy foods into a healthful eating plan!

One cup (250 mL) of milk provides about 300 mg of calcium. As a teen, you need about 1,300 mg of calcium daily. Do you get enough servings from the Milk, Yogurt, and Cheese Group? You'll get ideas on how to make sure you do as you read this chapter.

INFOLINK

For more information on bone health, turn to Chapter 6, page 96.

To learn about options for people with lactose intolerance (difficulty digesting milk), see Chapter 10, page 142.

Chapter 24 *Milk, Yogurt, and Cheese* • **321**

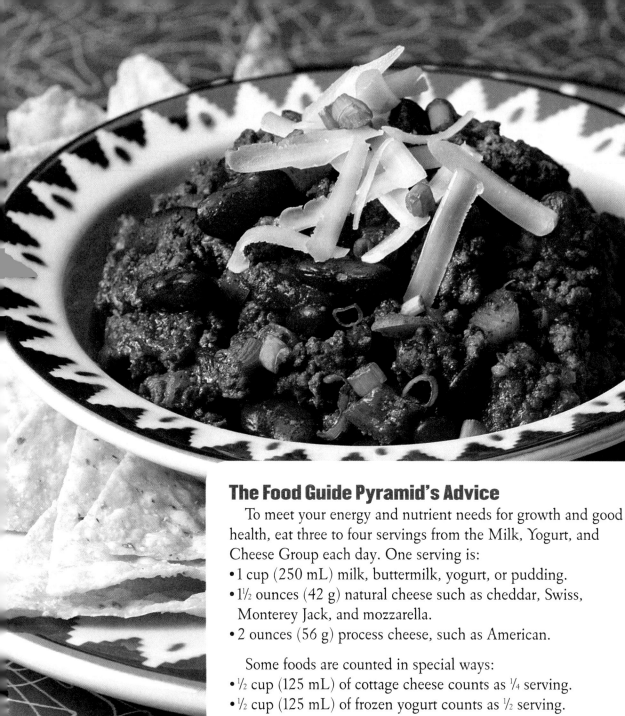

The Food Guide Pyramid's Advice

To meet your energy and nutrient needs for growth and good health, eat three to four servings from the Milk, Yogurt, and Cheese Group each day. One serving is:
- 1 cup (250 mL) milk, buttermilk, yogurt, or pudding.
- 1½ ounces (42 g) natural cheese such as cheddar, Swiss, Monterey Jack, and mozzarella.
- 2 ounces (56 g) process cheese, such as American.

Some foods are counted in special ways:
- ½ cup (125 mL) of cottage cheese counts as ¼ serving.
- ½ cup (125 mL) of frozen yogurt counts as ½ serving.
- ½ cup (125 mL) of ice cream counts as ⅓ serving.

Although it's not a dairy food, calcium-fortified soy milk fits into this group, too. It's a good way for vegetarians who don't eat dairy foods to get the calcium they need.

Butter, cream, sour cream, and cream cheese are mostly fat. These "extras" belong in the Pyramid tip. Use them in small amounts to add flavor to your meals and snacks.

Activity: Make a meal plan that includes three to four servings from the Milk, Yogurt, and Cheese Group each day. Compare plans.

Adding cheese to a mixed dish is a tasty way to meet Pyramid serving recommendations. How much cheese is one serving?

Ways to Enjoy Dairy Foods

It's easy to add a variety of flavorful dairy foods to your daily eating plan! Try these quick and tasty ideas at meals or snack time.

- Top fresh or frozen fruit yogurt with crunchy breakfast cereal.
- Put cheese and apple slices on crackers.
- Create your own flavored milk: blend in pureed fruit, peanut butter, or almond extract.
- Make a refreshing smoothie: whirl yogurt with fruit and ice in a blender.
- Stir dry Italian dressing mix—or herbs—into ricotta cheese or whipped cottage cheese. Use as a dip for veggies or bagel chips or as a baked potato topping.
- Make instant pudding with fat-free milk.
- Pour yourself a tall glass of ice-cold, refreshing milk.
- Sip a steaming mug of hot cocoa, made with milk.
- Blend ice cream or frozen yogurt with milk for a rich and creamy milkshake.
- Use plain yogurt as a calcium-rich substitute for sour cream. It's great on a baked potato or in dips.
- Slip a slice of cheese into a sandwich.
- Sprinkle shredded cheese on salads and soups.

Activity: Write an article for a newspaper foods section on interesting and unusual ways to enjoy dairy foods.

Check This Out!

"I'D DRINK MORE MILK, BUT..."

Have you ever heard teens give reasons like these for not eating dairy foods? They might change their minds if they knew all the facts.

"I'm not a kid anymore." Dairy foods aren't just for children. Even when you reach your adult height, your bones continue to grow stronger and more dense—important jobs that depend on the nutrients in dairy foods.

"It'll make me fat." No single food will make you fat—what you eat overall is what counts. However, if you're watching calories, choose fat-free and low-fat dairy products. These contain the same bone-building nutrients as the varieties with more fat.

"My friends don't drink milk." Be a trendsetter! Start drinking milk, and your friends may follow your lead. Milk goes great with a burger or pizza!

"I don't like the taste." Try flavored milk or a fruit smoothie. Make sure milk is ice-cold so that it's more refreshing. You can also get plenty of calcium from yogurt and cheese.

It's Your Turn!

Think of some other reasons teens might give for not drinking milk. Pick one of the excuses and create an advertising campaign or web site to help encourage teens to get the recommended daily servings from this food group.

Activity: In small groups, develop skits to illustrate the excuses teens use to not drink milk (include excuses that are not valid).

Teaching With Visuals: Compare the nutrients listed in all the milk choices. What are the similarities and differences? (*The amount of protein and calcium is basically the same in all the milk choices. The number of calories and the fat content vary.*)

Shopping for Dairy Foods

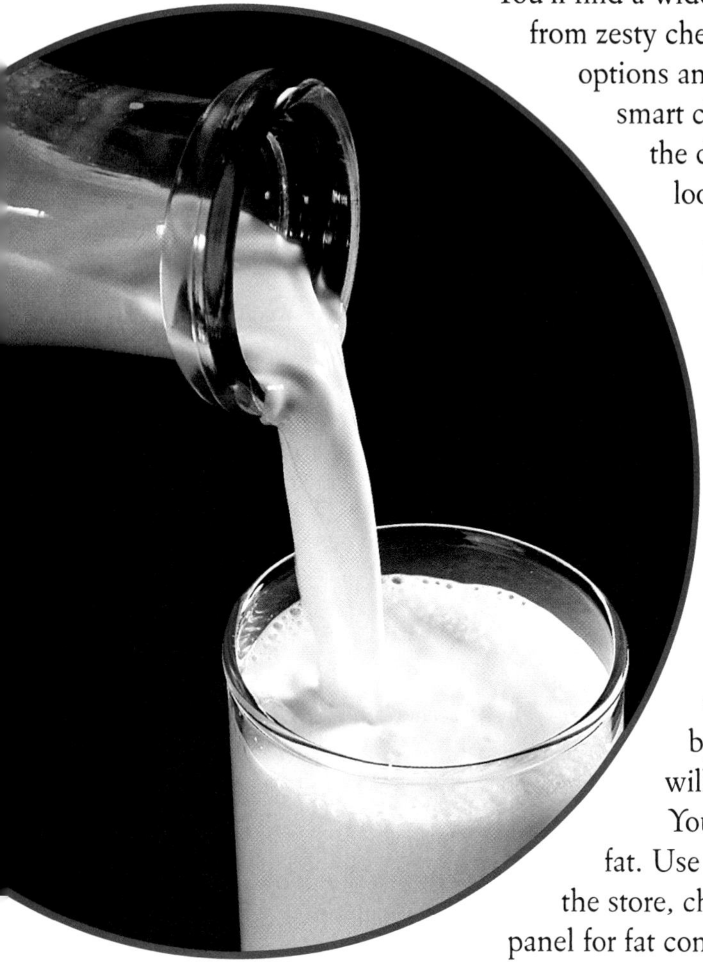

You'll find a wide variety of milk and milk products ranging from zesty cheese to sweet frozen yogurt. Knowing your options and the qualities to look for helps you make smart choices. You might be surprised to discover that the dairy case and freezer aren't the only places to look for dairy foods.

Milk for All Tastes

Most milk sold in the United States is cow's milk. Before it reaches the store, milk is pasteurized and homogenized. **Pasteurized** milk has been *heat-treated to destroy bacteria that could cause disease or spoil the milk.* **Homogenized** milk is *processed so that the fat is evenly distributed.* Otherwise, the cream would rise to the top.

You can buy fresh milk in paper cartons, plastic jugs, and sometimes glass bottles. Be sure the carton or jug isn't leaking. The "sell by" date is the last date the milk can be sold. It will keep in your refrigerator several more days.

You can choose milk with different amounts of fat. Use the chart below to compare milk choices. In the store, check the product name and Nutrition Facts panel for fat content.

Comparing Milk Choices

PRODUCT NAME	CALORIES PER SERVING	FAT (g)	CALORIES FROM FAT	PROTEIN (g)	CALCIUM (mg)
Whole milk	150	8	72	8	291
Reduced-fat milk (2% milk)	120	5	45	8	297
Low-fat milk (1% milk)	100	3	27	8	300
Fat-free, or nonfat, milk (skim milk)	80	0	0	8	302

For a change of taste, you can buy flavored milk, such as chocolate or fruit-flavored. This can be made from whole, reduced-fat, low-fat, or fat-free milk. Calories are usually higher than in the same type of unflavored milk because of added sweeteners.

Buttermilk has "friendly" bacteria added to fat-free or low-fat milk. This gives it a tangy flavor. Despite the name, butter isn't added! Buttermilk is a good thirst quencher.

Convenience Forms of Milk

Fresh milk is convenient because it's ready to drink. You can also buy other kinds of milk that are more convenient to store.

Nonfat dry milk can be mixed with water and used as you would fresh milk. You can also use it dry in recipes, such as for creamy soups or casseroles, or add it to fresh milk to boost the calcium.

UHT milk has been treated with a special process (called ultra-high temperature). It doesn't need refrigeration until after it's opened. Like dry milk, it's handy to have when you run out of fresh milk.

Evaporated milk comes in cans. It's made by removing some of the water from milk. This makes it thick—great for soups and sauces.

Sweetened condensed milk is similar to evaporated milk but with an important difference. It has added sugar. You may need it for some dessert recipes.

Activity: Visit a local supermarket. Find and list all the different forms of milk available.

Activity: Find out about the process involved in producing UHT milk. Report your findings to the class.

Evaporated milk is a great way to add extra nutrients to your favorite recipes. In what types of recipes would you add sweetened condensed milk?

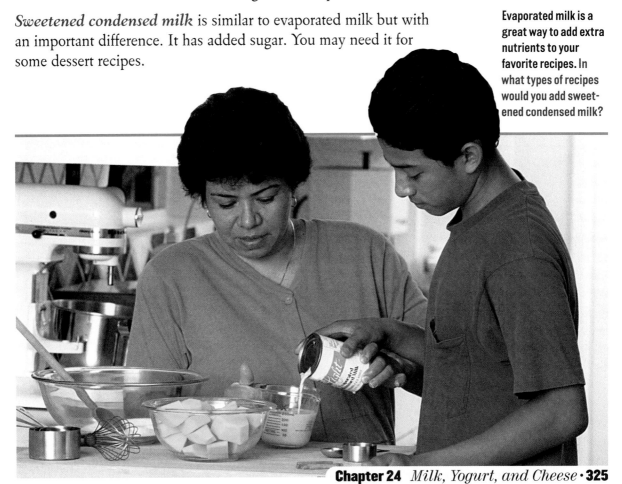

Yogurt

Like buttermilk, yogurt is another cultured dairy food with added "friendly" bacteria. This gives yogurt its distinctive flavor.

With so many kinds of yogurt on store shelves, how can you find what you want? Reading labels is the key. You can find yogurt in fat-free, low-fat, and whole-milk varieties. Some yogurts have fruit added. Flavored yogurts may be high in sugar. Try buying plain yogurt and adding your own fruit.

Cheese

When you shop for cheese, look at all the variety in cheese flavors and textures—from soft, mild, and creamy to hard, pungent, and crumbly. Natural cheeses are made by adding ingredients to milk that cause it to thicken and separate. It separates into whey, the liquid portion, and curds, the solid portion. Hard cheeses, such as cheddar, contain mostly curds, and soft cheeses, such as mozzarella, have some whey. Cottage cheese contains all of the curds and whey. Cheeses are aged for varying times depending on the kind of cheese being made.

- Unripened cheeses—sometimes called fresh cheeses—are not aged. These include ricotta, cottage cheese, and mozzarella.
- Ripened (or aged) varieties include brick, Muenster, cheddar, Gouda, Colby, and Parmesan—to name just a few.
- **Process cheese** is *a pasteurized blend of two or more ripened or unripened cheeses.* Process American cheese is an example.

Most cheese is sold in bricks or wedges. You'll also find grated, sliced, and shredded cheese, as well as cheese spreads. These convenience options add to the cost.

Activity: Sample various kinds of cheeses. Describe each cheese using elements such as texture, flavor, and color. As class, combine your descriptions in a pamphlet titled "All Kinds of Cheeses."

Cheese appears in every shape, size, and form imaginable—and with differences in flavor. Visit a supermarket and write down at least ten cheeses you could purchase.

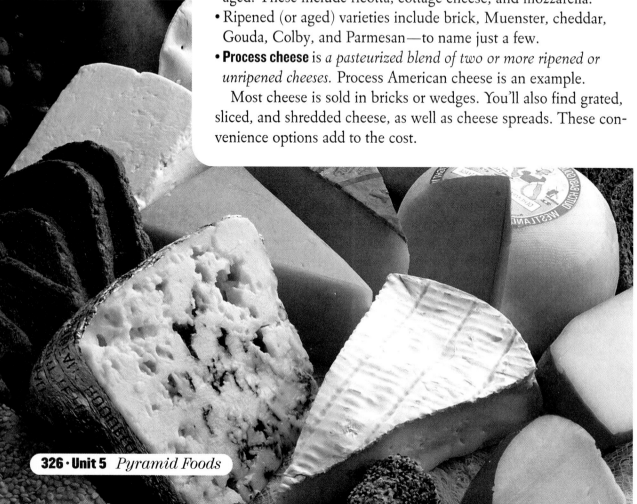

Frozen Dairy Foods

Frozen dairy foods—ice cream and frozen yogurt—are cool, creamy, and refreshing options from the Milk, Yogurt, and Cheese Group. They get their sweet flavor from added sugars. The sugar and fat content can vary. Use the Nutrition Facts panel to compare.

Look for solidly frozen cartons that are not dented or discolored. Discoloration often means melting occurred and then the products were refrozen.

INFOLINK

For more about frozen desserts, turn to Chapter 32.

More About Storing Milk: Why is milk packaged in opaque containers? (Artificial light and sunlight destroy riboflavin.)

Storing Dairy Foods

To keep your dairy purchases fresh-tasting and safe to eat, store them properly.

- Refrigerate fresh milk, yogurt, and cheese as soon as possible. For peak flavor, keep most perishable dairy foods no longer than a week. Most cheeses—except for ricotta and cottage cheese—last longer.
- Keep dairy foods tightly closed, covered, or wrapped so that they retain nutrients and quality. This also prevents them from picking up flavors from other foods in your refrigerator or freezer.
- After opening canned or UHT milk or adding water to dry milk, store these dairy foods as you would fresh milk. Store open canned milk in a covered pitcher rather than in the can to avoid a flavor change.

You can add dairy foods in many creative ways to your eating plan to meet your daily needs. How many servings have you had today?

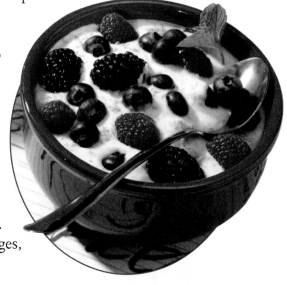

Preparing Dairy Foods

Many dairy foods need no special preparation. You can enjoy these "fast foods" just as they are! You'll find, however, that dairy foods show up in all sorts of recipes. They provide rich flavor and a creamy texture in beverages, soups, sauces, casseroles, desserts, and more.

Cooking with Milk

When heating milk for hot beverages or other uses, follow the guidelines on the next page. They will help keep the milk from scorching, curdling, or foaming over. Scorched milk has a burnt taste. Curdled milk has tiny solid particles (curds) in it. Milk that foams over makes a mess!

INFOLINK

To learn why milk curdles, see Section 4-5 of the Food Preparation Handbook.

Emphasize: Don't pour milk from a serving glass back into the original container. Discard if left out more than two hours.

A skin can form on cooked milk products, such as puddings and sauces, as they cool. To prevent this, place a piece of plastic wrap on the surface of the milk product before cooling.

Discuss: What problems have you experienced when cooking with milk? How might you have avoided the problems?

Cook cheese at low temperatures. What happens to cheese if it is cooked at a high temperature?

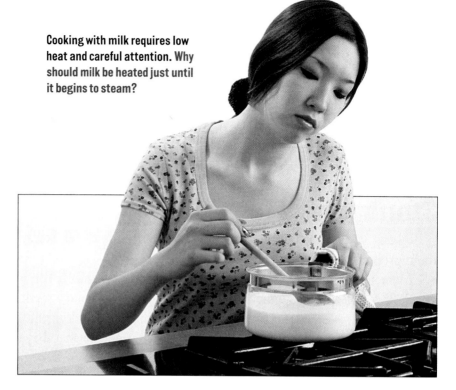

Cooking with milk requires low heat and careful attention. Why should milk be heated just until it begins to steam?

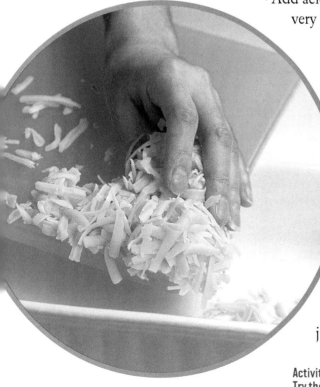

• Use low heat on the range. In the microwave oven, use the power level given in the recipe or instructions.
• Stir frequently.
• Watch carefully. Heat just until the milk begins to steam.
• Add acidic ingredients, such as lemon juice or tomato sauce, very slowly while stirring. They can cause milk to curdle.

Cooking with Cheese

Many snacks and main dishes—such as nachos and pizza—call for cooking with cheese. To help cheese keep its texture and flavor, cook at low temperatures for a short time. High heat and long cooking make cheese tough and rubbery and may cause the fat in cheese to separate out.

• For sauces, add cheese in small pieces or shreds near the end of cooking time. Then heat just until melted.
• Add cheese toppings at the end of baking or broiling time.
• If you microwave cheese, cook at medium power just until it begins to melt.

Activity: Find recipes that include cheese. What cooking methods are used? Try the recipe and share with the class.

NOW *You're* COOKING!

SKILL

Cooking with Milk

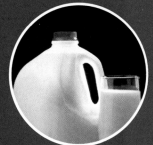

*I*n cold, wintry months, this chocolate-flavored milk recipe tastes great when it's hot. Serve it over ice on a summer day. You can use any type of milk—from whole to nonfat. Drinking hot chocolate almondine is a wonderful way to get the calcium you need.

RECIPE

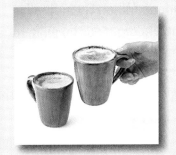

Hot Chocolate Almondine

CUSTOMARY	INGREDIENTS	METRIC
⅓ cup	Sugar	75 mL
3 Tbsp.	Unsweetened cocoa powder	45 mL
4 cups	Milk	1 L
1 tsp.	Almond extract	5 mL

Yield: 4 servings, 1 cup (250 mL) each

1. Combine sugar and cocoa in medium saucepan. Slowly add milk while stirring.
2. Over medium heat, stirring constantly, heat just until little bubbles form around the edge of the pan. Do not boil.
3. Add almond extract; beat with electric mixer or whisk for 30 to 45 seconds or until mixture foams. Ladle into mugs.

Per Serving:* 152 calories, 9 g protein, 28 g carbohydrate, 0.6 g fat, 126 mg sodium, 0 g fiber (* based on nonfat milk)

Percent Daily Value: vitamin A 15%, vitamin D 25%, riboflavin 20%, vitamin B_{12} 15%, calcium 30%, phosphorus 26%

More Ideas For more fun and flavor:

- Experiment with different extracts or different spices to change the flavor of the cocoa-milk mixture.
- For wintertime fun, stick a candy cane in each cup or drop in a few red hot candies.

Your Ideas Flavored milk makes a great snack or meal beverage. What other ingredients can you blend with milk to make a refreshing or wintertime warming beverage? Look through cookbooks for ideas. Prepare one of these drinks for your friends or family.

LOOKING BACK

- Dairy foods are good sources of many important nutrients, including protein, calcium, and vitamin D.
- Eat three to four servings from this food group to help meet your energy and nutrient needs.
- You can choose from a wide variety of fresh and convenience dairy products.
- To keep dairy foods fresh-tasting, appealing, and safe to eat, store them properly.
- Cook milk and cheese carefully to retain their texture and flavor.

UNDERSTANDING KEY IDEAS

1. What might happen to your bones if you don't eat dairy foods during the teen years?
2. What types of fresh milk are available? What types of milk are convenient to store?
3. What is the difference between unripened and ripened cheeses? Name two of each.
4. Based on the Pyramid, list dairy foods you might choose to include in meals and snacks over a three-day period.
5. How would you properly store a half-eaten container of yogurt? An opened can of evaporated milk?
6. If you were heating milk on the range for hot cocoa, what steps would you follow?

DEVELOPING LIFE SKILLS

1. **Leadership:** What advice would you give to a younger sister who doesn't drink milk because she doesn't like the taste? How could you be a good role model for her?
2. **Management:** After dinner, Ryan's father asked Ryan to go buy a gallon of milk. On the way home from the store, Ryan stopped at his friend Guillermo's house to shoot some hoops. When Ryan finally returned home and opened the milk, he discovered that it wasn't cold anymore. Did Ryan practice good management? Explain. What would you have done in this situation?

Wellness Challenge

During summer vacation, Tracy and her family are planning to go on a four-day camping trip in the mountains. They'll be sleeping outdoors in a tent and most likely no electricity will be available. They usually eat three to four servings each day from the Milk, Yogurt, and Cheese Group. Tracy wants to create an eating plan that will allow her and her family to eat dairy foods on the camping trip.

1. What challenges might Tracy face?
2. What are some possible solutions?

APPLYING YOUR LEARNING

1. **Promoting Dairy Foods:** In recent years, a variety of humorous ads have promoted milk. Create an advertisement with your own catchy slogan for a different dairy product, such as yogurt or cheese. Describe the nutritional qualities of the product in your advertisement.

2. **Yogurt Variety:** Choose at least five different varieties of yogurt, such as plain, regular fruit-flavored, low-fat, no-sugar, and fat-free. Compare the cost, ingredients, and nutrient content per serving. Compile your findings in a chart. Why do you think so many varieties are available?

EXPLORING FURTHER

1. **Milk Processing:** Find out more about how milk is processed. How did pasteurization get its name? When was it invented? How does pasteurization differ from UHT processing? Present your findings to the class.

2. **Cheese Choices:** Learn more about different varieties of cheese from around the world. Create a chart describing their appearance, texture, and flavor. Also include suggestions for how each might be used, such as pairings of cheese and fruit for appetizers or desserts.

Making CONNECTIONS

1. **Science:** Create a presentation that explains how "friendly" bacteria are used to make buttermilk and yogurt. What types of bacteria are used? What role do the bacteria play? How does this process relate to biology? To chemistry?

2. **Math:** Compare the prices of several sizes of fresh milk— quart, half-gallon, and gallon. What is the cost per serving for each size? Is the gallon always the most economical choice? When might a smaller size be more economical?

FOODS LAB

Cut a chunk of hard cheese, such as cheddar, into two halves. Put each half in a microwave-safe bowl. Melt one piece of cheese in the microwave on low power for a short time. Melt the other piece on high power for a longer time. Compare the appearance, texture, and flavor of the cheese in each bowl. Which one is more appealing? Why?

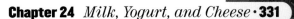

CHAPTER 25

Meat, Poultry, and Fish

Objectives

After studying this chapter, you will be able to:

- Explain how the nutrients in meat, poultry, and fish contribute to good health.

- Identify ways to include a variety of meat, poultry, and fish choices in your eating plan.

- Summarize tips for selecting lean meat, poultry, and fish.

- Describe how to store and prepare meat, poultry, and fish for quality and safety.

Do You Know...

...how to save money when you buy meat, poultry, and fish?

...why removing poultry skin gives you a lean advantage?

...how to prepare hamburgers so that they're juicy *and* safe to eat?

If not, you'll find out in this chapter!

Look for these TERMS

finfish	lean meat
shellfish	marbling
cut	marinade

Think of how

versatile meat, poultry, and fish are! They often take center stage in lunch and dinner meals. They can be a main dish in themselves or harmonize with other foods in soups, stews, casseroles, pizza, or sandwiches. However they are eaten, meat, poultry, and fish can add to the enjoyment and satisfaction of meals—and to their nutrition, too.

Meat, Poultry, and Fish— Packed with Protein

Roast beef . . . a pork chop . . . chicken stir-fry . . . turkey cold cuts . . . tuna salad . . . grilled shrimp. No matter how you slice them, the meat, poultry, and fish in these choices provide important nutrients for growth and good health!

Protein power. Meat, poultry, and fish are well known for the high-quality protein they provide. You need protein to help build and repair the tissues in your body and keep them healthy. Getting enough protein is especially important when you're growing, like now in your teen years.

Vitamins and minerals. Meat, poultry, and fish supply B vitamins, including thiamin, niacin, vitamin B_6, and vitamin B_{12}. They're also important sources of iron and zinc. Fish with edible bones, such as sardines and canned salmon, can supply calcium, too.

What about fat? The choices in this food group have different amounts of fat, but all can be part of a healthful eating plan. In this chapter you'll learn how the fat content of meat, poultry, and fish varies. That will help you make the best choices for you!

You have many different choices with this food group. No matter what your choice, these foods provide important nutrients. What vitamins and minerals are supplied by chicken salad?

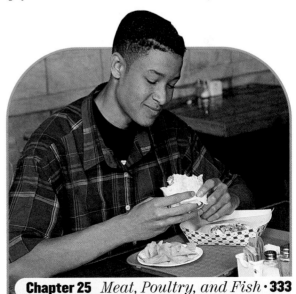

Discuss: How many portions of meat, poultry, and fish do you eat daily? Are your portions larger than those in the chart? The average American eats more than needed. Extra protein is changed into sugar and can be stored as body fat.

The Food Guide Pyramid's Advice

Meat, poultry, and fish are grouped in the Food Guide Pyramid with other protein-rich foods—dry beans and peas, tofu, eggs, nuts, and seeds. Although many people eat more, you need just two to three servings from this food group each day. One serving of meat, poultry, or fish is 2 to 3 ounces (56 to 84 g)—about the size of a deck of cards.

Your servings for the whole day should add up to 5 to 7 ounces (140 to 196 g), or the equivalent in helpings of eggs, dry beans or peas, tofu, or nuts. You can eat all of your daily servings from this group at one or two meals or spread them out among more meals and snacks.

INFOLINK

To learn how to count servings of dry beans, tofu, eggs, and nuts, see Chapter 26.

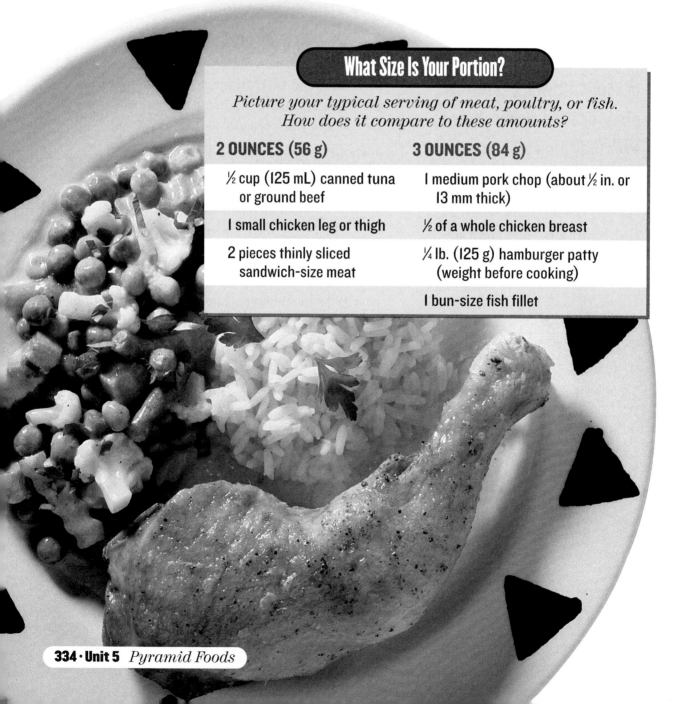

What Size Is Your Portion?

Picture your typical serving of meat, poultry, or fish. How does it compare to these amounts?

2 OUNCES (56 g)	3 OUNCES (84 g)
½ cup (125 mL) canned tuna or ground beef	1 medium pork chop (about ½ in. or 13 mm thick)
1 small chicken leg or thigh	½ of a whole chicken breast
2 pieces thinly sliced sandwich-size meat	¼ lb. (125 g) hamburger patty (weight before cooking)
	1 bun-size fish fillet

Sensational Selection

As with other food groups, you have plenty to choose from when it comes to meat, poultry, and fish. How many of these have you tried?

- Meat, or "red meat," includes beef, veal (meat from a calf), pork, and lamb.
- Organ meats include liver, kidney, and tongue.
- Poultry includes chicken, turkey, duck, Cornish hen, and goose.
- Giblets are poultry parts such as the heart, liver, and gizzard. Giblets are sometimes used to flavor soups and stuffing.
- Processed or cured meat and poultry products range from ham to sausage to many types of cold cuts.
- **Finfish** are *fish with fins, backbones, and gills.* Choices include catfish, flounder, haddock, perch, red snapper, salmon, and tuna.
- **Shellfish** *have a shell instead of bones and fins.* Shellfish choices include crab, lobster, shrimp, clams, oysters, scallops, and snails.

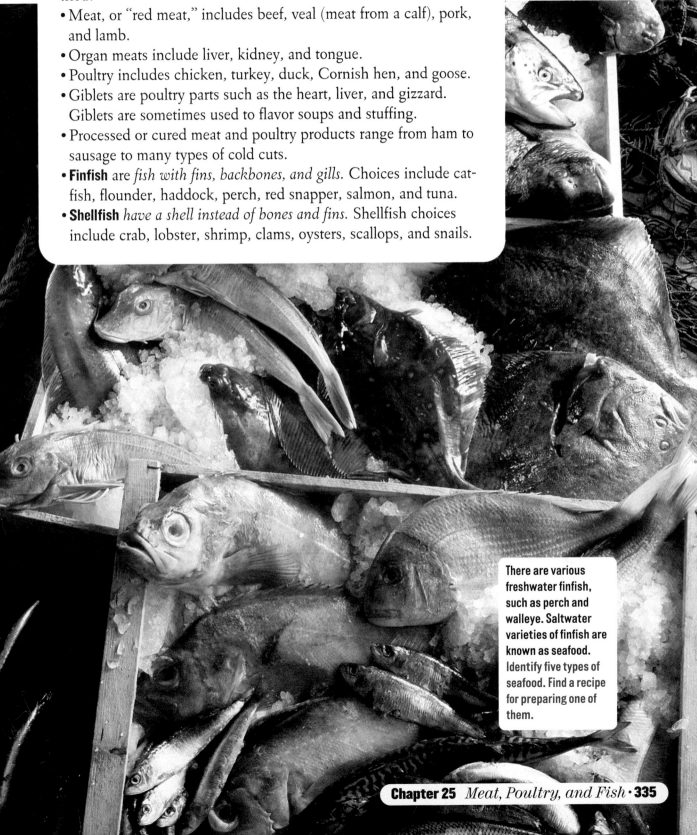

There are various freshwater finfish, such as perch and walleye. Saltwater varieties of finfish are known as seafood. Identify five types of seafood. Find a recipe for preparing one of them.

THE Cutting Edge

What's the difference between a roast and a steak? To keep your knowledge "a cut above," take a look at the options you'll find in most supermarkets. Retail **cuts** are *sections of meat divided into sizes that are purchased by the consumer.*

BEEF AND PORK
- **Roasts.** Cuts that are more than 2 inches (5 cm) thick.
- **Steaks and chops.** Cuts that are less than 2 inches (5 cm) thick.
- **Ground meat.** Fat content varies depending on the cut from which meat was ground.

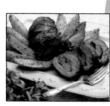
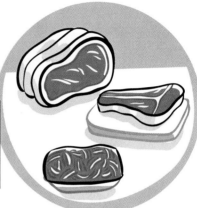

FINFISH
- **Dressed.** Fish with the head, tail, fins, scales, and internal organs removed.
- **Fillets.** Sides of the fish cut from the bones and backbone. Usually boneless.
- **Steaks.** Cross sections cut from a dressed fish. May contain bones and backbone.

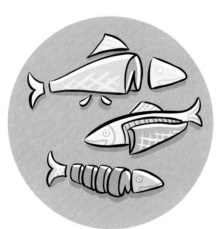
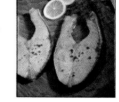

POULTRY
- **Whole.** May include giblets. Select a broiler-fryer for tenderness.
- **Parts.** Can be a cut-up whole chicken or packages of specific parts, such as wings or legs and thighs.
- **Boneless, skinless.** Poultry breasts with all the bone and skin removed. Also called cutlets.
- **Ground poultry.** For leaner choices, look for the word "meat" on the label, which means no skin is included.

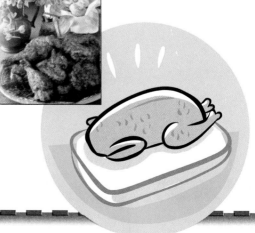

Check This Out!

WEIGHING THE CHOICES

Which meat, poultry, and fish choices have less fat than others? How about cholesterol? Here are some rules of thumb to guide you.

- Most fish is lower in fat than poultry or meat.
- The fat in fish and chicken is less saturated than the fat in beef, pork, lamb, and veal.
- Light-meat poultry (such as turkey breast or chicken breast) has less fat than dark meat (such as legs and thighs).
- Finfish with light-colored flesh usually have less fat than finfish with darker flesh, such as salmon and mackerel.
- Most shellfish are quite low in fat but may be relatively high in cholesterol.
- Organ meats are often higher in fat and cholesterol.
- Processed meats vary in fat and sodium content. Check the labels to find lean options.

It's Your Turn!

Explain how you would apply this information when planning meals.

Planning Meals with Meat, Poultry, and Fish

Before you set out to buy meat, poultry, or fish, have a plan for what you'll look for. What do you have in mind for your meal—fajitas, a seafood salad, a hearty stew? No matter what the menu, you have many options to choose from when buying. A plan will help you get good nutrition, make the most of your time and money, and enjoy flavorful meals prepared well.

Planning for less fat. Within this food group, choices vary in the amount of total fat, saturated fat, and cholesterol per serving. To fit your strategy for healthful eating, balance your choices. Enjoy lower-fat choices most often. Have higher-fat meat, poultry, and fish less often or in smaller amounts. Remember, the choice of cooking method affects the fat content. Broiled fish, for example, has less fat than fried fish.

Critical Thinking: Why is it good to substitute dry beans or peas one or more times a week in place of meat, poultry, or fish?

INFOLINK

To review the chart comparing different cooking methods, turn to page 194 in Chapter 14.

To learn more about tenderness in meat, read Section 4-6 of the Food Preparation Handbook.

Planning your cooking method. Deciding on your cooking method can help you know what kind of meat to put on your shopping list. Why? Meat choices can vary in how naturally tender they are. Certain cooking methods work best with tender meats; others, with less tender meats. Match the meat to the method! The chart below shows tender and less tender choices and how to cook them.

Planning to save money. Tender cuts of meat usually cost more than less tender ones. You can save money by planning ways to use less tender cuts. Another way to cut costs is by planning meals that "stretch" your meat, poultry, and fish purchases. That means using smaller amounts and combining them with other foods. For instance, you can stir-fry chicken strips with fresh vegetables. How about using just a small amount of cooked ground beef in chili or spaghetti sauce for flavor and texture? Besides saving money, this is a good way to reduce fat, add variety, and keep serving sizes from the meat and beans group within bounds.

Tenderness and Cooking Methods

WITH THESE CUTS...	...USE THESE COOKING METHODS
Tender meats: • Loin, sirloin, and short loin cuts • Rib cuts • Leg, round, and ham cuts	**Dry heat:** • Grilling • Broiling • Baking • Roasting • Stir-frying • Microwaving
Less tender meats: • Shoulder • Chuck • Flank • Short plate • Brisket	**Long, slow cooking in moist heat:** • Stewing • Braising
Poultry	**Dry or moist heat**
Fish	**Dry or moist heat**

Go beyond burgers and hot dogs! Team your meat choices with foods from other food groups to expand your taste options and boost nutrition. Try combining lean beef or chicken strips, stir-fried vegetables, and tortillas. In what other ways can you make your meat, poultry, and fish purchases go further?

Activity: Find recipes in cookbooks or food magazines for stewing or braising meats. Share your recipes with the class.

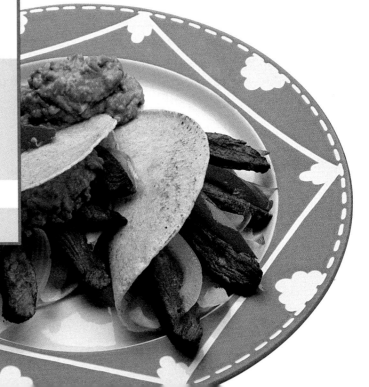

Shopping for Meat, Poultry, and Fish

Once you're at the store, knowing what to look for in meat, poultry, and fish will help you make smart choices.

Label Lingo

A meat, poultry, or fish label gives you several kinds of helpful information.

Activity: Look in a cookbook for recipes for preparing a sirloin steak and a chuck roast. How do they compare?

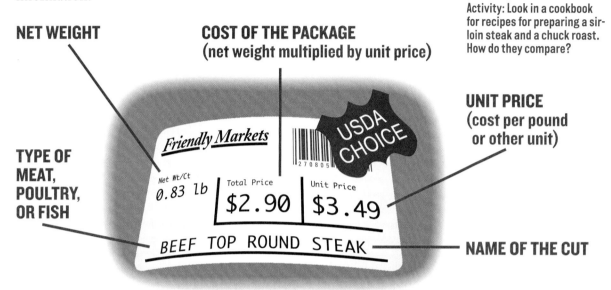

NET WEIGHT

COST OF THE PACKAGE (net weight multiplied by unit price)

UNIT PRICE (cost per pound or other unit)

TYPE OF MEAT, POULTRY, OR FISH

Friendly Markets

USDA CHOICE

270805

Net Wt/Ct 0.83 lb | Total Price $2.90 | Unit Price $3.49

BEEF TOP ROUND STEAK

NAME OF THE CUT

Signs of Quality

How can you tell whether fresh or frozen meat, poultry, or fish is of good quality?

- Check the "sell by" date on the package.
- Look for beef that is bright red. Young veal and pork should be grayish pink, and lamb can be light to darker pink.
- Look for poultry that's meaty, with creamy white to yellow skin. The skin should be free of bruises and tiny feathers and not torn or dry.
- Fresh finfish have a mild aroma, firm and moist flesh, shiny skin, and no browning around the edges.
- Fresh shellfish are often sold live. When you tap the shells of fresh live clams, mussels, and oysters, they should close tightly. Choose crabs that move when they're touched and lobsters whose tails curl when they're picked up.
- Buy packages that are well wrapped and do not leak. Frozen packages should be frozen solid and free of ice crystals.

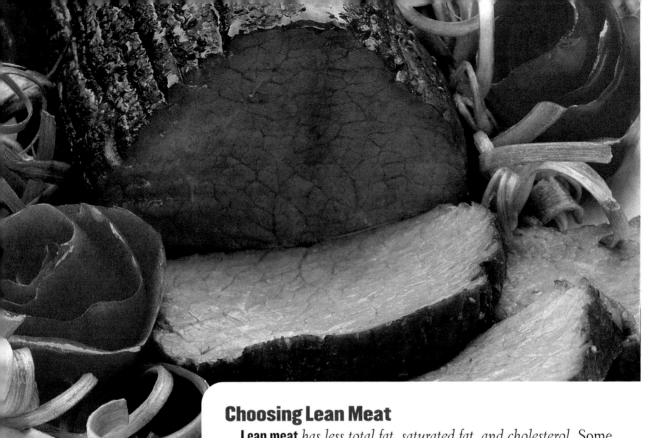

For meat that is lower in fat, select cuts with less marbling. What are other methods of selecting a leaner cut of meat?

Tip

For less fat, look for tuna canned in water, not oil.

Choosing Lean Meat

Lean meat *has less total fat, saturated fat, and cholesterol.* Some cuts of beef, pork, lamb, and veal are leaner than others. Use the following clues for choosing lean cuts.

- Look for information about fat and cholesterol on the Nutrition Facts panel. It may be on packages or in posters or brochures posted near the meat counter.
- Look at the meat's appearance. Lean cuts of meat have less **marbling**—*the thin streaks and flecks of fat that you can see in a piece of meat.* Usually, lean meats are also trimmed, so there's very little fat around the edges.
- Choose mostly beef graded "Select" and veal and lamb graded "Good." These grades have less marbled fat and often cost less than "Choice" or "Prime." (Pork cuts are not graded.)
- Check the name. Cuts of beef with the words *round* or *loin* in the name are lean. For pork and lamb, look for *loin* or *leg* in the name.

Emphasize: Trimming meat removes much of the fat. Cholesterol and fat are also found in the muscle. For ground poultry, look for ground breast meat; it's comparable to lean ground beef.

How Much to Buy?

Suppose you plan to braise a pork roast. How large a roast do you need to put on your shopping list? The answer depends on how many people you are serving and whether you want leftovers for another meal. Did you know it also depends on whether the roast is boneless? The chart on the next page can help you determine the right amount to buy.

How Much Will You Buy?

FORM OF MEAT, POULTRY, OR FISH	NUMBER OF COOKED, 3-OZ. (84 g) SERVINGS PER POUND
Boneless or ground meat and poultry, fish fillets, scallops, peeled shrimp	4
Meat with a small amount of bone (steaks, roast, chops)	2–3
Meat with a large amount of bone (shoulder cuts, short ribs)	1–2
Whole chicken or turkey	2
Fish steaks with bone	2
Live clams and oysters	2–3

Activity: Calculate how much of each form of meat, poultry, or fish listed in the chart you need to buy to serve eight people.

Activity: Suppose boneless sirloin steak costs $4.98 per pound and whole chicken costs $2.29 per pound. Calculate the cost per serving for each. (Steak: $1.25; Chicken: $1.15)

Comparing Costs

To be a smart shopper, base your purchase on cost per serving rather than cost per pound. Why? The cost per pound is based on the entire weight—including parts you won't eat, such as bones or fat you're going to trim off. To find out the cost per serving:

1. Refer to the chart above to find the number of servings per pound.
2. Multiply by the number of pounds in the package. This gives you the number of servings in the package.
3. Divide the total price by the number of servings in the package.

Comparing the cost per serving can help you find bargains. For example, you may find that whole poultry costs less than a cut-up bird. In that case, you can save money by buying the whole poultry and cutting it up yourself.

Convenience Options

For meat, poultry, or fish that's easy to store or quick to prepare, you can turn to convenience options. They range from meat that's already cut up for stir-frying to canned tuna, ready-to-eat cold cuts, roast poultry from the deli counter, and frozen main dishes to pop in the microwave oven. What are some of the pros and cons of these choices?

Activity: Compare the Nutrition Facts labels of ready-to-eat ham and turkey ham. Which has less fat?

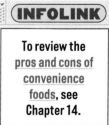

Tip

In many recipes, you can substitute one type of fish for another. Choose from what's available based on freshness and cost per serving.

INFOLINK

To review the pros and cons of convenience foods, see Chapter 14.

INFOLINK

For more guidelines on storing foods, see Section 1-2 of the Food Preparation Handbook.

Emphasize: Refrigeration does not stop the growth of bacteria in food—it merely slows it. Meat, poultry, or fish kept in the refrigerator longer than the recommended amount of time will start to spoil.

Storing Meat, Poultry, and Fish

If you plan to use fresh meat, poultry, or fish within a few days, store it in the refrigerator. Make sure the package is wrapped tightly. Place it in a pan or on a plate to keep raw juices from spreading bacteria to other foods.

Freeze any purchases you don't plan to use right away. Wrap them tightly in freezer paper or store in airtight plastic bags or containers to protect their quality.

Preparing Meat, Poultry, and Fish

Juicy, tender, and full of flavor—these are qualities of properly cooked meat, poultry, and fish. Nutrition and food safety are also important to consider when cooking.

Keep It Lean

You can keep the fat content in bounds when cooking, just as you do when planning meals and shopping. Here's how.

- Trim visible fat before cooking.
- Remove the skin from poultry before eating. You can do this before or after cooking. A lot of the fat is just under the skin.
- Use lean cooking methods that allow fat to drain off, such as grilling, broiling, and roasting.
- Go easy on rich, high-fat sauces and gravies.

Many choices in this food group are low in fat. How can the preparation method also affect the fat content?

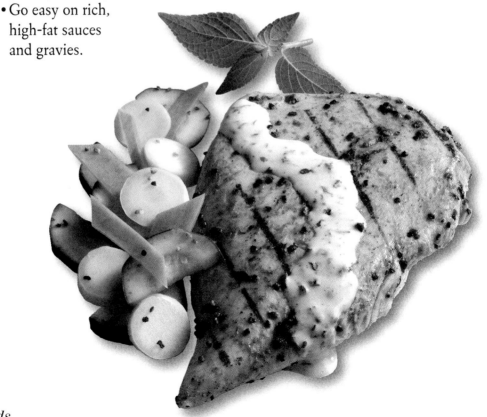

When Is It Done?	INTERNAL, COOKED TEMPERATURE	
	°F	°C
Fresh Beef, Veal, Pork, and Lamb		
Ground products	160	71
Roasts, steaks, or chops:		
medium	160	71
well done	170	77
Ham		
not precooked	160	71
precooked	140	60
Poultry		
Ground products	170	77
Whole chicken or turkey	180	82
Breasts, thighs, roasts	170	77
Fish	145	63
Leftovers (reheating)	165	74

Emphasize: Cook meat, poultry, and fish until it is done. Never partially cook meat and finish cooking it later. Even if it is refrigerated, harmful bacteria will not have been destroyed and will continue to multiply in the partially cooked food.

Cooking to Safe Temperatures

Meat, poultry, and fish must be cooked thoroughly to destroy harmful bacteria that could cause foodborne illness. Remember, you can't always tell by looking whether food has cooked long enough to be safe. Use a thermometer to check the internal temperature. With roasts and whole poultry, you can use an ovenproof thermometer that you leave in while cooking. For smaller cuts, such as burgers or fish, use an instant-read thermometer after cooking. Be sure the food reaches at least the temperature shown in the chart above.

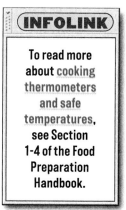

INFOLINK

To read more about cooking thermometers and safe temperatures, see Section 1-4 of the Food Preparation Handbook.

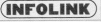
Tip

Measure fish at its thickest point to estimate cooking time. Cook fish for approximately 10 minutes per inch (2.5 cm) of thickness (20 minutes per inch if fish is frozen). Fully cooked fish flakes when you test it with a fork.

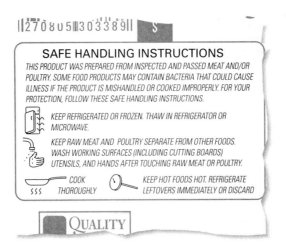

‖2‖70805‖30338 9‖   S

SAFE HANDLING INSTRUCTIONS

THIS PRODUCT WAS PREPARED FROM INSPECTED AND PASSED MEAT AND/OR POULTRY. SOME FOOD PRODUCTS MAY CONTAIN BACTERIA THAT COULD CAUSE ILLNESS IF THE PRODUCT IS MISHANDLED OR COOKED IMPROPERLY. FOR YOUR PROTECTION, FOLLOW THESE SAFE HANDLING INSTRUCTIONS.

KEEP REFRIGERATED OR FROZEN. THAW IN REFRIGERATOR OR MICROWAVE.

KEEP RAW MEAT AND POULTRY SEPARATE FROM OTHER FOODS. WASH WORKING SURFACES (INCLUDING CUTTING BOARDS) UTENSILS, AND HANDS AFTER TOUCHING RAW MEAT OR POULTRY.

COOK THOROUGHLY

KEEP HOT FOODS HOT. REFRIGERATE LEFTOVERS IMMEDIATELY OR DISCARD

QUALITY

To help avoid foodborne illness, cook ground beef properly. Use a meat thermometer to check the internal temperature. Why is it important to follow safe handling instructions?

INFOLINK

For more tips on using specific cooking methods, see Section 3-6 of the Food Preparation Handbook.

To learn why a roast browns in dry heat, see Section 4-6 of the Food Preparation Handbook.

Cooking Principles

When properly cooked, meat, poultry, and fish are not only safe to eat but also tender and juicy. If overcooked, they can become dry and tough. A basic cookbook is a good source of instructions for cooking meat, poultry, and fish in different ways.

Adding Flavor

You can find many recipes that give meat, poultry, and fish a special flavor. You can also rely on your own creativity to add flavor when using basic cooking methods. For example:
- Gently rub the surface with a blend of herbs and spices before cooking.
- Baste (brush the surface) with a prepared sauce, such as barbecue or soy sauce, mustard, or chutney.
- Soak meat, poultry, or fish in **marinade**, *a flavorful liquid,* before cooking. Most marinades contain acidic ingredients, such as citrus juice, salsa, or salad dressing, that help tenderize meat. Discard leftover marinade that the raw food soaked in.

INFOLINK

To learn how marinade can tenderize meat, see Section 4-6 of the Food Preparation Handbook.

Activity: Devise your own recipe for a dry rub or marinade for meat, poultry, or fish. Try it out and report the results.

Emphasize: Discard leftover marinade in which raw food was soaked; it may contain bacteria that cause foodborne illness.

For a flavor sensation, rub on your favorite herbs and spices—perhaps a blend of garlic, basil, thyme, and lemon peel. When would you use a dry spice rub, and when would you choose to marinate meat?

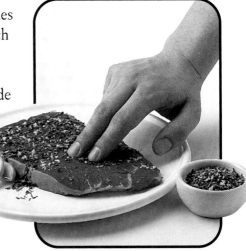

NOW You're COOKING!

Broiling Poultry

*F*or a fast and convenient way to prepare a meal, try broiling. Almost any type of food—from poultry, fish, and tender cuts of meat to fruits and vegetables—can be cooked under a broiler. Keep the broiler rack about 5 to 8 inches (13 to 20 cm) from the heat source so the food doesn't brown too fast or get charred.

RECIPE

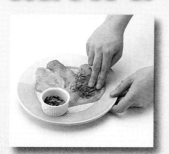

Rosemary Chicken

CUSTOMARY	INGREDIENTS	METRIC
4	Boneless, skinless chicken breasts, pounded to ¼-inch (6-mm) thickness	4
	Vegetable oil cooking spray	
1 tsp.	Dried rosemary leaves	5 mL
½ tsp.	Ground black pepper	2 mL

Yield: 4 servings

❶ Lightly spray grid of broiling pan and both sides of chicken with vegetable oil spray.

❷ Combine rosemary and pepper. Rub half of rosemary mixture over chicken. Broil 4 to 5 minutes or until chicken is lightly browned on top.

❸ Turn chicken over; rub with remaining rosemary mixture. Broil 4 to 5 minutes longer or until juices are clear when pierced with a fork and meat is lightly browned. Check for doneness; the internal temperature should be 180°F (82°C).

Per Serving: 189 calories, 35 g protein, 0.4 g carbohydrate, 4 g fat, 83 mg sodium, 0 g fiber

Percent Daily Value: niacin 77%, viamin B$_6$ 33%, phosphorus 25%

More Ideas Try these other flavorful ways to season broiled chicken:

• Rub with ground ginger and garlic powder, or lemon peel mixed with pepper.

• Brush with a special mustard, pesto sauce, or barbecue sauce before broiling.

Your Ideas Make a list of the herbs and spices in your kitchen. Which ones could you use as a rub on poultry, seafood, or meat?

LOOKING BACK

- Eat two to three servings each day from the Meat, Poultry, Fish, Dry Beans, Eggs, and Nuts Group to get important nutrients for growth and good health.

- Planning ahead before you buy meat, poultry, and fish can help you make the best choices based on your nutrition needs, desired cooking method, and budget.

- Smart shopping for meat, poultry, and fish will help you get the most for your money.

- Store and prepare meat, poultry, and fish properly to ensure quality, good taste, and food safety.

UNDERSTANDING KEY IDEAS

1. What nutrients do meat, poultry, and fish provide? Why are these nutrients important?

2. Suppose you have eaten ground beef three times this week. What choices of meat, poultry, and fish could add variety to your menu?

3. If you were shopping for a lean steak to serve for dinner, what would you look for?

4. How would you store fresh fish that you'll cook tomorrow? Chicken for next week?

5. To what internal temperature would you cook a roast for medium doneness? Why is it important to use a thermometer when cooking meat, poultry, and fish?

DEVELOPING LIFE SKILLS

1. **Critical Thinking:** Why do you think many people eat more servings from the meat and beans group than they need? What are some possible negative effects?

2. **Management:** What are some ways in which time management relates to buying, storing, and preparing meat, poultry, and fish?

Wellness Challenge

As class president, Monisha is responsible for planning the end-of-the-year picnic. She would like to hold the picnic in a nearby county park. Since the park has barbecue facilities, Monisha plans to serve hamburgers and boneless chicken breasts.

1. What are some challenges Monisha will face if she plans to serve beef and poultry at the picnic?

2. How might she go about finding solutions?

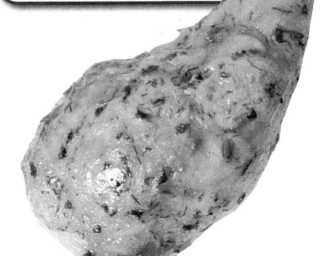

APPLYING YOUR LEARNING

1. **Menu Planning:** Imagine that you're planning a dinner party for 12 people. Select a type of meat, poultry, or fish to serve. Explain how you would select and prepare it. How might you make lean choices when buying? How much would you buy and why? What pre-preparation and cooking methods would help you prepare your choice without too much fat? What other foods would you serve in the meal and why?

2. **Protein Promotion:** Create a magazine ad or a script for a radio spot about the nutritional qualities of beef, poultry, and fish. Include money-saving tips and quality guidelines, too.

EXPLORING FURTHER

1. **Local Fish:** Find out what fish are caught or raised in your state or region. What fish are shipped in from other areas? What kinds of frozen fish are available? Compare the cost of fresh and frozen fish in your local store.

2. **The Use of Technology:** Investigate the process of food irradiation for beef, pork, and lamb. How does it work? Why is it done? What are the food safety advantages?

Making CONNECTIONS

1. **Health:** Research an outbreak of illness caused by harmful bacteria in meat, poultry, or fish. How did people contract the illness? What steps were taken to prevent further outbreaks? Report your findings to the class.

2. **Career Connections Experience:** Find a nonprofit group in your community that serves meals as a service to the needy or as a fundraiser. Work as a volunteer preparing food. Write a report about the experience, including how you applied the knowledge and skills you have learned in this course.

FOODS LAB

In groups of four or five students, broil one ground beef patty. Pan-fry a second one. Cook both to 160°F (71°C), checking with an instant-read thermometer. Compare the appearance, texture, and flavor of the two. What can you conclude?

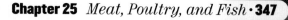

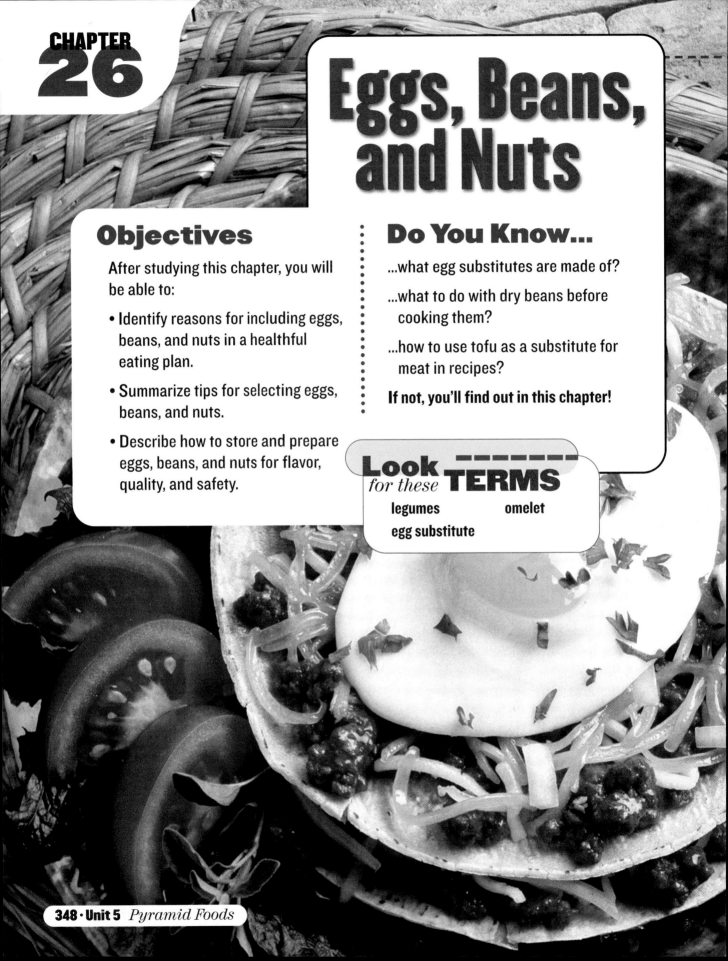

Eggs, Beans, and Nuts

Objectives

After studying this chapter, you will be able to:

- Identify reasons for including eggs, beans, and nuts in a healthful eating plan.

- Summarize tips for selecting eggs, beans, and nuts.

- Describe how to store and prepare eggs, beans, and nuts for flavor, quality, and safety.

Do You Know...

...what egg substitutes are made of?

...what to do with dry beans before cooking them?

...how to use tofu as a substitute for meat in recipes?

If not, you'll find out in this chapter!

Look *for these* TERMS

legumes   omelet
egg substitute

Have you ever

enjoyed a breakfast bean burrito, a spinach quiche, or a vegetable stir-fry with toasted almonds? Nutrient-packed beans, eggs, and nuts in these dishes are tasty, convenient ingredients. Enjoy them at any meal or as a snack.

INFOLINK

To review the difference between complete and incomplete protein, see Chapter 6.

Eggs, Beans, and Nuts— Nutritious Choices

What do eggs, beans, and nuts have in common? These foods—along with meat, poultry, and fish—all fit into the same food group in the Food Guide Pyramid. The beans in this food group are specific kinds called legumes. **Legumes** (leg-yooms) are *edible seeds that grow in pods*. Besides dry beans (but not green beans), they include dry peas—the kind in split pea soup—lentils, and peanuts.

All these different foods are grouped together mainly because they're high in protein. They provide many other valuable nutrients, too!

Protein. Eggs—like meat, poultry, and fish—are a good source of complete protein. Legumes and nuts deliver plenty of the amino acids that make up protein. With enough variety, these and other plant-based foods can help you meet your protein needs!

Vitamins and minerals. Eggs, legumes, and nuts are loaded with vitamins and minerals. Eggs supply folate and other B vitamins, vitamins D and E, and iron. Legumes bring you folate and other B vitamins, iron, potassium, and small amounts of calcium. Nuts offer folate, vitamins A and E, and phosphorus. Both legumes and nuts supply small amounts of zinc.

Legumes offer another choice from the Meat, Poultry, Fish, Dry Beans, Eggs, and Nuts Group. What serving size of beans equals I ounce (28 g) from the meat and beans group? What other food group do legumes fit in?

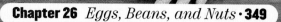

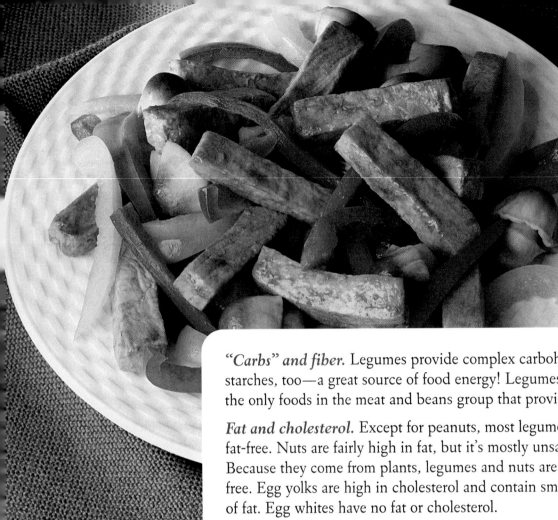

"Carbs" and fiber. Legumes provide complex carbohydrates from starches, too—a great source of food energy! Legumes and nuts are the only foods in the meat and beans group that provide fiber.

Fat and cholesterol. Except for peanuts, most legumes are nearly fat-free. Nuts are fairly high in fat, but it's mostly unsaturated. Because they come from plants, legumes and nuts are cholesterol-free. Egg yolks are high in cholesterol and contain small amounts of fat. Egg whites have no fat or cholesterol.

The Food Guide Pyramid's Advice

You need about two to three servings per day from the Meat, Poultry, Fish, Dry Beans, Eggs, and Nuts Group. Because this group includes so many different kinds of foods, counting servings is a little tricky! To count servings of eggs, legumes, and nuts, first "convert" them to what they equal in ounces (or grams) of meat. Then add up those amounts—plus your actual servings of meat, poultry, and fish—for the whole day. The total should be 5 to 7 ounces (140 to 196 g).

The following amounts are typical helpings of eggs, legumes, and nuts. Each counts as 1 ounce (28 g) from the meat and beans group.

- 1 egg
- ¼ cup (50 mL) egg substitute
- ½ cup (125 mL) cooked dry beans, peas, or lentils
- ⅓ cup (75 mL) nuts
- 2 tablespoons (30 mL) peanut butter
- 4 ounces (112 g) tofu (soybean curd)

Give tofu a try sometime. It's rich in high-quality protein and B vitamins, and it's low in sodium. Some varieties provide calcium—check the label. What are some ways you might eat tofu?

More About Cholesterol: One egg yolk has more than 200 mg of cholesterol. To put that in perspective, the recommended daily limit of cholesterol is 300 mg.

Remember that beans and other legumes do double duty. You can count them toward a serving from either the Vegetable Group or the Meat, Poultry, Fish, Dry Beans, Eggs, and Nuts Group. Choose one, since the same serving can't count toward both groups.

Choices for Variety

Eggs, beans, and nuts can take center stage in a meal—or add variety to side dishes and snacks.

- Get the low-fat, fiber-rich benefits of beans or other legumes several times a week. Besides adding texture and nutrition, beans come in many colors and shapes that make foods look and taste appealing.
- Go easy on eggs since they're high in cholesterol. Try to eat no more than four egg yolks a week. Since egg whites have no cholesterol, you can eat more of them. An **egg substitute**, which is *made from egg whites and contains very little fat and no cholesterol*, is also an option.
- Enjoy nuts and peanut butter in small amounts. They're convenient choices with flavors that go a long way!

Shopping for Eggs, Beans, and Nuts

When it comes to price and nutrition, eggs and legumes are usually a bargain. Along with nuts, they're convenient to keep on hand.

Choosing eggs. The color of the shells, white or brown, has no effect on the taste or nutrition of eggs. Look for a "sell by" date for freshness. Open the carton and make sure the eggs are clean and not cracked. You'll find pasteurized frozen egg products in the freezer case, and egg substitutes in either the refrigerator or freezer case.

Check This Out!

TOFU— A VERSATILE FOOD

Tofu, sometimes called soybean curd, is a soft, cheese-like food made from soybeans. Tofu has a wonderful ability to soak up the flavors of other foods and seasonings.

Types of tofu. Firm tofu is dense and solid. It keeps its shape when it's prepared. Soft and silken tofu are good choices when you want to blend tofu with other ingredients.

Storing tofu. Tofu is perishable, so store it in the refrigerator or freezer. Once it's opened, rinse leftover tofu and cover it with fresh water to store. Change the water daily and use the tofu within one week.

Preparing tofu. Add cubes of firm tofu to soups, stir-fry dishes, and stews. Cut back on meat by mixing crumbled tofu into meat loaf or adding it to the ground beef you use in tacos or spaghetti sauce. Blend soft tofu with seasonings for a vegetable dip or salad dressing. Use silken tofu as a substitute for part of the mayonnaise, sour cream, cream cheese, or ricotta cheese in a recipe.

It's Your Turn!

Find a recipe for tofu and give it a try. Report the results to the class.

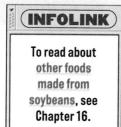
INFOLINK

To read about other foods made from soybeans, see Chapter 16.

Discuss: Are you eating the recommended number of servings from the Meat, Poultry, Fish, Dry Beans, Eggs, and Nuts Group? How often do you eat eggs, beans, and nuts? What are your favorite foods from this group? Your least favorite?

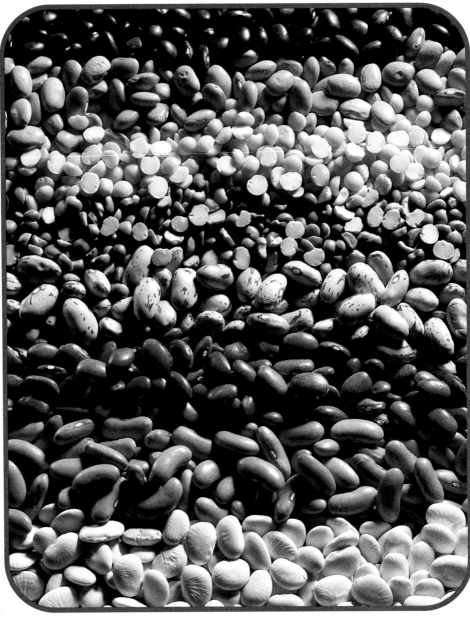

BLACK BEANS

PINK BEANS

YELLOW SPLIT PEAS

GREEN SPLIT PEAS

PINTO BEANS

RED BEANS

KIDNEY BEANS

WHITE BEANS

Beans, peas, and lentils are common varieties of legumes. Peanuts are also a type of legume, although they're eaten like nuts. Visit a supermarket and identify all the ways you can buy legumes. Share your findings with the class.

Looking for legumes. Look in the grocery aisles for dry legumes in bags or boxes. Canned beans are ready to heat and serve. They may have ingredients that add salt or fat, so check the ingredient list and Nutrition Facts panel to compare. Tofu is often sold in the produce department.

Picking nuts. You'll find nuts in jars, bags, and sometimes in bulk bins. Nuts may be sold with or without the shell, salted or unsalted. In the baking aisle, you can buy whole, ground, sliced, or chopped nuts. Peanut butter and nut butters are convenience options that are great for making sandwiches.

Storing Eggs, Beans, and Nuts

To keep eggs, beans, and nuts fresh and safe to eat, store them properly. Refrigerate fresh eggs in their carton. Keep pasteurized eggs and egg substitutes refrigerated or frozen—check the package directions. Store legumes and nuts in airtight containers in a cool, dry cabinet. After cooking legumes, refrigerate leftovers and use them within three to four days.

Discuss: Do hard-boiled eggs, with shells removed, have the same storage longevity as fresh eggs? Why or why not?

INFOLINK

For more guidelines on storing foods, see Section 1-2 of the Food Preparation Handbook.

Cooking Eggs

To keep eggs tender, tasty, and safe, cook them at low temperatures just until done. Eggs are fully cooked when the white and yolk are completely set and no visible liquid egg remains. High heat and overcooking make eggs shrink and become tough. Don't eat raw or undercooked eggs because of the danger of foodborne illness. That means skip the urge to eat cookie dough you make with eggs, too!

Eggs for Quick Meals and Snacks

When you have eggs on hand, you're only minutes away from a meal! Try these types for breakfast, lunch, dinner, or snacking.

Scrambled. Beat eggs with a little milk or water, then cook in a hot skillet. For the best texture, don't stir during cooking— just gently draw a turner across the pan. For more flavor and nutrients, add extras like chopped vegetables, shredded cheese, or diced ham.

Omelet—a dish made by cooking beaten eggs without stirring. Start the same as for scrambled eggs, but let the mixture set into a flat shape, like a pancake. Before you fold it over, you can tuck veggies, cheese, meat, chicken, or seafood inside.

Activity: Unlike an ear of corn or a steak, these dishes don't fully resemble their ingredients. Find pictures of the ingredients in these dishes and of the finished products for comparison. Create posters that present this information.

Check This Out!

HAVE YOU TRIED THESE?

As ingredients in mixed foods, eggs and legumes belong in dishes from all over the world!

- *Huevos rancheros*, a Mexican dish, combines scrambled eggs with onions. Salsa, refried beans, and tortillas are served on the side.
- Succotash is a Native American side dish of corn and lima beans.
- Hummus is a Middle Eastern spread made with mashed chickpeas and flavored with garlic and other seasonings.
- Quiche is a rich egg mixture baked in a pie shell. This French dish can be flavored with ingredients such as cheese, bacon, spinach, ham, and shellfish.
- Beans and rice is a combination dish with many variations: Southern Hoppin' John (black-eyed peas and white rice), Cuban *Moros y Cristianos* (black beans and rice), Puerto Rican *asapao de gandules* (pigeon peas and rice), and Indian *kitchri* (rice and lentils).
- Hearty bean soups, such as Dutch pea soup, are flavored with ham.

It's Your Turn!

Find an egg or legume recipe you would like to try. Share it with the class.

Check This Out!

LIGHTEN UP YOUR EGGS

For less fat and cholesterol . . .

- When you fry eggs, use a nonstick skillet and vegetable oil cooking spray—or no fat at all.
- Try egg substitutes for scrambling.
- Make quiche using nonfat condensed milk instead of cream.

- In baked goods and mixed dishes, substitute two egg whites or $^1/_4$ cup (50 mL) egg substitute for each whole egg.
- Look for specialty eggs with altered fat content at your local supermarket. Check the label for nutrient facts.

It's Your Turn!

What other ways can you think of for reducing fat and cholesterol in egg dishes?

Critical Thinking: Research the incidence of cholesterol-related health problems in children. Should children "lighten up" their eggs? Should you wait until you have a health problem to reduce fat and cholesterol? Is it easy to change eating habits?

Tip

Crack an egg by tapping its side firmly on a hard, flat surface. Pull the shell apart using your thumbs. Crack each egg into a small bowl before adding it to the pan or the recipe. That way you can check for problems, such as a broken yolk or stray bits of shell, before using the egg.

Poached. Bring a saucepan of water to a boil, then reduce to a simmer. Break the egg into a bowl and gently slip the egg into the water. Simmer the egg until it's cooked.

Hard-cooked or soft-cooked. Place eggs in their shell in a pan of water, bring the water to a boil, and turn off the heat. Let the eggs stand in hot water for about 5 minutes (soft-cooked) or 15 minutes (hard-cooked).

Fried. Gently break the eggs into a bowl and slip them into the heated skillet with a small amount of fat. Cover the pan and cook slowly. "Over-easy" means the eggs are turned over during cooking. "Sunny-side up" means the eggs are not turned. In either case, be careful not to break the yolks.

Baked. Break the eggs into a bowl, then slip them into a greased dish. Bake at 325°F (160°C) until done.

In the microwave oven. You can make scrambled or "baked" eggs in the microwave oven. Check a cookbook for power level and time. Pierce the yolk before "baking" the eggs to prevent the yolk from bursting. Don't cook eggs in the shell in the microwave oven—they'll explode!

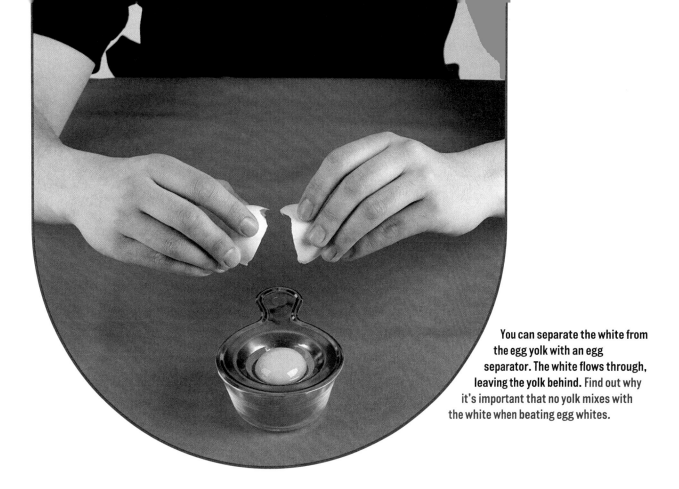

You can separate the white from the egg yolk with an egg separator. The white flows through, leaving the yolk behind. Find out why it's important that no yolk mixes with the white when beating egg whites.

Using Eggs in Recipes

Eggs serve many important roles in recipes. For instance, you can use eggs to thicken sauces, hold ingredients together (as in meat loaf), and give structure to batter and dough for baked goods.

Preparing Legumes

You can enjoy beans and other legumes lots of ways—in chili, Mexican dishes, hearty soups, salads, seasoned baked beans, casseroles, and more! Will you use dry or canned legumes? That depends on how much time you have. Either way, it's easy. The flavors and textures of beans, peas, and lentils combine well with other foods.

Quick ways with beans. You can put a quick and easy meal together using canned beans. Combine them with a few other ingredients, and they're ready to enjoy! For example, to make a breakfast burrito, wrap refried beans, scrambled eggs, and cheese in a flour tortilla. Add a can of kidney or other beans to canned chili or pasta sauce to make a quick, hearty main dish with protein, other nutrients, and fiber.

INFOLINK

To learn about beating egg whites, see Section 4-7 of the Food Preparation Handbook.

Activity: Examine the nutrition labels of a package of dry legumes and the same legume in a can. Is there a difference in nutritional value? In cost? In ease of use and preparation?

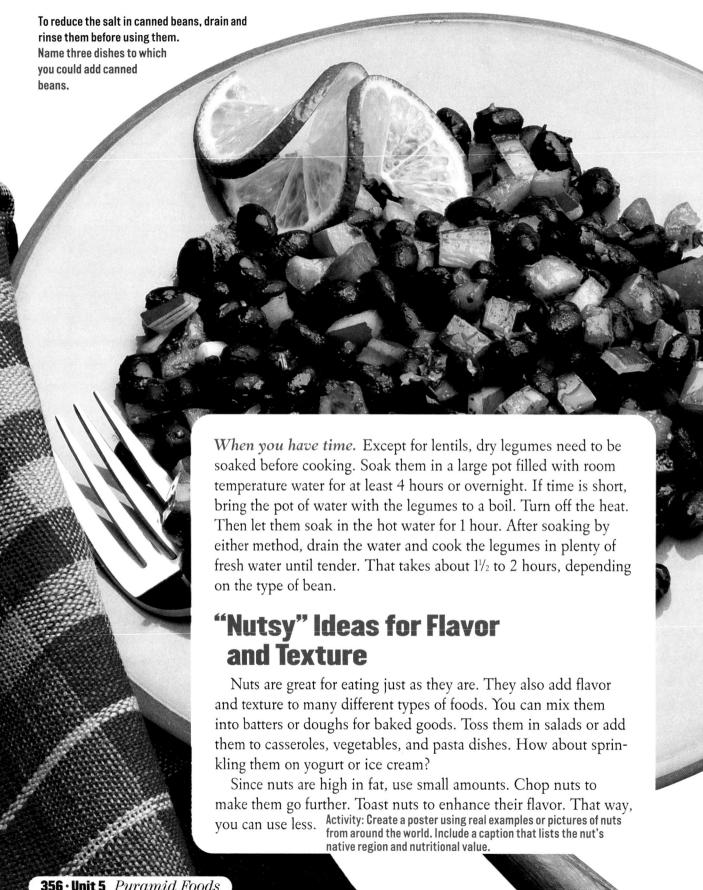

To reduce the salt in canned beans, drain and rinse them before using them. Name three dishes to which you could add canned beans.

When you have time. Except for lentils, dry legumes need to be soaked before cooking. Soak them in a large pot filled with room temperature water for at least 4 hours or overnight. If time is short, bring the pot of water with the legumes to a boil. Turn off the heat. Then let them soak in the hot water for 1 hour. After soaking by either method, drain the water and cook the legumes in plenty of fresh water until tender. That takes about 1½ to 2 hours, depending on the type of bean.

"Nutsy" Ideas for Flavor and Texture

Nuts are great for eating just as they are. They also add flavor and texture to many different types of foods. You can mix them into batters or doughs for baked goods. Toss them in salads or add them to casseroles, vegetables, and pasta dishes. How about sprinkling them on yogurt or ice cream?

Since nuts are high in fat, use small amounts. Chop nuts to make them go further. Toast nuts to enhance their flavor. That way, you can use less. Activity: Create a poster using real examples or pictures of nuts from around the world. Include a caption that lists the nut's native region and nutritional value.

NOW You're COOKiNG!

SKILL
Making an Omelet

Want to make a perfect omelet? Try these tricks: have the eggs at room temperature, use a nonstick pan coated with vegetable oil cooking spray or a small amount of margarine or butter, and get the pan hot before adding eggs.

RECIPE

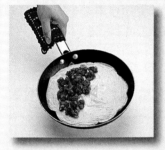

Mexican Omelet

CUSTOMARY	INGREDIENTS	METRIC
	Vegetable oil cooking spray	
3	Large eggs, at room temperature	3
1 Tbsp.	Water	15 mL
2 Tbsp.	Prepared salsa	30 mL

Yield: 2 servings

❶ Lightly spray a 10-inch (25-cm) nonstick skillet with vegetable oil cooking spray. Preheat skillet over medium-high heat.

❷ In small bowl, mix eggs and water together with a fork. Pour egg mixture into pan.

❸ As eggs begin to set, lift the edge with a turner, allowing the uncooked portion to flow underneath. Continue cooking until eggs are set and no visible liquid egg remains, about 1 ½ to 2 minutes.

❹ Spread salsa over half of omelet. Flip unfilled half over other half with turner. Cut into two pieces and slide one piece onto each plate.

Per Serving: 157 calories, 10 g protein, 3 g carbohydrate, 12 g fat, 312 mg sodium, 0 g fiber
Percent Daily Value: vitamin A 19%, vitamin D 12%, riboflavin 23%, vitamin B_{12} 11%, phosphorus 16%

More Ideas | Fill your omelet with other food-group ingredients: shredded cheese, steamed chopped vegetables, small pieces of cooked meat or fish, or even pizza sauce.

Your Ideas | Choose a combination of omelet fillings that sounds great to you. Prepare one version with whole eggs and another with egg substitute. How do they compare?

LOOKING BACK

- Eggs, beans, and nuts are high in protein and also provide many other valuable nutrients.
- Eat about two to three servings each day from the Meat, Poultry, Fish, Dry Beans, Eggs, and Nuts Group.
- Eggs and many varieties of beans and nuts are convenient to keep on hand.
- Store eggs, beans, and nuts properly for freshness and food safety.
- Eggs are great for quick meals and snacks and serve many functions in recipes.
- The flavors and textures of legumes and nuts combine well with other foods.

UNDERSTANDING KEY IDEAS

1. What are the benefits of including eggs, beans, and nuts in your eating plan?
2. What should you look for when selecting fresh eggs? Canned legumes?
3. How should you store fresh eggs? Legumes and nuts?
4. How can you tell when eggs are fully cooked? What happens if they're over-cooked?
5. If you had only a few hours before dinner, how would you cook dry legumes?

DEVELOPING LIFE SKILLS

1. **Critical Thinking:** Compare and contrast shell eggs with egg substitutes. In what ways are they similar? In what ways are they different? Why might some people prefer one over the other?
2. **Creative Thinking:** How might you use walnuts, pecans, cashews, and almonds in cooking? Without looking in a cookbook, think of as many ideas as you can. Share them with the class.

Wellness Challenge

Some of the students have been asked to plan the menu for a new food stand at the Saturday football games. They have decided the menu should include several main dish choices that are nutritious and low in cost. Once the menu is chosen, the school will sign a contract with a supplier that will be in effect for the entire football season.

1. What items featuring legumes might the students consider for their menu? Why?
2. Besides nutrition and cost, what else should the students consider before deciding on the menu items? Why?
3. How might the students address these considerations?

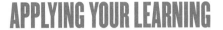

APPLYING YOUR LEARNING

1. **Adapting Recipes:** Show how you could substitute tofu for a traditional ingredient in recipes for an appetizer, main dish, side dish, and dessert. How would the substitution affect the nutrient and calorie content? Share your recipes with the class.

2. **Egg Promotion:** Imagine you have been hired by a company to promote eggs. Think of five ways you could encourage consumers to enjoy the versatility and nutritional advantages of eggs. Get feedback on your ideas from a classmate, then choose the best idea to develop into an ad campaign. Present it to the class.

EXPLORING FURTHER

1. **The Growing Process:** Learn where and how dry beans and peas are grown. How are they processed after harvesting?

2. **Egg Safety:** Find out more about why cooking eggs completely is so important. What foodborne illness is the main concern? Why? Have incidents of this illness increased or decreased in the last ten years? What are some possible reasons?

Making CONNECTIONS

1. **Social Studies:** Identify a country where legumes are a main source of protein. Determine why they are popular. How are they prepared and in what types of dishes are they used? Report your findings to the class.

2. **Technology:** Several new types of eggs and egg products have been developed recently. Some of these include organic eggs, vegetarian eggs, and eggs with less fat. Using library or Internet sources or by visiting a store, find out more about these new eggs. What are the advantages and disadvantages? Which ones are available in your area?

FOODS LAB

Choose one of the basic egg preparation methods described in this chapter to try in the foods lab. Time how long it takes you to prepare an egg using this method. Would you choose this method again for a quick meal or snack? Why or why not?

CRAVING THE CRAWLIES

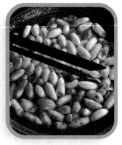

▲ Silkworms are boiled in their cocoons.

Come and get 'em. Bugs are the new culinary item in Thailand. "They have a rich texture, and the flavors are like nothing you've ever tasted," says Nusara Thaitawat, author of *Cuisine of Thailand*. The meat and potatoes, so to speak, of the insect biz are grasshoppers, beetles, and bamboo worms. "They're good food, but bugs have bad public relations," says Thaitawat.

Lots of people eat insects: nearly 3,000 ethnic groups in 113 countries. In fact, some 1,400 kinds of bugs are known to be edible. Considering that Earth may have millions of insect species, there may be many more ripe for the munching. ■

Insects Are Good For You

This chart shows how some species of insects compare to eggs, pork, and chicken.

FOOD	PROTEIN (per 100 g)	FAT (per 100 g)	ALSO RICH IN
Giant water bug (*Mang da*)	19.8 g	8.3 g	Calcium and iron
Grasshopper (*Takkatan*)	20.6 g	6.1 g	Calcium and niacin
Silkworm pupae (*Dakdae*)	9.6 g	5.6 g	Calcium and riboflavin
Chicken eggs	12 g	10 g	Calcium
Roast chicken	31.4 g	3.5 g	Niacin and phosphorus
Pork	14.1 g	3.5 g	Thiamin and niacin

Source: *Creepy Crawly Cuisine* by Julieta Ramos-Elorduy, professor of biology at the National University of Mexico

NOODLE NATION

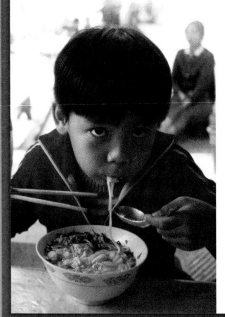

Visitors to Vietnam are often surprised to discover that rice isn't the only staple of Vietnamese diets. The people who live there are crazy about noodles. Noodles are often on the menu for the three main meals of the day. Noodles are also popular snacks. Unlike pasta with which Americans are familiar, Vietnamese noodles are made from many ingredients. You can dine on wheat, rice, and mung bean noodles. The noodles are often served in soup or are pan-fried. They can also be mixed with meats, herbs, and vegetables.

It's common to see Vietnamese stopping their bicycles or motor scooters at roadside stands for a fast-food meal of noodles and a quick chat with friends. According to Jackie Passmore, an author of Asian cookbooks, "Perhaps no one in the world eats as many noodles as the Vietnamese." ■

BREAKFAST IS SERVED

Here are some typical breakfasts for several East and Southeast Asian nations. How do they compare with your typical breakfast?

Indonesia: Fried rice mixed with thin strips of cooked egg; sliced cucumber, fried shallots, rice crackers, and coffee or sweet iced tea.

China: Rice, vegetables, meat dishes, dim sum.

Philippines: Rice, salty fish, fried egg.

tidbits

In primarily Muslim countries such as **Indonesia**, don't pick up or pass food with your left hand. In **China**, leave the bowl of rice served at the end of the meal unfinished (to show the host that you couldn't eat one more bite). In **Malaysia**, it is polite to leave the table once you have finished eating. In **Japan**, hosts never fill your teacup to the top. That way, you'll come back again for more.

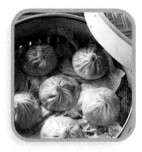

Dim sum means "touch the heart" in Chinese. These dumplings (photo above) trace their roots to Guangzhou (gwahn-zhow), a province in China. ■

teatime

In Asian societies, green tea is drunk about as much as coffee is in the West. Green tea is loaded with natural chemicals that may be good for the body. Studies suggest that one group of chemicals in green tea may help prevent cancer by depriving early tumors of nourishment. Studies from Japan show that drinking 10 cups a day may lower the risk of heart disease. If that much tea seems hard to swallow, consider using it as a mouthwash! Reports suggest that swishing green tea around the mouth may slow cavity-causing germs. What about black tea? It may be equally beneficial, scientists suspect. All in all, it seems that whatever the color, a cup of tea is absolutely TEA-RIFFIC! ■

> Green tea may reduce heart disease and cancer risk, but you will have to swallow a lot of it.

Southeast & East Asia

Even floods ▶ won't keep people away from outdoor markets in the Philippines.

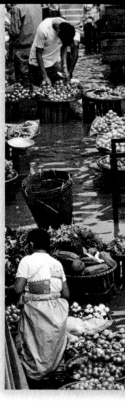

The foods of East and Southeast Asia have several things in common. Rice and noodles are the main attractions at most meals, while hot chilies, garlic, ginger, cilantro, and other bold-tasting foods add flavor. Fresh vegetables and small portions of meat are often cut up in bite-size pieces and cooked quickly on a hot wok. Tofu (a soft or firm cheese-like product made from soy milk) is found in many of the Pacific Rim nations. Of course, each country has its own individual cuisine. Different local spices, vegetables, and seafood make a nation's food as unique as a fingerprint.

China Throughout China, as well as many of the other nations in this area of the world, cooks try to balance textures, colors, temperatures, and tastes. A well-balanced meal provides a combination of five tastes: sour, salty, bitter, hot (spicy), and sweet.

Soy sauce, tofu, ginger, dumplings, and pork-filled steamed buns—these are just some of the foods asso-

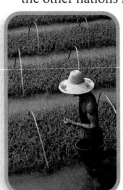

▲ A man works in a rice field in China. Rice is a staple of most Asian nations.

ciated with Chinese cooking. China is made up of many regions, and each has its own style of preparing foods. The south is the home of Cantonese cooking, which uses oyster sauce, fermented soybean sauce, lard, sugar, and vinegar. Canton dishes are fairly mild, but their ingredients can be wild—from birds and snakes to rodents and insects.

In the western part of China, the cuisine is hot! It uses lots of chilies to make fiery dishes like kung pao (gong-baow) chicken, which is fried with peanuts and chili pepper.

In the southern region of the Yangtze (yang-see) River, people eat lots of fish and shellfish such as stewed crab and crisp eel. In the north, lamb is often cooked in a Mongolian fire pot—a hot pot full of broth. Instead of rice, people eat bread and noodles.

Japan Japanese food is influenced by the seasons. In the autumn, oden is popular. This is a stew made of fish dumplings, fried tofu, eggs, and vegetables. In winter, people eat nabemono (nah-bee-moh-noh) dishes—raw foods that are placed by the eater in a boiling pot of liquid. Ingredients range from oysters and scallops to chrysanthemum leaves.

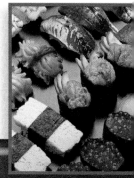

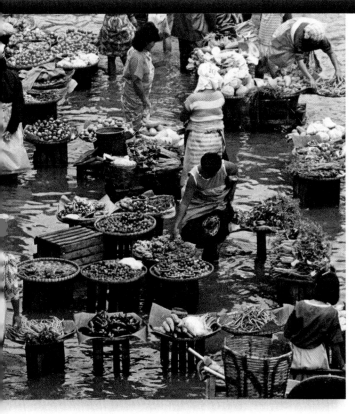

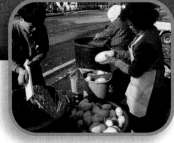

A family in Korea works together to make kimchi.

The most recognizable Japanese food is sushi, which is seasoned rice often topped with raw seafood such as tuna or with cooked foods and vegetables. In one type of sushi, the rice is layered with seaweed, seafood, and vegetables, rolled up and cut into slices. Sashimi (sah-SHEE-mee) is raw seafood sliced thin and served with soy sauce, pickled ginger, or wasabi, a type of horseradish.

Korea

North and South Korean cuisine is influenced by the other Pacific Rim nations. Foods are cooked with seasonings such as hot red peppers, green onion, soy sauce, soybean paste, mustard, and vinegar, which are combined in different ways. There are almost 200 varieties of kimchi (gim-chee), Korea's fiery national dish. It may be made of cabbage and white radishes, turnips, potatoes, or other vegetables, blasted with hot red peppers and garlic, and left to ferment in clay pots. Many types of hot and pickled vegetables are often served as side dishes.

Koreans eat three meals a day, with breakfast traditionally the biggest. Breakfast usually consists of boiled rice, soup, kimchi, and a small portion of meat, poultry, or fish. For most meals, rice is the main course, with bits of vegetables or small amounts of meat added. Special herbs and spices—such as small amounts of mugwort, aralia shoots, and shepherd's purse—may also be included. Soups, noodles, and cheong-po (chung-poh), a tofu-like product made from mung beans, are all important foods in Korea.

Philippines

Whether Filipinos are eating chicken, pork, or fish, they like their food flavored by strong seasonings, such as fermented fish or shrimp sauce. Food is also dipped in sauces made of mustard, chili, garlic, vinegar, and soy sauce.

Many dishes are made with coconut, which grows everywhere. The national dish is adobo—chicken or pork stewed in vinegar and soy sauce.

The Chinese have influenced Filipino food: Noodle dishes, known as pancit (PAHN-seet), are a staple, as are steamed buns. The United States has given Filipinos fried chicken, but the Filipinos have given it their own twist. Before it's fried, the chicken is marinated in soy sauce, vinegar, and garlic. ■

◄ Japanese sushi comes in many varieties.

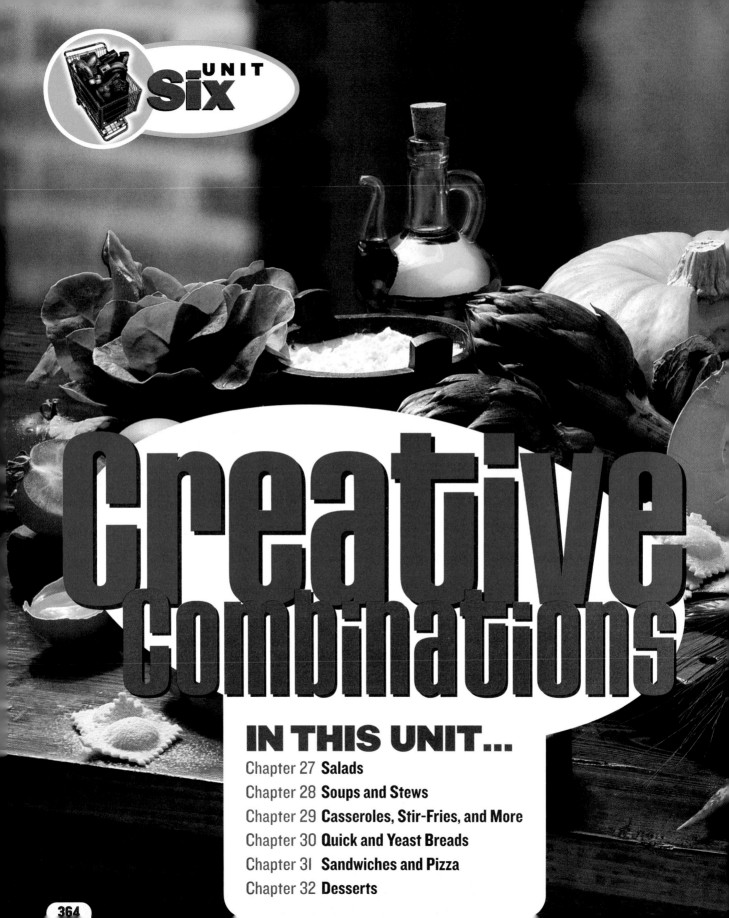

Creative Combinations

IN THIS UNIT...

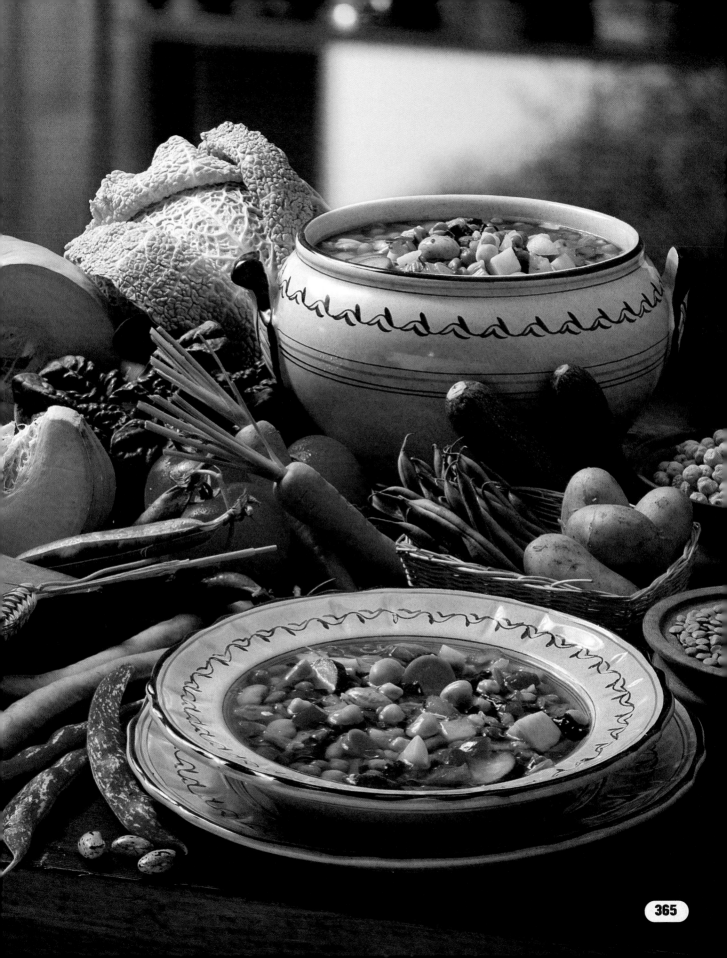

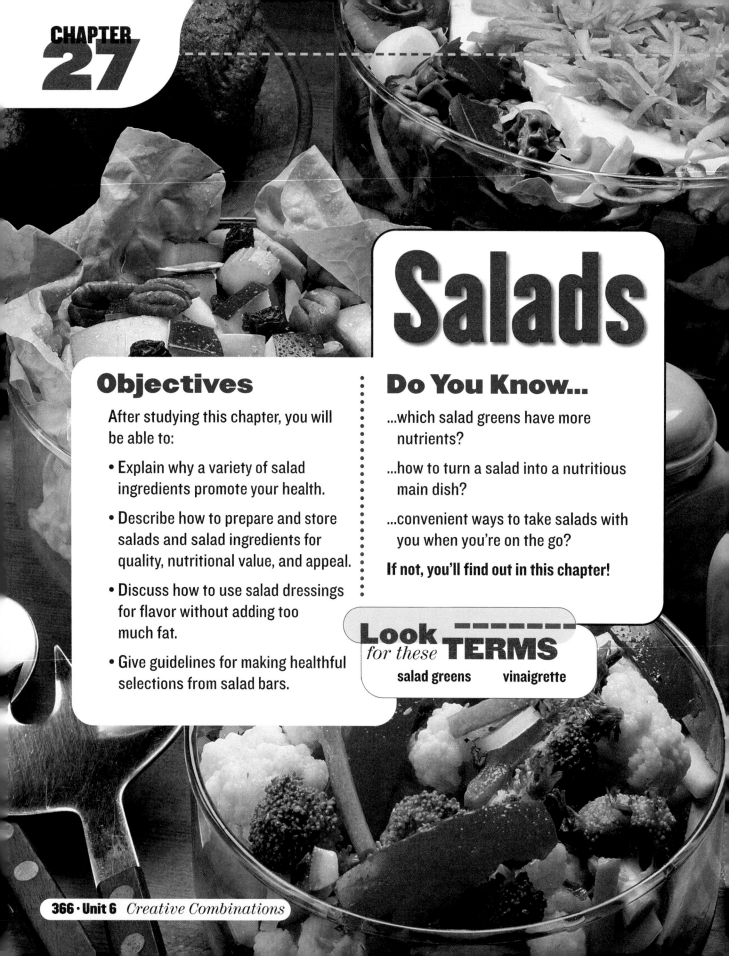

CHAPTER 27

Salads

Objectives

After studying this chapter, you will be able to:

- Explain why a variety of salad ingredients promote your health.

- Describe how to prepare and store salads and salad ingredients for quality, nutritional value, and appeal.

- Discuss how to use salad dressings for flavor without adding too much fat.

- Give guidelines for making healthful selections from salad bars.

Do You Know...

...which salad greens have more nutrients?

...how to turn a salad into a nutritious main dish?

...convenient ways to take salads with you when you're on the go?

If not, you'll find out in this chapter!

Look for these TERMS

salad greens   vinaigrette

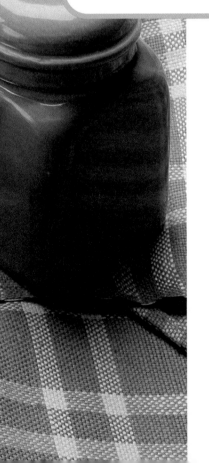

Salads are an

easy, tasty way to include a variety of foods in your eating plan. You can eat salads at any time of day. Think of fruit salad for breakfast, a seafood salad on greens for lunch, a spinach salad with dinner, a pasta salad for a potluck meal, or even a taco salad folded in a tortilla to eat on the run!

What's in Your Salad?

The nutritional benefits of salads come from the mix of ingredients. You can choose ingredients from any of the five food groups and the Pyramid tip and get flavor benefits.

Grain products. Rice, pasta, bulgur wheat, and couscous are just some of the grain products that add complex carbohydrates, B vitamins, and perhaps fiber to a salad.

Vegetables and fruits. Go for variety with vegetables and fruits. Among other nutrients, they provide vitamins A and C, folate, potassium, and fiber. Hint: the darker the salad greens, the more nutrients they have!

Dairy products. Cheese, cottage cheese, and yogurt supply calcium, protein, and riboflavin.

Meat, poultry, fish, dry beans, eggs, and nuts. Many salads include these high-protein foods. Besides protein, they give you iron, zinc, and B vitamins. Beans add fiber, too!

Salad dressings. These add flavor to your salads. Many contain large amounts of fat, so use them in moderation. Remember, these dressings belong in the tip of the Food Guide Pyramid.

Salads can add eye appeal and boost the nutrition on your dinner plate. What nutrients will this salad contribute to the meal?

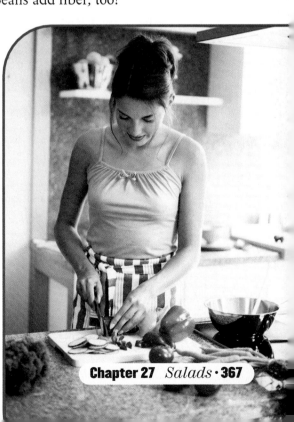

Making Salads Great!

The beauty of salad making is that you can come up with new combinations every time! Variety and versatility add up to convenience, interest, and great taste.

Making a Mixed Greens Salad

When making a tossed salad, many people think only of iceberg lettuce. However, there are many other **salad greens**, or *edible leaves*, that can add variety of color, flavor, and texture to your salad. Have you tried using spinach, watercress, Boston, butterhead, romaine, or red or green loose-leaf lettuce? Many of these choices are more nutritious than iceberg lettuce. Look at the chart below to compare the nutrients in different greens.

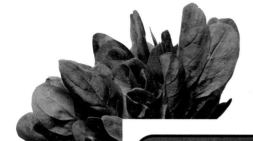

Teaching with Visuals: Compute the amount of the greens you would have to eat to get 100% of the vitamins and minerals listed. Why is variety from the five food groups an important part of meal planning?

Rate Your Salad Greens	PERCENT DAILY VALUE per 1 cup (250 mL) serving			
	Vitamin A (%)	Vitamin C (%)	Folate (%)	Potassium (%)
Boston lettuce	11	7	10	4
Iceberg lettuce	4	4	8	2
Romaine lettuce	15	11	9	5
Spinach (raw)	40	14	15	5

Source: USDA Nutrient Database for Standard Reference.

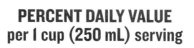
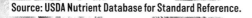

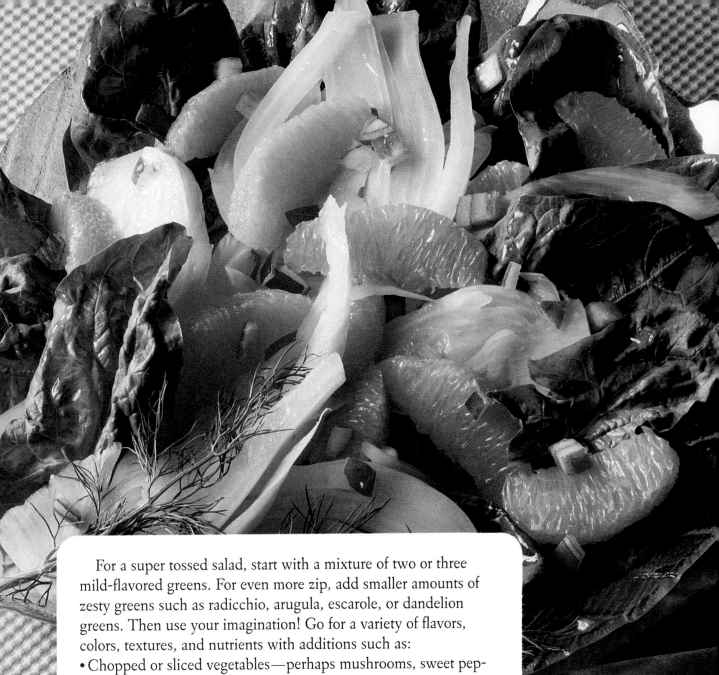

For a super tossed salad, start with a mixture of two or three mild-flavored greens. For even more zip, add smaller amounts of zesty greens such as radicchio, arugula, escarole, or dandelion greens. Then use your imagination! Go for a variety of flavors, colors, textures, and nutrients with additions such as:

- Chopped or sliced vegetables—perhaps mushrooms, sweet peppers, cauliflower, celery, tomato, artichoke hearts, or jicama.
- Alfalfa, bean, or broccoli sprouts.
- Shredded cheese.
- Drained canned garbanzo or kidney beans.
- Citrus slices, chopped apples, berries, raisins, or dried cranberries.
- Sunflower seeds or toasted chopped nuts.
- Croutons—crunchy dried bread cubes, plain or seasoned.

Depending on what you put in it, a mixed greens salad can be light or hearty. To turn it into a main dish, just include protein foods such as sliced meat or poultry, drained canned beans, or cubed firm tofu.

Selecting nutritious ingredients for a salad can be easy and fun. Use a variety of textures, flavors, and colors for more interest. Name three ingredients you could combine with a lettuce salad to give you more protein.

Preparing Your Salad

Follow these tips to make mixed greens salads appealing.

- Choose crisp salad greens with evenly colored leaves and no wilting.
- Wash all salad greens under cool running water. Drain thoroughly. If needed, dry the greens by blotting gently with a paper towel or using a salad spinner.
- Tear rather than cut salad greens for best results. Cutting may brown the edges.
- Shred, slice, or cut other ingredients into bite-size pieces.
- Toss ingredients gently by turning them over several times with utensils to mix them.
- Toss the salad with the dressing just before you serve it. That way the greens won't wilt. You might also serve the dressing separately and let everyone add his or her own.
- Serve the salad on a chilled salad plate or in a chilled salad bowl.

Other Salad Ideas

If you browse through a cookbook, you can find many types of salads. Here are some examples.

Tossed or mixed salads. Besides mixed greens, you can toss together many other ingredients. You might enjoy pasta salad, potato salad, egg salad, cole slaw, carrot-raisin salad, or mixed fruit salad.

A salad means much more than just mixed greens. Combine colorful seasonal fruit for a nutritious mixed salad. What other kinds of mixed salad could you make?

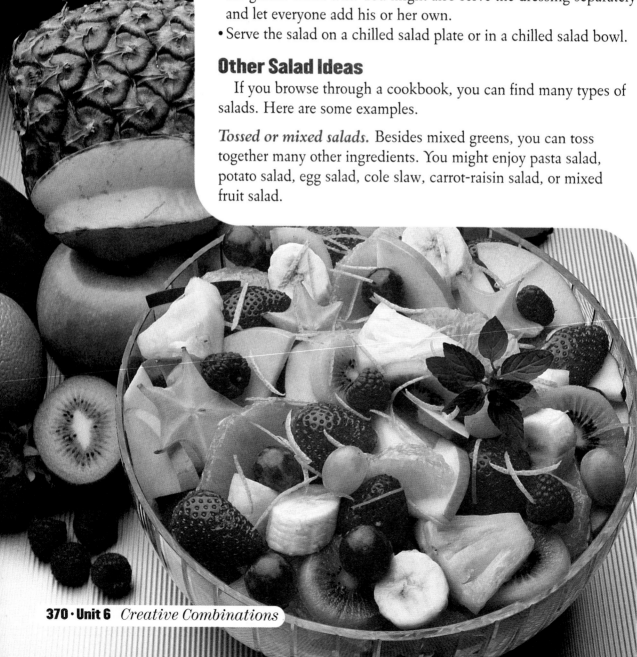

Arranged salads. These salads use colorful, flavorful ingredients that are artfully arranged on the plate. For example, you could start with a bed of lettuce as a base. Top with an arrangement of fresh fruit slices and a scoop of herbed cottage cheese.

Molded salads. Salad ingredients can be molded in a container to create a special shape. Most molded salads are made with gelatin. It's easy to work with gelatin—just follow the package directions. For extra flavor, you can use fruit juices such as apple, cranberry, or orange juice instead of the water called for in the directions. As the gelatin sets, fold in yogurt, sliced bananas, or drained canned fruit.

It's fun to try different salad recipes or use them for ideas as you create your own salads. Just as you do with a salad of mixed greens, look for ways to add color, flavor, texture, and nutrients with added ingredients. Use your imagination to give standard salad recipes new twists. For instance, you might add olives and capers to your potato salad for a flavor boost.

Tossing in Convenience

When you're at the grocery store, you can buy prepared salads from the deli department or salad ingredients from the salad bar. Many produce departments carry convenient bags of washed salad greens, slaw mixes, and cut-up veggies. Make sure you read the "sell by" date to buy the freshest. You may pay extra for the convenience. When would these foods be the best choices?

Planning ahead is another way to make salads convenient. Chop vegetables and cook chicken, hard-cooked eggs, or pasta ahead of time. Refrigerate until you're ready to make a salad. Keeping canned or frozen fruit on hand also helps you make a quick salad.

(**INFOLINK**)

To learn more about gelatin, see Section 4-8 of the Food Preparation Handbook.

Discuss: What steps can you take to be sure the salads you take along to eat later will remain fresh and unspoiled?

Check This Out!

TAKE-ALONG SALADS

Make these easy salads to eat when you are on the go!

- Stuff a garden salad or chicken salad in a pita bread.
- Roll a tortilla around carrot and raisin slaw.
- Fill a scooped-out hearty roll with Mexican bean salad.
- Pack a plain ice cream cone with cut-up, bite-size fruit.

It's Your Turn!

Look for ingredients in the supermarket that you could use for a take-along salad. Share your ideas with the class.

NOW *You're* COOKING!

Preparing a Mixed Salad

*T*his salad is nutritious as well as easy to prepare. Instead of peeling the carrots, save nutrients by simply scrubbing them with a brush under running water.

RECIPE

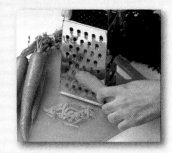

Carrot-Raisin Salad

CUSTOMARY	INGREDIENTS	METRIC
2 cups	Grated carrots	500 mL
½ cup	Raisins	125 mL
¼ cup	Mayonnaise	50 mL
½ tsp.	Dried mint leaves	2 mL

Yield: 4 servings, ½ cup (125 mL) each

❶ In medium bowl, stir together carrots and raisins.

❷ Add mayonnaise and mint leaves; stir until combined.

Per Serving: 135 calories, 1 g protein, 25 g carbohydrate, 5 g fat, 125 mg sodium, 3 g fiber

Percent Daily Value: vitamin A 155%, vitamin E 23%

More Ideas

- For less fat, use fat-free or light mayonnaise or plain yogurt.
- Try adding dried cranberries, chopped peanuts, drained pineapple tidbits, or grated cabbage for more flavor, color, and nutrients.
- You can substitute 1½ tsp. (7 mL) fresh mint leaves for the dried mint.

Your Ideas

Carrot salad can be a great take-along side dish for picnics. How could you change the recipe or handle the salad for an all-day family outing? Check Part I of the Food Preparation Handbook for tips on food safety. Then make a plan for a picnic carrot salad.

Make your own salad dressing using oil, vinegar or lemon juice, and other seasonings. How can you cut back on fat and calories when using salad dressings?

Salad Dressing Choices

A dressing adds moisture, holds ingredients together, and enhances flavor by lightly coating the ingredients. If you purchase bottled dressing, you'll find regular, low-fat, and fat-free varieties. You can also make your own dressing.

Oil dressings are often called by specific names such as French, Italian, or vinaigrette. **Vinaigrette** is *a mixture of oil and vinegar.* You can make your own by combining three parts oil and one part vinegar or lemon juice, then adding herbs. To cut fat and calories, use less oil. If you use a mild balsamic vinegar, you can skip the oil altogether.

Mayonnaise is often used as a dressing in mixed salads. Because mayonnaise is high in fat, use it sparingly. For some salads, low-fat yogurt is a good substitute. Add seasonings and herbs for extra flavor.

You can flavor your salad with other toppings, too. Try a squeeze of citrus juice, flavored vinegars, such as raspberry, and fresh herbs, such as chives or basil. What other low-fat alternatives to traditional salad dressing can you think of?

Storing Salads: Chill Out!

Keep salads and salad ingredients chilled for freshness and safety. Store salad ingredients in separate plastic bags or covered containers in your refrigerator. Refrigeration is especially important for protein foods such as meat, chicken, fish, eggs, and mayonnaise. If stored at room temperature, they could cause food-borne illness. Take salads to picnics in a chilled, insulated cooler.

Emphasize: If a salad has not been kept cold and there is any question about its food safety, do not take a chance—throw it out.

Tip

Dress lightly! Start with much less dressing than you think you'll need. Toss well. You'll be surprised how far a little goes.

INFOLINK

To learn more about food safety and storage, turn to Part 1 of the Food Preparation Handbook.

INFOLINK

To learn more about the science behind salad dressings, see Section 4-8 of the Food Preparation Handbook.

Salad Bar Savvy

Critical Thinking: Imagine that two of your classmates are going on a weight-loss diet and plan to eat nothing but salads for lunch and dinner. What advice can you give them about going on such a diet?

Salad bars in supermarkets, restaurants, fast-food places, and school cafeterias have lots of healthful food choices. However, you might be surprised to learn that the average salad from a salad bar is not always low-fat or low-calorie. In fact, it can have more than 1,000 calories! It's up to you to make wise choices.

• Fill your plate with plenty of fresh vegetables and fruits.
• If you're having salad from the salad bar as your main dish, include cooked dry beans, hard-cooked eggs, lean meat, turkey, or shrimp for protein.
• Go easy on mixed salads tossed in oil or mixed with mayonnaise.
• Have just a little salad dressing or choose the fat-free variety.
• To control portions, make just one trip to the salad bar.

Use your salad savvy to make healthful salad bar choices. What choices would you make for a side salad or a main dish salad?

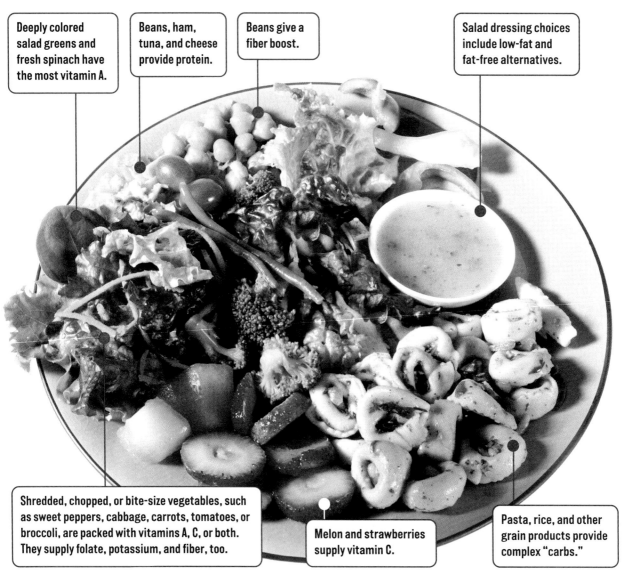

Deeply colored salad greens and fresh spinach have the most vitamin A.

Beans, ham, tuna, and cheese provide protein.

Beans give a fiber boost.

Salad dressing choices include low-fat and fat-free alternatives.

Shredded, chopped, or bite-size vegetables, such as sweet peppers, cabbage, carrots, tomatoes, or broccoli, are packed with vitamins A, C, or both. They supply folate, potassium, and fiber, too.

Melon and strawberries supply vitamin C.

Pasta, rice, and other grain products provide complex "carbs."

Leftover Lunches Help
People In Need

" **I** *'ll never work."*
"There's too much red tape."
That's what David Levitt heard when he told school officials about his plan to help people in need. Fortunately, David was not easily discouraged.

David, a student in Pinellas, Florida, had a simple plan. He wanted his school to give its surplus cafeteria food to local soup kitchens. Even after he was told the plan wouldn't work, David was determined to make it happen. He wrote a report and presented it to the school board, which voted to support David's plan.

In a recent year, the schools in David's district gave away more than 55,000 pounds of food. "It just took a kid to make them see this matters," Levitt says.

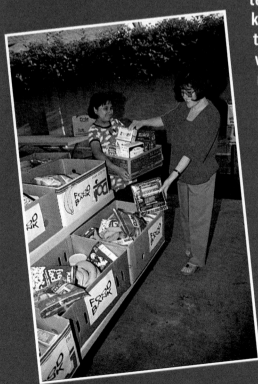

Take Action

How can your school help to feed the needy? Could you donate extra cafeteria food to a local food pantry? How about sponsoring a canned food drive for a homeless shelter? Choose a strategy that suits your community. Come up with a detailed plan for implementing the strategy. Write a report to describe your plan. Then put it into action.

LOOKING BACK

- Choose salad ingredients from any of the five food groups and the Pyramid tip.
- Creating new salad combinations will add convenience and taste to your eating plan.
- Salad types include tossed or mixed, arranged, and molded.
- Salad dressings add moisture, hold ingredients together, and enhance flavor.
- For freshness and safety, keep salads and salad ingredients chilled.
- When eating from salad bars, make healthful choices for good nutrition.

UNDERSTANDING KEY IDEAS

1. Why would a salad with ingredients from each of the five food groups be more nutritious than only iceberg lettuce? Be specific in your answer.
2. Describe the steps in preparing a salad of mixed greens, sweet peppers, and tomatoes.
3. How would you make your own vinaigrette dressing? How could you cut the fat?
4. How might you plan ahead when making egg salad? How would you safely store the ingredients?
5. If you were having a salad bar lunch, what are some healthful choices you could make?

DEVELOPING LIFE SKILLS

1. **Communication:** What communication methods might a produce department manager use to encourage sales of salad ingredients? What communication methods might you use to encourage a friend to try a new kind of salad? How are these methods similar and different?
2. **Creative Thinking:** Name four basic colors. (Example: green, yellow, red, purple.) How might you combine ingredients with those colors into a tasty, healthful salad?

Wellness Challenge

Consuelo and Matthew are organizing a Healthy Salads Day at school. Parents, students, and young children have been invited. Matthew and Consuelo want to offer salads that will appeal to everyone. They also want to promote the idea that all the food groups in the Food Guide Pyramid can be included in a salad.

1. What factors do Consuelo and Matthew need to consider when planning this event?
2. How might they display the food to show that all or most of the food groups may be included in a salad?
3. What salads would you suggest they serve?

APPLYING YOUR LEARNING

1. **Design a Salad:** Imagine you are a menu planner for a fast-food restaurant. You want to create a nutritious salad that goes well with burgers, grilled chicken sandwiches, and fish fillets. Write a description of the salad you would create. Include a list of ingredients you would use.

2. **Recipe Search:** Collect ten salad recipes that are made with different types of ingredients. Include at least one of each of the following: a tossed or mixed salad, an arranged salad, a molded salad, a layered salad, a hot salad, and a frozen salad. Share your recipes with the class.

EXPLORING FURTHER

1. **Great Greens:** Find out more about some interesting types of greens that can be used in a salad, such as arugula, radicchio, escarole, and curly endive. Create a chart that describes the color, texture, and flavor of each.

2. **Salad Origins:** Learn about how some well-known salads and salad dressings originated. For example, how did Caesar salad get its name? What changes have occurred in its ingredients and preparation method since it was introduced?

Making CONNECTIONS

1. **Science:** Plan and carry out an experiment related to the storage of salad ingredients. Describe it in a lab report. What was your hypothesis? How did you test it? What were the results? What conclusions do you draw?

2. **Foreign Languages:** Choose a country and find out about salads enjoyed there. Create a glossary that includes the native name of each salad, how it is pronounced, and a description of the ingredients and preparation. With your classmates, create an "around the world in salads" menu.

FOODS LAB

Make a small portion of vinaigrette salad dressing by combining three parts oil and one part vinegar. Add herbs of your choice. Next prepare the same vinaigrette but use less oil. Taste-test both on a small salad and compare the flavor.

Soups and Stews

Objectives

After studying this chapter, you will be able to:

- Identify typical ingredients used to prepare nutrient-rich soups and stews.

- Describe different kinds of soups and stews you can make or buy.

- Explain the ways to store soups and stews.

Do You Know...

...how to make soup out of fruit?

...how to make a healthful soup in less than five minutes?

...how to preserve nutrients when making a stew?

If not, you'll find out in this chapter!

Look *for these* TERMS

bisque   puree
broth   condensed
stock   soup
chowder

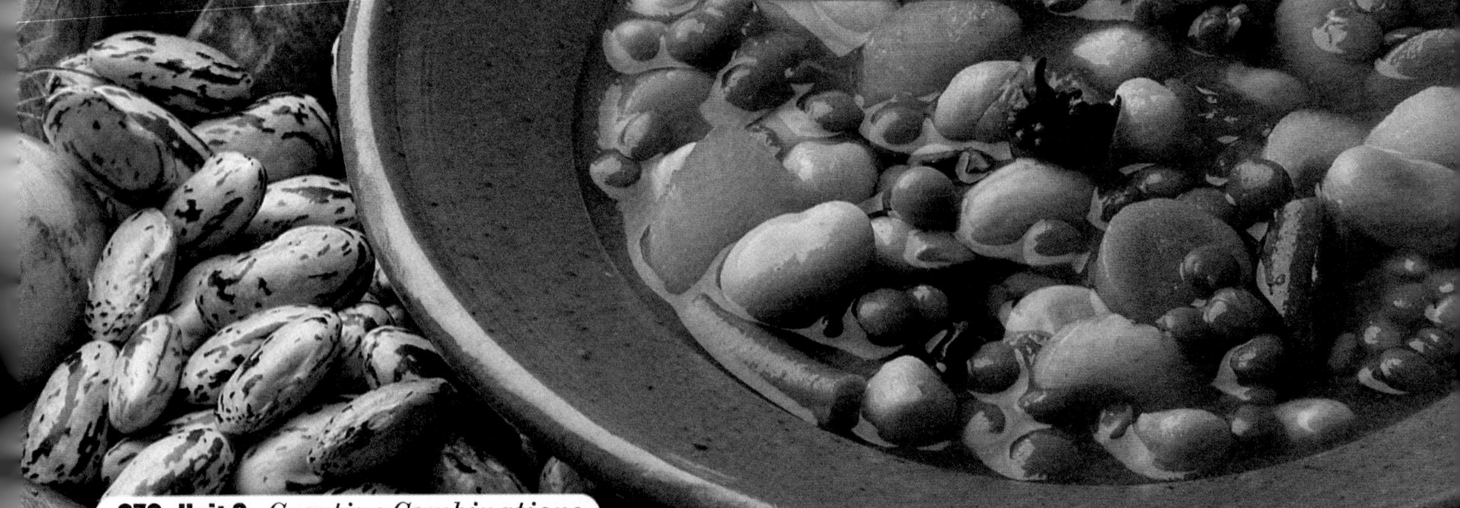

Soups and stews

are versatile! Soup partners perfectly with a sandwich or a salad. It's an ideal appetizer or main dish and even may be a refreshing dessert. Stew, usually heartier than soup, often serves as the meal's main dish. A small cup of chili or an Indian vegetable stew makes a super starter or satisfying side dish.

Soup or Stew for Variety

From avocado soup to zucchini-beef stew, an almost endless variety of soups and stews offer great flavors to try. Enjoy soup or stew at any time of the day, no matter what the weather. Buy it or make it! This glossary of soup and stew basics helps you make sense of the lingo.

Bisque is a *thick, rich soup made with finely mashed or ground seafood, poultry, or vegetables.* Bisques are traditionally made with butter and cream.

Broth, or **stock,** is *the seasoned liquid strained off after cooking meat, fish, or vegetables.* Bouillon and consommé are concentrated broth.

Chowder is a *thick, chunky soup.* Corn chowder, popular in the South, and clam chowder are among the best known. Creamy white New England clam chowder is made with milk or cream, and Manhattan-style clam chowder gets its red color from tomatoes.

Fruit soups are chilled, sweet, and refreshing. Strawberries, peaches, and melons make delicately flavorful soups to start or end a meal.

Stew is a thick, hearty mixture of chunky vegetables and perhaps meat, poultry, or fish cooked slowly in liquid.

Soup and a sandwich is a popular special on restaurant menus. It's an easy meal to prepare at home, too. Plan three or four tasty soup-and-sandwich combinations.

Activity: Visit a grocery store and list the variety, with respect to ingredients, of prepared soups and stews that are available. Compare your list with the variety in a soup cookbook.

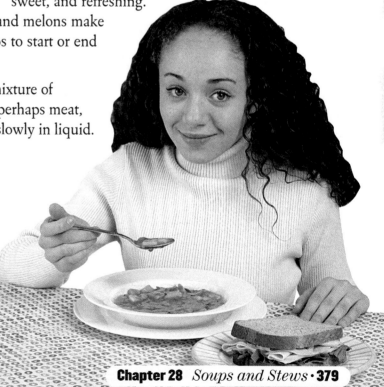

More About Thickeners: Cornstarch, available in stores in powder form, can be a convenient additive to thicken soups and stews. It contains no fat or sodium.

(**INFOLINK**)

For more on using starches as thickeners, see Section 4-9 of the Food Preparation Handbook.

What's in the Bowl?

Soups and stews can be nutritious, convenient, and economical. Take a look at the Food Guide Pyramid. Then create your own nutritious soup or stew combination with foods from two or more food groups. Nutrients in soups and stews depend on the ingredients.

Grain products. Rice, barley, pastas such as noodles or couscous, and other grain products make hearty additions to soups. Think of the many shapes and colors of pasta available, too! Besides providing B vitamins and iron, grain products are high in complex carbohydrates. Brown rice, barley, and other whole grain products add fiber. Grain products act as thickeners because their starch absorbs water and swells as it cooks.

Veggies and fruits. Vegetables and fruits make flavorful, colorful soup and stew ingredients, offering interesting texture, too. They contribute vitamins, minerals, and fiber, and most are fat-free.

Dairy foods. Creamy soups, such as bisques and chowders, are made with dairy products. Adding milk, yogurt, or cheese to soups and stews helps you meet your day's bone-building need for calcium—and supplies protein, too. Top lentil soup, chili, or other soups with grated cheese.

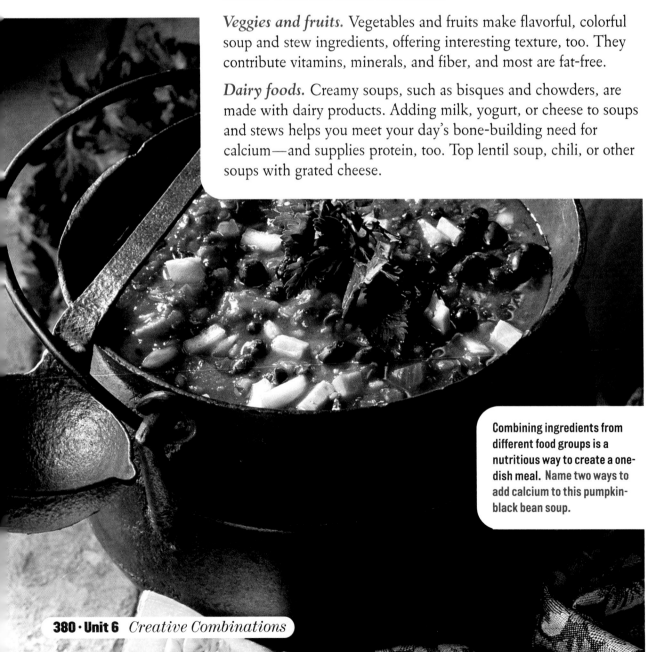

Combining ingredients from different food groups is a nutritious way to create a one-dish meal. **Name two ways to add calcium to this pumpkin-black bean soup.**

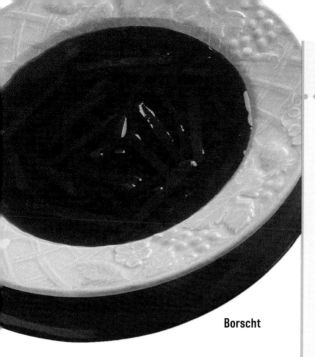

Borscht

Meat and beans group.
Turn simple soup into a hearty, protein-rich meal by adding meat, poultry, fish, cooked dry beans, or tofu. You can use less expensive cuts of meat because the slow, moist cooking helps tenderize meat. What other nutrients do these ingredients provide?

Create a Soup or Stew

When you want to go beyond a can opener, make soups and stews from scratch. Some take time to make, so you need to plan ahead. Others you can put together more quickly.

Make Your Own Stock

Although you can buy canned broth, or stock, you can make your own, too. Cook less expensive and less tender meat or poultry—such as a whole stewing chicken or pork or beef shoulder—slowly in a covered pot of liquid. Add onion, celery, carrots, herbs, and spices. Bring it to a boil, lower the heat, and cook gently until the meat is tender or the chicken falls from the bones. Allow the

Check This Out!

GREAT SOUPS AND STEWS AROUND THE WORLD

People in cultures all over the world make great-tasting, nutrient-rich soups and stews.
- *Gumbo,* the spicy Creole specialty, is made with okra, tomatoes, onions, and meat or fish.
- *Gazpacho* (gah-SPAH-cho), a chilled soup from Spain, is made with chopped or pureed fresh tomatoes, cucumbers, onions, and peppers.
- *Callaloo soup* is made with callaloo greens (the large edible greens of the taro root) from the Caribbean. The soup is also flavored with coconut milk, okra, yams, and chilies.
- *West African peanut soup* combines chicken, tomatoes, peanut butter or peanuts, and spices.
- *Egg drop soup* from China is made with chicken stock, spices, green onions, and, of course, an egg.
- *Borscht* is a classic soup of Russia. Its main ingredient, beets, gives it a deep red color.
- *Avgolemono* is a lemon and egg soup with rice that's a favorite in Greece.

It's Your Turn!

Describe some soups or stews from your family's heritage. To learn about the recipe, talk to a family member or check a cookbook.

Tip

To prevent foodborne illness, divide the stock into small batches and cool it in the refrigerator.

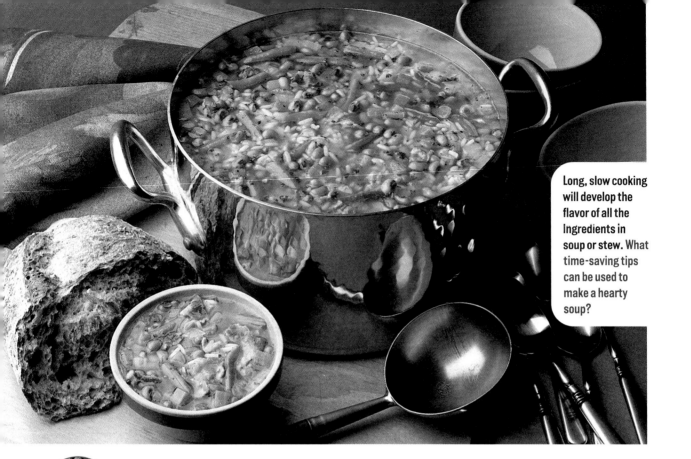

Long, slow cooking will develop the flavor of all the Ingredients in soup or stew. What time-saving tips can be used to make a hearty soup?

Tip

Have you added too much salt to your soup? You can rescue it by simmering a peeled, raw potato in it for about 10 minutes. The potato absorbs some of the salt. Remove the potato before serving.

Emphasize: If the heat under a soup or stew is too high, the liquid will boil off even if the pot is covered. Check the soup periodically.

broth to cool, strain it, and skim the fat off the top. You can use some of the meat or poultry in the stew or soup and save some for a salad or casserole.

Simmering Ingredients

Most soups and stews develop their flavor from long, slow cooking. Adjust the heat to keep the liquid below the boiling point so the soup or stew simmers. Use a regular pot, a slow cooker, or a pressure cooker. Start with your stock. Cut ingredients into uniform-sized pieces. First add the ingredients that require the longest cooking time. Add ingredients that require less time near the end of the cooking to prevent overcooking. That includes cut or sliced potatoes, carrots, and other vegetables, rice, and noodles, as well as herbs. Keep the soup covered while simmering to preserve nutrients and keep moisture in the pot.

Quick Tricks for Homemade Soups and Stews

When your time is short, these tips can help you make speedy soups and stews.

• Use canned broth or bouillon cubes in place of homemade stock.
• Use canned, frozen, or leftover cooked veggies or fruit to cut down on cooking time.

- Use leftover meat or poultry. Don't have any leftovers? Buy a slice of lean ham or turkey, cut it into chunks, and add it to your soup.
- Cook part or all of the recipe in the microwave oven. Keep in mind, however, that this won't tenderize less tender cuts of meat.
- Make big batches of your favorite recipes. Freeze them in small, individual containers. For a quick meal, pop one into the microwave oven.

Try It Cold!

You can add pizzazz to your menu with chilled fruit soups! Start with fresh, canned, or frozen fruits. Use a blender or food processor to **puree**—*finely mash or grind*—the fruits. Add juice, yogurt, or milk, plus spices such as cinnamon, nutmeg, or cloves. Fish and meat make fruit soups heartier.

Convenience Soups and Stews

No time to cook a pot of soup? Check out the supermarket aisles and freezer cases for convenience soups. For quick meals, keep some on hand in your kitchen. Look for canned and frozen heat-and-eat soups and stews, dehydrated soup mixes, and microwavable cups of soup. Canned **condensed soup** *has some of the water removed in processing*. To prepare it, just add liquid before heating. Keep in mind that prepared soups and stews can be high in fat and sodium. Check the Nutrition Facts panel on food labels!

Activity: Inventory the foods in your refrigerator or cupboards and create an original soup recipe.

Enjoy a chilled fruit soup when the weather's hot. Look for a fruit soup recipe. Share it with the class. Decide which one is the most appealing. Why?

Check This Out!

PUT A PERSONAL TOUCH IN CONVENIENCE SOUPS

For new tastes and easy, quick meals, combine convenience soup with one or more additional foods. For example, you can:
- Serve canned chili over cooked, boil-in-the-bag rice. Look for fat-free chili.
- Add canned minced clams to frozen clam chowder.
- Add your favorite herbs and spices. Celery seed, marjoram, and garlic are some herbs that add flavor to vegetable soup.
- Top canned tomato soup with packaged croutons and dill.
- Make chicken and vegetable soup heartier by adding leftover vegetables, pasta, or rice.
- Add sliced baby carrots to chicken noodle soup.
- Combine two different soups—perhaps beef-barley soup and vegetable soup.

It's Your Turn!

Try one of the above suggestions or create your own. Report the results to the class.

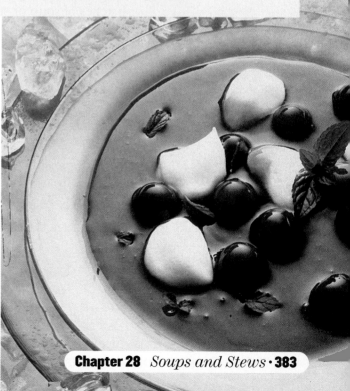

Keeping Nutrition High

Soups and stews provide nutrients from their flavorful food-group ingredients. To add nutrients and variety yet keep the fat and sodium low, follow these tips.

- To lower the fat in creamed soups, use fat-free evaporated milk or buttermilk instead of cream.
- For extra calcium, stir in nonfat dry milk or add low-fat or nonfat yogurt to creamed soup.
- Dilute condensed soups with milk, perhaps low-fat or fat-free, instead of water.
- Thicken soups with pureed vegetables or other starchy foods such as legumes, potatoes, pasta, barley, or rice. Using these foods as thickeners adds more nutrients and less fat than thickening with a mixture of butter and flour.
- Chill homemade stock or soups overnight. The fat will rise to the top and become firm. Just lift it off and discard.
- Use herbs and spices to add flavor without adding salt.
- Save the liquid from cooking vegetables for your soup. You get nutrient and flavor benefits!

Storing Soups and Stews

Store soups and stews properly so illness-causing bacteria don't have a chance to multiply. Promptly refrigerate leftovers in covered containers. If you have a large batch to store, divide it into several smaller containers so they chill quickly. You can also freeze small batches of soup or stew in covered plastic bowls or freezer bags for up to three months.

Activity: Look in a newspaper or cooking magazine for soup recipes with nutritional information. Compare the fat and sodium content of at least three prepared soups and three made from scratch.

INFOLINK

For more on storing foods safely, see Section 1-2 of the Food Preparation Handbook.

Emphasize: Prevention of illness-causing bacteria is important when thawing soups and stews, too. Food should be thawed in a refrigerator overnight, or on the defrost cycle in a microwave. Do not thaw foods for hours at room temperature.

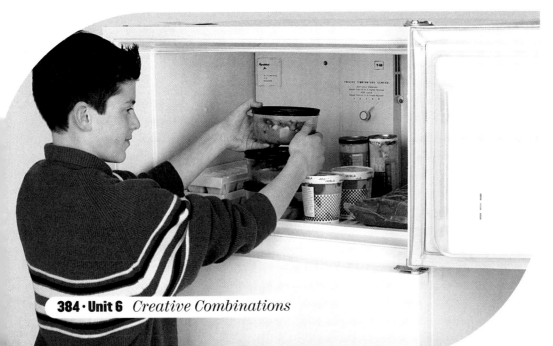

Why is it important to store any left-over soup or stew in the refrigerator or freezer quickly? How can you cool stock quickly?

NOW *You're* COOKING!

SKILL
Creating a Speed-Scratch Soup

S Soup can be quick and easy to prepare the speed-scratch way—using convenience foods to speed up your homemade cooking. In this recipe, canned broth gives you a head start. Check the the Nutrition Facts label to find varieties with less fat and sodium.

RECIPE

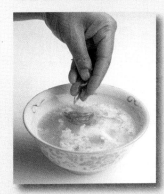

Egg Drop Soup

CUSTOMARY	INGREDIENTS	METRIC
2 (14.5 oz.) cans	Chicken broth	2 (411 g) cans
1 Tbsp.	Low-sodium soy sauce	15 mL
1	Large egg	1
1 Tbsp.	Thinly sliced green onion, green part only (optional)	15 mL

Yield: 4 servings, 1 cup (250 mL) each

1. In medium saucepan, bring broth and soy sauce to a boil.
2. Beat egg with a fork until yolk and white are combined.
3. Slowly pour egg over prongs of fork into boiling soup. Cook 30 seconds or until egg is set. Ladle into bowls. Garnish with onion, if desired.

Per Serving: 54 calories, 6 g protein, 1 g carbohydrate, 3 g fat, 738 mg sodium, 0 g fiber

Percent Daily Value: niacin 15%

More Ideas

- Add a package of frozen or canned vegetables, shredded cooked chicken, rice, or pasta to broth to create a nourishing soup.

- Use seasoned broth to add additional flavor to any soup, stew, or chowder.

Your Ideas
Do you have a favorite soup recipe? Bring one in to share with the class. Check cookbooks for other variations of your recipe. Make one of them at home.

LOOKING BACK

- You can buy or make soups and stews in a variety of flavors to enjoy any time of day and in any weather.

- Following the Food Guide Pyramid, you can create nutritious soups and stews with foods from two or more food groups.

- You can create soups and stews from scratch by making a stock and adding other foods.

- Convenience soups and stews are good for quick meals.

- Store soups and stews properly to keep illness-causing bacteria from multiplying.

UNDERSTANDING KEY IDEAS

1. Why are grain products and dairy foods nutritious additions to soups and stews?

2. Describe how you would make chicken stock using a whole stewing chicken.

3. If you were in a hurry, what type of soup would you make? How could you add more flavor?

4. How would you store a large batch of stew that you planned to use over the next month?

5. If you wanted to use some extra tomatoes from your garden, which international soup or stew might you make? What other ingredients would you need?

DEVELOPING LIFE SKILLS

1. **Management:** In what ways is making soup or stew an example of good management?

2. **Creative Thinking:** What combinations of two or more different canned soups might be appealing? What else might you add to jazz up your soup combo and boost its nutrition?

Wellness Challenge

After her friend Shandell had surgery, Becca and her father brought Shandell some homemade soup. That gave Becca an idea. She'd like to organize a group of student volunteers who will prepare and freeze batches of soup, then deliver them to families that are facing health problems or other crises.

1. How might Becca recruit volunteers for this project?

2. What should the teens take into consideration when deciding who will receive the soup?

3. Besides volunteers, what other resources will be needed to carry out this project? How might they be obtained?

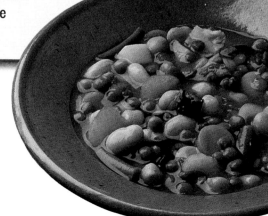

APPLYING YOUR LEARNING

1. **Computer Lab:** Design a database or table listing various types of soups and stews with information about their nutrition. You might show how the ingredients in one serving of each contributes servings from the Pyramid food groups, and/or identify the foods' significant contributions of vitamins and minerals. Think of ways to distribute your work in the community.

2. **Recipe Comparison:** Obtain recipes for similar stews that use different preparation methods, such as beef-vegetable stew prepared on the cooktop, in the oven, and in a slow cooker. Analyze their similarities and differences. How do the recipes compare in cooking time? In proportion of liquid? What conclusions can you draw?

EXPLORING FURTHER

1. **Clarifying Stock:** Learn what the term "clarify" means in regard to cooking stock. How is it done? Why?

2. **Comfort Food:** Many people think of soup as a comfort food. Survey family and friends to find out which soups people think of first when they want a comfort food. Share your findings in class.

Making CONNECTIONS

1. **Math:** Shop for two or more convenience forms of the same type of soup. For example, you might choose vegetable soup as canned heat-and-eat soup, dehydrated soup mix, and a microwavable cup of soup. How many servings does each one make? What is the cost per serving for each? Which one provides the most nutrients for your money?

2. **Language Arts:** Using library or Internet resources, look up the Stone Soup folktale. Find out about its origins. What does the story tell you about making a tasty soup? What does it tell you about working with others? Invent your own soup recipe based on the story.

FOODS LAB

Prepare the convenience soups you compared in the math activity on this page. Rate the flavor, texture, and color of each. Which would you choose again? Why?

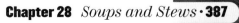

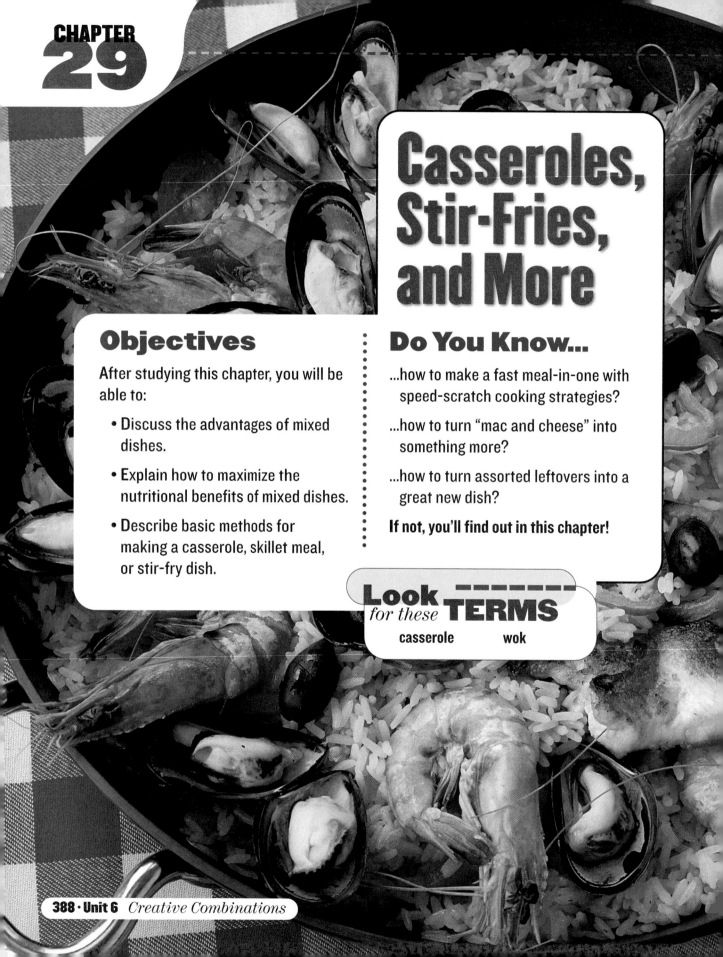

Casseroles, Stir-Fries, and More

Objectives

After studying this chapter, you will be able to:

- Discuss the advantages of mixed dishes.

- Explain how to maximize the nutritional benefits of mixed dishes.

- Describe basic methods for making a casserole, skillet meal, or stir-fry dish.

Do You Know...

...how to make a fast meal-in-one with speed-scratch cooking strategies?

...how to turn "mac and cheese" into something more?

...how to turn assorted leftovers into a great new dish?

If not, you'll find out in this chapter!

Look *for these* **TERMS**

casserole   wok

Make a meal-in-one!

In the last two chapters you've learned about salads, soups, and stews. When you include ingredients from several food groups, these dishes can become almost meals in themselves. That's also true of other great mixed dishes, from chicken potpie and vegetable lasagna to all kinds of ethnic dishes. See how many creative combinations you can invent!

Marvelous Mixtures

What types of hearty mixed dishes do you enjoy? The main dish at one meal might be a **casserole**, *a mixture of cooked foods heated in a baking or casserole dish.* Another time it might be a quick meal made in a skillet or a stir-fry served over rice. These types of mixed dishes can offer several advantages.

Flexibility. Casseroles, stir-fries, and many other mixtures can be made with just about any foods you like. The result is a meal with a unique blend of flavors and textures. Inventing new combinations is part of the fun!

Time management. With some mixtures, you need only one pan or skillet for the whole meal. That saves on cleanup time! You can make and freeze casseroles ahead of time—good for busy schedules and easy entertaining. For stir-fries, you can slice the ingredients ahead or buy them presliced.

Economy. Casseroles and other mixtures can be easy on the budget. They're a great way to use leftovers that might otherwise go to waste. Just a small amount of meat, poultry, or fish goes a long way when combined with other foods.

Nutrition and appeal. Mixed dishes can include foods from any food group. You get a variety of taste, texture, color, and nutrients—all in one dish!

Casseroles and other mixtures can feature foods from a variety of food groups. Which food groups might be represented in each of these dishes?

> **INFOLINK**
>
> To review how food combinations fit in the Food Guide Pyramid, see Chapter 8, page 151.

Boosting Nutrition and Variety

The variety of nutrient-dense foods in mixed dishes can add up to a powerful nutrition profile! High-carbohydrate foods such as pasta and rice are especially good sources of food energy. Vegetables contribute fiber and nutrients such as vitamins A and C. Cheese boosts the calcium. Lean meats, fish, poultry, beans, tofu, eggs, and cheese add protein and other nutrients.

Round out the meal with variety from the food groups. For instance, you might serve a chicken-rice casserole with a tossed mixed greens salad, crusty whole grain bread, low-fat milk, and sliced fruit for dessert.

Emphasize: Most casseroles are easy to reheat in a conventional oven or a microwave. That makes them a good meal choice for days when family members may eat at different times due to scheduled activities.

Casserole Creations

With a little imagination, you can create a tasty casserole even without a recipe! Just follow these steps.

Plan. Check your kitchen to see what canned, frozen, or leftover foods might be the start of your dish. Use the chart on page 391 as a guide and add your own ideas. Choose ingredients that you'll enjoy and will harmonize in flavor, texture, and color.

Precook. Unless you're using leftovers or convenience foods, you'll need to precook ingredients such as pasta, rice, meat, poultry, and fish. Defrost solid blocks of frozen vegetables in the microwave oven.

Tip

Go easy on high-fat sauces in casseroles. Mix in low-fat, creamy canned soups instead. For a calcium boost, mix in some dry milk.

Tip

Frozen vegetables that pour easily from the package don't need to be thawed first. Just mix them into the casserole before baking.

Give your family a new flavor sensation by combining ingredients into your own original casserole. How can casseroles help save on the family budget?

Casserole Mix and Match

To create a casserole, choose one or more ingredients from each row. The suggested amounts are for a 1½ quart (1.5 L) casserole dish, which makes about four servings.

TYPE OF INGREDIENT	TOTAL AMOUNT TO USE	EXAMPLES
Cooked grain products These give the casserole its body and contribute complex carbohydrates, B vitamins, and perhaps fiber.	2–4 cups (500 mL–1 L)	Spaghetti, noodles, macaroni, couscous or other pasta, brown or white rice, barley
Vegetables These contribute to the flavor and appearance as well as add fiber and nutrients, such as vitamins A and C.	1–2 cups (250–500 mL)	Any cooked, canned, or thawed frozen vegetables, such as corn, green beans, peas, carrots, zucchini or yellow squash, broccoli, eggplant, mushrooms, onions, and bell peppers
Lean meats, fish, poultry, beans, tofu, eggs, or cheese These add protein as well as other nutrients. They also contribute to the casserole's body and appeal.	1–1½ cups (250–350 mL)	Cut-up leftover meat, poultry, or fish; cooked, drained ground beef; canned tuna or salmon; cubed, sliced, or shredded cheese; firm tofu cubes; canned kidney, pinto, or other beans; diced, hard-cooked eggs
Liquid This holds the ingredients together. Different liquids supply different nutrients.	1–1½ cups (250–350 mL)	Broth; fruit or vegetable juice; milk; spaghetti sauce; canned soup such as asparagus, celery, chicken, mushroom, shrimp, tomato, or pea
Toppings These enhance flavor, appearance, and texture.	To taste	Fresh or dry bread crumbs; cracker crumbs; crispy, canned noodles; crushed flake cereal; chopped, toasted nuts; Parmesan cheese; grated cheese
Seasonings These add flavor.	¼–½ tsp. (1–3 mL)	Dried, crushed oregano, basil, thyme, or marjoram; ground ginger, mace, cinnamon, chili powder, cayenne or black pepper

Activity: Refer to the chart and create your own casserole. Choose two ingredients from each category. Give your creation a name and share your ideas with the class.

Check This Out!

A WORLD OF MIXED DISHES

You can bring the flavors of the world to your family dinner table.

- *Pancit*—Filipino dish that combines rice noodles with sliced, stir-fried vegetables; cooked chicken, pork, and shrimp; soy sauce; and patis (fish sauce), served with chopped, hard-cooked eggs sprinkled on top.
- *Risotto*—Italian dish in which Arborio rice and chopped onions are sautéed in butter or oil and then cooked in a hot broth. Chicken, shellfish, sausage, vegetables, or cheese is often added.
- *Jambalaya*—Creole mixture of cooked rice, tomatoes, onions, green peppers, and almost any kind of meat, poultry, or shellfish.
- *Enchiladas*—Mexican specialty featuring a soft tortilla rolled around a meat, chicken, vegetable, bean, or cheese filling and topped with salsa and grated cheese.
- *Pastitsio*—Greek casserole dish with pasta, ground beef or lamb, grated cheese, tomatoes, seasonings, and a white sauce.
- *Jollof rice*—West African dish with steamed, then browned, meats, layered with rice, tomatoes, hard-cooked eggs, and vegetables.
- *Perok*—The Aleuts of Alaska use halibut or salmon, cooked rice, onions, and hard-cooked eggs in this pie.

It's Your Turn!

How many of these mixtures from around the globe have you tried?

Teaching With Visuals: Search magazines or the Internet for pictures of these mixed dishes and other international mixed dishes. Bring your photos to class and tack them on the appropriate locations on a world map.

Assemble. Combine the ingredients in the baking dish, then sprinkle on the topping.

Bake. Baking time varies depending on the number of servings, the size of the dish, and the ingredients. Typically, it's about 30 minutes in a 350°F (180°C) oven for a 1½ quart (1.5 L) casserole if all the ingredients are precooked. In a conventional oven, cover the casserole until the last 15 minutes, then remove the cover for browning. In a microwave oven, leave the cover on. Use the power level and cooking time recommended in the microwave oven owner's manual or cooking guide.

Simple Skillet Meals

For a quick and easy meal, you can combine ingredients in a skillet rather than baking them in a casserole. Try these ideas.

- Brighten up macaroni and cheese by stirring in cooked broccoli, sweet red peppers, or other vegetables as the cheese melts.
- Prepare a packaged mix for seasoned rice, noodles, or couscous. Stir in leftovers such as cooked vegetables and meat or poultry. Heat and eat!
- Combine uncooked rice with broth. (Check the rice package for amount of rice and liquid.) Add other ingredients—perhaps cut-up leftover beef, mushrooms, asparagus, and a dash of teriyaki sauce. Cover and simmer until the rice is cooked.

More About Skillets: The skillet, also called a frying pan, was important to the pioneers who settled the American West. Miners used their cast iron skillets to scoop gold-laden water (or so they hoped) into their sorting screens. A skillet was an essential cooking tool for people in wagon trains.

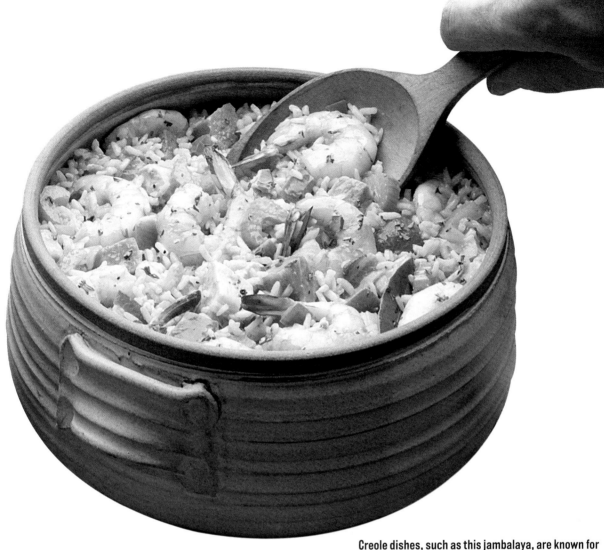

Creole dishes, such as this jambalaya, are known for their blending of flavors. **Find another Creole recipe you would like to try. What flavors are combined?**

Super Stir-Fries

Stir-frying is another fun way to create your own mixture. Remember, stir-frying means cooking small pieces of food quickly in a little oil over high heat—stirring as you cook. Vegetables that work well in a stir-fry dish include snow peas, celery, sliced carrots, broccoli, bamboo shoots, and many others. Add a protein food to make it a main dish. Meat, poultry, or fish can be raw when you stir-fry it or already cooked. Firm tofu also works well. The finished stir-fry is often served over rice.

The traditional utensil for stir-frying is a wok. A **wok** is *a special pan with a narrow, round bottom and a wide top designed for stir-fry cooking.* If you don't have a wok, you can stir-fry in a skillet.

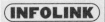

For more about stir-frying, see **Section 3-6 of the Food Preparation Handbook.**

Critical Thinking: Compare the amount of meat in one serving of a typical stir-fry dish with that of the average steak.

A wok allows you to cook cut-up pieces of food quickly over high heat. When stir-frying, why does the preparation usually take longer than the actual cooking?

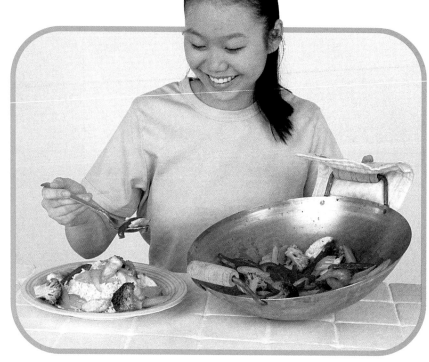

Tip

With a stir-fried dish, slicing can take longer than cooking! For speed-scratch cooking, use a frozen stir-fry vegetable mixture or buy already cut-up vegetables from the super-market salad bar.

Tip

To make a small amount of oil go further, use a nonstick wok or skillet.

INFOLINK

To learn about thickening with starches, read Section 4-9 of the Food Preparation Handbook.

These tips will help you turn out delicious stir-fried dishes.

- Have all your ingredients ready and waiting before you begin to cook. Once you start stir-frying, you won't have time to stop and chop!
- With each ingredient, keep pieces the same size and shape for even cooking.
- Use only a small amount of oil. Heat it before you add ingredients.
- If you're cooking raw meat, poultry, or fish, stir-fry it separately before the other ingredients. Then take it out and put it on a clean plate.
- Add other ingredients in the order of how long they take to cook. Start with those that take the longest, such as carrots. Leave them in the skillet or wok as you add the quicker-cooking ingredients, such as snow peas.
- When the vegetables are done, add the cooked meat, poultry, or fish or the tofu back to the wok or skillet.
- Add liquids and seasonings last. You might use broth, fruit juice, or vegetable juice, perhaps with a little soy sauce or mustard for flavor. If you like, you can thicken the liquids with cornstarch to make a sauce.

Emphasize: The oil in the wok must be very hot before adding ingredients. If it isn't hot, the food will sit in the oil too long and absorb it, adding more calories to the meal and giving the food a greasy texture.

NOW You're COOKING!

SKILL
Making a Casserole

For an attractive presentation of your casserole, wipe the edges of the dish before putting it in the oven so there will be no browned areas after baking. Fresh parsley leaves sprinkled over the baked casserole make an attractive garnish.

RECIPE

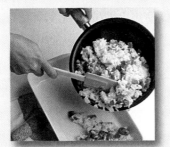

Creamy Rice Casserole

CUSTOMARY	INGREDIENTS	METRIC
1 cup	Instant rice (uncooked)	250 mL
½ lb.	Light turkey/pork sausage	250 g
1 can (10 ¾ oz.)	Low-fat condensed cream of mushroom soup	305 g
½ cup	Chopped green or red bell pepper	125 mL

Yield: 4 servings, ¾ cup (175 mL) each

❶ Preheat oven to 350°F (180°C).

❷ Prepare rice according to package directions using only water.

❸ Heat a medium skillet; add sausage and cook, stirring frequently, for 4 to 5 minutes or until browned. Drain in a colander. Return sausage to pan; add rice, soup, and green pepper. Stir until combined.

❹ Pour rice mixture into a shallow 1-quart (1-L) casserole. Bake 15 to 20 minutes or until hot.

Per Serving: 315 calories, 13 g protein, 33 g carbohydrate, 8 g fat, 928 mg sodium, 1 g fiber

Percent Daily Value: vitamin C 16%, thiamin 25%, riboflavin 12%, niacin 17%, phosphorus 11%

More Ideas

• Add a dash or two of hot pepper sauce, a teaspoon of Italian seasoning, or your favorite herb.

• Leftover, canned, or frozen vegetables may be added for greater flavor, nutrition, and color.

Your Ideas
With help from your friends and family, see how many different casseroles you can list that use rice as a base. Look at international cookbooks for some new ideas you might not have thought about.

LOOKING BACK

- Mixed dishes offer several advantages, including flexibility, time management, economy, nutrition, and appeal.

- Combining nutrient-dense foods in mixed dishes provides variety and good nutrition.

- You can create a tasty, nutritious casserole by following these steps: plan, precook, assemble, and bake.

- Skillet meals and stir-fries are other ways to create quick, easy mixed dishes.

UNDERSTANDING KEY IDEAS

1. How do mixed dishes offer flexibility, nutrition, and appeal?

2. Imagine that you want to make a tuna casserole. What nutrients does tuna provide? What other ingredients could you add for maximum nutrition?

3. Describe the steps you would take to make a casserole if you didn't have a recipe.

4. How could you create a skillet meal by starting with a packaged couscous mix? With uncooked rice and broth?

5. Describe how you would prepare and cook a stir-fry meal of chicken, snow peas, and sliced carrots in a wok.

DEVELOPING LIFE SKILLS

1. **Leadership:** Suppose you have a little brother. When it's his turn to clear the table after a meal, he throws away extra food from serving dishes because he doesn't like leftovers. How could you use leadership skills to encourage him to save the leftovers for use in mixed dishes?

2. **Creative Thinking:** If you were inventing a stir-fry dish for your own fast-food restaurant chain, what would you put in it? Why?

Wellness Challenge

Every year the high school celebrates a Multicultural Day with a variety of activities, including a mixed-dish dinner. This year Courtney and Diego are responsible for planning the menu and staying within the allowed budget.

1. What types of information would help Diego and Courtney plan the menu? Where might they find it?

2. What criteria might Courtney and Diego use to choose dishes for the dinner?

3. What strategies could help them stay within their budget?

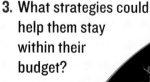

APPLYING YOUR LEARNING

1. **Mix and Match Dishes:** Write down five foods you could use in a mixed dish. Trade your list with a classmate. Using the ingredient list you are given, write instructions for preparing a mixed dish. You may add other ingredients and herbs and spices as necessary. Share your creation with the class.

2. **Homemade or Convenience Food?** Find a recipe for a popular casserole or other mixed dish, such as lasagna or chicken pot pie. Then find a prepackaged version of the same dish in the supermarket. Compare the ingredients, nutrient content, and preparation times. When might you choose each method? Why?

EXPLORING FURTHER

1. **Buffet Line:** Mixed dishes are often served buffet-style in places such as cafeterias, supermarket salad bars, and restaurants. Consult the manager of one such buffet and find out how he or she chooses the dishes that are served.

2. **Then and Now:** Find out how mixed dishes have changed over the past 40 years in ingredients, preparation, and nutrient content. (Hint: Interview an older relative or neighbor, or research old cookbooks and magazines at the library.)

Making CONNECTIONS

1. **Social Studies:** Research the origins of stir-fry cooking. How does it relate to the availability of resources in the place and time it was invented? Report your findings to the class.

2. **Language Arts:** An analogy is a comparison based on similarity. For example: "Love is like the measles; we all have to go through it" (Jerome K. Jerome). Write a paragraph that uses the characteristics of a casserole (based on what you've learned in this chapter) to make an analogy.

FOODS LAB

Prepare two samples of stir-fry vegetables. For one sample, cut the vegetables into uniform sizes. For the other, cut the vegetables into varying sizes and shapes. Stir-fry both for the same amount of time. Compare the texture, flavor, and appearance. What can you conclude?

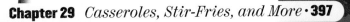

Quick Breads and Yeast Breads

Objectives

After studying this chapter, you will be able to:

- Identify the basic ingredients in breads.
- Explain the differences between quick breads, yeast breads, and flat breads.
- Give guidelines for making quick and yeast breads.
- Explain how to store homemade breads.

Do You Know...

...why pita bread is flat but bagels aren't?

...shortcuts to use when making homemade bread?

...what ingredients you can add to make breads more interesting, flavorful, and nutritious?

If not, you'll find out in this chapter!

Look for these TERMS

batter	yeast bread
dough	quick bread
shortening	flat bread
leavening agent	knead

You probably

enjoy eating many kinds of breads, but have you tried making your own? Bread making can be satisfying and fun. You might cook up a stack of hot blueberry pancakes for breakfast or bake a batch of whole wheat muffins to enjoy with soup for lunch. Homemade rolls fresh from the oven can turn an ordinary dinner into a special occasion!

What Are Breads Made Of?

The basic ingredients of bread include flour, liquid, and fat. Many breads also have an ingredient that makes them rise and perhaps eggs, sugar, or other flavorings, too. Together, these ingredients affect the appearance, texture, flavor, and nutrition of breads.

Flour

Flour, the main ingredient in many baked products, gives them their structure. Since it's milled from grain, flour is a source of complex carbohydrates. Barley, buckwheat, corn, rice, and rye are all milled to make flour and used to make bread. However, the most commonly used types of flour are made from wheat.

All-purpose flour, the white flour from just the grain's endosperm, gives good results for most baked products.

Whole wheat flour, milled from the whole grain, has more fiber than all-purpose flour. In baking, you can often replace two-thirds of the all-purpose flour with whole wheat flour.

Self-rising flour includes salt and baking powder, so you don't have to add them to the recipe separately. Use this flour only when the recipe calls for it.

Bread flour is designed to give bread a strong structure.

More about White Flour: White flour is usually enriched with riboflavin, thiamine, niacin, and iron to make its nutrients equal to those in whole wheat flour, except for fiber.

Baking bread can be a good way to express your creativity in the kitchen. For what special occasions could you bake bread?

INFOLINK

To learn about gluten in flour and how it affects the structure of bread, see Section 4-10 of the Food Preparation Handbook.

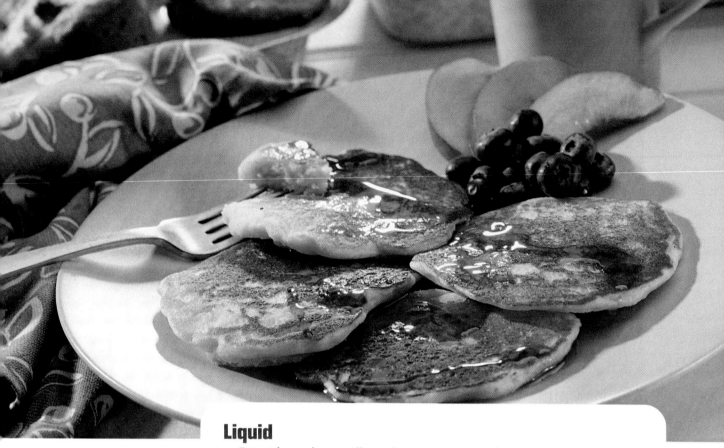

Basic pancake batter can be varied by adding fruit, nuts, and different types of flour. Besides syrup, think of two other toppings from the food groups that you could use on your pancakes.

Liquid

Liquids such as milk and water moisten the dry ingredients and help bind them together. Depending on the amount of liquid compared to flour, the mixture of ingredients is called a batter or a dough. A **batter** *is thin enough to be poured or dropped.* A **dough,** because it has less liquid than a batter, *is stiff enough to be molded or rolled on a board.*

Fat

Fat adds flavor and richness to breads and also helps give a tender texture. Some recipes use vegetable oil as the fat. Others call for a solid fat such as butter, margarine, or shortening. **Shortening** is *a solid fat made from vegetable oil.*

Leavening Agents

Have you ever looked closely at a slice of bread and noticed the many tiny holes in it? They were caused by a leavening agent. A **leavening agent** *makes a baked product rise by causing pockets of gas to expand in the batter or dough as it bakes.* This process lightens the texture and increases the volume of bread and other baked goods.

Ingredients that act as leavening agents include baking soda, baking powder, and yeast. Some baked goods are leavened by trapped air or steam.

Emphasize: All breads contain flour, liquid, and fat, and most breads contain a leavening agent such as yeast, baking powder, or baking soda.

INFOLINK

To learn more about how leavening agents work, see Section 4-10 of the Food Preparation Handbook.

Breads fall into three basic categories depending on their leavening agent. In **yeast breads,** *the leavening agent is yeast.* Whole wheat bread, bagels, and breadsticks are all yeast breads. In **quick breads,** *the leavening agent is baking powder or baking soda.* Quick breads—which include pancakes, muffins, and biscuits—get their name because they rise faster than yeast breads. **Flat breads,** such as tortillas and pita bread, *are made with little or no leavening agent.* They are part of the cuisine of many cultures. For example, *naan* is an East Indian flat bread that puffs slightly when baked.

Other Ingredients

Extra ingredients can enhance a bread's flavor and appearance. Depending on your choices, they can also boost fiber and nutrition. Eggs, nuts, dried fruits, pureed fruits or vegetables, onions, cheese, herbs, and spices are some ingredients that can be found in breads. Have you ever tried apricot-nut muffins, cheddar-herb bagels, or pumpkin bread? You might enjoy Swedish *limpa,* a rye bread flavored with anise, cumin, and orange peel. Italian focaccia (foh-KAH-chee-uh) is a round yeast bread brushed with olive oil, often flavored with rosemary.

INFOLINK

To review the nutrients in breads, turn to pages 281-282 in Chapter 21.

Discuss: What are some other kinds of breads, including muffins and pancakes, that you've tasted with added ingredients? How did you like these breads?

Breads come in all shapes and sizes, from quick breads to yeast breads to flat breads. Think of the breads you have eaten in the last two days. Categorize them as quick, yeast, or flat breads.

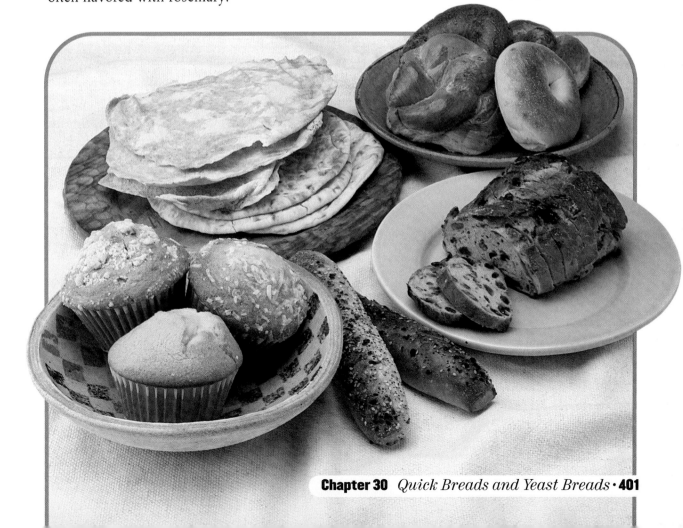

Making Quick Breads

The secret to making delicious quick breads with good texture is to follow the recipe instructions carefully. The mixing method depends on what kind of quick bread you're making.

Muffins and More

To make many quick breads—including muffins, loaves such as banana bread, and pancakes—mix the batter this way.

- Sift together all dry ingredients. Sifting makes sure these ingredients are combined evenly.
- Blend liquid ingredients together.
- Add the liquid ingredients to the dry ingredients. Stir just until the dry ingredients are moistened, leaving some lumps in the batter. Overmixing will give the baked product an uneven texture.

After mixing, spoon muffin batter into muffin cups or loaf batter into the pan. Be sure to divide the batter evenly among the muffin cups. Bake according to recipe directions. For pancakes, pour the batter onto a lightly greased hot skillet or griddle. You might use about ¼ cup (50 mL) batter per pancake. You can tell when they're ready to be flipped over—the tops are bubbly and the edges appear dry. The cooked side should be golden brown. Flip the pancakes with a turner and cook them briefly on the other side. Enjoy them while they're hot!

Activity: Prepare a chart of the important steps in making good quick breads. Include key words and a simple illustration for each step.

Quick breads are fun to make. Add extras such as fruit or nuts to increase flavor and nutrition. Find a muffin recipe you would enjoy making. What "extras" would you like to add?

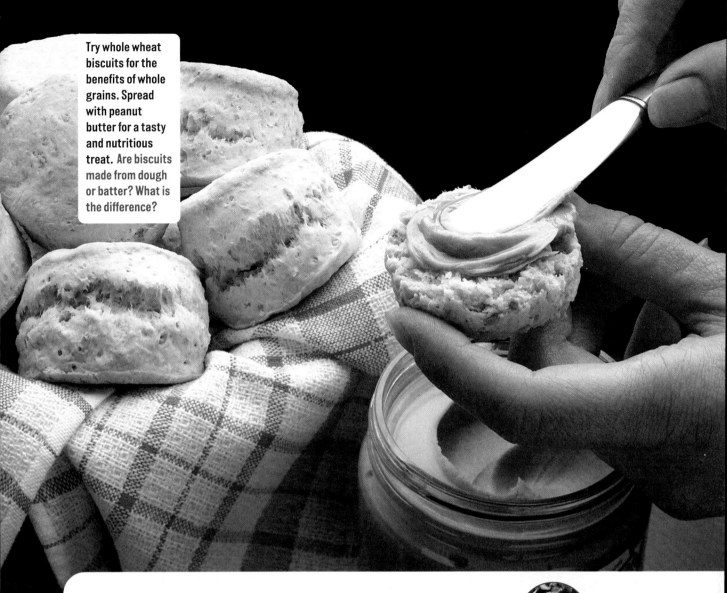

Try whole wheat biscuits for the benefits of whole grains. Spread with peanut butter for a tasty and nutritious treat. Are biscuits made from dough or batter? What is the difference?

Biscuits

Biscuits are usually made from a dough that you mix this way.

• Sift together all dry ingredients.

• Cut fat into the dry ingredients. To do this, use a pastry blender or fork and mix the ingredients with a cutting motion. Keep going until the particles are pea-sized.

• Add the liquid ingredients and stir just until blended.

After the biscuit dough is mixed, the recipe may tell you to **knead** it, or *work and press it with the hands.* Put the dough on a lightly floured surface and press it with the heels of your hands. Fold the dough over, give it a quarter turn, and press it again. Continue for as long as the recipe says. Finally, roll the dough out to an even thickness, cut out the biscuits, and put them on a baking sheet—ready for the oven! Bake as directed in the recipe.

Tip

When quick breads and yeast breads are finished baking, remove them from the pans to a wire rack for cooling. That way, the bread won't get soggy on the sides and bottom.

Making Yeast Breads

If you plan to make yeast bread from scratch, set aside several hours. You won't be working on the bread all this time. Most of the time the dough is rising before baking. A typical recipe for making yeast bread from scratch follows the steps shown on page 405.

Faster Bread Making

Speed up homemade bread with a few nifty tricks. Lots of convenience products in the supermarket can help you fill your home with the wonderful aroma of fresh-baked goods.

- Use a dry bread mix. All you usually have to do is stir in a liquid and finish the preparation.
- Buy frozen or refrigerated dough for breads and rolls. Just follow the directions on the package, and bake.
- Brown-and-serve products need only be opened and heated to brown them.
- Use a bread machine. It will mix, knead, and bake the dough for you.

Check This Out!

ADD PIZZAZZ TO YOUR BREADS

Give your breads interesting shapes and great flavor:

- Knead nuts, onions, sun-dried tomatoes, grated cheese, or herbs into homemade or store-bought dough.
- Before baking, top the dough or batter with chopped nuts, seeds, coarse salt, or herbs.
- Shape bread dough into breadsticks and roll in grated Parmesan cheese or poppy seeds.
- Cut pizza dough in small rounds or squares. Top one side of each round or square with lean ham and low-fat cheese. Fold over and bake.

It's Your Turn!

Try one of these creative ideas or invent your own. Report the results to the class.

Activity: Think of and describe breads that would be unusual in shape or ingredients or both. Give names to your creations.

STEPS TO
Great Yeast Bread

*M*aking bread can be a cozy way to spend a rainy Saturday afternoon. Follow these steps to make a well-textured yeast bread.

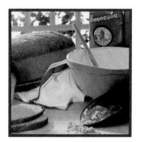

❶ *Mix the dough* using the method given in the recipe. Before you begin, be sure the ingredients are at room temperature and the liquid is warmed to the temperature given in the recipe so that the yeast will grow.

❷ *Knead the dough* by hand, with a food processor, or with a mixer that has a dough hook. Knead until the dough becomes satiny and elastic and has little bubbles under the surface.

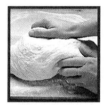
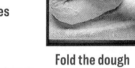

Fold the dough   Press with heel of hand   Rotate dough one-quarter turn and repeat folding, pushing, turning

❸ *Let the dough rise* in a warm place until it doubles in size (about 1 to 2 hours).

❹ *Punch down the dough* by gently pressing your fist in the center. Pull the dough from the sides of the bowl and press down again. This works out the large air bubbles.

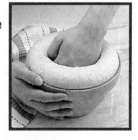

❺ *Shape the dough* into loaves or rolls. Place the dough into a pan or onto a baking sheet. Let the dough rise a second time.

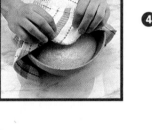

❻ *Bake* according to the recipe.

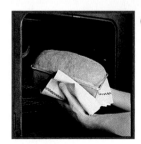

Investigate Further

What happens to yeast if the water you add is too hot?

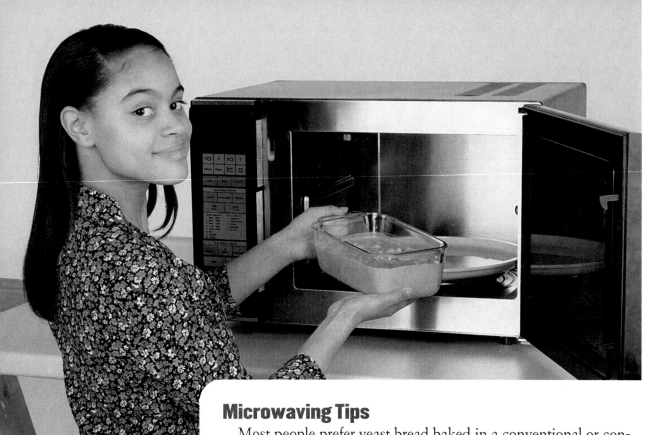

Using a microwave oven can speed cooking time. Describe the advantages and disadvantages of baking quick breads in a microwave oven.

Microwaving Tips

Most people prefer yeast bread baked in a conventional or convection oven. However, a microwave oven can be handy for defrosting and warming yeast breads and reducing the rising time.

Quick breads baked in a microwave oven don't brown. However, they're more moist, rise higher, and bake more quickly than in a conventional oven. Remember these hints when baking in a microwave oven.

• Fill containers half full.
• Put containers on a rack or inverted saucer to let the air circulate underneath.
• Rotate containers during cooking for even baking.
• To make up for lack of browning, use batters with color—pumpkin bread, for example—or add a topping.

Keeping in Quality

To keep your homemade breads fresh and appealing, store them properly. Remember, many store-bought breads have additives to help preserve them. Your homemade breads won't stay fresh as long. You can store them for several days in airtight containers, aluminum foil, or plastic bags in a cool, dry place. In hot weather, when heat and humidity encourage mold growth, store baked goods in the refrigerator.

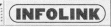

INFOLINK

For more tips on storing foods, see Section 1-2 of the Food Preparation Handbook.

NOW *You're* COOKING!

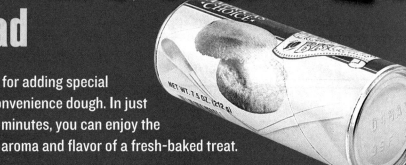

Baking Bread

*T*ry this recipe for adding special touches to convenience dough. In just minutes, you can enjoy the aroma and flavor of a fresh-baked treat.

RECIPE

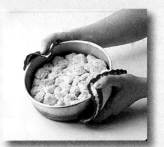

Pull-Apart Parmesan Dill Bread

CUSTOMARY	INGREDIENTS	METRIC
2 Tbsp.	Parmesan cheese	30 mL
½ tsp.	Dried dill weed	2 mL
1 package (12 oz.)	Refrigerated biscuits	340 g
1 Tbsp.	Margarine or butter, melted	15 mL

Yield: 8 servings, ⅛ of recipe each

❶ Preheat oven to 400°F (200°C). Lightly grease an 8-inch (20-cm) round cake pan.

❷ In small bowl, stir cheese and dill until combined.

❸ Cut biscuits in quarters. Add a few biscuits at a time to margarine, separating pieces with fingers. Add cheese mixture and toss with fingers until all pieces are coated. Arrange in one layer in prepared pan.

❹ Bake 12 to 14 minutes or until golden brown. Turn upside down on serving plate. Pull apart to serve, or cool for 5 minutes before cutting into 8 wedges.

Per Serving: 70 calories, 2 g protein, 9 g carbohydrate, 3 g fat, 216 mg sodium, 0 g fiber

More Ideas

• For a breakfast bread, try using sugar and cinnamon in place of the Parmesan and dill.

• For an easy snack or appetizer, press each biscuit into a 4- to 5-inch (10- to 13-cm) circle. Add 1 to 2 Tbsp. (15 to 30 mL) of cooked meat, vegetables, or cheese. Fold in half, press edges together, and bake.

Your Ideas

Packages of refrigerated dough make bread baking easy. Create other speed-scratch ways to use a package of refrigerated biscuits for breakfast, snacks, or dinner. Check recipes from cookbooks, magazines, or the Internet.

LOOKING BACK

- Breads are made of flour, liquid, fat, and often a leavening agent.
- Breads fall into three basic categories: yeast breads, quick breads, and flat breads.
- The mixing method for quick bread depends on the kind of quick bread you're making.
- When making yeast bread from scratch, allow several hours for the dough to rise.
- Using convenience products or a microwave oven saves time when making homemade bread.
- Store homemade breads properly to keep them fresh and appealing.

UNDERSTANDING KEY IDEAS

1. What is the purpose of each of the three basic ingredients of bread?
2. What leavening agent is used in yeast breads, quick breads, and flat breads? What are two examples of each type of bread?
3. How would you mix dough for biscuits?
4. Describe the steps you would take to make yeast bread from scratch.
5. What convenience products could you use to make homemade bread quickly?
6. Why won't homemade breads stay fresh as long as store-bought breads? How would you store homemade breads?

DEVELOPING LIFE SKILLS

1. **Communication:** Leon has agreed to give a talk about bread making to the 8- and 9-year-old girls in his sister's scout troop. What information should Leon provide? How can he keep the children's attention?
2. **Critical Thinking:** Jason's family enjoys homemade bread. They have decided they can afford to buy either a bread machine or an electric mixer with a dough hook, but not both. What factors do you think should enter into their decision? What are some possible pros and cons of each choice?

Wellness Challenge

The marching band is using a variety of fundraisers to pay for new uniforms. Hahn, one of the flute players, suggested they hold a "Breakfast Bake Sale" in the cafeteria one morning before school. She explained that band members could sell nutritious homemade muffins, quick bread loaves, and biscuits. The fundraising committee liked the idea and put Hahn in charge of organizing the bake sale. However, she's never done anything like this before and isn't sure where to begin.

1. Where might Hahn turn for advice?
2. What are some aspects of the event that Hahn will need to organize?
3. What could Hahn do that might help boost the nutrition of the foods offered at the bake sale?

APPLYING YOUR LEARNING

1. **Baking Comparison:** Find a quick bread recipe that provides directions for both a conventional oven and a microwave oven (or choose two similar recipes, one conventional and one microwave). How do the directions differ? Are there any differences in ingredients? Share your findings.

2. **Math:** Find a bread recipe that uses all-purpose flour only. Revise the recipe to use two-thirds whole wheat flour and one-third all-purpose flour. Explain how your changes affect the bread's nutritional value.

EXPLORING FURTHER

1. **Breads and Celebrations:** Matzo, an unleavened bread, is usually eaten to celebrate the Jewish Passover. Report on the special meaning of this bread. What role does matzo play in the ceremonial feast called the Seder?

2. **Bread Additives:** Most store-bought bread contains substances to improve the quality of the bread. Learn about these additives. What are they? What functions do they serve?

Making CONNECTIONS

1. **Social Studies:** Learn about pueblo bread. What culture does it come from? How was it made? How does the baking method relate to other aspects of that culture? Write a report on your findings.

2. **Career Connections Experience:** Write the script for a TV cooking show in which you'll demonstrate how to make yeast bread. Plan to show loaves in different stages of preparation, since time will not permit you to show making one loaf from start to finish. Videotape your show or present it to the class live.

FOODS LAB

Prepare two batches of muffins, one by mixing the muffin batter just until the flour is moistened and the other by mixing the batter until it has a smooth consistency. Bake both batches and compare your results. What differences do you note in the appearance, texture, and flavor? What can you conclude?

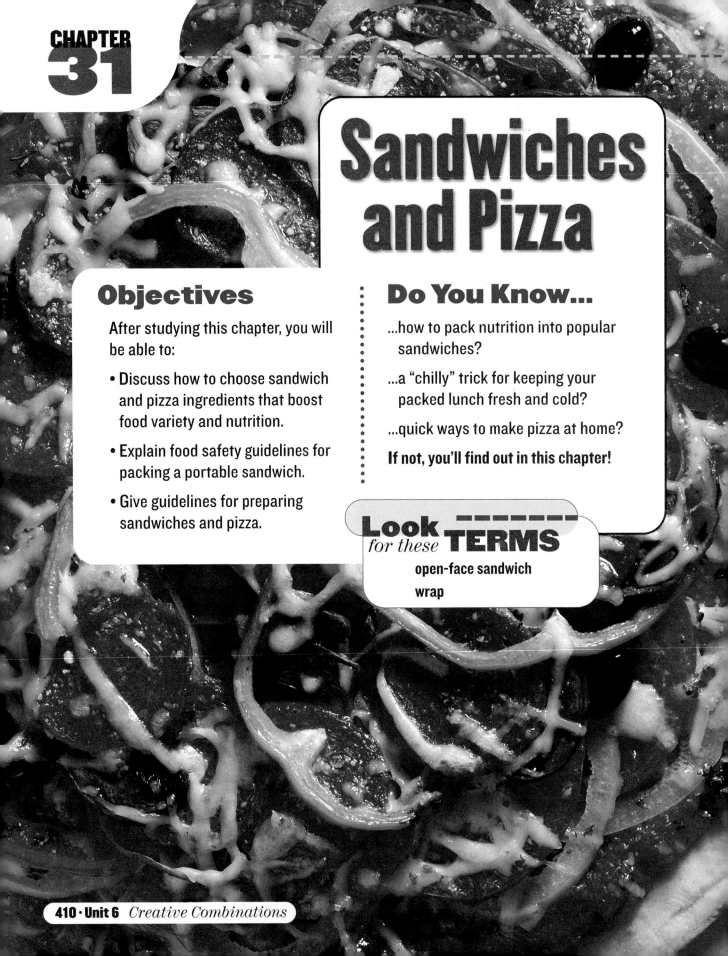

CHAPTER 31

Sandwiches and Pizza

Objectives

After studying this chapter, you will be able to:

- Discuss how to choose sandwich and pizza ingredients that boost food variety and nutrition.

- Explain food safety guidelines for packing a portable sandwich.

- Give guidelines for preparing sandwiches and pizza.

Do You Know...

...how to pack nutrition into popular sandwiches?

...a "chilly" trick for keeping your packed lunch fresh and cold?

...quick ways to make pizza at home?

If not, you'll find out in this chapter!

Look *for these* **TERMS**

open-face sandwich

wrap

Chances are

your list of favorite foods probably includes at least one sandwich or pizza choice. Sandwiches are easy and convenient whether you're at home or on the go. Pizza is another all-time favorite with traditional toppings or inventive new combinations. Both sandwiches and pizza can be as varied as you are creative!

Sandwiches for the Health of It

In a sandwich, you can enjoy a variety of foods all in one bite—and get the nutrients from each ingredient! A sandwich can give you complex carbohydrates and B vitamins from bread (fiber, too, if it's whole grain); calcium, some vitamins, and protein from cheese; vitamins from vegetables; and protein and iron from foods such as lean meat, turkey, tuna, or beans.

You can make a sandwich to eat anytime—at any meal or snack! For a quick breakfast, add sliced banana or apple to a peanut butter sandwich. Enjoy it with a glass of milk. At lunch or dinner, sandwiches pair well with soup, a salad, or fresh fruit.

Discuss: What are the favorite sandwiches of your family or friends? Do they eat a variety of sandwiches?

Stocking Up for Sandwiches

What goes in a sandwich? Your choice of ingredients is limited only by your imagination. Be adventurous! For a quick meal or snack, keep a variety of sandwich fixings on hand.

Bountiful breads. To make sandwiches more interesting, vary your bread choices. Breads come in all shapes and sizes—regular loaves, French or Italian breads, pitas, bagels, corn or flour tortillas, chapatis, focaccia, and English muffins, to name just a few. Can you name others? For flavor variety, try whole wheat, multigrain, rye, or oatmeal bread for your sandwich. Choose whole grain breads often for their fiber.

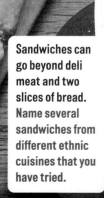

Sandwiches can go beyond deli meat and two slices of bread. Name several sandwiches from different ethnic cuisines that you have tried.

Check This Out!

A SANDWICH BY ANY OTHER NAME

Do you think of burritos, tacos, and spring rolls as sandwiches? They are—if you define a sandwich as any filling put in or on some kind of bread or other wrapper. How many of these sandwich variations from around the world have you tried?

- A *gyro* (YEE-roh *or* ZHEE-roh) is a Greek sandwich. It's a mixture of seasoned cooked lamb, chopped tomato, and cucumber-yogurt dressing stuffed in a pita pocket.
- *Calzone* (kal-ZOHN) originated in Italy. It's a handheld variation of pizza—the dough is folded over the fillings and sealed.
- *Spring rolls* from China are made with assorted vegetables, meat, poultry, or seafood rolled in a pastry wrapper.
- *Empanada* (em-pah-NAH-dah), from Spain and South America, is a single-serving turnover. It's made with a pastry crust enclosing a meat and vegetable filling. A similar food from England is called a *Cornish pasty* (PASS-tee).

It's Your Turn!

Find a recipe for preparing one of these foods or another sandwich from around the world. Share it with the class.

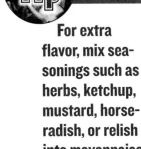

Tip

For extra flavor, mix seasonings such as herbs, ketchup, mustard, horseradish, or relish into mayonnaise. With more flavor, you may decide to use less spread.

Fabulous fillings. Sliced deli meats, cheeses, canned tuna or salmon, and canned refried beans are convenient for making sandwiches. Look for lean and low-fat choices when you shop. Use leftover meat such as meat loaf, poultry, and fish as is or in filling mixtures such as chicken salad.

Excellent extras. Add flavor and nutrients to your sandwiches with fresh vegetables and other extras. Tomatoes, green or red peppers, onions, and lettuce are popular choices. Would you have thought of using zucchini, avocado, shredded carrots, or sunflower seeds in a sandwich? How about adding "zing" with pickles or hot peppers?

Super spreads. Spreads add flavor and moisture to a sandwich. They can also protect the bread so that it doesn't get soggy. Mayonnaise, butter, and pesto sauce are high in fat and calories, so spread them on sparingly. Try some tasty low-fat alternatives. Besides using low-fat or fat-free mayonnaise, you might spread your sandwiches with hummus, chutney, fruit spreads, cranberry relish, or mustard.

Building Great Sandwiches

Most sandwiches don't need directions for preparation. Just choose your ingredients, then spread, stack, stuff, or roll and go! Other sandwiches, especially hot ones, take more cooking skills.

- An **open-face sandwich** *has only a bottom slice of bread*. For an open-face tuna melt, spread tuna salad on an English muffin half. Top with cheese and broil just until the cheese melts.

Teaching with Visuals: List the ingredients of your favorite sandwich. Combine your list with your classmates' and divide the ingredients into the categories shown on pages 411-412. Now create new sandwiches from those ingredients.

Sandwich Makeovers

SANDWICH	TRADITIONAL WAY	LIGHTER WAY
Club sandwich	Three slices of toasted bread layered with turkey, ham, or other meat, lettuce, tomato, mayonnaise, and bacon.	Scale back the size. Use less bacon or a leaner variety. Use reduced-fat or fat-free mayonnaise or other fat-free spread, such as chutney.
Grilled cheese sandwich	Made with full-fat cheese. Cooked in butter or margarine.	Toast the bread first, rather than grill it in fat. Layer in sliced tomato and low-fat cheese. Heat in the toaster oven or under the broiler to melt the cheese.
Tuna or chicken salad sandwich	Cooked chicken or tuna and other ingredients (such as diced celery, pickles, and onion) mixed with mayonnaise.	Add more veggies. Use less mayonnaise or use the reduced-fat or fat-free version. Another option: moisten the salad with yogurt.

- Grilled sandwiches traditionally are cooked in a skillet. Use vegetable oil spray, or spread a light coating of margarine or butter on the outside of the sandwich. Cook one side until golden brown, then do the flip side. For a lighter version, see "Sandwich Makeovers" above.

- To make sloppy joes or barbecued meat sandwiches, brown ground beef or turkey, drain, then simmer it in a spicy sauce. You can buy ready-made sauce or create your own.

- Pan-broil burgers in a skillet without added fat. Even better, broil them so that the fat drains off. Remember to check the internal temperature with an instant-read thermometer—they're done at 160°F (71°C).

Critical Thinking: Find advertisements from fast-food restaurants that offer a variety of sandwiches, including chicken, fish, and vegetarian. Why are there more sandwich choices in restaurants today than there were 40 years ago?

Sandwiches on the Go

Need a portable meal? Sandwiches are easy to pack and take along. You can prepare most cold sandwiches ahead, then refrigerate or freeze them. So that they won't dry out, wrap them tightly in plastic or foil. With a few exceptions, refrigerate sandwiches for no more than a day or freeze them for up to a week. Egg salad, lettuce, tomatoes, and mayonnaise lose their quality when they're frozen, so add them only to refrigerated sandwiches.

Tip

Pack ingredients such as lettuce and tomato separately so that they stay fresh and the sandwich doesn't get soggy. Add them just before eating.

Check This Out!

COOL TIPS AND HOT IDEAS FOR SANDWICHES

Hot or cold, light or hearty—you can be creative when you make a sandwich.

- *Have a hero.* Whether you know them as heroes, subs, hoagies, grinders, or poor boys, these long sandwiches piled with meats, cheeses, and sliced veggies are a hit. What do you like on yours?
- *Pick a pita.* Pita bread is great filled with a variety of ingredients. Try mashed avocado topped with lettuce, slices of red onion and tomato, a few sunflower seeds for crunch, and some shredded cheese.
- *Wrap it up.* A **wrap**—*flat bread rolled around a filling*—is easy and portable. Try spreading Scandinavian flat bread with mustard and rolling it around sliced ham and cheese. Roll lean turkey, Monterey Jack cheese, shredded lettuce and carrots, and salsa in a corn tortilla for a Mexican wrap.
- *Spread out.* Invent your own spreadable fillings. Try cottage cheese or thick yogurt mixed with chopped fruits, vegetables, or herbs. Make a hearty spread of mashed cooked beans, cilantro or parsley, and other seasonings.
- *Build a better burger.* Season uncooked meat—ground beef, turkey, or a combo—with an Italian or Mexican herb blend, chopped parsley, shredded carrot, or chopped onion. Cook through. Then serve it on a whole grain bun or English muffin, layered with your favorites: lettuce, sprouts, tomato, sliced peppers, portobello mushrooms, other veggies, or cheese.

It's Your Turn!

Design your own sandwich creation. Write a taste-tempting description of your sandwich that could be used on a restaurant menu. Share it with the class.

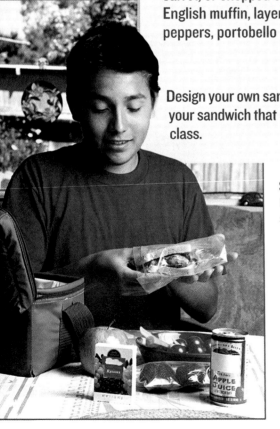

Sandwiches complement an on-the-go lifestyle. Name three ways to add additional food-group servings to your sandwiches.

Keep sandwiches cold so that they stay fresh and safe to eat—especially in hot weather when foods spoil easily. An insulated bag, with a frozen juice can or cold pack tucked inside, can help keep your sandwich cold for several hours. You can also pack a frozen sandwich in your lunch bag and it will thaw out in time for lunch. For food safety, use a fresh sandwich bag or wash your insulated lunch bag before packing your sandwich.

Activity: Break out of the "burger rut" and try a turkey burger or veggie burger. Report your impressions to the class.

NOW You're COOKING!

Creating a Quick Sandwich

*S*andwiches are an on-the-go type of food. Fillings can be rolled on a tortilla or a piece of lettuce, stuffed in a pita pocket, or placed in a roll or a bagel.

RECIPE

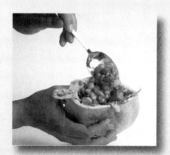

Chili Pitas

CUSTOMARY	INGREDIENTS	METRIC
1 can (15 oz.)	Prepared chili con carne	425 g
4 rounds	Whole wheat pita bread	4 rounds
2 cups	Shredded lettuce	500 mL
½ cup	Chopped tomatoes	125 mL

Yield: 4 servings each, 1 pita (2 halves) with filling.

1. Pour chili into a medium microwave-safe dish. Microwave, covered with waxed paper, on 100% power for 2 minutes or until hot, stirring every minute.
2. Cut each pita round in half to form two pockets.
3. Fill each pocket with lettuce and chili. Garnish with tomatoes.

Per Serving: 254 calories, 12 g protein, 35 g carbohydrate, 7 g fat, 783 mg sodium, 3 g fiber
Percent Daily Value: thiamin 15%, niacin 14%, phosphorus 18%

More Ideas

- Fill pita bread halves with tuna salad, chicken salad, or grilled vegetables.
- Use pita bread as the base for a quick pizza.
- Try vegetarian chili instead of the chili with meat.

Your Ideas

Pita bread is common in many countries in Southwest Asia. Find out about the fillings commonly served in pita bread. Then create your own pita pocket with your favorite fillings.

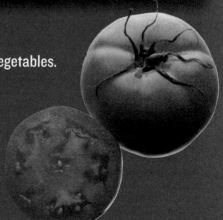

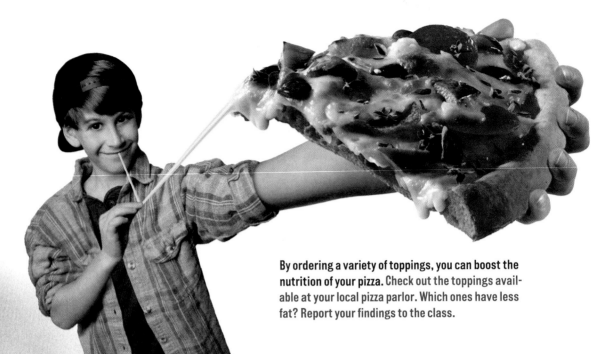

By ordering a variety of toppings, you can boost the nutrition of your pizza. Check out the toppings available at your local pizza parlor. Which ones have less fat? Report your findings to the class.

Pizza for Meals and Snacks

Pizza can pack a lot of nutrition into one slice. You can enjoy pizza for breakfast, lunch, or dinner, or as a snack. Too tired to fix yourself breakfast? Enjoy a slice of leftover pizza, either hot or cold, with your orange or grapefruit juice.

Pizza with Pyramid Power

Pizza's another food that can pack Pyramid power! Boost its nutritional value by selecting a variety of foods from different groups in the Food Guide Pyramid. As with other combination foods, the nutrients and calories in pizza depend on what goes in it. Whether you buy it or make your own, keep these tips in mind for a nutrition-wise pizza.

- Choose a whole-grain crust for more fiber. For fewer calories, try a thin crust.
- Pile on the veggie toppings—and give fruit toppings a try—for vitamins A and C, folate, potassium, and fiber.
- For toppings from the Meat, Poultry, Fish, Dry Beans, Eggs, and Nuts Group, select mostly lower-fat options such as lean ham, lean ground beef, grilled chicken, or refried beans with no added fat.
- For less fat, consider using lower-fat cheeses. Remember, cheese is a good source of calcium and protein from the Milk, Yogurt, and Cheese Group.

Discuss: Why would pizza be a good choice for breakfast? What nutrients would it supply?

Tip

Pizza freezes well and reheats easily in a conventional oven, toaster oven, or microwave oven. When reheating pizza in the microwave oven, lay the pizza on a paper towel so that the crust doesn't get soggy.

Making Your Own Pizza

You know you can buy frozen pizzas, order pizza when you eat out, or have one delivered to your door. Have you tried making your own pizza? It's fun, and you can make it just the way you like!

Base. Traditional pizza calls for a yeast bread crust. You can make your own or save time by using a ready-made crust. For easy individual pizzas, you might use halved English muffins, sliced French bread, or pita bread.

Sauce. Pizza sauce from a jar is convenient. For variety, try canned pasta sauce, taco sauce, spaghetti sauce, enchilada sauce, salsa, or even a little pesto sauce. When you're in the mood for a refreshing pizza, use pureed fruit for the sauce and top with fruit slices.

Seasonings. You can flavor your pizza with anything from the traditional oregano to chopped fresh garlic and basil to chili powder to cinnamon.

Toppings. What combination of toppings would you and your family enjoy? Be creative! Try any chopped or sliced vegetables, such as tomatoes, mushrooms, broccoli, eggplant, bell pepper, zucchini, or spinach. How about pineapple with Canadian bacon, or refried beans with taco meat? Leftovers make great pizza toppings, too!

Cheese. Pick a cheese to match your creation—mozzarella, cheddar, Swiss, feta, and Gouda are a few possibilities, or create your own cheese "combo." Packaged shredded or crumbled cheese will save you time.

How you bake your pizza depends on what ingredients you use. With individual English muffin pizzas with pre-cooked toppings, for instance, just heat them briefly in the microwave or toaster oven until the cheese melts. Pizza with a yeast dough crust needs to be baked longer. Check a cookbook for directions.

When you have an urge for a special pizza, try making it yourself. Ready-made crusts and canned sauce cut down on preparation time. Think of a pizza combination that would provide foods from all five food groups.

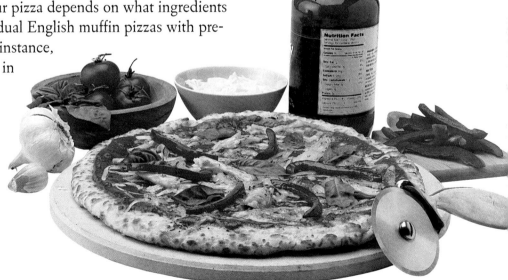

LOOKING BACK

- A sandwich can provide a variety of nutrients depending on ingredients used.
- For a quick meal or snack, keep a variety of sandwich fixings on hand.
- Most sandwiches don't require preparation directions; however, hot sandwiches require some cooking skills.
- You can prepare most cold sandwiches ahead, then refrigerate or freeze them.
- Whether you buy pizza or make it, boost its nutrition with a variety of ingredients.

UNDERSTANDING KEY IDEAS

1. What sandwich fixings might you choose to boost nutrition? Which breads and spreads might you use for flavor variety?
2. If you were making your own pizza, what steps would you follow?
3. How might you safely pack a sandwich?
4. What sauce and cheese choices could you make for variety on a pizza?
5. Describe how to make a grilled cheese sandwich with less fat and fewer calories.
6. Suppose you and your friends are ordering pizza from the local pizza restaurant. Name two ways to increase its nutritional value.

DEVELOPING LIFE SKILLS

1. **Creative Thinking:** Suppose you're making a peanut butter sandwich. What spreads other than the traditional jam or jelly could you add to it? What other foods might you pair with peanut butter for more nutrients?
2. **Leadership:** How might you apply the principles of reducing, reusing, and recycling when packing a sandwich for your lunch at school? How would these actions show leadership?

Wellness Challenge

One of the most popular items on the school lunch menu has always been pepperoni pizza. To meet nutrition guidelines, the menu is being changed. Pizza will still be offered, but it will be lower in fat and include a variety of fresh vegetable toppings. The cafeteria manager has asked for help from a committee of students. Their job is to help determine what vegetable toppings would appeal to students, and then to encourage students to try the new pizza offerings.

1. Since the menu will be changed in any case, why do you think the staff wants the committee's help?
2. How might the committee find out which toppings students prefer?
3. How might they promote the new pizza menu?

APPLYING YOUR LEARNING

1. **Sandwich Savvy:** Adriana has kept track of her daily meals and notices that she is not getting enough servings from the Milk, Yogurt, and Cheese Group and the Vegetable and Fruit Groups. Describe five sandwiches that would each contain ingredients from all three of these groups.

2. **Menu Planning:** Imagine you're in charge of making the family dinner. You've decided that your main course will be a sandwich or a pizza. You want the dinner to be fairly easy and quick to prepare and offer servings from all five food groups. Make a list of the ingredients will you use for your pizza or sandwich. What will you serve with your meal? If possible, carry out your plan by preparing the dinner.

EXPLORING FURTHER

1. **Then and Now:** In Philadelphia, the hero sandwich is known as a hoagie. Find out the history of this sandwich. Why is it called a hoagie? By what names is it known elsewhere? What are the most common ingredients?

2. **A Slice of History:** Learn about the history of pizza. How did it originate in Italy? How did it become popular in the United States? How do the Italian and American versions differ?

Making CONNECTIONS

1. **Child Development:** Plan a sandwich or pizza you could make with a four-year-old child. Why would it be a good choice? Describe activities for fun and learning that you and the child could share while preparing or eating the food. How do the activities fit the child's development level?

2. **Math:** Imagine you're going to invite 15 friends to your house for a Super Bowl party. Would it be more economical to buy deli meats and cheeses, breads, and spreads to make sandwiches yourself or to order prepared sandwiches from the deli? Calculate the cost per serving for each option.

FOODS LAB

Conduct a taste test of white, whole wheat, and oatmeal bread spread with regular, low-fat, and fat-free mayonnaise. Compare the texture and flavor. How do the nutrients compare? Create a nutrient-rich sandwich with your choice of bread and spread.

Desserts

Objectives

After studying this chapter, you will be able to:

- Explain how desserts fit into a healthful eating plan.

- Identify ways to make desserts that are lower in fat and calories.

- Distinguish between various types of milk-based desserts, cookies, cakes, and pies.

- Describe how to store desserts for food safety.

Do You Know...

...the difference between sorbet and sherbet?

...which type of cake has no fat?

...how to make baked desserts with nutrition in mind?

If not, you'll find out in this chapter!

Look for these TERMS

custard	chiffon cake
shortened cake	pastry dough
foam cake	cobbler

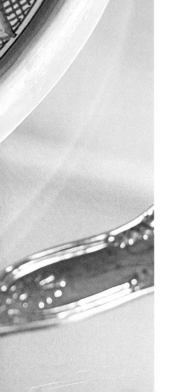

Desserts end

a meal with a festive touch and a sweet flavor. Like any other part of the meal, they can contribute toward servings from the five food groups. Think about oatmeal cookies, warm fruit cobbler, and creamy pudding. Where do their main ingredients fit on the Pyramid? Desserts aren't essential but a choice—one that can fit into a healthful eating plan!

How Desserts Fit In

Desserts not only satisfy your "sweet tooth." When they contribute toward food-group servings, they help balance your whole day's food choices. For instance, bread pudding is cubes of bread soaked in a milk, egg, sugar, and spice mixture and then baked. It counts toward your day's servings from the Bread, Cereal, Rice, and Pasta Group. What desserts contribute servings from the Fruit Group or Milk, Yogurt, and Cheese Group?

It's true that some desserts are high in fat, added sugars, and calories. Just remember—in your nutrition-wise eating plan, any food can fit! It's okay to have rich desserts occasionally or to enjoy them as snacks. In fact, on very active days you may need the extra food energy they provide. Just make sure your overall day's food choices match Pyramid guidelines, without going over your fat and calorie budgets.

When you're not so active, think of ways to trim fat and calories in your dessert choices.
• Eat a small portion of a rich dessert or share it with a friend.
• Choose or prepare dessert options with less fat and less added sugar, such as the ones you'll read about in this chapter.
• Look for alternatives with less fat and fewer calories when you shop or eat out. Just remember, "fat-free" doesn't mean "calorie-free"! Reading the Nutrition Facts panel on food labels will help you.

Discuss: Is fresh fruit a "fun" dessert? This chapter will show you how to turn fruit into a tasty dessert.

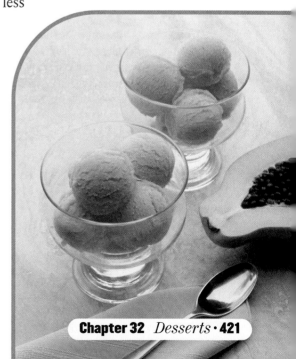

A fruit sorbet is a low-fat, low-calorie dessert. Find a sorbet recipe you would like to make.

Light and Easy Desserts

Are you looking for a dessert on the lighter side? Try one of these ideas. They're not only low in fat and calories but quick and simple to prepare.

Fresh fruit is sweet and satisfying. Enjoy a dish of fresh peach slices or berries with milk. Try combining mixed fruits with chopped mint, grated citrus rind or ginger, chopped nuts, a splash of fruit juice, and a sprinkling of cinnamon or nutmeg.

Baked apples can be ready in a flash. Core an apple, then fill it with cinnamon, raisins, and brown sugar mixed with a bit of butter or margarine. Microwave until tender, about 5 to 10 minutes.

Angel food cake is fat-free, and you can buy it already made. Top with sliced or pureed fresh fruit, or drizzle it with a little chocolate sauce.

Frozen fruit tidbits are cold and crunchy. Just freeze peeled, sliced bananas or washed grapes to enjoy later!

Flavored gelatin, often mixed with chopped fruit and chopped nuts, can be a dessert as well as a salad.

INFOLINK

For more about gelatin, see Chapter 27 and Section 4-8 of the Food Preparation Handbook.

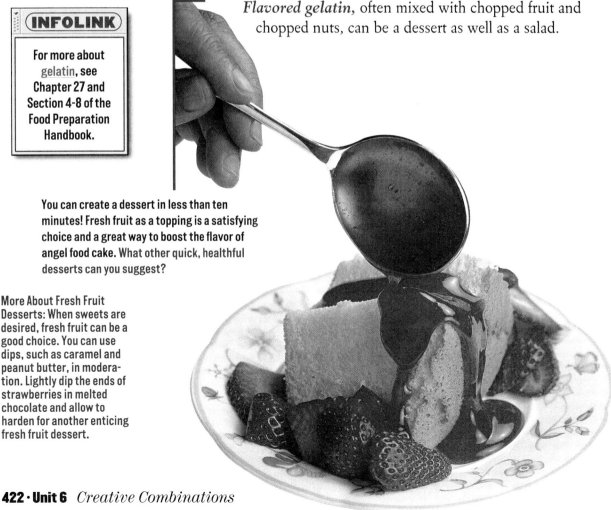

You can create a dessert in less than ten minutes! Fresh fruit as a topping is a satisfying choice and a great way to boost the flavor of angel food cake. What other quick, healthful desserts can you suggest?

More About Fresh Fruit Desserts: When sweets are desired, fresh fruit can be a good choice. You can use dips, such as caramel and peanut butter, in moderation. Lightly dip the ends of strawberries in melted chocolate and allow to harden for another enticing fresh fruit dessert.

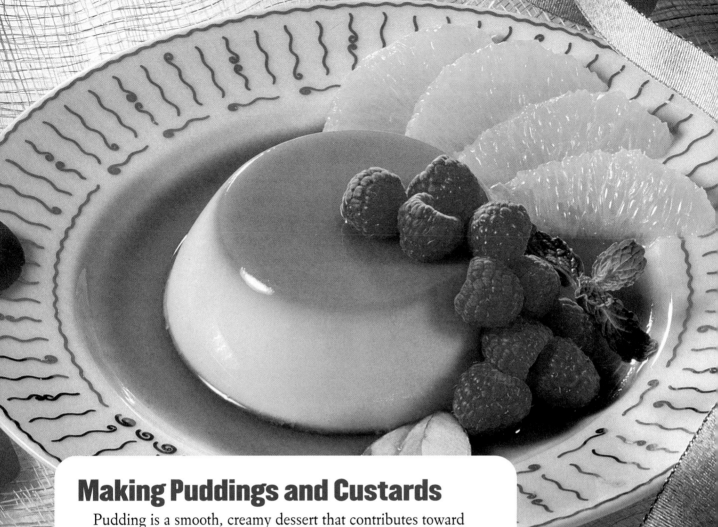

Making Puddings and Custards

Pudding is a smooth, creamy dessert that contributes toward servings from the Milk, Yogurt, and Cheese Group. Packaged instant pudding mix is simple to prepare—just add milk to the mix, beat, and chill. Homemade pudding is made with milk, sugar, and perhaps eggs. Most recipes are thickened with cornstarch. The mixture is cooked gently, then chilled.

Custard is *a cooked mixture of milk and eggs prepared on the range top or baked in the oven.* The eggs thicken the custard and give it a rich flavor. Sweeteners and other flavorings turn it into a dessert. Some recipes make a creamy, stirred custard that's thin enough to use as a sauce. Other recipes make a firmer custard that's baked in the oven. You can also use packaged mixes to make a no-bake firm custard.

Add your own spark of creativity to pudding or custard.
• Slice a banana into a dish before pouring in the pudding.
• Use stirred custard—warm or chilled—as a sauce over fresh berries or angel food cake.
• Drizzle a little maple syrup over vanilla pudding or custard.

More About Puddings: Rice or bread in puddings expand the dessert beyond the Milk, Yogurt, and Cheese Group. Raisins are commonly added to both types of puddings and some bread puddings may contain apples and nuts.

Custard with caramel sauce is a dessert with flair. In France, this dessert is called crème caramel, while in Spain and Latin American countries, it's called flan. Find a recipe for crème caramel or flan. How is the caramel sauce made?

INFOLINK

To learn more about thickeners, see Section 4-9 of the Food Preparation Handbook.

HERE'S THE SCOOP ON FROZEN DESSERTS

Whether they're served in a cone or a dish or as a topping for fruit or baked foods, frozen desserts offer a refreshing flavor. Do you know the differences between these frozen dessert choices?

- *Ice cream* is made with cream or milk, sugar, and sometimes eggs. Besides the many flavors, you'll find choices ranging from fat-free to low-fat to premium (higher butterfat) ice cream.
- *Frozen yogurt* is like ice cream but with added yogurt cultures. It's often, but not always, low-fat or fat-free.
- *Sherbet* is a frozen mixture of sweetened fruit juice, water, and often milk.
- *Sorbet* (sor-**BAY**) is a frozen fruit treat that's similar in texture to sherbet but has no milk.

Enjoy frozen desserts just as they come from the carton, or jazz them up by topping them with sliced fresh fruit, crunchy cereal, or wheat germ.

It's Your Turn!

Check the Nutrition facts panel on the label of several different frozen desserts. Compare the nutrients and calories in one serving.

INFOLINK

To learn about leavening agents, see pages 400-401 in Chapter 30 and Section 4-10 of the Food Preparation Handbook.

Making Baked Desserts

Want to bake a sweet treat? You might enjoy the satisfaction of making cookies, cakes, and pies from scratch. To save time, you can use convenience products and add your own personal touches. Either way, the best tip for success is to follow recipe or package directions carefully. If you do, your creations will be as enjoyable to make as they are to eat!

Cookies

How many kinds of cookies can you think of? Hundreds have been invented. Have you ever tried granola-pecan cookies, gingersnaps, cinnamon-flavored snickerdoodles, or peanut butter bars?

Cookie dough is made with flour, fat, sugar, perhaps eggs, and a leavening agent to add volume. Beyond those basics, a variety of ingredients gives the different kinds of cookies their distinctive flavors. Ingredients such as oatmeal, nuts, dried fruits, and pureed pumpkin contribute nutrients, too.

The way you shape the dough before baking depends on the type of cookie.

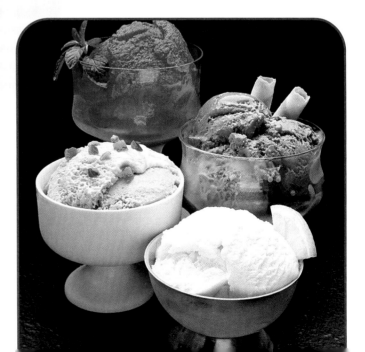

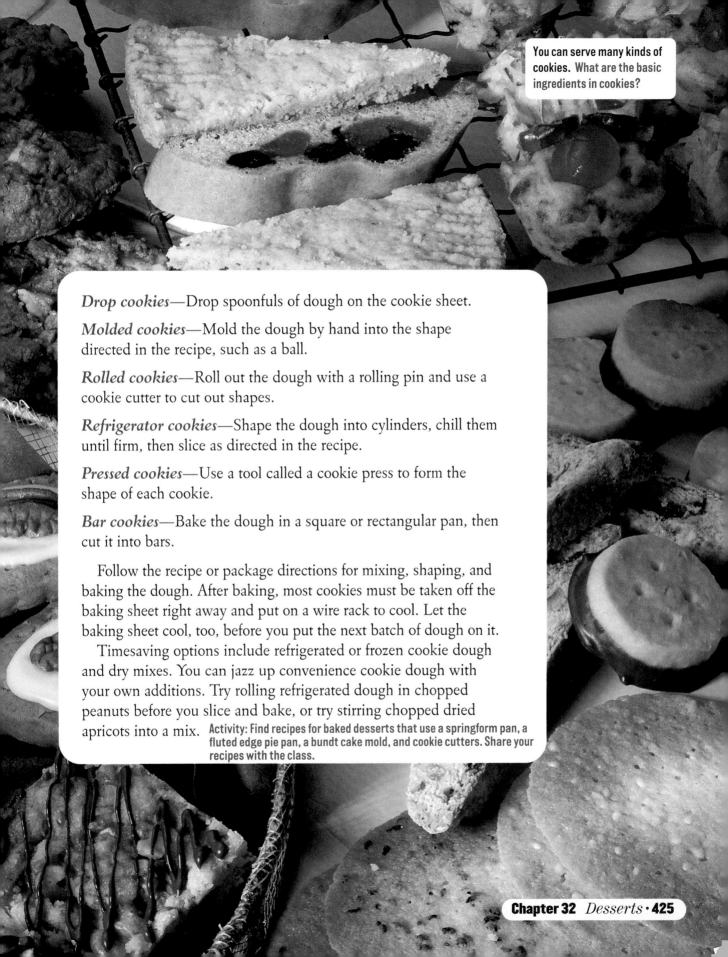

You can serve many kinds of cookies. What are the basic ingredients in cookies?

Drop cookies—Drop spoonfuls of dough on the cookie sheet.

Molded cookies—Mold the dough by hand into the shape directed in the recipe, such as a ball.

Rolled cookies—Roll out the dough with a rolling pin and use a cookie cutter to cut out shapes.

Refrigerator cookies—Shape the dough into cylinders, chill them until firm, then slice as directed in the recipe.

Pressed cookies—Use a tool called a cookie press to form the shape of each cookie.

Bar cookies—Bake the dough in a square or rectangular pan, then cut it into bars.

Follow the recipe or package directions for mixing, shaping, and baking the dough. After baking, most cookies must be taken off the baking sheet right away and put on a wire rack to cool. Let the baking sheet cool, too, before you put the next batch of dough on it.

Timesaving options include refrigerated or frozen cookie dough and dry mixes. You can jazz up convenience cookie dough with your own additions. Try rolling refrigerated dough in chopped peanuts before you slice and bake, or try stirring chopped dried apricots into a mix.

Activity: Find recipes for baked desserts that use a springform pan, a fluted edge pie pan, a bundt cake mold, and cookie cutters. Share your recipes with the class.

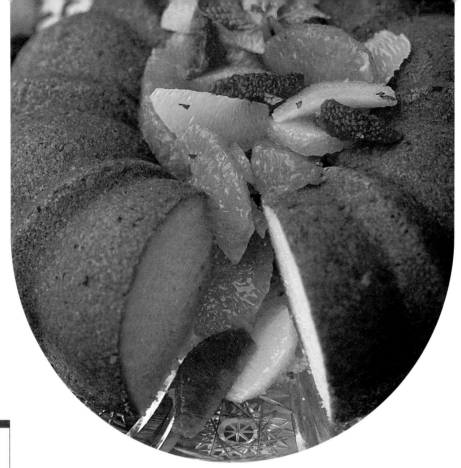

Cakes can be served with or without frosting. You could top a cake with fruit or dust it with confectioners' sugar for decoration. Why might you top a cake that way?

Tip

Shortened cakes are done baking when a toothpick stuck in the center comes out clean.

INFOLINK

To learn how to properly place more than one baking pan in the oven, see Section 3-6 of the Food Preparation Handbook.

Cakes

Plain or fancy, no matter what the flavor, cakes are often grouped into three general categories. The difference is in the ingredients, other than the basic ones of flour, sugar, and liquid.

• **Shortened cakes** *include a fat such as butter or shortening and use baking powder or baking soda as the main leavening agent.* Eggs— both yolk and white—are also mixed into the batter. Shortened cakes come in many flavors, such as white, chocolate, and spice.

• **Foam cakes** *do not include butter, shortening, or oil and use beaten egg whites as the main leavening agent.* The most common example is angel food cake, which is fat-free. Sponge cake is similar to angel food cake but has egg yolks in the batter.

• **Chiffon cakes** *include oil (or sometimes another fat) and egg yolks and are leavened with both beaten egg whites and baking powder.* They are almost like a cross between shortened and foam cakes.

You can make cakes from scratch or use a mix. Methods for mixing cake batter, baking cakes, and cooling them differ, so follow the recipe or package directions carefully.

Activity: Traditional icings can dramatically alter cake's nutritional content. Brainstorm alternatives.

Pies and Cobblers

Pies not only come in many varieties but can provide nutrients from their food-group ingredients. The filling of a pie might be made with fruits such as apples, berries, or cherries, vegetables such as pumpkin or sweet potato, milk-based pudding or custard, or nuts, as in pecan pie.

Most pie crust is made from **pastry dough**—*a blend of flour, fat, salt, and liquid.* Another type of crust is made of graham cracker crumbs mixed with melted butter or margarine and a little sugar. The crust often contains much of the fat in a pie. Here are some ways to cut down on fat.

- Instead of a two-crust pie (with crust both above and below the filling), make a one-crust pie (with only a bottom crust) or a deep-dish pie (made in a deep baking dish with only a top crust).
- Use less butter or margarine in crumb crusts, just enough to make the crust moist.

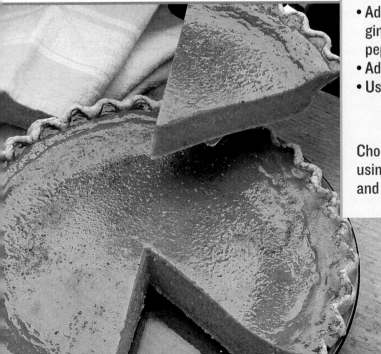

BAKING FOR MORE FLAVOR, BETTER NUTRITION

You can add flavor and nutrients while reducing fat, sugar, and calories when you bake. When you make changes, expect the new version to differ somewhat in flavor and texture from the original. Experiment to create the right recipe for you. Try these ideas.

For less fat and cholesterol
- Use half the amount of fat (butter, margarine, shortening, or oil) called for in your cake and cookie recipes. Substitute an equal amount of applesauce, mashed ripe banana, canned pumpkin, or baby food fruits. You'll add vitamins and minerals, too!
- Use ¼ cup (50 mL) egg substitute or two egg whites in place of one whole egg.
- Use mini chocolate chips to spread out the flavor and reduce the amount called for in the recipe.

For less sugar
With many recipes, you can cut sugar by one-fourth to one-third. Experiment to find out. To boost the flavor, you also might:
- Add "sweet spices" such as ground cinnamon, ginger, or nutmeg or extracts such as vanilla or peppermint.
- Add dried or chopped fresh fruits to the recipe.
- Use apple juice for some of the liquid in the recipe.

It's Your Turn!

Choose a recipe for cake or cookies and revise it using one of the above ideas. Try the new recipe and share the results with the class.

Pies can be made quickly and easily with convenience options. Check the grocery shelves, refrigerated cases, and freezer section for options such as pie crust mix, pastry dough sticks, rolled-out pastry dough circles, and prepared pie shells. Easy fillings include instant pudding, custard mix, and canned fruit filling. With a little imagination, you can come up with other quick ways to make pies. How about filling a prepared graham cracker crust with frozen yogurt and sliced fresh fruit?

A **cobbler** is *a cooked fruit dessert with a sweetened biscuit-dough topping.* You can make it with fresh or canned fruit, such as peaches, blueberries, or cherries. With most recipes, you cook the fruit with sugar and other flavorings to make a thick mixture. After pouring the hot fruit mixture into a baking dish, spoon the biscuit dough on top. Then bake the cobbler until the topping is browned. Fruit crisp is similar to cobbler but without the biscuit dough. Instead, it's topped with a mixture of oats, flour, sugar, spices, and a little butter or margarine.

Keeping Desserts Fresh

Proper storage keeps desserts appetizing and safe to eat. For food safety, the refrigerator is the place to keep desserts made with creamy milk or egg mixtures. This includes puddings, custards, custard sauces, cream pies, and custard or pumpkin pies. Fruit pies keep better when refrigerated, too.

Cakes and cookies will stay fresh at room temperature for a few days in a tightly covered container, a plastic bag, or aluminum foil. Cookies, unfrosted cakes, and cooked fruits keep their quality in the freezer for several months.

More About Keeping Desserts Fresh: Scientists in Antarctica don't need freezers. They just put the food outside!

Pudding is one of several desserts that must be kept chilled. What ingredient in pudding makes it perishable?

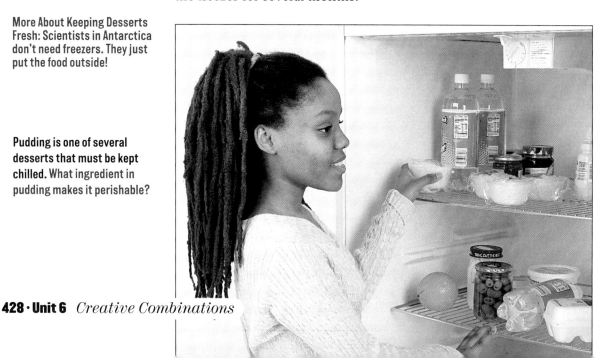

NOW *You're* COOKING!

(SKILL) Making a Nutritious Dessert

*M*any people enjoy ending a meal with something sweet. There are many ways to change a recipe to make it special or more nourishing. Have fun with this one!

RECIPE

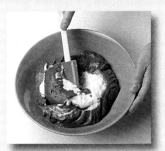

Chocolate Fudge Peanut Pudding

CUSTOMARY	INGREDIENTS	METRIC
2 Tbsp.	Chopped peanuts	30 mL
2 cups	Nonfat plain yogurt	500 mL
1 package (3.9 oz.)	Instant chocolate fudge pudding mix	110 g
¼ cup	Creamy or chunky peanut butter	50 mL

Yield: 4 servings, ½ cup (125 mL) each

1. Place peanuts in small skillet over medium heat. Stir frequently for 3 to 4 minutes or until toasted. Cool on a plate.

2. In medium bowl, beat yogurt, pudding mix, and peanut butter with an electric mixer or wire whisk for 2 minutes, scraping bowl every 30 seconds.

3. Spoon into dessert dishes. Sprinkle nuts over top of pudding to garnish. Refrigerate for 5 minutes or until ready to serve.

Per Serving: 270 calories, 14 g protein, 33 g carbohydrate, 10 g fat, 495 mg sodium, 1 g fiber

Percent Daily Value: vitamin E 15%, riboflavin 18%, niacin 14%, vitamin B_{12} 11%, calcium 25%, phosphorus 30%

More Ideas

- Try different flavors of pudding mix and top with fresh or canned fruit.
- Make a sauce from the pudding mix by adding extra yogurt or milk. It can be served with cake or fresh fruit.

Your Ideas
For additional flavor, color, and nutrition, name some foods that could be added when preparing a pudding. What flavors of pudding would you use with each new addition?

LOOKING BACK

- Desserts can fit into a nutrition-wise eating plan.

- Many desserts are not only low in fat and calories but are also simple to prepare.

- Puddings and custards contribute toward servings from the Milk, Yogurt, and Cheese Group.

- When making baked desserts, including cookies, cakes, pies, and cobblers, follow recipe or package directions carefully.

- Store desserts properly to keep them appetizing and safe to eat.

UNDERSTANDING KEY IDEAS

1. How can desserts fit into a healthful eating plan? When is it okay to have rich desserts?

2. When you're not especially active, how can you trim fat and calories in dessert choices?

3. Describe ways in which fruit can be used to make quick, simple, low-calorie desserts.

4. What is the difference between home-made pudding and custard?

5. For which type of cookies would you need a cookie press? A square or rectangular pan?

6. What are the three general categories of cakes? How is each one unique?

7. How would you store puddings and custards? Cakes and cookies?

DEVELOPING LIFE SKILLS

1. **Critical Thinking:** Many people seem to believe that desserts can't be part of a healthful eating plan. Where do you think they get this impression? How might you recognize misleading information about the nutritional role of desserts?

2. **Management:** Imagine that you're baby-sitting and you promised to bake cookies with the children. You want to make cookies that are fairly easy, won't take too long, and won't dirty too many utensils. If you decided to make cookies from scratch, which type(s) might be a good choice? Why? What convenience option(s) could you use instead?

Wellness Challenge

Malik's father has always enjoyed dessert with every evening meal. Recently, his doctor prescribed a low-fat, low-cholesterol, low-sodium diet. Malik's father thinks he will have to give up desserts from now on, and that's making him unhappy. Malik wants his father to understand that desserts can fit into a healthful eating plan.

1. If Malik's father tries to give up desserts entirely, what might happen as a result?

2. What could Malik do to help his father enjoy desserts within his new eating plan?

APPLYING YOUR LEARNING

1. **Recipe File:** Find one recipe for each general type of dessert in the chapter (such as rolled cookies and shortened cake). For each type of dessert, how many variations did you and your classmates find? What are the similarities and differences in the recipes?

2. **Job Interview:** Imagine that you own a restaurant and want to hire a new dessert chef. Make a list of questions you could ask in an interview to find out what the job candidates know about making desserts. With a partner, take turns asking and answering the interview questions.

EXPLORING FURTHER

1. **Mixing Methods:** Investigate the different methods used to mix cake batter. (You might survey recipes and compare the methods used.) How many basic methods can you identify? When is each used? Present your findings to the class.

2. **Local Treats:** Visit a local bakery. Find out how the owners determine what desserts they offer and what ingredients they use. Look for baked goods made with whole grains, fruits, shredded or pureed vegetables, milk or cheese, and eggs or nuts. Report your findings to the class.

Making CONNECTIONS

1. **Math:** Choose a dessert that can be purchased ready-made, made from convenience products, or made from scratch. (Apple pie is one example.) How does the cost per serving compare? Make sure the serving sizes are the same when comparing. What nutritional differences are there? Explain if and when you would choose to serve each form of the dessert.

2. **Social Studies:** Select a foreign country. Choose a holiday that is celebrated there and research what desserts are served for the occasion. Share your findings with the class.

FOODS LAB

Find a recipe for homemade pudding or custard. Prepare two samples: one by following the recipe directions carefully and the other by cooking it at a higher temperature than the recipe calls for. Compare the texture and flavor of each. What can you conclude?

What's in a Name?

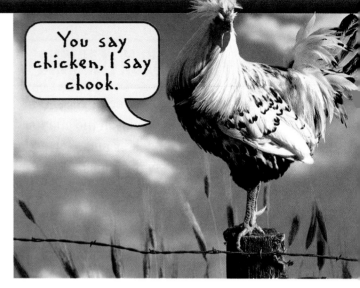

You say chicken, I say chook.

new Zealand is famous for the kiwi fruit. But "kiwi" wasn't the fruit's first name, and New Zealand wasn't its first home. The kiwi fruit was originally called yang tao, or Chinese gooseberry, and had been grown in China for centuries. In 1906, New Zealand also began growing this slightly sweet, slightly tart fruit. After a few years, it was renamed kiwi. The kiwi bird is the symbol of New Zealand, and many New Zealand objects are called kiwi. The fruit may have gotten its name for another reason: Its not-so-perfect oval shape and fuzzy brown skin make it look a bit like the bird. With its subtle taste (a combination of strawberries, nectarines, and melons) and high amount of vitamin C, kiwi has become one of the most popular fruits throughout the world. Kiwi now comes in two colors—traditional green and the new, sunny golden. ■

AUSSIE SPEAK

Even though Australians speak English, they have some terms that are unknown to people in the United States. Take a look.

Anzac Biscuits: crisp biscuits (cookies) made from wheat flour, rolled oats, dried coconut, and maple syrup. Reportedly made for the ANZACS (Australian and New Zealand Army Corps) during World War I.

Barbie: a barbecue, which is very popular in Australia.

Bickie: a biscuit or cookie.

Chips: French fries or potato chips. To "spit chips" means you are very angry.

Chook: chicken.

Lolly: candy or boiled sweet. Lolly water is the term for a soft drink.

Sanger: sandwich. Also called sango.

Snag: sausage.

Vegemite: a brown yeast extract that is spread on toast and sandwiches. Many Australians consider this their national food.

PUT A 'ROO ON THE BARBIE

Anew food is hopping into Australia's kitchens: kangaroo. Recently, meat from kangaroos and emus (large, flightless birds similar to the ostrich) has begun showing up in restaurants and food stores. The meat from both animals is very low in fat and cholesterol.

Other native bush foods that are gaining in popularity include bush tomatoes, paperbark (used to wrap foods to keep them moist while cooking), wattleseed (roasted and ground seeds used in coffee, gravy, or bread), and possibly the world's richest natural source of vitamin C, kakadu plum. ■

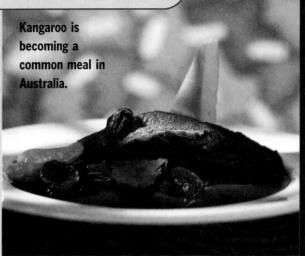

Kangaroo is becoming a common meal in Australia.

FISH STORY

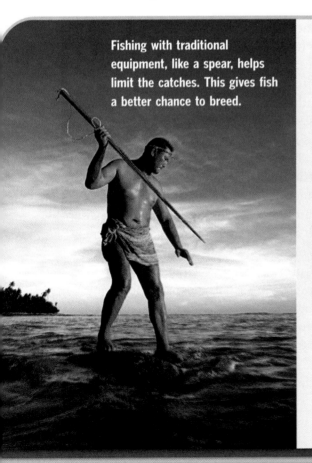

Fishing with traditional equipment, like a spear, helps limit the catches. This gives fish a better chance to breed.

fish are making a comeback in Samoa. For years, the sea provided unlimited fish to people on these South Pacific islands. Fish are vital to their existence. What people catch in nearby lagoons and reefs they share with relatives and neighbors; some is sold to add to their small incomes. Until 1995, fish were plentiful in Samoa. Then people noticed a change—their catches began shrinking. Says one Samoan: "We used to fish for two hours and have enough for our families and neighbors. Then we started staying out for six hours and still came back with fewer fish."

The problem was that fishers had begun catching fish with modern equipment. Fishing was so easy, there weren't many fish left. Now, villagers are creating rules to limit fishing, so the lagoons are filling up with fish again. Villagers plan to keep protecting this special resource. Says one Samoan, "We love the sea as our ancestors did. And we want to preserve it this way for our children." ■

Australia, New Zealand & Oceania

New Zealand's food is a reflection of the ethnic makeup of its people: There are about 3 million people of British descent, about 280,000 native Maori (MAU-ree), and about 250,000 Pacific Islanders. Most of the country's dishes are British in flavor, but other groups have brought their own influence to New Zealand's cuisine.

New Zealand is a land of plenty. Dairy products, world-famous lamb, and the kiwi fruit are just a few of its many delicious food products. Beef, chicken, and sausages are plentiful. Hot pastry-covered meat pies filled with beef or lamb and topped with gravy are practically a national dish. New Zealand is made up of islands, so saltwater and freshwater fish and shellfish are plentiful. Fish and chips—

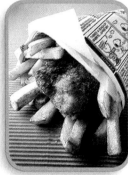

▲ Fish and chips are traditionally sold wrapped in newspaper.

fried pieces of fish and french fries—are a quick lunch.

Fresh fruits and vegetables grow throughout the year. The traditional dessert, pavlova, is made from meringue (sugar and egg whites) filled with whipped cream and fresh fruit. This dessert is also claimed by Australia, New Zealand's neighbor across the Tasman Sea.

Australia In fact, there isn't much difference in food likes and dislikes between Australians and New Zealanders. Both like meat and lamb dishes, chicken, and foods that were brought over from Great Britain. Barbecues are very popular with Australians, many of whom prefer a casual lifestyle and enjoy eating outdoors.

Cooking methods in both New Zealand and Australia have changed in the past 15

Traditionally dressed men from the Fiji Islands get ▶ ready to cook a pig in an underground oven. These ovens are used throughout the South Pacific islands.

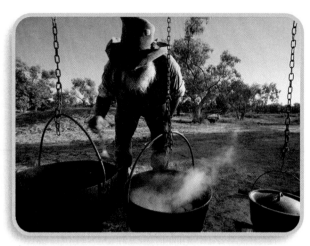

◀ Aborigines have been eating native plants for thousands of years. The plants can be highly nutritious.

years or so, partly because of the increasing numbers of European and Asian immigrants who have brought their cooking traditions to their new home. Meals tend to be a bit lighter with fewer heavy sauces. Japanese, Thai, and Chinese dishes are gaining in popularity, so meat is often stir-fried or served yakitori (yah-kih-TOH-ree) style (skewered).

More recently, Australians have been discovering foods that have been eaten by Aborigines (a-boh-RIDJ-uh-nees)—the first inhabitants—for thousands of years. Australians are using the enormous variety of native herbs, spices, fungi, fruits, vegetables, insects, and animals in their cooking. There's even a term for this kind of food: bush tucker.

Meat and fish dishes are seasoned with certain kinds of ground-up flowers. Wild tart berries soaked in honey are served with meat dishes, and a wild peach, called quandong, is used in flavoring ice cream.

Like many people around the world, the Aborigines eat grubs and insects. The best known is the witchetty grub. This fat creature lives in the roots of gum trees. It is a staple among Aboriginal women and children. These grubs taste something like almonds.

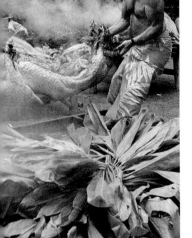

▲ An Australian in the outback prepares food the "old-fashioned" way.

South Pacific Islands On special occasions, islanders enjoy feasting the way their ancestors did. A traditional feast features foods that were mainstays before the Europeans arrived: fish and shellfish from the Pacific; pork and chicken; fruits such as bananas, coconuts, and breadfruit; and starchy root vegetables such as taro and yams.

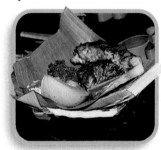

▲ A meal in the Cook Islands consists of fish and vegetables steamed in a banana leaf.

Besides the food itself, what makes an island feast special is the way it's cooked. Heated stones are placed in a pit, forming an underground oven. Meats, fish, and vegetables are wrapped in leaves, placed on the stones, and covered with more leaves and dirt. After several hours, the food is ready to unwrap and eat. This is a great way to enjoy the tastes of the South Pacific. ■

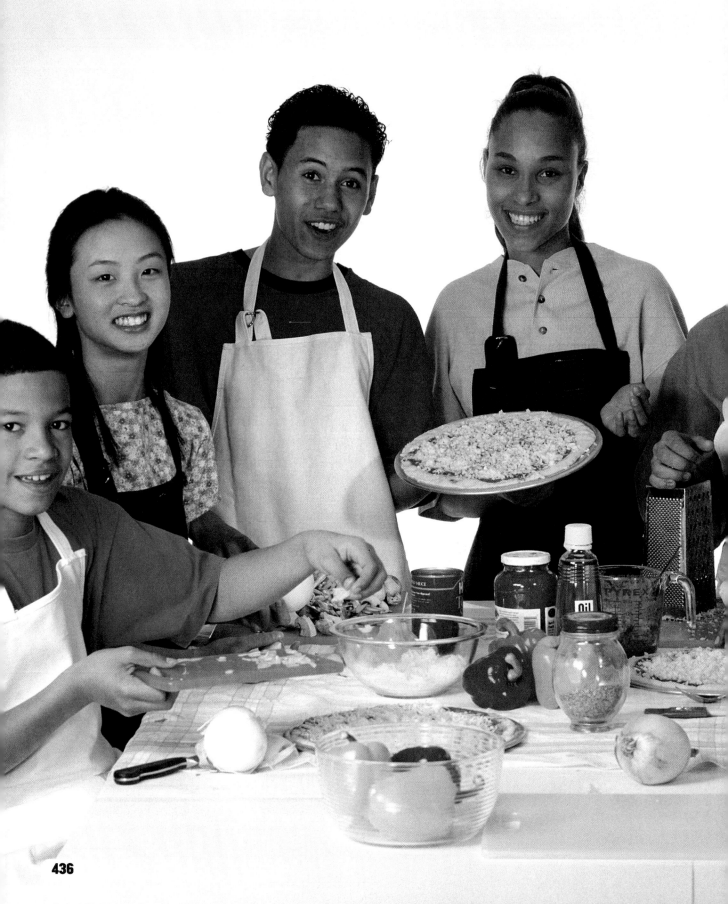

FOOD PREPARATION HANDBOOK

PART 1	Preparing Food Safely
PART 2	Kitchen Equipment
PART 3	Skills for Preparing Food
PART 4	The Science of Preparing Food
PART 5	The Art of Preparing Food

PART 1

Preparing Food Safely

Objectives

After studying pages 439-46l, you will be able to:

- Describe the causes of foodborne illness.

- Explain principles of food storage and handling, cleanliness, and temperature control that can reduce the risk of foodborne illness.

- Identify ways to prevent kitchen accidents.

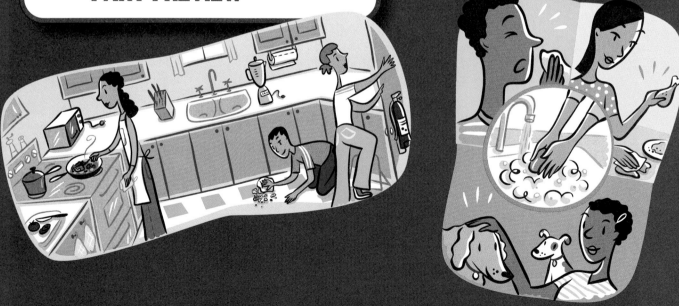

Look *for these* **TERMS**

foodborne illness
microorganisms
danger zone

What Is Foodborne Illness?

"I think I'm coming down with the flu." "There's a stomach bug going around." "It must have been something I ate." Although these three people have different explanations for the way they feel, it's possible that all three have a **foodborne illness.** That means *sickness resulting from eating food that is not safe to eat.* Foodborne illness can range from mild illnesses to very serious—even fatal—ones. That's why following safe food practices is extremely important!

Meet the Microorganisms

Microorganisms—*tiny, living creatures that can be seen only with a microscope*—cause most cases of foodborne illness. Microorganisms include different kinds of bacteria, parasites, and viruses.

Not all microorganisms are harmful—in fact, some are helpful. For instance, certain "friendly" bacteria are used to make yogurt, vinegar, and some cheeses. Even harmful microorganisms don't always cause illness. The human body usually can handle some of them in small amounts. However, when you eat food contaminated with large numbers of harmful microorganisms, foodborne illness may result.

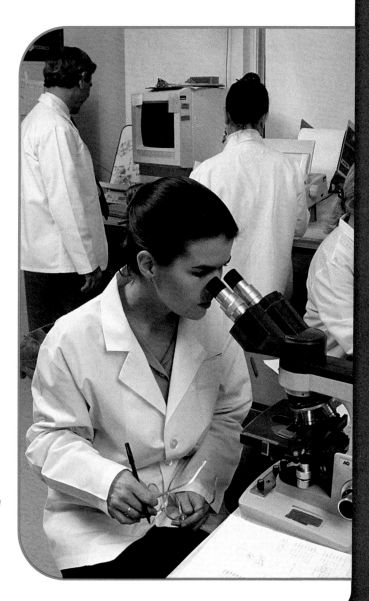

Scientists at the Centers for Disease Control and Prevention track outbreaks of foodborne illnesses. Find out more about what steps are taken when a large outbreak of foodborne illness occurs.

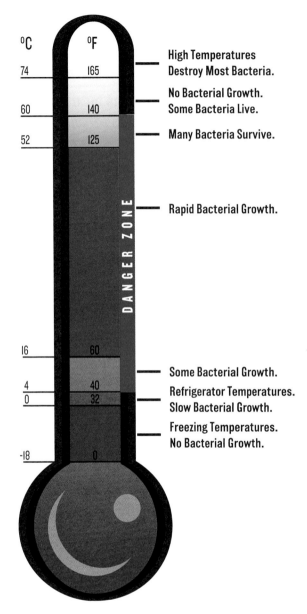

°C	°F	
74	165	High Temperatures Destroy Most Bacteria.
60	140	No Bacterial Growth. Some Bacteria Live.
52	125	Many Bacteria Survive.
		DANGER ZONE — Rapid Bacterial Growth.
16	60	
4	40	Some Bacterial Growth. Refrigerator Temperatures.
0	32	Slow Bacterial Growth.
		Freezing Temperatures. No Bacterial Growth.
-18	0	

Temperature is an important factor in food safety. When certain foods are kept at temperatures in the danger zone, bacteria can multiply rapidly. How would you apply this information when planning a picnic or party?

Teaching With Visuals: Discuss which temperatures are best in preventing bacterial growth.

How Is Food Contaminated?

You can't see, smell, or taste microorganisms, but they're all around you. They're on your skin, in the air you breathe, in the soil, and in the intestines of animals. They may be present on foods when you purchase them. They can get into food during preparation, serving, or storage.

When harmful bacteria get into food, they can multiply to dangerous levels—if they have the right conditions. To survive and multiply, bacteria need food, moisture, and the right temperatures.

To see how different temperatures affect bacteria, study the thermometer diagram on the left. Notice the area labeled the **danger zone**. That's *the temperature range in which bacteria grow fastest—between 40° and 140°F (4 and 60°C)*. In fact, at room temperature bacteria can double their numbers every 30 minutes!

When Foodborne Illness Strikes

What are the symptoms? Foodborne illness can be hard to diagnose. The symptoms vary, and many of them are similar to those of other illnesses, such as influenza. They can occur from 30 minutes to two weeks after eating food containing harmful microorganisms. Most often, however, symptoms appear within 4 to 48 hours. The chart on page 442 lists some bacteria that can cause foodborne illness and their symptoms.

Who is at risk? Anyone can suffer from foodborne illness. Some people—infants, young children, pregnant women, older people, and those with a weakened immune system—are at greater risk of becoming sick after eating contaminated food.

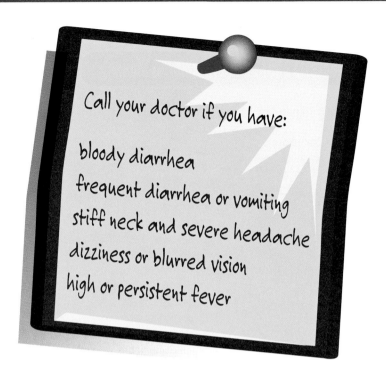

Call your doctor if you have:

bloody diarrhea
frequent diarrhea or vomiting
stiff neck and severe headache
dizziness or blurred vision
high or persistent fever

What should you do? If you think you have a foodborne illness, follow these steps:

1. Rest and drink plenty of fluids. If symptoms last more than a day or two or if they match any of those listed above, call your doctor right away.

2. If a portion of the suspect food is available, wrap it securely, label it "Danger," and refrigerate it. If it was packaged, save the can, carton, or other packaging materials.

3. Call your local health department to report the incident if the suspect food was:
   • from a restaurant or other food service facility, or...
   • a packaged food sold at stores, or...
   • eaten at a large gathering, such as a wedding reception, family reunion, or community food event.

Preventing Foodborne Illness

You can fight bacteria and other microorganisms that cause foodborne illness. How?

• By taking steps to keep harmful microorganisms from getting into food or spreading from one food to another.

• By not giving bacteria the time and conditions they need to multiply.

• By destroying harmful bacteria through proper cooking.

As you read on, you'll learn more about what you can do to help prevent foodborne illness. It's everyone's responsibility!

Activity: Call the local health department to find out what precautions it takes to prevent the spread of bacterial infection in the community.

Some Bacteria That Cause Foodborne Illness

BACTERIA	POSSIBLE SOURCES	SYMPTOMS	TIMING
Campylobacter jejuni Disease: campylobacteriosis	Raw or undercooked poultry, unpasteurized milk, untreated water (perhaps from a stream or river).	Diarrhea; may also include fever, abdominal pain, nausea, headache, muscle pain.	Symptoms begin 2 to 5 days after eating contaminated food; may last 7 to 10 days.
E. coli 0157:H7 Disease: hemorrhagic colitis (caused by a toxin that the bacteria produce)	Raw or undercooked ground meat, unpasteurized milk, unchlorinated water, unwashed produce, unpasteurized apple cider.	Severe abdominal pain, diarrhea (often bloody), sometimes vomiting. More serious symptoms can occur in children, the elderly, and people with weakened immune systems.	Symptoms begin 2 to 5 days after eating contaminated food; last about 8 days.
Listeria monocytogenes Disease: listeriosis	Raw or undercooked meat, poultry, or fish; unwashed produce; unpasteurized milk; ready-to-eat foods contaminated during or after processing, such as soft cheeses and hot dogs.	Fever, muscle aches; sometimes nausea, diarrhea, vomiting. May spread to nervous system, causing headache, stiff neck, confusion, loss of balance. Mainly affects pregnant women, newborns, the elderly, and people with weakened immune systems.	Varies
Salmonella Disease: salmonellosis	Raw and undercooked eggs, poultry, meat, fish; unpasteurized milk.	Nausea, vomiting, abdominal pain, diarrhea, fever, headache. Symptoms are most severe in elderly or infirm people and those with weakened immune systems.	Symptoms begin 6 to 48 hours after eating contaminated food; may last 1 to 2 days or longer.
Clostridium botulinum Disease: botulism (caused by a toxin that the bacteria produce)	Canned foods that aren't processed or stored properly.	Double vision; droopy eyelids; difficulty speaking, swallowing, and breathing. Can be fatal if not treated immediately and properly.	Symptoms can appear 4 hours to 8 days after eating contaminated food (usually 18 to 36 hours); may last years.
Staphylococcus aureus Disease: staphylococcal food poisoning (caused by a toxin that the bacteria produce)	Prepared foods left too long at room temperature. Typical sources: meat; poultry; egg products; mixtures such as tuna, chicken, potato, or egg salad; cream-filled pastries.	Nausea, vomiting, abdominal pain, exhaustion; sometimes headache and muscle pain.	Symptoms begin 30 minutes to 8 hours after eating contaminated food; usually last about 2 days, but sometimes longer.

Shop Safely & Store Food Right!

Your role in keeping food safe to eat begins when you put the food in your shopping cart or basket. Learn how to handle food right when you shop and after you bring it home!

INFOLINK

For more about freshness dates, see Chapter 13, page 181.

Food Safety When You Shop

- Look at the dates on packages that tell you about a food's freshness.

- Choose canned goods that are free of dents, bulges, rust, or leaks.

  Activity: Create a poster that promotes or explains about food safety when shopping for food.

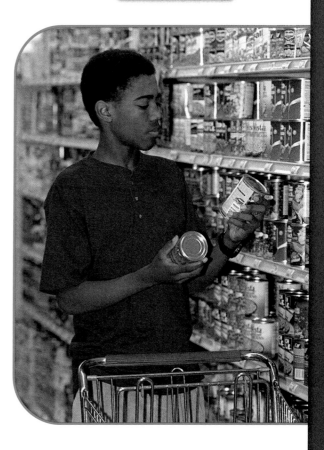

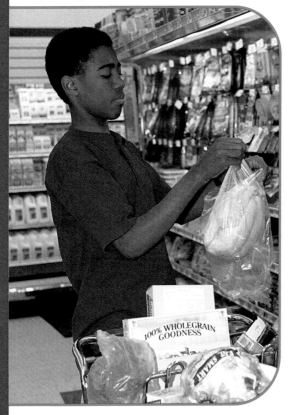

100% WHOLEGRAIN GOODNESS

- Place raw meat, poultry, and fish in plastic bags to keep their juices from dripping on other foods in your shopping cart.

- Make sure food packages don't have holes, tears, open corners, or broken safety seals.

- Check that refrigerated foods feel cold and frozen foods feel solid. Avoid frozen food packages with ice crystals or discoloration—they may have thawed, then refrozen.

- Plan your shopping so that you select refrigerated foods, frozen foods, and hot items from the deli last. That way they're at room temperature for as short a time as possible.

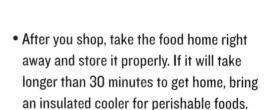

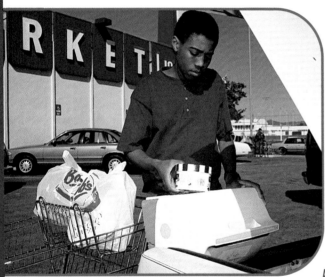

- After you shop, take the food home right away and store it properly. If it will take longer than 30 minutes to get home, bring an insulated cooler for perishable foods.

Activity: Make a sketch of the kitchen in your home or an imaginary kitchen. Show where you would store a variety of foods.

Storing Food

To keep food safe and fresh at home, know how to store it! The three basic food storage areas are dry storage, the refrigerator, and the freezer. If you're not sure where to store your food purchases, check the label for instructions.

Dry Storage

What it means: A cabinet or other area that's clean, dry, dark, and cool (below 85°F or 29°C). Don't store foods under the sink or in cabinets next to heat-producing appliances (including the refrigerator). Also, don't store household cleaning products or trash in the same cabinet as food.

What to store here: Foods such as canned goods, cereal, crackers, pasta, dry beans, baking mixes, vegetable oil, and peanut butter. Check labels for foods that should be refrigerated after they're opened.

Storage tips: Rotate canned and packaged goods by putting new purchases behind the older ones. That way you'll remember to use the older items first.

Refrigerator Storage

Proper temperatures: Between 32 and 40°F (0 and 4°C). Use a refrigerator thermometer to check.

What to store here: Perishables such as meat, poultry, fish, dairy foods, eggs, fresh fruits and vegetables, and leftovers. Check package labels for other foods that need refrigeration before or after opening.

Storage tips:

- To keep foods from drying out, use foil, plastic wrap, plastic bags, or airtight containers. This will also keep odors from transferring to other foods.

- Leave space between foods to allow room for cold air to circulate.

- Wipe up spills immediately and remove spoiled foods.

- Use door shelves for foods that aren't highly perishable, such as condiments. Interior shelves and drawers—which stay colder than the door shelves— are the place for meat, poultry, fish, milk, and eggs.

Adjust the refrigerator temperature control to keep food safe. How can you be sure the refrigerator is cold enough?

Activity: Check the temperature of the refrigerator and freezer in the foods lab or at home. Report the results.

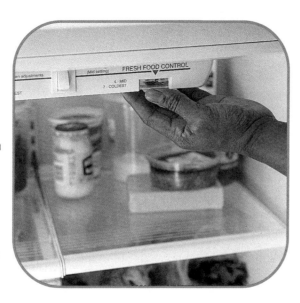

Freezer Storage

Proper temperatures: 0°F (-18°C) or less— for the longest storage or to freeze foods at home. Check with a freezer thermometer. If your freezer can only get as cold as 10 to 15°F (-12 to -9°C), you can use it to store already-frozen foods for a few weeks.

What to store here: Food purchased frozen, as well as foods that can be frozen for longer storage (including meat, poultry, fish, breads, and home-prepared foods such as casseroles).

Storage tips:

- Store foods purchased frozen in their original packages.

- Wrap other foods properly to avoid **freezer burn**, *changes in color, flavor, and texture that result when food loses moisture in the freezer.* Food with freezer burn has areas that look white and dried up. It isn't harmful, but it's not appealing either. To prevent freezer burn, use freezer paper, heavy-duty foil, plastic freezer bags, or airtight containers.

- Label foods you freeze yourself with the name of the food, date frozen, and number of servings.

- Rotate foods as you store them, putting oldest foods toward the front where you'll be more likely to use them.

Activity: Demonstrate how to wrap food with foil to prevent freezer burn.

How Long Will Food Keep?

Even when foods are stored properly, they won't stay fresh forever! The following charts show how long you can keep some common foods.

Shelf Storage Chart

Teaching With Visuals: Devise a way to keep track of how long food is stored in your home.

FOOD	STORAGE AT 70°F (21°C) (UNOPENED)	STORAGE AT 70°F (21°C) (OPENED)	IN REFRIGERATOR AFTER OPENED
Beans, dry	12 months	12 months	
Bread	2-4 days	2-4 days	7-14 days
Canned goods, high acid (juices, fruit, pickles, sauerkraut, tomatoes, tomato soup)	1½ -2 years		3-4 days
Canned goods, low acid (meat, poultry, fish, soups, beans, most vegetables)	5 years		3-4 days
Cereal, ready-to-eat	6-12 months	3 months	
Cornmeal	6-12 months		12 months
Flour, white	6-12 months	6-8 months	
Flour, whole wheat	1 month		6-8 months
Lentils, dry	12 months	12 months	
Milk, canned evaporated	12 months		4-5 days
Oils, olive and vegetable	6 months	4-6 months	
Onions	2-3 weeks	2-3 weeks	
Pasta, dry	2 years	1 year	
Peanut butter	6-9 months	2-3 months	
Potatoes	1-2 months	1-2 months	
Rice, brown	12 months		6 months
Rice, white	2 years	1 year	
Salad dressings	10-12 months		3 months
Shortening, solid	8 months	3 months	
Sugar, granulated	2 years		
Sugar, brown	4 months		
Tea bags	18 months	12 months	
Vinegar	2 years	1 year	

Cold Storage Chart

FOOD		IN THE REFRIGERATOR	IN THE FREEZER
Beverages	Fruit juice in cartons, fruit drinks, or punch, opened	7-10 days	8-12 months
Condiments and Salad Dressings	Ketchup, opened	6 months	Don't freeze
	Mayonnaise, opened	2 months	Don't freeze
	Mustard, opened	12 months	Don't freeze
	Salad dressing, opened	3 months	Don't freeze
Dairy Products	Milk	1 week	3 months
	Yogurt	7-14 days	1-2 months
	Cheese, hard, opened	3-4 weeks	6 months
	Cheese, soft	1 week	6 months
Eggs	Fresh in shell	3 weeks	Don't freeze
	Hard-cooked	1 week	Don't freeze well
Fish, Fresh	Lean fish	1-2 days	6 months
	Fatty fish	1-2 days	2-3 months
Fruits and Vegetables, Fresh	Most fruits	3-4 days	Some don't freeze
	Leafy greens	1-2 weeks	Don't freeze well
	Most other fresh vegetables	varies, 3 days-2 weeks	Some don't freeze
Hot Dogs and Lunch Meats	Hotdogs, opened	1 week	1-2 months
	Lunch meats, opened	3-5 days	1-2 months
Leftovers	Leftovers, cooked	3-4 days	2-3 months
Meat, Fresh	Beef, steaks	3-5 days	4-12 months
	Pork or veal chops	3-5 days	4-12 months
Meat, Ground & Stew Meats	Hamburger and stew meat	1-2 days	3-4 months
	Ground pork, veal, or poultry	1-2 days	3-4 months
Poultry, Fresh	Chicken or turkey, whole	1-2 days	12 months
	Chicken or turkey, pieces	1-2 days	9 months
Sauces	Salsa, opened	1 month	Don't freeze
	Spaghetti sauce, opened	5-7 days	Don't freeze
Soups and Stews	Vegetable or with meat added	3-4 days	2-3 months

When Food Spoils

When food has been stored improperly or too long, a number of things can happen to it. Some foods, such as fresh fruits and vegetables, lose nutrients. Changes in moisture content can make foods less appealing—as in the case of stale bread, freezer-burned meat, or wilted celery. Even in properly stored food, microorganisms can grow slowly. Some can eventually cause food to look or smell bad. With others, the food may look and smell normal—even though it can cause illness. How do you know whether food should be thrown away? Use the following list as a guide. *Never taste foods that you suspect are spoiled!*

Discard without tasting:

• Canned goods that leak, bulge, have a foul odor, or are badly dented.

• Jars that are cracked or have loose or bulging lids.

• Any container that spurts liquid when you open it.

Activity: Brainstorm ways to ensure that perishable foods and leftovers get used before they spoil.

Discuss: Why is it important to clean the storage area thoroughly after discovering spoiled food?

Activity: Use empty food packages, food storage containers, and wraps or bags to show how you would store, label, and rotate various types of food, including leftovers.

• Food that is slimy, mushy, discolored, or just doesn't look or smell right.

• Moldy foods—except as explained under "Dealing with mold" below.

• Leftovers that have been in the refrigerator more than 4 days—and those "mystery foods" that are who-knows-how old!

• Any food you're not sure of. Remember: *When in doubt, throw it out!*

Dealing with mold:

• On hard cheeses, such as cheddar, you can safely cut away small areas of mold. Cut away at least 1 inch (2.5 cm) around the moldy area. Put the remaining cheese in a clean, fresh wrapper or container.

• Discard all other foods that are moldy.

• Mold gives off invisible spores—that's how it spreads. Wrap moldy food well before you discard it. Check other foods for mold, too. Clean the container and the refrigerator well.

Activity: Team up with classmates and create skits in which the characters share their experiences with spoiled foods. Present the skits in class.

Keep It Clean!

From the supermarket to your table, one way to prevent foodborne illness is by following rules of sanitation. **Sanitation** means *preventing illness through cleanliness.* Keeping yourself and the kitchen clean helps get rid of some microorganisms. It also helps keep the ones that remain from multiplying and from getting into food.

Personal Cleanliness

Remember, *you* can be a source of bacteria. Keeping yourself clean when you handle food helps prevent the spread of illness-causing bacteria.

Wash Your Hands

Wash your hands the right way! Wash them vigorously with warm, soapy water—front and back, between your fingers, under your fingernails—for at least 20 seconds.

When do you need to wash your hands? More often than you may think!

- Before you begin preparing food.

- After handling raw food.

- Between handling different kinds of food.

- After using the toilet or changing a diaper.

- After touching pets.

- After touching your mouth, nose, hair, or other parts of your body while handling food.

More Ways to Keep Clean

- Don't handle food if you have diarrhea, a fever, or other symptoms of illness.

- Before you begin to prepare food, tie back long hair.

  Activity: While a classmate observes, prepare yourself as if you were going to work in the kitchen. Rate one another's cleanliness.

- Wear clean clothing. An apron will help protect you against spills and spatters.

- Cover any cuts or sores on your hands with a clean waterproof bandage—or wear clean plastic or rubber kitchen gloves. Wash gloved hands as often as you would bare hands.

- Don't sneeze or cough over food.

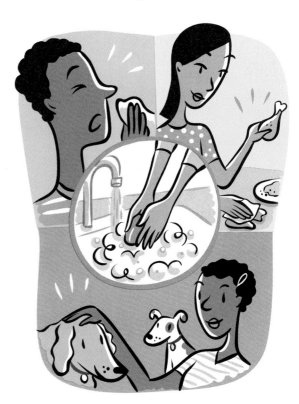

Washing your hands is an important step in preventing foodborne illness. Time yourself the next time you wash your hands. Are you scrubbing long enough?

The Clean Routine

- Clean kitchen surfaces and appliances—outside and inside—on a regular basis. Use hot, soapy water, a disinfectant cleaner, or a mixture of bleach and water.

- Keep the kitchen clean as you work. Wipe up spills right away.

- Consider using paper towels to clean kitchen surfaces. If you use cloth towels or sponges, rinse them well between uses. Wash them often in the hot cycle of a washing machine.

- Always use clean utensils and dishes.

- Keep dirty dishes away from food preparation areas. Wash dishes promptly.

- Wipe the tops of canned foods before opening them. Clean the blade of the can opener after each use.

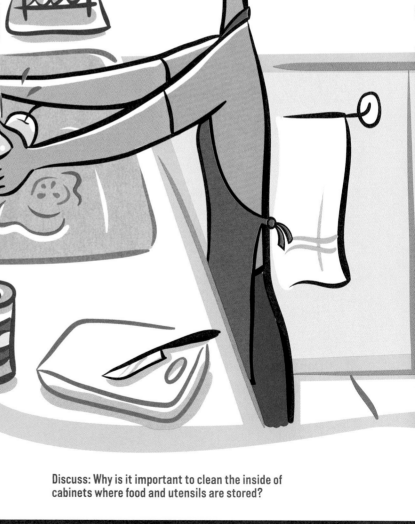

Activity: Work in pairs to create a skit that demonstrates the correct way to clean a kitchen.

Activity: Demonstrate how to clean the can opener blade.

Discuss: Why is it important to clean the inside of cabinets where food and utensils are stored?

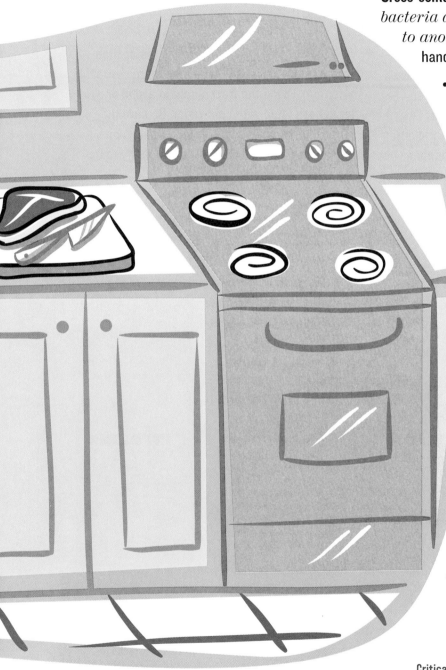

Avoid Cross-Contamination

Cross-contamination occurs *when harmful bacteria are transferred from one food to another.* Be especially careful when handling raw meat, poultry, and fish.

- Keep raw meat, poultry, and fish and their juices away from ready-to-eat foods—in your shopping cart, grocery bags, refrigerator, and while preparing foods.

- If possible, use one cutting board for meat, poultry, and fish and another one for other foods.

- Use plastic or other non-porous cutting boards. Make sure they're free of cracks and crevices—those are hiding places for bacteria.

- Wash everything that comes in contact with raw meat, poultry, or fish in hot, soapy water before it's used again. This includes cutting boards and other utensils, dishes, the counter, and your hands.

- Never place cooked or ready-to-eat food on an unwashed plate or cutting board that previously held raw meat, poultry, or fish.

Critical Thinking: What are some situations in which cross-contamination is possible? How can these situations be avoided?

Activity: Demonstrate how to practice sanitation when choosing, using, and washing cutting boards.

Control Temperatures!

Don't give bacteria the temperatures they need to thrive! To defend against foodborne illness, control the temperature of food when you thaw it, cook it, and serve it.

Thawing Food Safely

Some frozen foods—including uncooked frozen meat, poultry, and fish—need to be thawed before you cook them. If these foods are allowed to thaw at room temperature, the outer surface temperature may reach the danger zone. Bacteria on the surface can grow while the center of the food is still thawing. Use one of these safe methods for thawing frozen food:

In the refrigerator. Place frozen foods on the lowest shelf in a plastic bag to collect any juices. This method requires some advance planning, since many frozen foods take a full day or longer to thaw in the refrigerator.

In cold water. This method is faster than refrigerator thawing but requires more attention. Place the frozen item in a sink or large bowl filled with cold water. Be sure the food is wrapped in a leak-proof package or plastic bag. Change the water frequently to be sure it stays cold.

In the microwave oven. Place the item in a microwave-safe container and defrost on the "low" or "defrost" setting. Check the owner's manual for specific directions. If you use this method, always cook or reheat the food right away. Why? Some areas of the food may begin to cook during microwave thawing, and it's not safe to cook a food only partially. Read on to learn why!

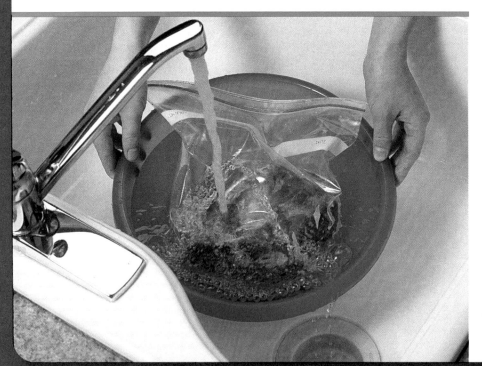

INFOLINK

Review the diagram showing the danger zone, on page 440.

When thawing food in cold water, test the water often to make sure it remains cold. Why shouldn't the water be warm?

Cooking Food Thoroughly

Foods are properly cooked when they are heated for a long enough time and at a high enough temperature to destroy harmful bacteria. Always cook food thoroughly, and finish cooking once you start. Don't try to roast your turkey for half the cooking time today and the rest tomorrow—that won't do the job!

The best way to determine whether foods are properly cooked is by measuring the internal, or inside, temperature with a clean meat thermometer. Color and texture changes are not always reliable signs, so use a thermometer whenever possible. Some microwave and convection ovens also have a temperature probe you can use. The probe shuts off the oven when the food reaches the right internal temperature.

The chart below shows safe internal temperatures for different foods.

When Is It Done?

	SAFE INTERNAL TEMPERATURE	
	°F	°C
Fresh Beef, Veal, Lamb, and Pork		
Ground products	160	71
Other cuts: medium	160	71
well done	170	77
Poultry		
Ground products	170	77
Breasts, thighs, roasts	170	77
Whole chicken or turkey	180	82
Stuffing (cooked alone or in bird)	165	74
Fish	145	63
Eggs		
Egg dishes	160	71
• Cook eggs until whites and yolks are firm		
Ham		
Precooked (to reheat)	140	60
Not precooked	160	71
Leftovers (reheating)	165	74
• Boil sauces, soups, and gravies for at least 1 minute before eating		
• When microwaving, cover leftovers, stir, and rotate for thorough heating		

Types of Meat Thermometers

Different types of meat thermometers can be used, depending on the type of food and the cooking method. You may want to have more than one type on hand.

Oven-proof. Place this thermometer in sturdy foods, such as roasts or poultry, at the beginning of cooking and let it remain there throughout cooking.

Microwave-safe. This type of thermometer is made of materials that are safe to use in a microwave oven while it's operating. Other thermometers made of metal are not safe to use in a microwave.

Instant-read. Not intended to stay in food while it's cooking, an **instant-read thermometer** *gives you a quick reading of a food's temperature.* Insert the stem of the thermometer about 2 inches (5 cm) into the food. Insert it sideways into thin foods such as hamburgers or fish.

Pop-up. This type of thermometer is already inserted into some poultry. The center of the thermometer pops up when the food is cooked to the proper temperature. It's a good idea to double-check the temperature with another type of thermometer.

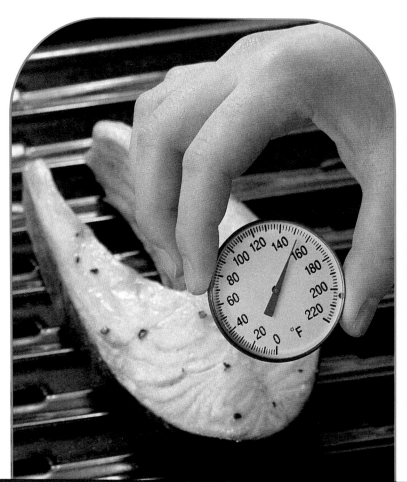

Fish, meat, or poultry may look done on the outside before the inside reaches a temperature that destroys harmful bacteria. What is the safe internal temperature for a hamburger?

Activity: Bring each of the four types of meat thermometers to class for students to see. Review how each thermometer is used and discuss students' experiences with these thermometers.

Serving Food Safely

Controlling temperatures is just as important once food is ready to eat. To keep the food safe, follow these three basic rules. They apply to any situation where food is served—including everyday and holiday meals, buffets, potlucks, picnics, and take-out foods.

Keep hot foods hot. If there will be a delay in eating hot food, keep it at a temperature higher than 140°F (60°C). At a party, for instance, you might use a slow cooker to keep foods hot at the buffet table. If you're waiting to eat take-out food, you could keep it warm in the oven.

Keep cold foods cold. Refrigerate cold take-out foods until you're ready to serve them. For buffets, keep platters of cold food on ice. If you'll be transporting food for a picnic, store it in an insulated cooler with ice or freezer packs.

Follow the two-hour rule. Perishable foods that contain meat, poultry, fish, eggs, or dairy products should not be allowed to sit at room temperature longer than two hours. If the air temperature is over 90°F (32°C), the time limit is one hour. The clock starts as soon as food is set out for serving! Remember, harmful bacteria can multiply rapidly in the danger zone of 40 to 140°F (4 to 60°C). Refrigerate perishable foods and leftovers as soon as possible after the meal is finished. Don't cool leftovers first—just divide them into small portions in shallow containers for faster cooling. For safety, discard food that has been sitting at room temperature too long.

Activity: Write a rap or poem describing proper ways of serving food safely.

Activity: Demonstrate how to pack hot food and cold food for a picnic.

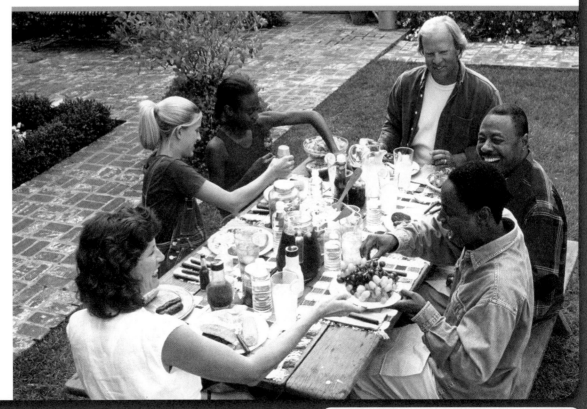

Prevent Accidents!

Accidents in the kitchen often can be prevented—because they're usually caused by carelessness. Take steps to make sure you don't hurt yourself or others when working in the kitchen. Play it safe!

Basic Kitchen Safety Rules

For general safety:

- Don't let hair, jewelry, sleeves, or apron strings dangle. They could catch fire or get tangled in appliances.

- Pay attention to the task you're doing.

- Use the right tool for the job.

To prevent cuts:

- Store knives in a knife block, rack, or special drawer divider.

- Don't soak knives or other sharp utensils in a sink where you may not see them.

- Use a cutting board—don't hold foods in your hand while you cut them.

- Clean up broken glass carefully. Use a broom and dustpan or a wet paper towel.

To prevent bruises, falls, and back injuries:

- Close drawers and cabinet doors after you open them.

- Wipe up spills, spatters, and peelings on the floor immediately.

- Use a sturdy stepstool to reach higher shelves.

- Store heavy items within easy reach. Lift them with care.

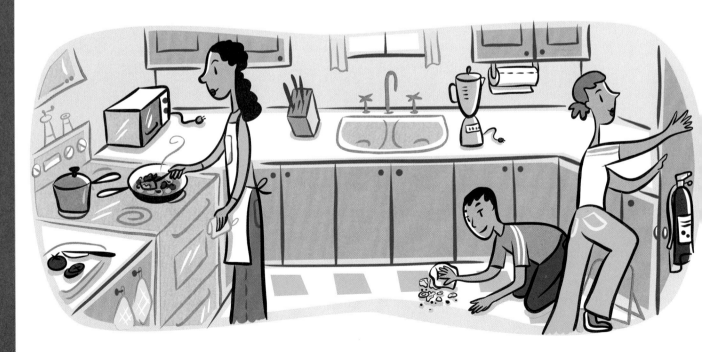

To prevent electrical shock:

• Keep small electrical appliances away from water. Don't use them when your hands are wet or you're standing on a wet surface.

• Keep electrical cords away from the range and other heat sources.

• Unplug small appliances before cleaning them. Don't put any electrical appliance in water unless the label reads "immersible."

• Never insert a fork or other object into a toaster or other electrical appliance.

• Don't plug too many appliances into one outlet.

To prevent burns:

• Keep pot holders and oven mitts within easy reach. Use them whenever you handle hot items. Be sure they're dry.

• Turn the handles of pots and pans toward the inside of the range to prevent accidental spills.

• When lifting the cover of a hot pan, tilt it so the steam flows out the back, away from you.

• If you spill something on a hot appliance, wait until it cools before wiping up the spill.

To prevent fires:

• Keep flammable items, such as paper towels and food packages, away from the range.

• Watch foods while they're cooking on the range.

• Store aerosol cans away from heat.

• Keep a fire extinguisher handy. Make sure you know how to use it.

Activity: Inspect the kitchen at home or school and identify potential safety hazards.

Activity: Working in teams, choose an area of the kitchen. Demonstrate how to practice safety when working with tools, equipment, and food in that area.

To prevent poisoning:

• Store household chemicals—such as detergents and other cleaning products, pest control products, and drain cleaners—away from food and out of children's reach. Keep the chemicals in a locked cabinet, if possible. Be sure containers are clearly labeled.

• Follow label directions when you use household chemicals. Never mix two chemicals together.

Handling Kitchen Emergencies

No matter how careful you are, an accident may still happen. It will be easier to handle if you're prepared.

To prepare yourself for emergencies:

• Keep a list of emergency telephone numbers near each phone. Include the number of the nearest poison control center.

• Keep a first aid kit and book of instructions handy.

• Learn life-saving techniques. Everyone should know how to perform the **Heimlich maneuver**—*a first aid technique for choking*—and **CPR**—*first aid to use when someone's breathing and heartbeat have stopped.* For training, contact your local Red Cross.

In an emergency:

• Stay calm so you can think clearly and respond quickly.

• Call for help if you need to.

• In case of poisoning, immediately call the nearest poison control center. Be ready to report the kind of poison, amount swallowed, when it was swallowed, and any symptoms. Follow the instructions you are given.

Putting Out a Kitchen Fire

Never pour water on a kitchen fire—that would cause grease to spatter and give you serious burns. Here's what to do instead.

For a fire on the range top or in an electric skillet:

1. Turn off the heat.

2. Put the cover on the pan—or pour salt or baking soda on the flames.

For a fire in the oven, broiler, microwave oven, or toaster oven:

1. Turn off or disconnect the appliance.

2. Keep the appliance door closed. The fire will go out when it runs out of oxygen. Make sure nothing else around it can catch fire.

Kitchen Safety for Children

If you're caring for young children, take these extra precautions to prevent accidents in the kitchen.

- Use safety latches on drawers and cabinet doors.
- Always stay with children when they're in the kitchen.
- When children help in the kitchen, set up a sturdy stepstool or child-size table. Give children simple tasks right for their age and abilities, such as stirring or mashing.
- Keep young children away from knives, the range, and appliances with moving parts.
- Set a good example by always following basic kitchen safety rules.

Discuss: What precautions would you have to take in your home to prevent kitchen accidents involving young children?

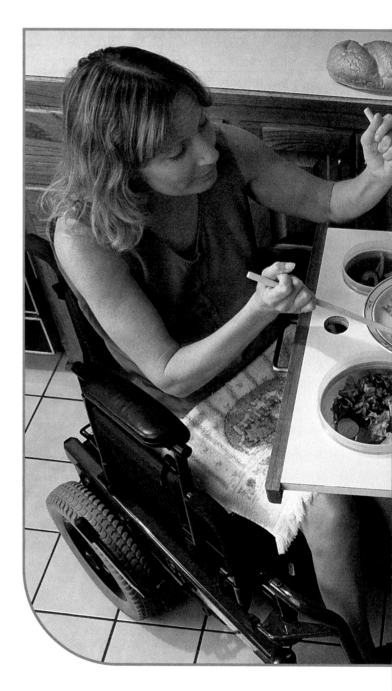

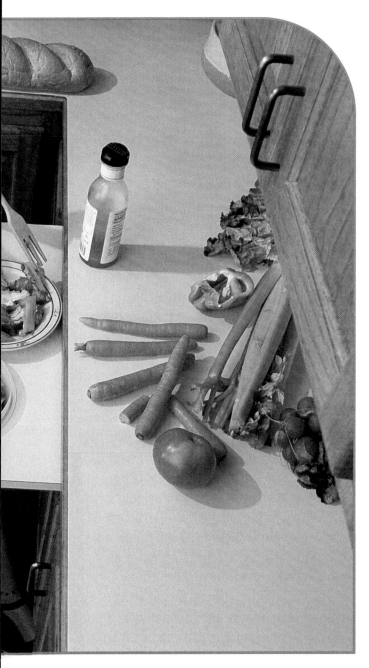

This kitchen work surface is at a convenient height for a seated user. What other features does it offer?

For Those with Physical Challenges

Almost everyone has a physical challenge sometime in life. Think of an elderly person who has trouble seeing, a teen with a broken arm, or someone who uses a wheelchair. What simple changes could make a kitchen safer and more convenient for them? Here are some ideas.

For a person with impaired vision: Add more or better lighting. Relabel food containers in large letters. Make countertop edges and other boundaries more visible with bright, contrasting paint or tape.

For a person with limited hand strength: Replace cabinet door and drawer pulls with large, easy-to-grasp handles. Put suction cups or wet dishcloths under mixing bowls and cutting boards to hold them in place. Attach a looped strap to the refrigerator or oven door handle. Provide a potato masher or other device for turning knobs.

For a person who stands or walks with difficulty: Provide a chair or stool for working while seated. Eliminate throw rugs. Provide a sturdy rolling cart for transporting items.

For a wheelchair user: Store items in accessible places. Provide long tongs for reaching items. Set up a sturdy table or other work surface at wheelchair height. Attach a sturdy wooden tray to the wheelchair for safely transporting hot pans and dishes.

Activity: Find magazine or Internet articles that discuss ways of making the kitchen safe and accessible for physically challenged people.

LOOKING BACK

- Eating food contaminated with large numbers of microorganisms can cause foodborne illness. You can take steps to fight against this problem.

- Keep food safe to eat by handling it right when you shop and when you store it.

- Keep yourself and the kitchen clean to help prevent foodborne illness.

- Control food's temperature from purchasing through serving so bacteria can't thrive.

- You can prevent most kitchen accidents by following basic kitchen safety rules.

UNDERSTANDING KEY IDEAS

1. Define foodborne illness. How can microorganisms cause it?

2. How can you handle refrigerated food safely when you shop?

3. If you were making lunch, when would you need to wash your hands?

4. If you were preparing flounder for dinner, how could you avoid cross-contamination?

5. How would you safely thaw a frozen steak?

6. Name at least five guidelines for handling leftovers safely.

7. How can you prevent cuts in the kitchen?

DEVELOPING LIFE SKILLS

1. **Leadership:** Now that you've learned basic facts about preparing food safely, do you have a responsibility to help others learn them too? Why or why not? What would you do if you were at someone else's home and saw food being handled in ways that aren't safe? Why?

2. **Critical Thinking:** Taylor has invited some friends over for grilled hamburgers. She puts the raw hamburger patties on a plate to carry them outside. She puts the cooked burgers back on the same plate to serve them. What might happen as a result of this practice? What might Taylor have done instead?

Wellness Challenge

Selena and Eric are members of the high school chapter of a national environmental group. The group is holding a benefit concert. Student volunteers will sell food and drinks all day. Eric and Selena know the importance of controlling the temperature of food. They want to make sure that the concert offerings will not be a breeding ground for bacteria.

1. How can Selena and Eric make the student volunteers aware of food safety?

2. What steps for safety can they take?

APPLYING YOUR LEARNING

1. **Quiz Show:** Hold a classroom quiz show. Choose three rules of kitchen safety and rewrite them so they are incorrect. As a class, divide into two teams. When it's your team's turn, read one of your incorrect rules. The other team's goal is to decide why it is incorrect.

2. **Household Safety:** Imagine that you're a newspaper writer working on a kitchen safety article. You want to alert readers to potential hazards in the home. Write your article. Trade with a classmate and edit the work you are given.

EXPLORING FURTHER

1. **Is it Safe?** Raw seafood in the form of sushi is becoming increasingly popular in the United States, but is it safe to eat? Learn more about how you can protect yourself from foodborne illness and still enjoy sushi.

2. **Local Incidents:** Find out about an incident of foodborne illness in your area in the past two years. What type of bacteria caused this illness? Did the problem occur at a restaurant, home, or store? How could it have been avoided? (Hint: call your county health department, check back issues of newspapers, or do Internet research.)

Making CONNECTIONS

1. **Health:** Learn about antibacterial hand soaps. How do they fight bacteria? Are they better at removing bacteria from hands than other soaps? What are some possible disadvantages of these soaps? Present your findings to the class.

2. **Science:** Learn what epidemiologists do. Who employs them? How do they carry out their jobs? What science and other courses would someone need to prepare for this career? Report to the class.

FOODS LAB

Obtain two ripe fruits, such as peaches, nectarines, or strawberries. Label each "Do Not Eat." Put one fruit in a plastic bag on the counter and one in the refrigerator. After 5 days, record the changes in each fruit. What can you conclude about bacterial growth?

PART 2

Kitchen Equipment

Objectives

After studying pages 463-477, you will be able to:

- Identify and explain the uses of some basic kitchen tools.

- Distinguish between different items of cookware and their uses.

- Explain the use and care of basic kitchen appliances.

- Describe how to organize a kitchen for efficiency.

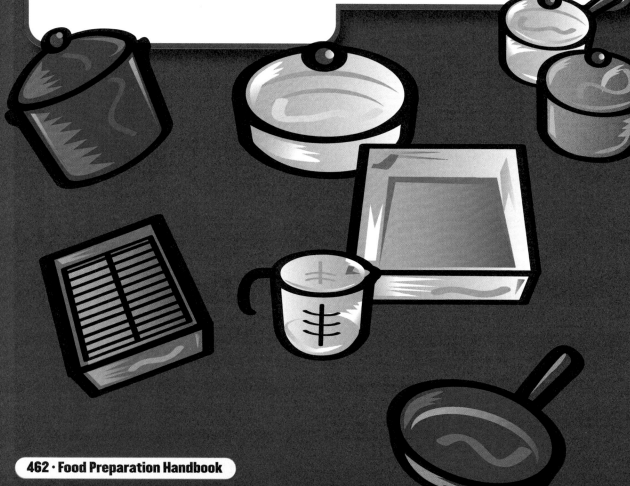

Kitchen Tools

Having the right tool for the job helps you prepare foods easily and successfully. A few tools are essential, while others are useful but not necessary. You have a tremendous variety of kitchen tools to choose from. Most of the basics are relatively inexpensive.

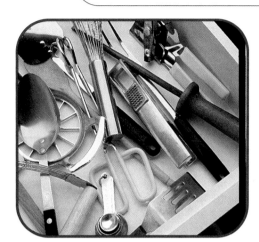

Measuring Tools

Because measuring tools have standardized sizes, they help you accurately measure the amounts called for in recipes. You can buy equipment for customary units of measure (those most commonly used in the United States) or metric units (those used in most other parts of the world).

Activity: List the kinds and amount of foods you would measure with each tool.

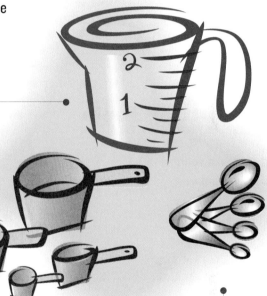

Liquid measuring cup.
Made of glass or plastic. Extra space at the top lets you carry liquids without spilling. Has a spout for easy pouring. Usually marked with both customary and metric measurements. Comes in I cup (250 mL), 2 cup (500 mL), and other sizes.

INFOLINK

You'll learn more about <u>units of measurement</u> in Section 3-1 of the Food Preparation Handbook.

Dry measuring cups.
Used to measure dry and solid ingredients. A basic customary set includes I cup, ½ cup, ⅓ cup, and ¼ cup sizes. A metric set includes 250 mL, 125 mL, and 50 mL sizes.

Measuring spoons. Used to measure small amounts of liquid and dry ingredients. Most customary sets include I tablespoon, I teaspoon, ½ teaspoon, and ¼ teaspoon sizes. A metric set includes 25 mL, 15 mL, 5 mL, 2 mL, and I mL sizes.

Knives

Properly sharpened knives cut better and cause fewer accidents.
Each type of knife has its special use.

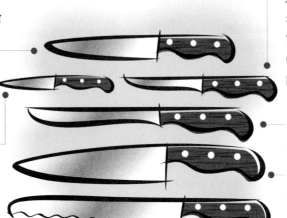

Utility knife. **All-**purpose knife used to cut and slice many foods.

Paring knife. **Used** to peel, cut, and slice small fruits and vegetables.

Bread knife. **Has a** **serrated,** or *sawtooth,* edge that makes cutting bread and cake easy.

Boning knife. **Has a** strong tip and narrow, flexible blade to make it easy to separate meat or poultry from the bone.

Slicing knife. **Used to** slice meat and poultry.

Chef's knife. **Used for** cutting, slicing, and chopping.

Teaching With Visuals: Identify the knives you are familiar with and describe how you have used them.

Other Cutting Tools

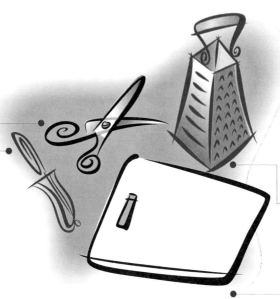

Kitchen shears. Used for tasks such as cutting dried fruit, parsley, or chives, or snipping skin from poultry.

Peeler. Used to remove a thin outer layer from vegetables and fruits.

Activity: Show students how to properly sharpen kitchen knives. Then have students demonstrate that they know how to use the technique safely.

INFOLINK

The meaning of food preparation terms is explained in Part 3 of the Food Preparation Handbook.

Grater. **Used to shred** cheese, potatoes, and carrots and to grate citrus peel and nutmeg.

Cutting board. **Comes** in a variety of sizes. Protects the counter or table while you're cutting.

Mixing Equipment

Pastry blender. **U**-shaped wires capped with handle. Used to cut fat into flour for making pastry dough.

Rotary beater. **Used to** blend, whip, and beat ingredients more quickly than using a spoon or whisk.

Wire whisk. **Flexible wires held together by the handle. Used to blend, stir, and beat. Whisks with a rounder, bulb-like shape can be used to beat egg whites.**

Sifter. **A container with a blade that forces dry ingredients, such as flour, through a fine wire screen. Used to get rid of lumps or to mix dry ingredients thoroughly.**

Mixing spoon. **Used to mix, beat, and stir.**

Mixing bowls. **Can be made of glass, plastic, or metal. Often sold in sets of different sizes.**

Activity: Beat eggs with each of the following: mixing spoon, wire whisk, rotary beater. Which tool do you think is most effective? Why?

Cooking and Baking Tools

Teaching with Visuals: Display each of the cooking and baking tools shown here. Call on volunteers to demonstrate how to use each tool.

Utility fork. Has long, strong tines that aid in lifting or carving roasts and turning steaks or chops.

Meat thermometer. Used to measure the internal temperature of meats and poultry for food safety.

Tongs. Used to turn foods or to transfer them to another container.

Slotted spoon. Used to lift solid pieces of food from cooking liquid or sauce.

Basting spoon. Large, shallow spoon with long handle used to baste, stir, and spoon up sauces.

Ladle. Used to spoon soup or stew from cooking pan to serving bowl.

Colander. Used for draining liquid from foods such as cooked pasta.

INFOLINK

Read about other types of meat thermometers on page 454.

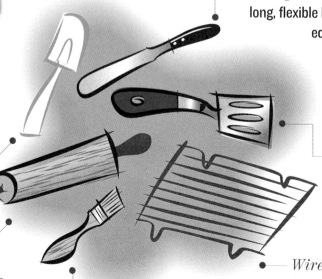

Rubber scraper. Has a flat, flexible blade. Used to scrape batter and other foods from containers. Also used to fold one ingredient into another.

Rolling pin. Used to roll out pastry, biscuit, or cookie dough.

Pastry brush. Used to brush sauces or glazes on food.

Straight-edge spatula. Has a long, flexible blade with straight, dull edges. Used to level off ingredients when measuring, loosen baked goods from pans, and frost baked foods.

Turner. Used for turning foods such as fried eggs and pancakes and to remove food from baking sheets.

Wire racks. Used as place to cool cookies and other foods.

Cookware

Cookware refers to *the wide variety of pots and pans used for cooking and baking.* Today, the sizes and types of cookware available are almost limitless. Many different materials are used, including aluminum, stainless steel, cast iron, glass-ceramic, heat-resistant glass, enamel, and ceramic. Many types of pots and pans are available with a non-stick finish. The best cookware heats evenly and is durable and easy to clean.

Cookware for the Range

Saucepans. **Have one long handle. Come in various sizes, usually with covers. Used for cooking foods on top of the range.**

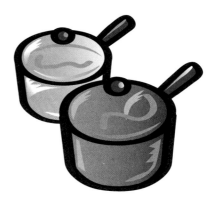

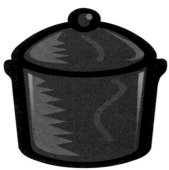

Pots. **Have two small handles and are generally larger than saucepans. Come in various sizes, usually with covers. Used for cooking foods on the range. Some can be used in the oven, too.**

Skillets. **Also called frying pans. More shallow than a pot or saucepan; may have slanted sides. Some come with covers. Size is usually measured by the diameter. Used for browning and frying foods.**

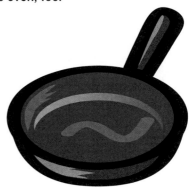

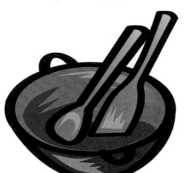

Wok. **A pan designed for stir-frying. Deeper than a skillet. Slanted sides are wider at the top than the bottom, which may be rounded or flat.**

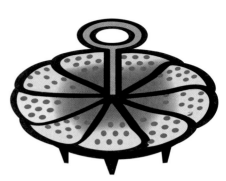

Steamer basket. Used for steaming foods, such as vegetables. It's inserted in a saucepan to hold the food above the boiling water. Small holes allow steam to pass through to cook the food.

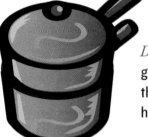

Double boiler. A two-part saucepan for gently heating delicate foods without burning them. Boiling water in the lower compartment heats food in the upper compartment.

Casserole dishes. Covered or uncovered containers used for baking mixed dishes and some desserts. Usually made of heat-resistant glass, pottery, or ceramic. Measured by quart or liter size.

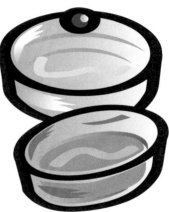

More About Cookware: Cast-iron cookware was first used in China over 3,000 years ago. Cast-iron cookware is strong and inexpensive and adds iron to the food that is being cooked.

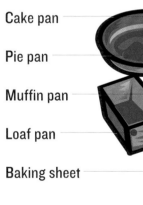

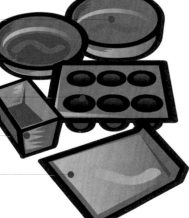

Cake pan

Pie pan

Muffin pan

Loaf pan

Baking sheet

Baking pans. Usually made of metal or heat-resistant glass. Come in a wide variety of shapes and sizes.

Roasting pan. Shallow pan used for roasting meat and poultry. Usually has a rack on the bottom to keep meat separate from its juices.

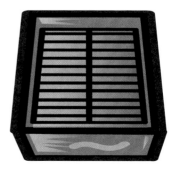

Cookware for the Microwave Oven

You can use many kinds of containers in the microwave oven, including some that can't be used in a conventional oven. Other materials, however, aren't meant for microwaving—they could get damaged, damage the oven, or even start a fire. Play it safe—know your microwave-safe materials!

Activity: Make a display of items, categorizing those that are safe to use in the microwave oven and those that are not safe to use.

Safe for Microwaving

- Heat-resistant glass containers such as casserole dishes, baking dishes, and liquid measuring cups
- Cookware especially designed for microwave oven use
- Plastic items labeled microwave-safe
- Paper plates and towels labeled microwave-safe

Not for Microwaving

- Metal cookware
- Aluminum foil (except small amounts used according to the instructions for the oven)
- Pottery with metallic glazes
- Plastic containers from dairy foods and take-out foods
- Brown bags
- Products made of recycled paper
- Wooden containers
- Straw baskets or plates
- Materials containing synthetic fibers, such as nylon or polyester

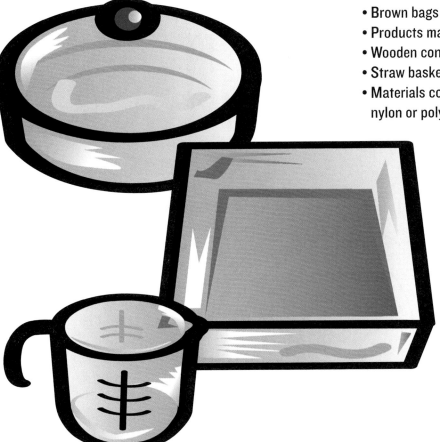

Appliances

Appliances bring convenience to the kitchen. Knowing some basic facts about them will help you put them to the best use!

Appliance Choices

Major appliances are large items such as ranges and refrigerator-freezers. The choices range from basic models to ones with all sorts of special features. Are these features worth the extra cost? That depends on your needs—and your budget.

Small appliances are portable items such as toasters, electric mixers, and waffle irons. Most perform specialized jobs, so choose them based on your needs. Weigh the cost of the appliance against how often you'll use it.

If you're shopping for appliances, take the time to compare prices and learn about the features of different models. Find out whether there's a warranty and what it covers. Look for a UL seal on electrical appliances or an AGA seal on gas appliances. These seals indicate that the product meets standards for safety and performance.

Safe Use and Care

Before using any appliance, read the owner's manual carefully. It will help you understand how the appliance works and how to use it with safety and energy efficiency in mind. You'll also learn what features the appliance offers and how to get the most benefits from it. Keep the owner's manual for later reference.

Discuss: Visit a local store and look for the safety seals on appliances. Report your findings to the class.

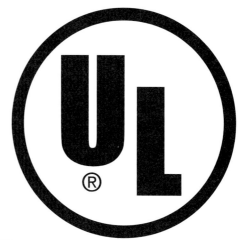

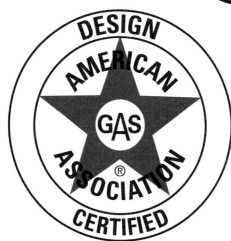

> **INFOLINK**
>
> For more about safety when using electrical appliances, see Section 1-5.

The Refrigerator-Freezer

Refrigerator-freezers keep perishable and frozen foods fresh and safe. Most refrigerator-freezers have two outer doors—one for the refrigerator compartment and the other for the freezer.

Activity: Use a refrigerator-freezer thermometer to check the temperature settings for the refrigerators and/or freezers in your homes as well as the ones in the foods lab. How many appliances are set properly?

Temperature. **Use a refrigerator-freezer thermometer to check the temperature in each compartment. For food safety, the refrigerator temperature should be between 32 and 40°F (0 and 4°C). Don't let it fall below 32°F (0°C). If possible, keep the temperature of the freezer at 0°F (-18°C) or less.**

Care tips. **If something inside the refrigerator-freezer spills or leaks, clean it up right away to prevent bacteria from multiplying. Regularly wipe the inside of the refrigerator with a solution of baking soda and water. If the freezer is not self-defrosting, defrost it when ¼ to ½ inch (6 to 13 mm) of ice has formed inside the freezer compartment. The owner's manual will tell you how.**

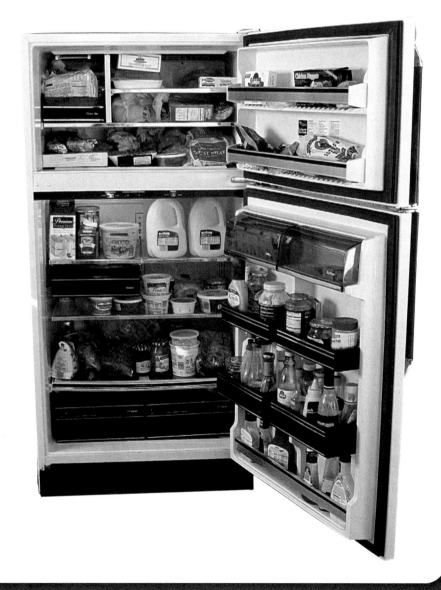

Major Cooking Appliances

In many kitchens, a range—gas or electric—is the main cooking appliance. It includes a cooktop, broiler, and at least one oven. In other kitchens, these components are separate items built into cabinets or walls, or portable models that sit on a countertop.

❶ *Cooktop.* A basic model has four heating units. These may be gas burners, electric coils, or various kinds of heating units hidden under a smooth surface. Controls for each unit let you adjust the heat from low to high.

❷ *Broiler.* The broiler lets you cook food by direct heat from above. In many broilers you don't adjust the level of heat. Instead, you adjust how far from the heat you place the food. Gas ranges usually have a separate broiler compartment. With an electric range, the oven compartment is used for broiling. Most electric ranges require that you leave the oven door slightly open when broiling food. Check the owner's manual for details.

❸ *Conventional oven.* Air inside a conventional oven is heated by gas or electricity. The hot air circulates naturally and cooks the food. The oven control lets you set an exact temperature.

Convection oven. This type of oven works like a conventional oven, except that a fan helps circulate the heated air. It cooks faster and more evenly than a conventional oven.

❹ *Microwave oven.* A microwave oven cooks faster than a conventional or convection oven, and therefore can save energy. Since microwaves don't heat the whole oven compartment, the kitchen stays cool.

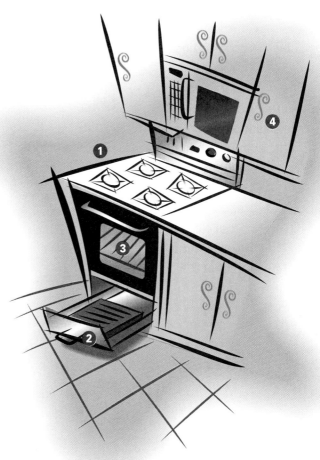

INFOLINK

To learn how a microwave oven heats food, turn to Section 4-2 in the Food Preparation Handbook.

Activity: Imagine you are an appliance designer. What feature would you like to see in a major cooking appliance? Describe what it is, how it works, and how it improves the appliance.

Small Cooking Appliances

At times you can use small appliances to do some of the same jobs as a range. Here are some examples.

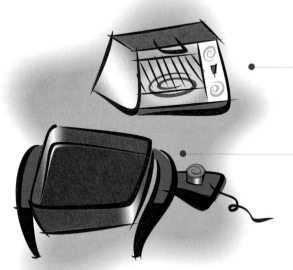

Toaster oven. Can toast, bake, and top-brown small amounts of food. Some models can also be used for broiling.

Electric skillet. Can fry, simmer, steam, roast, and bake. Has a temperature control.

Critical Thinking: At what age do you think children should be allowed to use each of the major and small cooking appliances listed on pages 472-473? What criteria should be used in determining the age?

Slow cooker. Cooks foods such as soups and stews at a low temperature over many hours. You can safely let it cook food all day while you're away from home.

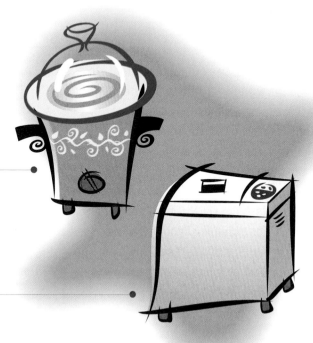

Breadmaker. Automatically mixes dough, lets it rise, and bakes loaves of bread.

Mixing and Cutting Appliances

Small appliances can make mixing and cutting jobs go more quickly and easily. Here are some of the more commonly used ones.

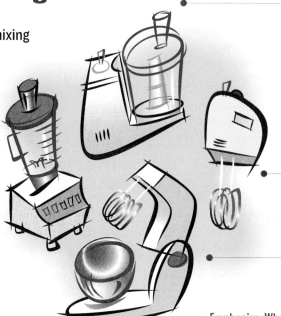

Food processor. Used to slice, grate, shred, chop, grind, and mix a wide variety of ingredients. Can also be used to knead dough.

Blender. Used for blending and liquefying foods. Can also grate, chop, and mince. Choices range from simple, two-speed types to ones with variable speeds.

Mixer. Mixes and beats ingredients. Lightweight, hand-held models and heavy-duty models attached to a stand are available.

Emphasize: When people follow energy-saving tips, they use less electricity, thereby decreasing the pollution.

Saving Energy

Appliances can save time and human energy, but they use energy from electricity or gas in the process. Following these energy-saving tips will lower your fuel bills—and help cut down on pollution, too!

- Keep the refrigerator or freezer door open for as short a time as possible.
- Keep the freezer full. In the refrigerator, allow enough room for air to circulate between items.
- Open the oven door as little as possible during oven cooking.
- When possible, bake several food items in the oven at one time. For example, if you're baking a meat loaf, take advantage of the remaining oven space to cook a vegetable dish and baked potatoes.
- On the range top, match the pan size to the size of the heating element.
- If you're cooking a small amount of food, consider using a small appliance. Instead of turning on a full-size oven just to bake one potato, use a microwave oven or toaster oven.

Refrigerator-Freezer
Capacity: 23 Cubic Feet

(Name of Corporation)
Model(s) AH503, AH504, AH507
Type of Defrost: Full Automatic

ENERGYGUIDE

Estimates on the scale based on a national average electric rate of 4.97¢ per kilowatt hour.

Only models with 2.5 to 22.4 cubic feet are compared in the scale

$91

Model with lowest energy cost
$68

THIS ▼ MODEL

Model with highest energy cost
$132

Estimated yearly energy cost

Your cost will vary depending on your local energy rate and how you use the product This energy cost is based on U.S. Government standard rates

How much will this model cost you to run yearly?

		Yearly cost
		Estimated yearly $ cost shown below
Cost per kilowatt hour	2¢	$36
	4¢	$73
	6¢	$109
	8¢	$146
	10¢	$182
	12¢	$218

Ask your salesperson or local utility for the energy rate (cost per kilowatt hour) in your area.

The Energy Guide label can help you buy an efficient appliance.

Organizing the Kitchen

A well-organized kitchen can save you time and energy in food preparation and cleanup tasks. You can organize storage and work areas to make the best use of whatever kitchen you have!

The imaginary lines that connect the three basic work centers form the work triangle. In an efficient work triangle, the three sides total 12 to 22 feet (4 to 7 meters).

Activity: Design a floor plan for the "ideal" kitchen. Display in class.

Work Centers

How can an organized kitchen help you work efficiently? The key is to store equipment and supplies where they'll be handy. Start by identifying **work centers**—*areas of the kitchen devoted to specific tasks.* Then store the items used for each task in or near the center where you'll use them.

The organization of work centers can vary, depending on the layout of the kitchen and the needs of the people who use it. The chart here describes three work centers that are basic to most kitchens. Can you think of other activities and items that might go with each work center? What other work centers might a kitchen have?

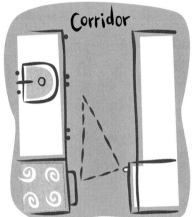
Corridor

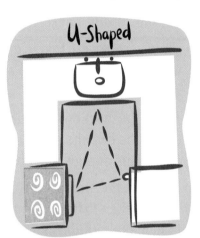
U-Shaped

Basic Kitchen Work Centers

WORK CENTER	LOCATION	ACTIVITIES	ITEMS TO STORE THERE
Cold Storage Center	Around the refrigerator-freezer	• Storing groceries • Storing leftovers	• Food storage containers • Foil, plastic wrap, and bags
Cooking Center	Around the range	• Cooking food	• Pots and pans • Cooking tools such as turners, ladles, and tongs • Small cooking appliances • Pot holders and oven mitts
Cleanup Center	Around the sink	• Washing fresh fruits and vegetables • Rinsing and washing dishes	• Vegetable brush, colander, peeler • Soaps, detergents • Dishtowels, dishcloths, other cleaning supplies

LOOKING BACK

- To prepare foods easily and successfully, use the right kitchen tools for measuring, cutting, mixing, cooking, and baking.

- Choose cookware that is appropriate for use on the range or in the microwave oven.

- To get the most out of your appliances, follow the owner's manual and keep safety and energy efficiency in mind.

- Organize the storage and work areas in your kitchen to help save time and energy in food preparation and cleanup tasks.

UNDERSTANDING KEY IDEAS

1. If you were preparing potatoes for potato salad, what kitchen tools would you use? Explain the purpose of each.

2. What are the similarities among saucepans, pots, and skillets? What are the differences?

3. What types of cookware are safe to use in the microwave oven? What types are not?

4. Imagine that your family just purchased a new refrigerator-freezer. What steps would you take to use and care for it?

5. What are work centers? How can they help you organize a kitchen for efficiency?

DEVELOPING LIFE SKILLS

1. **Critical Thinking:** If you could have only one of the following small cooking appliances, which one would you choose: toaster oven, electric skillet, slow cooker, or breadmaker? Why?

2. **Leadership:** Brianna is concerned about her family's refrigerator. Her younger brothers open the refrigerator door frequently and sometimes forget to close it. If they spill something inside the refrigerator, they don't always clean it up. It's packed with both new items and old leftovers, none of which seem cold enough. How can Brianna use leadership skills to help her family improve the safety and energy efficiency of the refrigerator?

Wellness Challenge

Kim's grandfather is having surgery and will be on a soft food diet for awhile. Kim wants to help out by preparing meals for him. She plans on making pureed vegetables, fruit sorbets, milkshakes and fruit smoothies, and nutritious soups.

1. What equipment might Kim need to make the foods she is planning?
2. What challenges might Kim face?
3. How can Kim meet those challenges?

APPLYING YOUR LEARNING

1. **Organization Is Key:** Imagine that you are a kitchen planner. You have been hired to design a kitchen in a new home. Draw a floor plan for the new kitchen. Locate the work centers and list items that the owners could store in each one. Include a summary describing why your plan is efficient.

2. **Tools of the Trade:** Find four recipes that require measuring, cutting, mixing, and cooking or baking. Explain which tools you would use for the tasks in the recipes and why. Make a three-column chart showing the task, the tool you would choose, and the reason for your choice.

EXPLORING FURTHER

1. **Then and Now:** Interview an elderly relative or friend. Find out what kitchen tools, cookware, and appliances were used in the past. How did these items affect the types of foods that were prepared? Report your findings to the class.

2. **Major Purchase:** Imagine that you are helping a relative purchase a new microwave oven. Research available models. Compare features, prices, and warranties. Which model would you purchase? Why?

Making CONNECTIONS

1. **Math:** Suppose you are comparison shopping for refrigerators. One sells for $700. The Energy Guide Label lists the operating cost as $100 a year. The second choice sells for $500 and costs $150 a year. Which refrigerator is a better buy if you keep it for 15 years? Why?

2. **Technology:** Find out which appliances today use microprocessors or computer chips. How does technology enable appliances to perform advanced functions? Are these appliances more efficient than those that do not use computers? If so, how?

FOODS LAB

Find a recipe that requires mixing and cutting. Prepare two samples. For one, use hand tools, such as a mixing spoon or rotary beater and a knife or peeler. For the other, use small appliances, such as a blender or food processor. Compare the two methods. What are the advantages and disadvantages of each? Which method did you prefer? Why?

Skills for Preparing Food

Objectives

After studying pages 479-505, you will be able to:

- Explain equivalent units of measure.

- Adjust recipes to change the yield.

- Measure ingredients accurately.

- Explain terms and techniques related to cutting, mixing, and cooking ingredients.

- Give guidelines for using a microwave oven properly.

- Describe management skills for working efficiently in the kitchen.

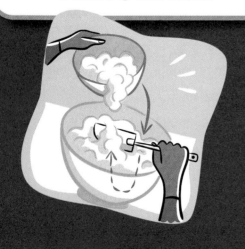

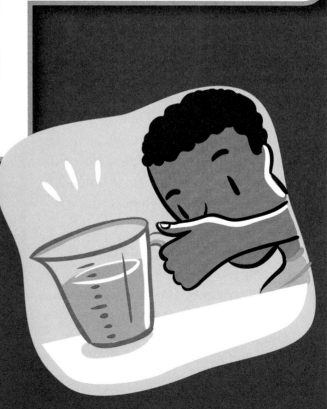

SECTION 3-1

Recipe and Math Skills

Look for these TERMS
- yield
- customary measurement system
- metric system

Recipes give you instructions for preparing certain foods or dishes. For good results, read and interpret recipes accurately, measure ingredients correctly, and understand the terms used in food preparation.

What a Recipe Tells You

Although recipes are written differently, most have the same basic information. Look for:

1. Ingredients and amounts. In a well-written recipe, these are listed in order of use.
2. Any pre-preparation needed. For example, in this recipe the cheese needs to be shredded before measuring.
3. The preparation steps.
4. The temperature and time of cooking.
5. The **yield**—*the amount the recipe makes.*
6. Information about nutrients and calories. Not all recipes provide this.

INFOLINK

For more about recipes and food preparation choices, see Chapter 14.

Activity: Choose a favorite recipe and identify any parts of the recipe that are missing.

Maple Baked Beans

(1)
- 2 12-oz. cans vegetarian baked beans
- ½ cup maple-flavored syrup
- ⅓ cup chopped onion
- ¼ cup ketchup
- 1 Tbsp. prepared mustard
- ¼ cup shredded (2) low-fat cheddar cheese (optional)

(3)
Preheat oven to 350°F. (4)
Mix all ingredients together. Pour into a greased casserole dish.
Bake, uncovered for 30 minutes or longer. (4)
Sprinkle cheddar cheese (optional) on top for the last ten minutes, baking until cheese is melted. Serve warm.
Yield: 6 (½-cup) servings (5)
Nutrition information per serving: 156 calories, 1g fat, 9g fiber (6)

Units of Measure

The amount of an ingredient may be given by:

- Volume, or how much space it takes up.

- Weight, or how heavy it is.

- A number of items, such as 2 bananas.

Critical Thinking: Find recipes in magazines or newspapers. Based on the information presented in the text, would you use the recipe? Why or why not?

The **customary measurement system** is *the system of measurement most commonly used in the United States.* The **metric system**, *based on multiples of 10,* is the system used in most countries.

Critical Thinking: What is the difference between an ounce and a fluid ounce?

Equivalent Measures

CUSTOMARY UNITS	CUSTOMARY EQUIVALENTS	APPROXIMATE METRIC EQUIVALENTS
Volume		
I teaspoon (tsp. or t.)		5 milliliters (mL)
I Tablespoon (Tbsp. or T.)	3 tsp.	I5 mL
I fluid ounce (fl. oz.)	2 Tbsp.	30 mL
¼ cup (C. or c.)		50 mL
⅓ cup		75 mL
½ cup		I25 mL
⅔ cup		I50 mL
¾ cup		I75 mL
I cup	8 fl. oz. or I6 Tbsp.	250 mL
I pint (pt.)	2 cups or I6 fl. oz.	500 mL
I quart (qt.)	2 pt. or 4 cups or 32 fl. oz.	I,000 mL or I liter (L)
I gallon	4 qt. or 8 pt. or I28 fl. oz.	4 L
Weight		
I ounce (oz.)		28 grams (g)
I pound (lb.)	I6 oz.	500 g
2 lb.	32 oz.	I,000 g or I kilogram (kg)

Changing the Yield

You may want to change a recipe's yield to make more or fewer servings. Here's how.

1. Decide how many servings you want. This is called the desired yield.

2. Use the following formula:
   desired yield ÷ original yield = "magic number"

3. Change each amount:
   original amount × "magic number" = new amount

Activity: Choose a recipe and double the yield, using metric measurements. Use the formula to determine the "magic number."

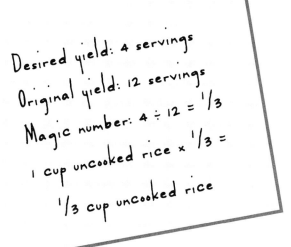

Desired yield: 4 servings

Original yield: 12 servings

Magic number: $4 \div 12 = 1/3$

1 cup uncooked rice $\times 1/3 =$

$1/3$ cup uncooked rice

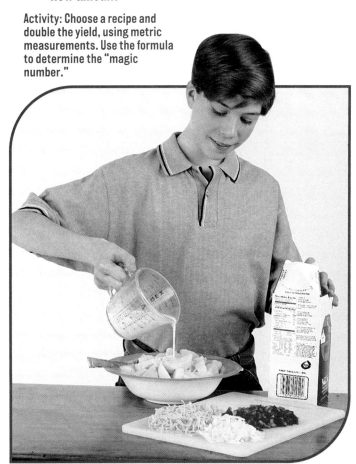

Tips for Changing the Yield

- Use the Equivalent Measures chart to convert hard-to-measure amounts, such as ⅛ cup, into easier ones, such as 2 tablespoons.
- Before you start to prepare the recipe, write down all the new amounts.
- For most casserole, stew, soup, and salad recipes, using exact amounts is often unnecessary. You can round them off if needed.
- For baked goods such as breads and cakes, using exact amounts is more critical. Instead of decreasing the yield, consider making the whole recipe and freezing portions of it.
- Remember to make changes in equipment sizes, too.

Some recipes are flexible, making it easier to change the ingredient amounts. If you want to change the yield for those recipes, what should you do?

Following a Recipe

Have you ever made chili that was too spicy or cookies that burned? What happened? Beginning cooks may make mistakes, but you can be successful if you follow recipes carefully. Here's how.

- Read the recipe carefully before you start. Is it clear and complete? Find out the meaning of unfamiliar terms. If the steps confuse you, choose another recipe.
- Assemble all the ingredients and equipment. Then you'll know if you have everything.
- If you're missing an ingredient, check the emergency substitution chart found in many cookbooks. Can you substitute an ingredient you have on hand? If not, you may need to shop for ingredients or find a new recipe.
- Measure carefully. This is especially true for many baked goods.

- Use the equipment named in the recipe. If a recipe calls for an 8-inch square pan, using an II- x 7-inch pan will give a different result!
- If you're a beginning cook, follow the recipe exactly. After you have gained experience, you can vary recipes to suit your needs and tastes.
- Reread the recipe as you work to be sure you didn't leave out anything.
- Pay attention to the signs of doneness. Checking meat, poultry, and fish with a meat thermometer helps ensure food safety.

Discuss: Why might a person change a recipe? (to account for the number of people, to reduce fat or sodium, to add fruit, vegetables, fiber, or flavor) Share experiences and give reasons for the changes.

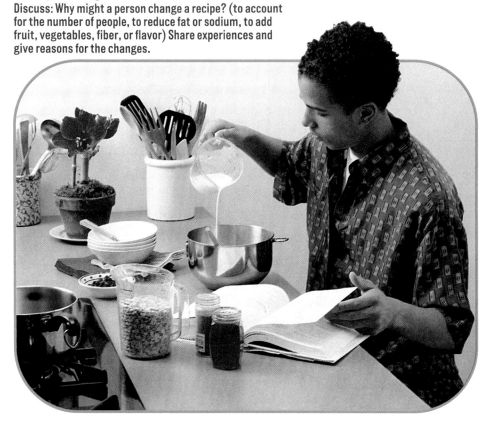

The first time you prepare a new dish, follow the recipe to produce good results. Then if you prefer, the next time you can personalize it. What recipes have you adapted to suit your own tastes?

Measuring Skills

Recipe success depends on accurate measuring. Use these methods to make sure your amounts measure up!

Measuring Liquids

- Use a glass or clear plastic measuring cup. Set the cup on level surface.
- Bend down to check the measurement at eye level.
- Fill the cup to the desired marking.

Activity: Practice measuring liquids in groups of three. One student fills a cup of water to ¼ cup, ⅜ cup, and ¾ cup. Have a second student read each measurement by looking down into the cup and have a third read the measurement at eye level. Compare the two readings.

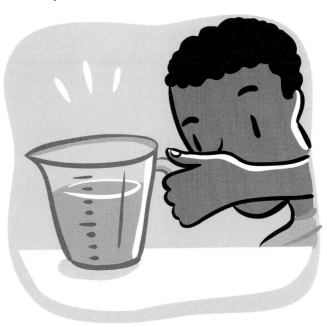

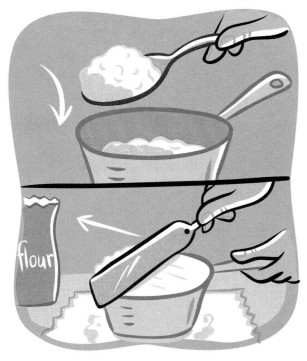

Measuring Dry Ingredients

Flour and white sugar are examples of dry ingredients.

- Use a dry measure or a measuring spoon. Choose the exact size for the amount you need.
- Spoon in lightly. Overfill slightly. Some recipes call for sifted flour. If so, sift the flour before measuring.
- Level off with a straight-edge spatula or the back of a knife.

Teaching With Visuals: Ask volunteers to demonstrate the proper way to measure dry ingredients.

Measuring Brown Sugar or Shortening

- Use a dry measure or measuring spoon. Choose the exact size for the amount you need.

- Pack in firmly by pressing with a rubber scraper or the back of a spoon. Leave no air holes.

- Fill level with the rim.

Discuss: Ask students to compare the method for measuring white sugar with the method for measuring brown sugar.

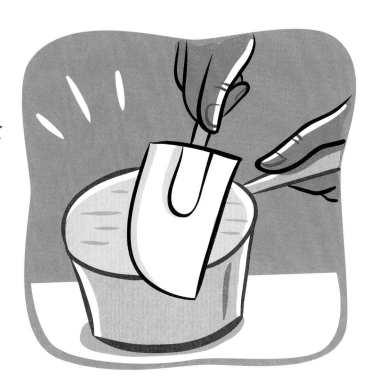

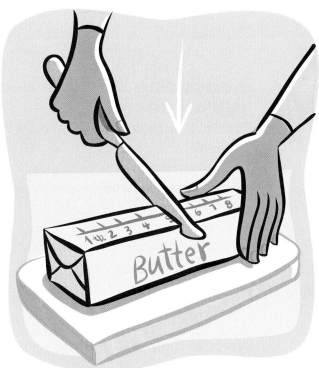

Measuring Stick Butter or Margarine

- Use the markings on the wrapper.

- Cut off the desired amount with a knife.

More About Measuring Fats: Another way of measuring fat is the water-displacement method, using a liquid measuring cup. Subtract the amount of fat needed from one cup. The difference is the amount of water to pour into the cup. To measure ½ cup of shortening, use ½ cup of water. Spoon the fat into the cup. When the water reaches the 1-cup level, you have the right amount of fat.

Cutting Skills

The words *chop*, *cube*, and *dice* all refer to cutting, but each one has a different meaning. By learning the terms and practicing a variety of cutting skills, your recipes will take shape!

chop To cut food with an up-and-down motion into small irregular pieces. *Also see mince.*

core To cut out the center part of a food, as to core an apple.

cube To cut into small square pieces that are ½ inch (or larger) on a side. *Also see dice.*

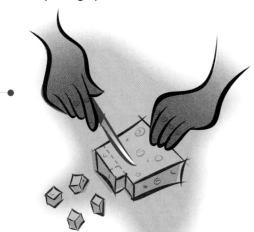

cut To divide food into pieces with a knife or scissors.

dice To cut into small square pieces that are ¼ inch (or less) on a side. *Also see cube.*

flake To break up a food into small pieces with a fork, as with canned tuna.

grate To break up food into small particles by rubbing over a rough surface, such as a grater, as with cheese or lemon peel. *Also see shred.*

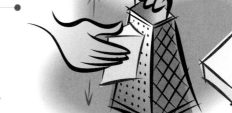

grind To reduce by crushing or cutting, usually in a food chopper. Meat is tenderized by grinding.

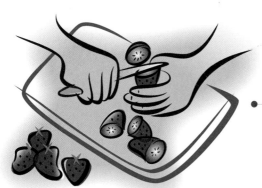

hull To remove the stem or outer covering of certain fruits and vegetables, such as strawberries.

Emphasize: When cutting food with a knife: keep fingers away from the sharp edge and never cut with the blade facing your body.

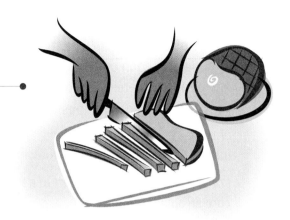

julienne To cut into thin matchlike strips, as with cheese or cooked meat.

mash To make a food soft and smooth by crushing or beating, as with cooked potatoes.

mince To cut with an up-and-down motion into very fine pieces, as with garlic or onion. *Also see chop.*

pare To cut off the outside skin or peel with a knife or other sharp tool, as with potatoes or apples. *Also see scrape.*

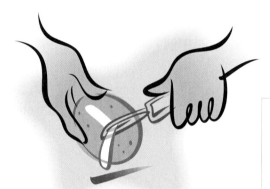

peel To strip off the outside skin or peel, as with oranges. Peeling may be done with the fingers.

pit To remove seeds or stones from fruit.

puree To force cooked food through a sieve, food mill, or strainer to make pulp, as with applesauce. Pureeing can also be done in a blender or food processor.

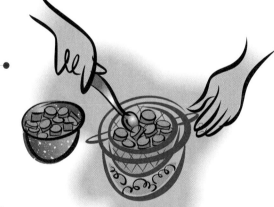

Activity: Provide a variety of vegetables and toppings for salads. Ask students to demonstrate cutting methods.

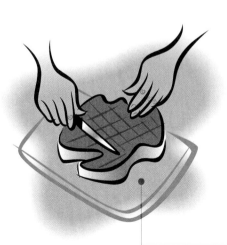

quarter To cut into four even pieces, as with round fruit.

score To cut the surface lightly with straight lines, as with ham.

scrape To remove the outside skin with a vegetable peeler, as with carrots. *Also see pare.*

section To separate the segments of a fruit from each other and from the fruit's membrane and skin, as with oranges or grapefruit.

shred To cut or tear into thin strips or pieces, as by grating cheese or by tearing salad greens with the hands. *Also see grate.*

slice To cut into thin, flat pieces, as with cucumbers. Food can be sliced straight up and down or on a slant.

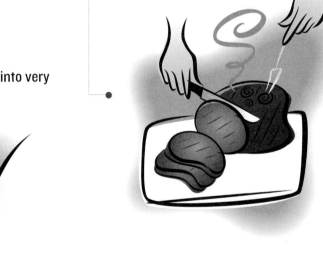

sliver To cut into long, thin pieces, as with almonds.

snip To cut with scissors or a knife into very small pieces, as with chives.

wedge To cut into a triangular shape, as with fruit, meat, or vegetables.

Activity: Find recipes that include various cutting techniques. Have students demonstrate.

Mixing Skills

Do you know why it's important to whip cream instead of stir it? Mixing ingredients properly is essential to a tasty finished product.

beat To make a mixture smooth either by using a brisk over-and-over motion with a spoon or a wire whisk or by using a rotary motion with an electric or hand mixer. *Also see blend, whip.*

blend To combine two or more ingredients until they are soft and smooth. *Also see beat.*

cream To soften a fat with a spoon or mixer, either before or while mixing it with another food (usually sugar), to make the mixture light and fluffy.

cut in To distribute solid fat in small pieces evenly through dry ingredients, using two knives, a fork, or a pastry blender in a cutting motion.

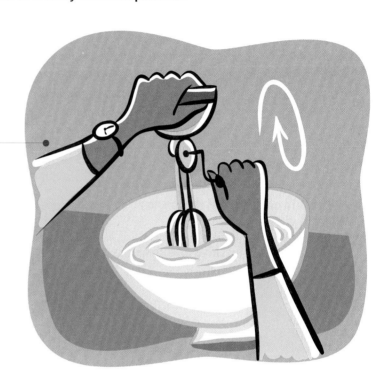

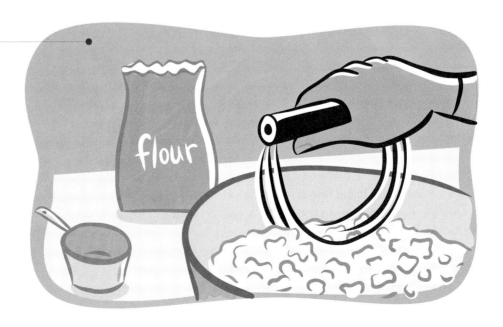

fold **To blend delicate ingredients, such as egg whites, gently using two motions, one to cut vertically through the mixture and the other to turn the mixture over. The bowl is rotated one-quarter and the procedure is repeated until the entire mixture has been lightly blended.**

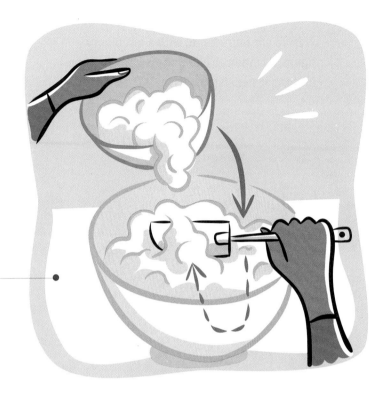

knead **To work dough with the hands by repeatedly folding, pressing, and turning it.**

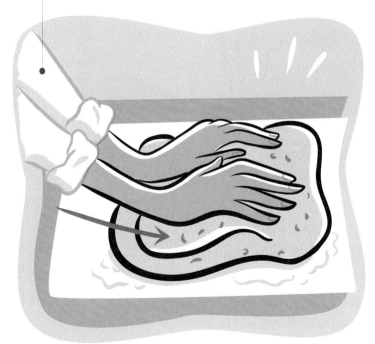

mix **To combine ingredients in any way that causes an even distribution of the ingredients.**

sift **To put dry ingredients through a flour sifter or fine sieve.**

Activity: Have students create a crossword puzzle, using the mixing terms and their definitions. Have students share and complete the puzzles.

stir To mix ingredients with a circular or figure-8 motion to blend them or make them uniform in consistency.

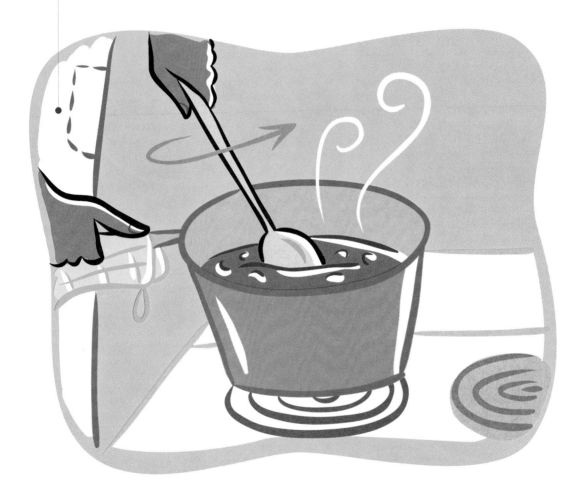

toss To mix ingredients lightly with a fork and spoon, as with salad greens.

whip To beat rapidly to incorporate air and increase volume, as with egg whites or whipped cream. *Also see beat.*

Microwave Skills

The microwave oven has become an important kitchen appliance! You can defrost, heat, reheat, and cook foods in a microwave oven. Microwaving is speedy and convenient. In many cases, you can save energy and nutrients because cooking time is short. Microwaving can reduce cleanup time, too. Microwave ovens do not give off heat, so the kitchen stays cool. Microwave ovens cook by vibrating food molecules.

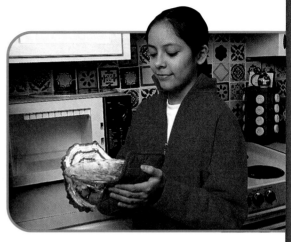

Microwave ovens offer the convenience of speedy cooking. Care must be taken when removing dishes from the microwave because the food and container can be very hot. What do you think are the most common uses of microwave ovens?

Choosing Containers

Be sure you use a container made of microwave-safe material, such as heat-resistant glass, glass-ceramic, microwave-safe plastic, china, or stoneware. Avoid containers that aren't made for microwave use, such as foam trays, butter tubs, some plastic containers, paper bags, paper plates, and metal utensils.

If you're cooking from a recipe, use the type and size of container the recipe suggests. For casseroles, cake batter, and other mixtures, round or oval containers work best. Food in the corners of square or rectangular containers tends to overcook.

Not all containers are suitable for use in a microwave oven. Which of those shown here should you avoid using?

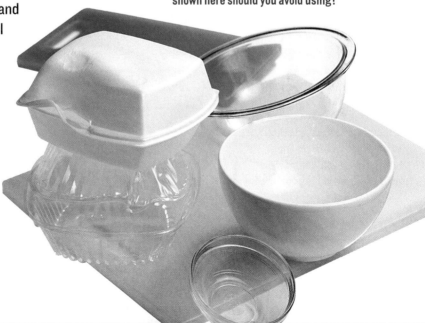

INFOLINK

For information on microwave cookware, see Section 2-2 of the Food Preparation Handbook.

Covering Food

When microwaving, covering the food helps keep moisture in. It saves cleanup time, too, because it keeps food from spattering onto the oven.

- When you want to retain moisture, use microwave-safe plastic covers that come with containers or use microwave-safe plastic wrap. Put the covers on loosely. When using plastic wrap, turn the wrap back on one corner or edge to leave a small opening. This vents it to let the steam escape. Don't let the plastic wrap touch the food.

- When you want moisture to evaporate, use waxed paper. Cover the dish loosely.

- When heating bread, wrap the items in paper towels to absorb moisture so that the bread does not get soggy. Also use paper towels to absorb the fat when cooking bacon in the microwave oven.

Activity: List the kinds of coverings used for microwaving various foods.

Cooking Time and Power Level

Before you push the Start button, think through the time and the power settings to use!

- Cook on the power level suggested in the recipe or instructions.

- Select the minimum time recommended in the recipe or the instructions. You can always add more time but do so in small amounts, such as 30 seconds. In a microwave oven, just a few seconds of overcooking can result in tough, dry food.

- Pay attention to differences in the oven wattage. Low-wattage ovens take more time to cook foods than higher-wattage ovens. If your oven uses less than 625 to 700 watts, you may need to add a little extra time or use a higher power setting.

- As you increase the amount of food you cook, cooking time also increases.

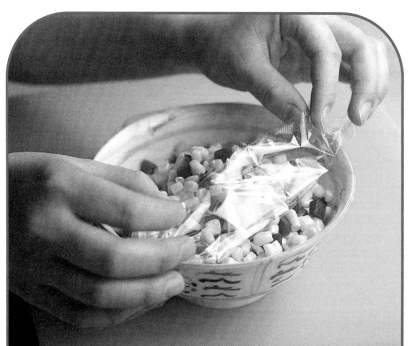

Covering foods with plastic wrap will hold in moisture during microwaving. Be sure to allow a way for steam to escape during cooking. What type of covering would you use if you wanted moisture to evaporate during cooking?

Critical Thinking: Describe situations in which the cooking time listed on labels or in recipes needed adjustment. Why was it necessary?

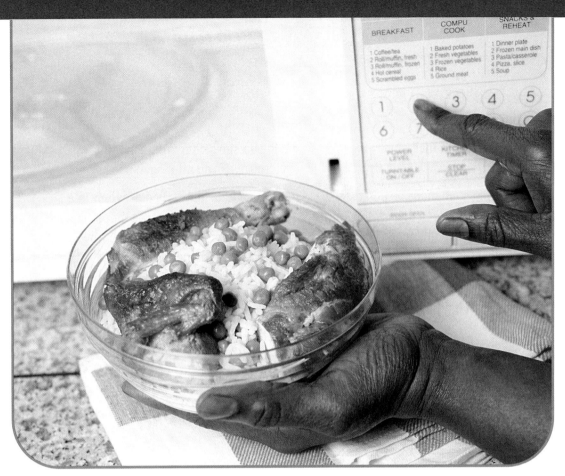

Arrange food so it will heat evenly. What is the advantage to arranging the chicken pieces this way?

For Even Cooking

The energy that cooks the food in a microwave oven isn't always distributed evenly. Take action to keep food from overcooking in some spots and undercooking in others! Depending on the type of food, you may need to:

- Place thicker or tougher parts of food toward the outside of the container.

- Stir foods during or after cooking.

- Rearrange pieces during cooking. Move outside pieces to the center and inside pieces to the outside.

- Turn foods over during cooking.

- Rotate the container during cooking or use a turntable.

When the microwave oven shuts off, food molecules continue to vibrate. *The period when the food continues to cook after being taken out of the microwave oven* is called **standing time.** Standing time lets heat penetrate all areas of the food. The internal temperature of food may go up during its standing time.

Discuss: Why is microwave cooking so popular today?

Microwave Oven Safety

Follow these tips and be safe!

- Do not microwave eggs in their shells; they will burst.

- Before microwaving such foods as potatoes, squash, and egg yolks, pierce them with a fork so that steam can escape and foods won't explode.

- Cook in small batches, which can be handled more easily and will cook faster than large batches.

- Use pot holders when removing food from the microwave oven. Heat from the food will pass into the cooking container and make it hot.

- When removing covers from cooking containers, watch out for steam. To avoid burns, remove covers *away* from your hands and face.

- Wipe up spills or splatters in the microwave oven after each use.

- Because food may not cook evenly in a microwave oven, make sure that it heats at a high enough temperature to destroy harmful bacteria. Determine if the food is cooked properly by measuring the internal temperature with a microwave-safe thermometer.

INFOLINK

For information on the safe internal temperatures of various foods, see the Food Preparation Handbook Section 1-4.

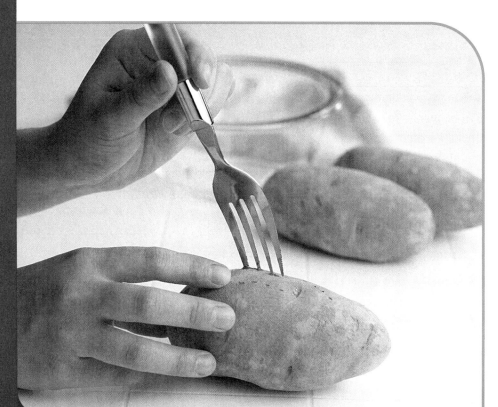

Some foods build up steam as they're cooking. Piercing them with a fork allows the steam to escape. What other foods should be pierced before cooking in a microwave?

Activity: In small groups, develop a pamphlet that illustrates the steps necessary for successful microwave cooking. Include safety tips to follow.

More Cooking Skills

The cooking skills you use will depend on the type of food you are cooking and the results you want to achieve. Here are some handy how-to tips.

Dry-Heat Cooking

With this cooking method, foods brown and develop a crisp or tender crust on the outside but stay moist and tender inside. Use a conventional oven or similar appliance, such as a toaster oven. Do not add liquid or fat. If cooking meat or poultry with a dry-heat method, use only tender cuts.

Baking and Roasting

- To roast meat or poultry, use an uncovered roasting pan with a rack. The rack allows the fat to drain away from the food.

- For baked goods such as breads and cakes, turn on the oven about 10 minutes before you are ready to bake.

- When baking several pans of food at one time, place them diagonally opposite one another, as shown below.

Broiling

- A broiler pan consists of a slotted grid, which holds the food, and a shallow pan that catches the drippings during cooking.

- Start with a cold pan to prevent foods from sticking. Pat the foods dry before cooking to make sure they become brown and crisp.

- For thick foods, place the pan farther from the heat and increase the cooking time so that the food is cooked thoroughly.

- Use tongs instead of a fork to turn foods while cooking.

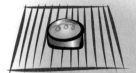
one pan

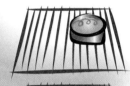
two pans

Discuss: Describe meals you have cooked or eaten that use the roasting method. What did you like or dislike about the meals? What are the advantages and disadvantages of this type of cooking?

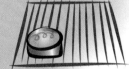

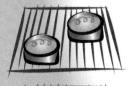
four pans

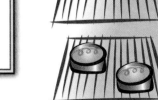
three pans

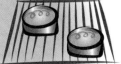

> **INFOLINK**
>
> For information on the types of foods and specific cooking methods for dry heat and moist heat cooking, see Chapter 14, page 194, and Units 5 and 6.

Moist-Heat Cooking

This means cooking foods in a hot liquid, steam, or a combination of both. You can tenderize less tender cuts of meat and poultry with this method. Moist heat is also used for foods, such as rice or dry beans, that must absorb liquid as they cook. Foods cooked in moist-heat do not brown. Moist-heat cooking may be done on a cooktop or in the microwave oven.

Boiling

- Use a saucepan or pot that is big enough to hold the liquid and the food.

- Bring the liquid to the boiling point, 212°F (100°C), and then add the food.

- Liquid should continue to boil as the food cooks.

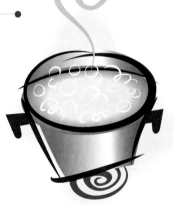

Steaming

- Use a steamer basket that fits inside a saucepan, or use an electric steamer. Allow enough space to keep the food raised over, not placed in, the boiling water.

- Cover the pan to keep in the steam.

- Keep the boiling water below the level of the food.

Activity: Find recipes that include each of the moist heat cooking methods. Share the recipes and explain the advantages and disadvantages of each method.

Simmering

- Use a saucepan or pot that is big enough to hold the liquid and the food.

- Bring the liquid to a boil and add the food. After the liquid returns to a boil, turn the heat down and cover the pan.

- Whenever possible, use the cooking liquid from vegetables and dry beans to preserve the nutrients.

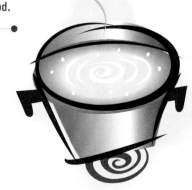

Frying

With this method, foods are cooked in a small or large amount of fat. Fat can be heated to a higher temperature than water. This gives the food a brown and crispy surface as well as flavor. Food may be coated with dry bread crumbs or cracker crumbs before frying. Remember, frying adds fat to food.

Stir-Frying

- Use a wok or a skillet.

- Cut food in small, uniform pieces before you start.

- Use a small amount of oil and high heat.

- Add the foods in order of the cooking time.

- Stir the food continuously.

Sautéing

- Use a small amount of fat in a skillet over low to medium heat.

- Stir or turn the food frequently.

Pan-frying

- Use a moderate amount of fat in a skillet over low to medium heat.

- Use larger pieces of meat, poultry, or fish than when sautéing.

- Turn the food if needed for complete cooking.

Emphasize: Food to be fried should always be dry, or the moisture could cause the fat to spatter and burn you.

Deep-Fat Frying

- Use an electric fryer or a large pot and a deep-fat or candy thermometer. Some pots have baskets for lowering the food into the fat.

- Cook the food in a large amount of fat until a brown crust forms and the center is done.

- Always use tongs to remove deep-fat-fried foods from the fat or oil.

- Do not overheat the fat or oil. Be prepared to act in case of a grease fire.

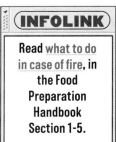

INFOLINK

Read what to do in case of fire, in the Food Preparation Handbook Section 1-5.

Critical Thinking: Review each of the frying methods. What method would add the least amount of fat to a food? Explain your reasoning.

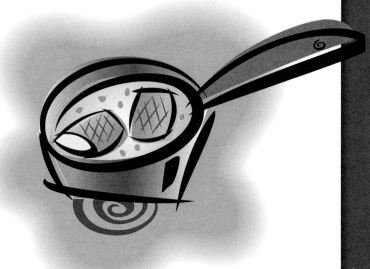

More Cooking Terms

Do you know the difference between *drain* and *strain*? If a recipe said to "dust" the food, would you know what to do? Check out these recipe terms related to cooking methods!

baste To moisten meat, such as turkey, or other food with cooking juices, fruit juice, melted fat, or a sauce while it cooks. Basting adds flavor and keeps the surface from drying.

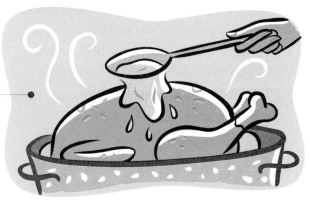

blanch To cook quickly in boiling liquid. Done to loosen the skin of fruit, nuts, and some vegetables; to set the taste and color of some vegetables for salads or to use with dips; or to prepare food for freezing.

bread (1) To coat the surface of food with fine, dry bread crumbs or cracker crumbs. (2) To coat with flour, then with milk or diluted, slightly beaten egg, and again with flour. Many fried foods are breaded before cooking because moisture can cause fat or oil to splatter.

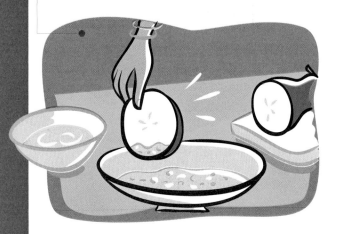

brown To make the surface of a food brown by frying, basting, baking, or broiling.

brush To coat lightly with another food, such as melted butter or egg white, usually with a pastry brush.

chill To refrigerate until cold.

drain To pour off a liquid from a food.

dust To sprinkle lightly, usually with flour, sugar, or powdered sugar.

garnish To add a small amount of one food to another for decoration, such as parsley or a lemon slice.

grease To rub a cooking utensil lightly with a fat, such as butter or shortening. For fewer calories, you can coat the utensil lightly with vegetable oil spray.

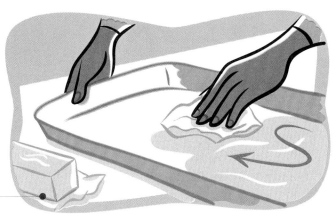

marinate **To let food stand in marinade for a certain length of time to tenderize it and develop its flavor. A marinade is a flavorful liquid such as French dressing.**

preheat **To heat an oven to a desired cooking temperature before putting in the food.**

reduce **To simmer or boil a liquid until it is half or less of its original volume to concentrate the flavor, as with sauces.**

roll **To make flat with a rolling pin or with the hands, as with dough.**

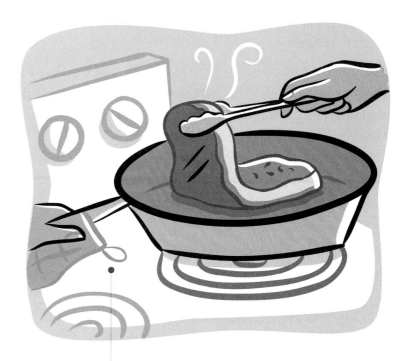

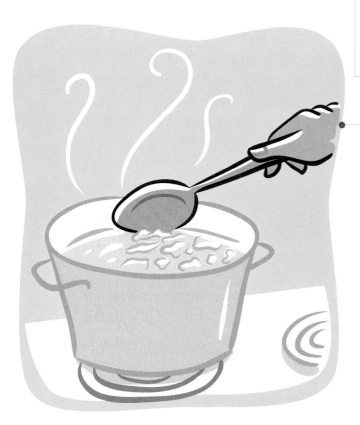

sear **To brown the surface of a meat quickly with very high heat.**

skim **To remove film from the surface of a liquid, such as gravy or pudding.**

strain **To separate liquid from solid food by passing the mixture through a sieve or strainer.**

toast **To brown a food by direct heat or in the oven.**

Activity: Refer students to the cooking methods listed on these pages. Ask students to choose one and create cartoons showing what would happen if the cooking methods they chose were used improperly.

Management Skills

You can use basic management skills to prepare a family dinner or a single recipe in your foods lab successfully. These skills include planning, scheduling, and working efficiently. Using these skills will save you time and energy in the kitchen!

Work Plan

Wash hands.
Gather food and equipment.

For risotto: Clean and slice mushrooms.
Chop onions and tomatoes.
Brown onions and mushrooms.
Add rice and broth.
Simmer 20-25 minutes.

For salad: Wash lettuce.

For risotto: Add tomatoes to rice mixture; heat 5 minutes.

For salad: Tear lettuce into bowl and add dressing.

For milk: Pour milk into glasses.

Serve.

Clean up.

Making a Work Plan

A **work plan** is *a list of all the steps you'll take to prepare the food*. Think about the order in which you'll do each task. You may need to include tasks not mentioned in the recipe directions, including some preparation steps.

The work plan at left is for a simple lunch of salad, Italian risotto with mushrooms and tomatoes, and milk.

Dovetailing

When you make your work plan, think about how you can dovetail tasks. **Dovetailing** is *keeping two tasks going at the same time*. It's like multitasking on a computer. For example, in this work plan, while the risotto is simmering, you can make the salad and pour the milk. Here are some other examples of dovetailing.

As bread toasts . . . pour juice in glasses.

As soup heats for lunch . . . make sandwiches or arrange salad.

As meat loaf bakes . . . prepare and cook vegetables, arrange salad, and set the table.

Activity: Ask students to work in pairs. Choose a recipe and work together to develop a work plan to prepare the food.

Making a Schedule

Here's how to use your work plan to make a schedule.

1. Estimate the time it will take you to complete each step in the work plan.

2. Calculate the total time needed for the recipe or meal. Remember, some tasks may be going on at the same time because of dovetailing.

3. Decide what time you want to serve the meal. Then "turn back the clock" to allow the amount of time needed for all the preparation.

That tells you what time to start! For example, if you want to serve lunch at noon and you estimate it will take 45 minutes to prepare, then you'll start to work at 11:15 A.M.

No schedule will be the same for everyone. People work at different speeds and may do tasks in a different order. The best schedules are flexible. They should be used as guides. Schedules also help by making you think ahead. What would your schedule for the work plan on page 500 look like? What tasks could you do at the same time?

When you prepare a schedule for a meal, remember that some tasks can be done at the same time. Why is flexibility important to a schedule?

Activity: Choose a main dish for a dinner party. Determine the time the dinner will be served. Develop a work plan and a schedule to insure dinner is served on time.

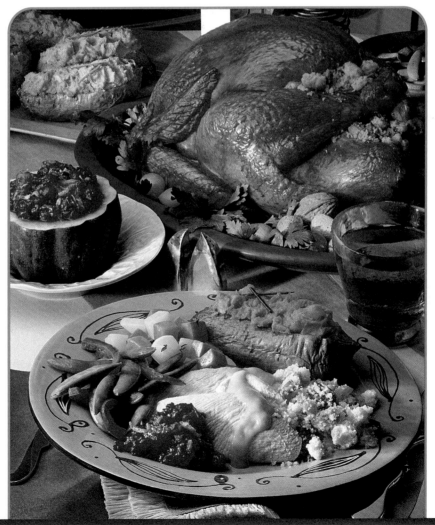

Working Efficiently

You can save even more time and energy by following these tips.

- Work in an orderly area. Have a place for everything and keep everything where it belongs.

- Know how to make the best use of your kitchen tools. Choose the right tool for the job. Which is the quickest way to chop onions? A food processor is one way. With practice, a chef's knife can work just as quickly and be easier to clean up.

- Clean up as you go along. You'll avoid mess and clutter, and you'll save time on cleanup later.

Cleanup Skills

After the meal, be sure to store leftover foods immediately and wash the dishes. To speed cleanup time, follow these tips.

- Scrape or rinse dishes and utensils immediately after using them.

- Wipe greasy pans with paper towels or newspaper before washing to remove excess oil.

- Arrange the dishes in the order they will be washed: glassware, flatware, dinnerware, and cooking utensils.

- Fill the sink or dishpan with hot, soapy water. Immerse a few dishes at a time.

- Wash dishes with a clean dishcloth or sponge.

- Rinse all washed dishes and cooking utensils in hot water.

- Put clean dishes in a dish drainer and let them air-dry or dry them with a clean towel.

- Clean the countertops and cooktop with hot, soapy water.

- Wipe off the dining table.

- Clean any food from the sink.

- Make sure there are no spills on the floor.

- Dispose of all garbage properly.

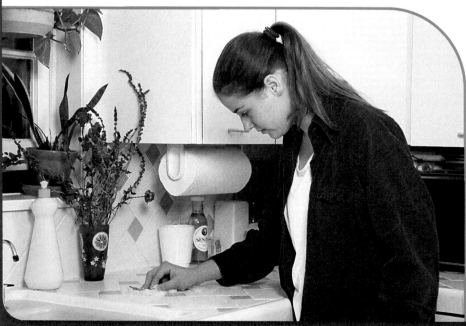

Save yourself the trouble of having a big kitchen task at the end of a meal by cleaning up as you go along. How could keeping a clean kitchen also make it a safer kitchen?

Critical Thinking: Using the right cooking tool helps prepare meals more efficiently. Choose a recipe and analyze whether the recipe could be simplified by using a substitute tool.

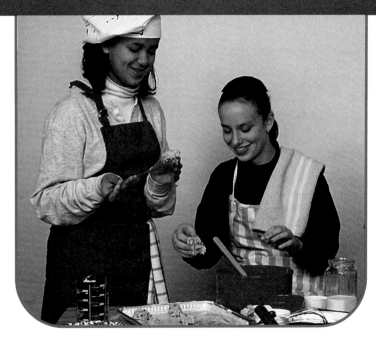

Teamwork goes a long way in getting a meal ready. Which jobs in the kitchen do you like to do best?

Working as a Team

Cooking successfully together with others, either at home or in your foods lab, takes teamwork. Just like a champion athletic team, you need to have your goal and game plan in mind. Members of the team need to know the rules, what each plans to do, and how to work together.

Working effectively as a team requires cooperation and responsibility. Cooperation means working together toward a common goal. Team members need to agree on their goal and their plan for achieving it. They must be considerate and willing to assist each other. Each team member, however, is responsible for his or her own work. You should carry out your assigned tasks to the best of your ability. Everyone needs to do his or her part for the team to reach its goal.

When working with others, you need to agree before you start who will do each job. Then prepare the work plan together. For example, one of you might gather the ingredients while the other sets the table. You might share the preparation steps.

When you work with others, your work plan will include:

- The different jobs to do for each menu item.

- The steps to follow for each job.

- Who will do each job.

- An estimate of the time each job will take.

Timing is usually very important in the foods lab. On your schedule, write down first when the food should be ready to eat and how long it takes to eat. Then write down how much time you'll need for cleanup. What remains is the time you have to prepare the food. If the food can't be prepared in that amount of time, you'll need to either choose another recipe or prepare part of the dish on the preceding day.

Discuss: How is food preparation at home similar to and different from food preparation in a school foods lab?

Activity: Brainstorm a list of ways to demonstrate cooperation and responsibility in the foods lab.

Activity: Draw a recipe at random. With two teammates, make a work plan and agree on each person's responsibilities.

LOOKING BACK

- You can change a recipe's yield to make more or fewer servings.
- Recipe success depends on accurately following the recipe.
- When cooking with a microwave oven, follow guidelines and use safety skills.
- Your choice of cooking methods depends on the type of food and the results you want.
- Basic management skills save time and energy in the kitchen.

UNDERSTANDING KEY IDEAS

1. A recipe calls for 30 mL of oil. You have only a standard measuring teaspoon. How can the Equivalent Measures chart help you?

2. What steps would you follow to alter a stew recipe from eight servings to four? What would you do if you couldn't reduce each ingredient exactly?

3. Compare and contrast the methods for measuring brown sugar and white sugar.

4. How does the technique for beating an egg differ from that for stirring a pudding mix?

5. When broiling, why might you need to move the pan farther from the heat?

6. Name four strategies for doing the dishes from a large family dinner.

DEVELOPING LIFE SKILLS

1. **Management:** Is it always good time management to use a microwave oven? Explain.

2. **Communication:** What makes a recipe easy to use and understand? Have you ever used a recipe that was hard to follow? Why was it confusing? How might you improve it?

3. **Critical Thinking:** Why isn't the metric system more widely used in the U.S.? What are the advantages of the metric system? The disadvantages?

Wellness Challenge

As part of Mrs. Brown's family and consumer sciences class, Tomás and three other students will work together in the foods lab. Mrs. Brown assigned them to make a work plan for each lab assignment so that each student in the group has a chance to learn the skills involved in preparing food.

1. How can the team members make sure that they will all have an equal chance to learn food skills?

2. How can the team members show cooperation and responsibility as they prepare the work plans? As they carry them out?

APPLYING YOUR LEARNING

1. **Skill Demonstration:** Imagine you are a restaurant chef. This week several students will join you to learn practical cooking skills. Choose a recipe for each day of the week and describe the skills in each. Give an oral presentation demonstrating three or more skills.

2. **Microwave Meals:** Choose one of your favorite hot meals. Describe ways you could use the microwave oven to speed its preparation. Write a menu, work plan, and schedule for the meal. Explain how you'd use principles of microwave cooking to get the best results.

EXPLORING FURTHER

1. **Occupational Outlook:** Learn more about high-school courses and activities that can help you prepare for a career in the culinary arts. Find out about programs in colleges and vocational schools. Report your findings.

2. **Beat the Clock:** Most managers look for ways to save time to increase productivity and profits. Using the Internet or library resources, find out more about the latest time management techniques used in business. How might you use some of these techniques in the foods lab or in your kitchen at home?

Making CONNECTIONS

1. **Math:** Fill several different mugs with water and measure the contents of each using a liquid measuring cup. Fill several different flatware teaspoons with sugar and measure the sugar again using a measuring teaspoon. What can you conclude about using standard measuring equipment?

2. **Science:** Plan and carry out an experiment to find out why it is important to follow recipes carefully. Choose a recipe for cupcakes. Fill the cupcake tins or paper cups to varying levels. Bake according to the recipe directions and judge the results. Write a report that includes your hypothesis, procedure, observations, and conclusions.

FOODS LAB

Peel two large potatoes. Cut them into big and small pieces. Microwave the pieces on high for one minute. Check the pieces to see whether they are done and add extra time in 30-second increments. Rotate the pieces frequently. Which pieces are done first? Last? What can you conclude?

PART 4

The Science of Food Preparation

Objectives

After studying pages 507-535, you will be able to:

- Relate basic science concepts to food.

- Describe the chemical structure of food's main components.

- Explain scientific principles related to the heat of cooking.

- Explain chemical and physical changes that occur during the preparation of grain products; vegetables and fruits; dairy foods; meat, poultry, and fish; and eggs.

- Describe scientific principles related to salad dressings, gelatin, and thickened foods.

- Explain the action of leavening agents and gluten.

Food Science: An Introduction

What did you have for breakfast this morning? Whatever you had, someone had to produce the ingredients, process and prepare them as necessary, and get them to your table. All of these activities are part of the study of food science.

What Is Food Science?

Food science is *the study of how food is produced, processed, prepared, and used.* It can help you understand the "why" and "how" of food preparation.

Food scientists are involved in all aspects of producing food products for sale to consumers. They work with plants to increase the amount of fruits or vegetables harvested or with animals to increase the meat yield. They help find better ways to dry, can, or freeze food. Some of these scientists test food to make sure it is safe to eat or work to make it more tasty and nutritious.

Food scientists are even employed by the space program. These scientists experiment with food products to decide which ones can be taken into space and how they should be packaged.

After studying this chapter, you may find that you are interested in a career as a food scientist. Whatever career you choose, learning about food science can help you to select and prepare foods that are healthful—and tasty!

Teaching With Visuals: Suggest ideas for space program foods. Explain why the food would be suitable.

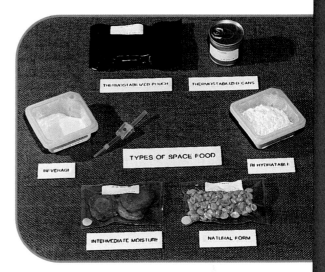

These foods were developed to suit the special conditions that astronauts encounter in space, while still meeting their need for nutritious and tasty food.

What Is Food Made Of?

Read the list of "ingredients" in these two mystery foods. Can you guess what they are?

Water, triglycerides of stearic, palmitic, oleic, and linoleic acids, myosin, actin, glycogen, collagen, lecithin, cholesterol, dipotassium phosphate, myoglobin, urea

Water, starches, cellulose, pectin, fructose, sucrose, glucose, malic acid, citric acid, succinic acid, anisyl propionate, amyl acetate, ascorbic acid, beta-carotene, riboflavin, thiamin, niacin, phosphorus, potassium

Food A is beef steak and Food B is cantaloupe. Surprised? Actually, every food is made up of chemicals that occur in nature. Chemicals can be natural or manufactured. They aren't necessarily good because they are natural, and they aren't necessarily bad because they are manufactured. Natural or manufactured, a chemical has basically the same structure.

The Building Blocks of Food

All foods are made of four basic chemical building blocks—water, proteins, carbohydrates, and fats—plus very small amounts of vitamins and minerals. These building blocks can be broken down still further into the parts from which they are made. Water, for instance, is a molecule made up of two elements: hydrogen and oxygen. It's also a compound.

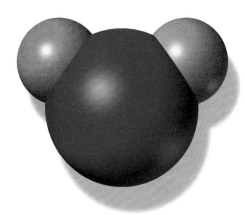

Water is a compound because water molecules are made from hydrogen and oxygen atoms.

Proteins are found in many foods, some from plants and some from animals. Protein molecules are made up of smaller units called amino acids, which are made of carbon, hydrogen, oxygen, and nitrogen. There are about 20 common amino acids. To make up all food proteins, these 20 amino acids are reused and arranged in different ways. One protein molecule might have thousands of amino acids in it.

SCIENCE CONCEPT:

Elements, Molecules, and Compounds

All visible matter can be classified as elements, molecules, and/or compounds. The first and simplest form of matter is the element. Elements are substances such as carbon, oxygen, iron, and potassium that cannot be further broken down. Each element comes in its own unique kind of atom.

Molecules form when two or more atoms stick together. A molecule is the smallest chemical unit of a substance that can exist independently. Molecules may be made up of one element, such as oxygen molecules (2 oxygen atoms), or of more than one element, such as water (2 hydrogen atoms and I oxygen atom).

When two or more elements join together, a compound is formed. Unlike an element, a compound can be broken down still further. For example, if you heat sugar in a test tube, it melts into a black substance—carbon—and water. Other compounds include table salt and vinegar.

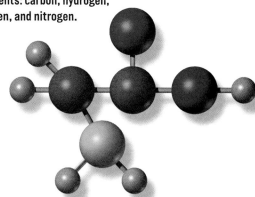

Proteins are made up of amino acids such as glycine. Each amino acid contains these elements: carbon, hydrogen, oxygen, and nitrogen.

Carbohydrates are found mostly in foods that come from plants. Carbohydrate molecules are simple sugars, such as glucose, or chains of simple sugars. They are made of carbon, hydrogen, and oxygen.

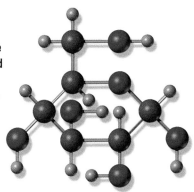

Glucose is a simple sugar that is a kind of carbohydrate. Carbohydrates are made up of hydrogen, oxygen, and carbon.

Fats and oils are found in both plant and animal foods. At room temperature, oils are liquid and fats are solid. A fat or oil is made up of one glycerol molecule and three fatty-acid molecules. A fatty-acid molecule is a chain of molecules made of carbon, oxygen, and hydrogen. The diagrams below show the middle of two fatty acids.

Discuss: What are other examples of physical change? List examples on the board.

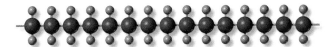

This molecule has the maximum number of hydrogen atoms for each carbon atom, making it a saturated fatty acid.

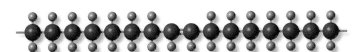

This molecule has fewer hydrogen atoms than the saturated fatty acid. This makes it an unsaturated fatty acid.

What Is a Chemical Reaction?

Did you have a slice of toast this morning? The bread you ate went through two kinds of changes—physical and chemical. Slicing a loaf of bread is a physical change. In a **physical change**, *the basic chemical nature of matter is not changed.* When you slice a loaf of bread, you change its shape and size. However, you don't change its identity—a slice of bread still tastes like bread.

Toasting bread produces a chemical change. When you toast bread, it becomes a new substance that looks, smells, and tastes different from untoasted bread.

SCIENCE CONCEPT:

Chemical Reaction

A chemical change, or **chemical reaction**, is *a process in which substances become new and different substances.* When you bake bread, many chemical reactions occur. The flour, fat, and other ingredients combine with one another to make a new substance—bread.

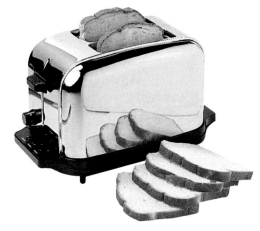

Which one is a physical change? What is the difference between a physical change and a chemical change?

The Science of Heat and Cooking

Imagine a world without cooked food. No more pizza—the dough couldn't be baked or the cheese melted. No more hamburgers and french fries or baked chicken and biscuits, either. Fortunately, people figured out a long time ago that cooked food tastes better. In fact, cooking affects food in other ways, too.

How Does Cooking Affect Food?

During cooking, heat energy is transferred from a heat source to the food. This heat energy affects food in a number of ways. Cooking...

• Improves food safety by destroying harmful bacteria.

• Allows you to digest some foods. For example, when you heat oatmeal grains in water, the starches in the oatmeal absorb water. The starches swell and soften, and the oatmeal becomes easier to digest.

• Affects texture—making a potato soft, bread dough firm, and bacon crispy.

• Affects color and flavor. Cook a green vegetable for a short time and the color changes to a bright green. Keep cooking, and its color changes from bright green to drab olive green. The flavor also changes—an overcooked vegetable may not be as tasty as one that was lightly cooked.

• Can cause nutrient losses. For example, boiling foods can cause some nutrients, such as vitamin C, to leach, or dissolve, into the cooking water. The vitamin C and water form a solution. When the cooking water is poured down the drain, the vitamins go with it.

Activity: Experiment with solutions. Create a solution of water and salt or one of eggs and sugar. How does it look?

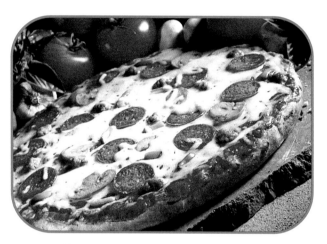

How does cooking affect the texture of a pizza?

SCIENCE CONCEPT:
Solutions

A **solution** is a *mixture in which one substance is dissolved in another*. To understand what this means, picture salt water. The salt is dissolved in the water, which means that salt molecules are floating around in the water, each molecule broken into two parts. You can't take salt water and separate it mechanically—that is, you can't pick the salt out of the water using your fingers or filter it with a machine. However, you can separate the molecules by boiling the water into vapor, leaving the salt behind. Many liquid foods are solutions, including iced tea (tea, water, and sugar) and soft drinks (water, sugar, salt, and flavor).

How Does Heat Transfer to Food?

When you cook your favorite dinner, you apply, or transfer, heat to food. Heat is a form of energy that makes molecules vibrate. The molecules move up and down and back and forth in one place very fast. They're so tiny, you can't see them vibrate, but you notice their vibration as heat.

Heat is transferred from a heat source to food by three processes.

Conduction. Energy is passed from molecule to molecule by conduction. Molecules transfer their heat energy to other molecules when they bump into each other. You can observe this happening when you fry an egg in a pan on an electric range. As the heating element heats up, its molecules begin to vibrate. These molecules touch the molecules on the bottom of the pan, and they begin to vibrate and heat up in turn. The heated molecules of the pan then bump into the molecules of the egg. The result: the egg cooks.

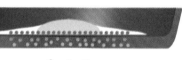

Conduction

Teaching With Visuals: Melt butter in a pan. Ask: What type of heat transfer are you observing?

Convection. In convection heating, heat is transferred through the flow of a heated material such as water or soup. For example, when you boil a pot of soup, the heat is first transferred to the bottom of the pan through conduction. As the molecules in the bottom of the soup are heated, convection begins. The molecules spread apart and become less dense. The heated liquid is now lighter than the cooler liquid above it, so it rises. The cooler liquid then sinks to the bottom where it is heated in turn. This continues until all the liquid reaches the same temperature. The entire pot of soup boils.

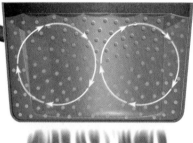

Convection

Air can also transfer heat by convection. In an oven, for example, the hot air helps heat the food being cooked.

Radiation. Heat energy can be transmitted by waves that travel through space. You may have seen warming lamps over the hot food on a restaurant buffet. If you move a hand under the lamp without touching it, you can feel the heat radiating out. The warming lamps put out heat as waves. When these waves reach the food, the molecules in the food vibrate and the food heats up. Grilling and broiling also transfer heat by radiation.

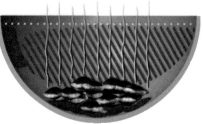

Radiation

How Does a Microwave Oven Work?

If you have a microwave oven, you probably like its speed and convenience. Food cooked in a microwave oven is hot and ready to eat in just a few minutes.

Microwave ovens cook by invisible waves of energy called microwaves. The main difference between microwaves and heat is that microwaves have the greatest effect on water molecules. Heat, on the other hand, affects all molecules equally.

When you cook food in a microwave oven, the microwaves cause the water molecules in the food to vibrate rapidly. This energy is transmitted to the other molecules, heating the food.

A microwave oven can cook foods in one-quarter to one-half the time that it takes with other cooking methods. Microwave cooking saves time because microwaves are absorbed by the food to a depth of 2 to 3 inches (5 to 7.5 cm). Heat from other sources is absorbed only at the surface, and then slowly moves through the food. So if you want a hot snack in a hurry, microwave cooking is the way to go!

Activity: Choose a food or recipe with microwave and range-top directions. Prepare both and compare cooking time and results.

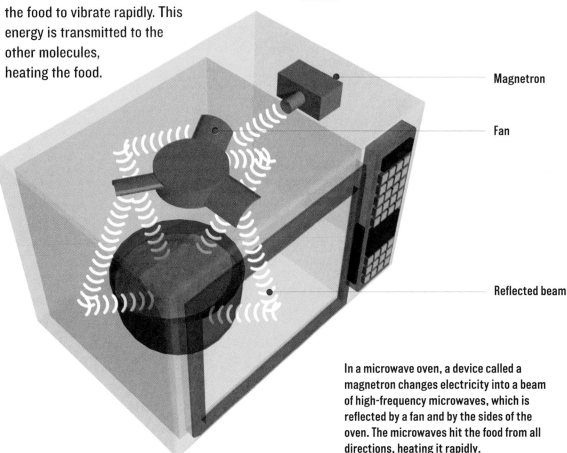

Magnetron

Fan

Reflected beam

In a microwave oven, a device called a magnetron changes electricity into a beam of high-frequency microwaves, which is reflected by a fan and by the sides of the oven. The microwaves hit the food from all directions, heating it rapidly.

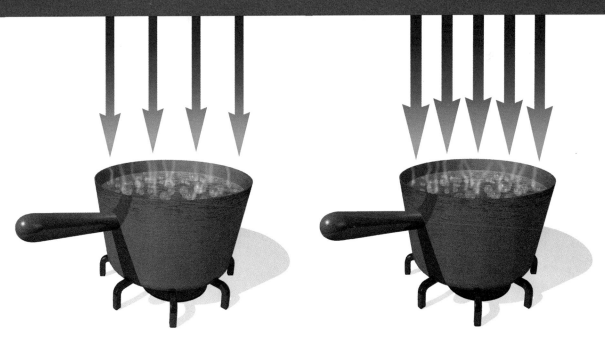

Less air pressure in Denver means that water boils at about 202°F (95°C). In Miami with more air pressure, water boils at about 212°F (100°C).

How Does Altitude Affect Cooking?

Just where you are, you can probably notice three different phases of matter: solid, liquid, and gas. This book and the chair beneath you are solids. Liquids include juice and water, and the air you're breathing is a gas. Heating or cooling a substance can cause it to change phases.

SCIENCE CONCEPT:
Phase Changes

A phase change occurs when a substance changes from one phase to another—from a solid to a liquid, from a liquid to a gas, or back again. You can watch water go through all the phase changes in just one day. On a cold morning, water starts out as ice, a solid. As the sun heats the ice, it melts to form liquid water. As temperatures continue to rise, some of the water becomes water vapor—a gas!

Activity: Read the directions on baking mixes and compare cooking directions for different altitudes.

The boiling point of water—the temperature at which it changes from a liquid to a gas—depends on the pressure of the air over it. The air above the liquid water pushes down, preventing the gas molecules from escaping into the air. Heating the water gives the molecules the necessary force to escape into the air as water vapor.

The higher the altitude, the lower the air pressure. As air pressure decreases, it becomes easier for water molecules to escape into the air. Air pressure can make a big difference—for each thousand feet above sea level, the boiling point of pure water drops almost 2°F (1°C)! So in the mile-high city of Denver, water boils at about 202°F (95°C), whereas in the coastal city of Miami, it boils at about 212°F (100°C).

What does this mean for cooks? It means a Denver cook must boil food longer—because of the lower boiling temperature—than a Miami cook.

The Science of Grain Products

How do you like your grains? Whether you enjoy pasta, rice, oatmeal, bread, or tortillas, you probably get a good part of your energy from the carbohydrates in cereal grains. You may not have realized, though, that cereal grains are actually seeds from grasses such as wheat, rice, oats, corn, rye, and barley. All cereal grains are processed and cooked to make them easier to eat and digest. Wheat, for example, is ground into flour, then baked into breads or cakes, or cooked as pasta or tortillas.

What Happens When Oatmeal Cooks?

A steaming bowl of oatmeal can taste good, especially on a cold morning. It's also a good demonstration of how grains change and become more digestible as they cook.

As you heat the oatmeal grains in water, the carbohydrates that make up the starch change. Some of the bonds between the atoms of the same molecule break and form new bonds with atoms of different molecules. The water molecules then get trapped in clusters of starch called granules. As the starch granules absorb the water molecules, they swell and soften. Eventually they break apart, releasing the nutrients inside. The oatmeal becomes softer and easier to digest.

Oatmeal that is started in cold water will taste creamier than oatmeal started in boiling water. This is because when you start cooking the oatmeal in cold water, it has more time to absorb the water.

Activity: Create a cartoon titled "What Happens When Oatmeal Cooks?" based on the text description. Display in the classroom.

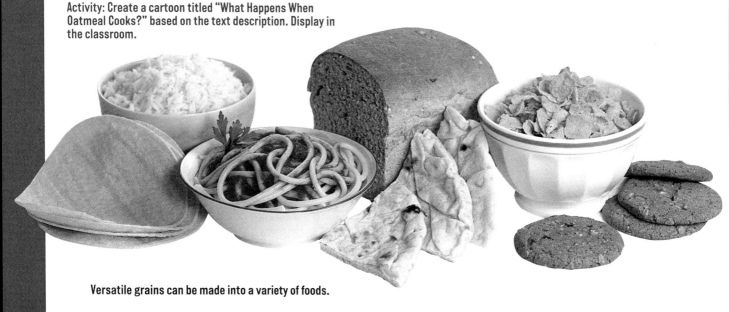

Versatile grains can be made into a variety of foods.

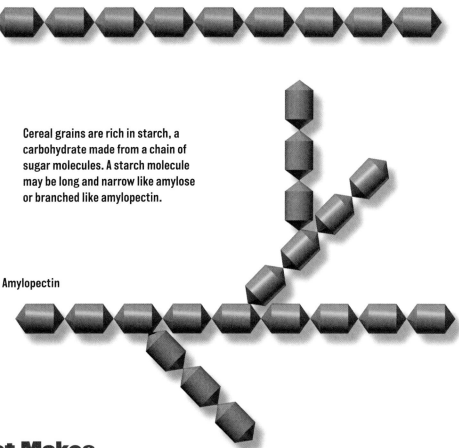

Amylose

Cereal grains are rich in starch, a carbohydrate made from a chain of sugar molecules. A starch molecule may be long and narrow like amylose or branched like amylopectin.

Amylopectin

What Makes Pasta Sticky?

If you don't prepare pasta noodles carefully, they may stick together into a large, unappetizing lump. Believe it or not, the noodles are actually "glued" together! When pasta cooks, the starch in the noodles dissolves into the cooking water and turns to a gluelike substance as it cools. This gluey starch attaches to the noodles, leaving them sticky.

How can you use science to avoid sticky noodles? First, you can use a lot of water for cooking pasta. The starch will be distributed through a larger amount of water, so less starch will be left on the pasta. If you're still getting sticky noodles, you can rinse the pasta after you cook it. (Don't worry about rinsing off the nutrients. Most nutrient loss happens as the pasta cooks, so rinsing only removes a slight bit more.) Another method is to add I tablespoon (15 mL) of oil or margarine per quart of cooking water. The oil coats the noodles, so the starch can't attach itself to them.

Discuss: What techniques do you use to avoid having sticky pasta? List ideas on the board.

Look *for these* **TERMS**

acid   enzyme

base

The Science of Vegetables and Fruits

You've probably heard this statement more times than you can count: "Eat your vegetables and fruits—they're good for you." But these members of the plant kingdom can be more than food you eat just because you're supposed to. If prepared properly, vegetables and fruits can be interesting and flavorful as well.

What Gives Vegetables and Fruits Their Color?

One enjoyable aspect of vegetables and fruits is their color. The color of these foods can be affected during the cooking process, making them dull and less attractive. Good cooks try to preserve the bright, natural colors found in these nutritious foods. Most of the different colors of vegetables and fruits come from three classes of pigments: chlorophyll, flavonoids, and carotenoids.

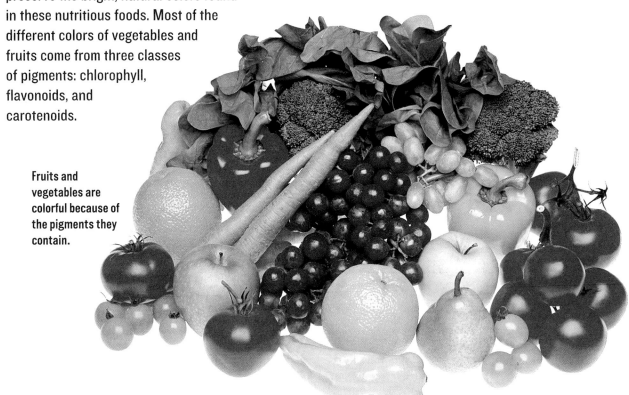

Fruits and vegetables are colorful because of the pigments they contain.

Chlorophyll

Green vegetables get their color from chlorophyll. When a green vegetable is cooked, its cells break down. Acid in the cells leaks out and comes in contact with the chlorophyll. The chlorophyll also comes in contact with the acid in tap water. (Although pure water is neutral—neither an acid nor a base—tap water is often slightly acidic.)

Acids and Bases

Acid is the name for *a group of chemicals that share certain characteristics*. Weak acids taste sour—but don't ever taste a chemical to test it. Many fruits contain weak acids. Oranges, lemons, and limes all contain citric acid, and apples contain malic acid. Some acids are poisonous—but foods don't contain them in harmful amounts. Strong acids can destroy skin and other body tissues on contact.

Base is the name for another group of chemicals. Bases are *the chemical opposite of acids*. They often feel slippery, and they have a bitter taste. Soap and detergent contain bases. Strong bases are as destructive as strong acids.

The longer you simmer a green vegetable such as broccoli or spinach, the longer its chlorophyll has time to react with its own acids and any acids in the cooking water. It's kitchen chemistry: through a chemical reaction, the chlorophyll reacts with the acids to form a new brown substance. The green vegetable turns a drab olive green or yellow-green.

The best way to prevent dull-colored vegetables is to add them to water after it is already boiling and to keep cooking time to under seven minutes. You can also steam your vegetables. Steaming works because the vegetable is held above the water, keeping it from contact with the acids in the water.

More About Bases: Bases are chemical substances that can react with acids to neutralize them—to decrease the acidic properties. A base is sometimes referred to as an *alkali*. When using a litmus paper test, solutions that include a base turn the paper blue.

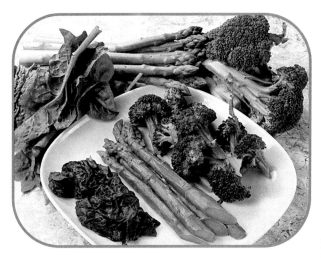

Steaming vegetables can help prevent them from turning brown because the vegetables are not in contact with the acids in the water.

Some cooks add baking soda to cooking water to help vegetables keep their bright color. This works but at a cost. Baking soda is a base, the chemical opposite of an acid. When baking soda is added to the water, it neutralizes some of the acids of the water, and the vegetable stays green.

Unfortunately, the baking soda also dissolves the vegetable's firm cell wall, making it too soft. It destroys vitamins, too. So the vegetable looks good, but it tastes soft and mushy and is less nutritious. That's a high price to pay for that bright green color!

Flavonoids

Flavonoids give many fruits and vegetables their beautiful red, purple, and blue colors, including eggplant, red cabbage, cherries, blueberries, and strawberries. These pigments dissolve in water. They easily leach out of the fruit or vegetable into the sauce or cooking liquid. Boil cherries and watch the water turn red.

Acid also affects these colors; they remain red as long as they are acidic. Red cabbage, for example, sometimes turns blue while cooking. That's because some of the natural acid in the cabbage escapes in the cooking steam during the first few minutes of boiling. You can prevent this by cooking red cabbage with something acidic such as an apple or a tablespoon of vinegar.

Carotenoids

Carotenoids, mostly yellow and orange but sometimes red, give color to tomatoes, squash, carrots, and sweet potatoes. Because carotenoids are very stable pigments, these vegetables don't lose their color unless they are badly overcooked.

Because of the color-keeping quality of these pigments, extracts of foods containing carotenoids are great for use as food coloring. For example, the pure form of one carotenoid—carotene—is bright yellow. It is used to color margarine, soft drinks, and cake mixes. Without carotene, you'd be spreading white margarine on your toast!

Why Does Cut Fruit Turn Brown?

Cut or peel a banana, pear, apple, avocado, or potato, and it starts to turn brown. Have you ever wondered why? The reason is a protein called an enzyme.

SCIENCE CONCEPT:
Enzymes

Enzymes are *special proteins that help chemical reactions happen.* Any chemical reaction needs energy to get started. Enzymes help chemical reactions by reducing the energy required to start the reaction.

In fruits, enzymatic browning occurs when the cells of cut, bruised, or peeled fruits are exposed to oxygen, or oxidized. Susceptible fruits contain a normally colorless compound that turns gray, brown, or black when oxidized, plus an enzyme that gets the reaction going. The darkened flesh of these fruits, although safe to eat, is unappetizing.

Cooking will destroy the enzyme responsible for enzymatic browning. You can also slow the browning by sprinkling the exposed surface of a cut fruit with lemon or orange juice. The citric acid in the juice slows the activity of the enzymes.

When the flesh of an apple is exposed to air, enzymes cause the flesh to darken.

Critical Thinking: Some detergents contain enzymes that are used to break down stains. Ask: What do you know about enzymes that would help to explain why they would be used in detergents?

The Science of Dairy Foods

Chances are that your refrigerator at home contains milk, cheese, or other dairy foods. Dairy foods are a good source of proteins, carbohydrates, fats, and certain vitamins and minerals. Milk is also a source of water—in fact, cow's milk is a solution that is 87 percent water!

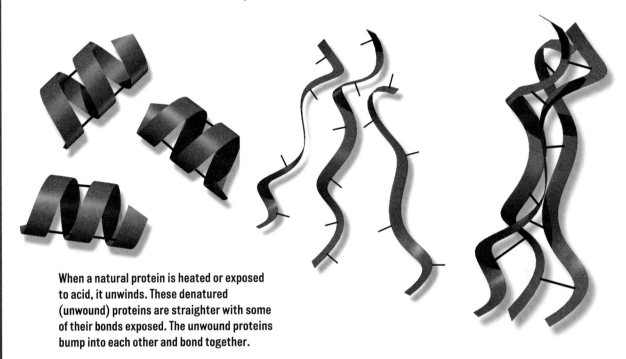

When a natural protein is heated or exposed to acid, it unwinds. These denatured (unwound) proteins are straighter with some of their bonds exposed. The unwound proteins bump into each other and bond together.

What Makes Milk Curdle?

Milk curdles because of the protein in it. About 80 percent of milk proteins are caseins. This protein can be coagulated by heat or acids.

SCIENCE CONCEPT:
Coagulation

Coagulation occurs when *a liquid changes into a soft semisolid or solid mass*. Natural proteins are in a formation of tight coils or loops. The particles in milk coagulate when the protein molecules unwind and become somewhat straighter. These proteins then bump into each other, joining tightly together into clumps. Sometimes coagulation is desirable. Cheeses, for example, are made by coagulating the casein protein in milk.

When cooking milk in sauces or puddings, coagulation is a problem caused by overheating. When proteins become too hot, they coagulate. Once it happens, no amount of stirring will get the lumps out of your sauce. You can avoid coagulation by heating milk either over low heat or in a double boiler. If you're following a recipe, stir the milk according to the directions. Stirring spreads the heat evenly through the milk, preventing overheating.

Milk will curdle at high temperatures only when other factors are also present. Acids such as vinegar or high levels of salt can cause milk to clot or curdle.

Add acidic mixtures to milk slowly, or they may cause curdling.

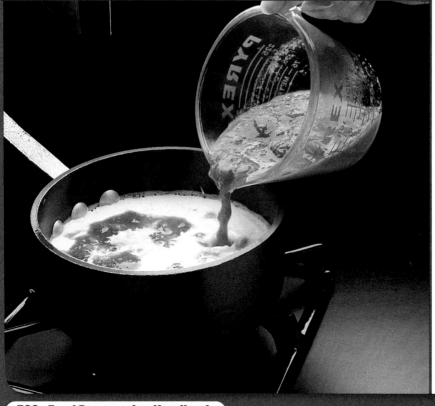

How Is Yogurt Made?

Yogurt is a tasty, easy-to-digest milk product. You can make yogurt at home by adding certain "friendly" bacteria, called lactic acid bacteria, to milk that has been heated. Heating the milk first kills unwanted bacteria. It also changes the structure of the whey proteins in the milk, increasing their capacity to bind water and promoting the growth of the "friendly" bacteria that ferment the milk.

SCIENCE CONCEPT:
Fermentation

Fermentation is *a chemical reaction that splits complex compounds into simpler substances.* Usually fermentation involves breaking down sugars into carbon dioxide and alcohol. In dairy foods, a sugar is broken down into lactic acid, which is very sour and gives foods such as plain yogurt and sour cream their sour taste.

The bacteria used to make yogurt grow best at temperatures between 106° and 113°F (41° and 45°C). To make yogurt at home, you must keep yogurt at that temperature for about eight hours to produce a smooth consistency. During that time, the bacteria produce acid and flavors that give yogurt its characteristic taste. After the yogurt is done, you can add fruit and sweetener.

Activity: Make your own yogurt using a small amount of commercial yogurt as the bacteria source to start the fermentation.

The Science of Meat, Poultry, and Fish

Cooking meat, poultry, and fish can be challenging. For example, when roasting a chicken, you have to make sure the dark thigh and leg meat are thoroughly cooked without overcooking the chicken to the point where the breast meat is dry and tough. Fortunately, food science can help you achieve success here as well.

What Affects Tenderness?

One of meat's most desirable qualities is tenderness. Tenderness is affected by a number of factors.

Connective Tissue

Tenderness depends on the amount and type of connective tissue in the meat. The main tissues in meat are skeletal muscles, the muscles that move the legs, wings, or other parts of the skeleton. Skeletal muscles are long fibers that are held in bundles by connective tissue. The more connective tissue a cut of meat has, the tougher it is. Cuts from shoulders, legs, and other muscles that do a lot of work contain more connective tissue, so these cuts are tough.

Two common types of connective tissue are elastin and collagen. The protein molecules that make up these connective tissues are shaped like a coiled metal spring. These form strong, ropelike fibers. Because the fibers are very strong, they serve as connective tissue, supporting and binding other tissues.

Elastin is also referred to as gristle. It does not break down during cooking. Since young animals

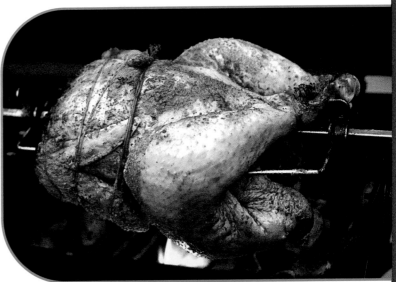

A whole chicken needs to be cooked to the proper internal temperature for food safety. Cooking skill helps you prepare the bird to perfection without drying out the white breast meat.

do not have much elastin, their meat is generally more tender than meat from older animals.

The other type of connective tissue is collagen. When collagen is heated in water, it disperses throughout the water. When cooled, it turns into a firm, semisolid mass called gelatin. Gelatin is much more tender than collagen and helps to give cooked meat its plump appearance.

Unlike meat and poultry, finfish and shellfish have very little connective tissue. These foods are naturally tender.

Emphasize: The fibers that serve as connective tissue in meats are not the same as dietary fiber.

Heat

Cooking also affects tenderness. When you cook meat and poultry, the proteins in the muscles unwind and join together with other proteins. However, if you overcook meat or poultry in dry heat, the proteins will shrink, becoming drier and tougher. This is why the secret to tender, juicy meat is careful control of heat.

You can also cook poultry or tough cuts of meat in moist heat with water or another liquid. Through long, slow cooking the liquid softens and dissolves the connective tissue, making the meat or poultry more tender.

Acids

Acids can break apart and unwind the large proteins in muscles. A marinade containing mild acids is actually a form of chemical tenderizer.

SCIENCE CONCEPT:
Acids

Acid is the name for a group of chemicals that share certain characteristics. Many fruits contain weak acids. Oranges, lemons, and limes all contain citric acid.

Because citrus juices are mild acids, soaking meat in a marinade containing orange, lemon, or lime juice will both tenderize it and add flavor.

Enzymes

Enzymes can be used to tenderize meat. Fruits such as papayas, pineapples, and figs contain enzymes that can break down muscle fiber and/or collagen. Enzyme-containing preparations are also sold as meat tenderizers.

Activity: Compare recipes for meat marinades. Determine which ingredients help to tenderize the meat.

SCIENCE CONCEPT:
Enzymes

Enzymes are special proteins that help chemical reactions happen. Any chemical reaction needs energy to get started. Enzymes help chemical reactions by reducing the energy required to start the reaction.

Both acid and enzyme tenderizers work only when they are in direct contact with meat. One way to increase the tenderizer's contact with meat is to inject the liquid into the meat.

Physical Methods

Muscle fibers can be as long as a foot. Meat can be tenderized by cutting or tearing the long fibers against the grain. To "cut across the grain" means to slice across the muscle fibers and connective tissue at a right angle. Thinly sliced meat seems tender because the thin slices contain only a tiny length of fiber. The thinner the slices, the shorter the segments and the less chewy the meat.

Think of roast beef or corned beef. Either meat can be tough when sliced thickly, yet when sliced thin as deli meat, they can be surprisingly tender and easy to chew.

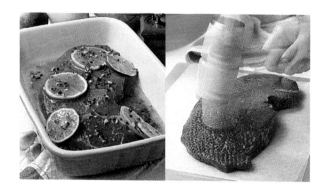

Tough cuts of meat can be tenderized by chemical reactions, such as marinades, or by physical methods, such as a tenderizing mallet.

Grinding, scoring, and pounding meat has a similar effect. The lengths of the muscle fibers and connective tissues are shortened, so the meat is easier to chew and more tender.

How Does a Roast Brown?

Have you noticed that the crust of roast meat or poultry is richer in color and flavor than the interior? That's because of a process called the Maillard reaction.

SCIENCE CONCEPT:
Maillard Reaction

The Maillard reaction—named for the French scientist who discovered it—is a type of browning reaction. It occurs when an amino acid from a protein reacts with a sugar at high temperatures. New substances are created and continue to change as the reaction goes on. The result: a deep brown color and rich flavor.

You may not think of meat as containing sugar molecules, but it does. The sugar and protein in the meat react in the high heat of the oven.

Why doesn't the inside of the meat get as brown as the crust? That's because the inside of the roast doesn't get as hot as the outside. On the inside, the meat's natural moisture limits how hot the roast can get. The outside, however, dries out in the dry heat of the oven, so it gets much hotter than the inside.

Now you know why meat doesn't brown in a microwave oven. The air in a microwave oven never gets hot enough for the Maillard reaction to take place!

Critical Thinking: Review the Maillard reaction with students. Ask: Why does moist-heat cooking not result in browned meats?

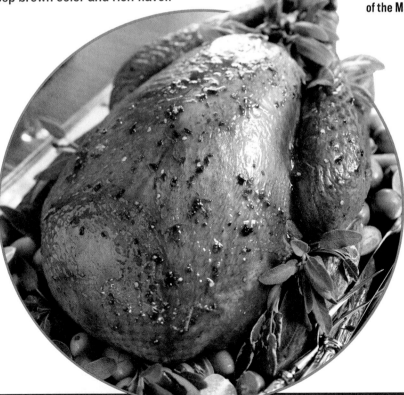

Grilled meat turns brown and gets its rich taste as a result of the Maillard reaction.

The Science of Eggs

How many different ways have you eaten eggs? Scrambled, fried, poached, hard-cooked, or deviled? Eggs are a versatile food. In recipes, they can be used to:

- Hold other ingredients together.
- Thicken foods such as custards and puddings.
- Help baked goods rise.
- Coat or glaze foods.

Eggs have so many uses because of their special properties. They combine protein, water, and fat in a complex package.

What Happens When an Egg Cooks?

When you fry an egg, the clear part turns white and the yellow part hardens. You can see the egg change from a liquid to a solid. Like curdled milk, this is an example of coagulation.

SCIENCE CONCEPT:
Coagulation

Coagulation occurs when a liquid is changed into a soft semisolid or solid mass. The particles in an egg coagulate when the protein molecules unwind and collide with one another. As the temperature rises, they bond and form into a solid. The egg is cooked.

Understanding how coagulation works can help you cook eggs to perfection. At first, the heat of cooking creates a weak, open network of protein molecules. The egg is still slightly liquid at that stage. For food safety, continue cooking until the egg has a more solid texture. Just don't cook an egg too long—overcooking squeezes out the water in the egg and tightens the bonds between proteins. The result? A dry or rubbery egg.

Activity: Diagram how protein molecules combine during cooking to form soft-cooked eggs and hard-cooked eggs.

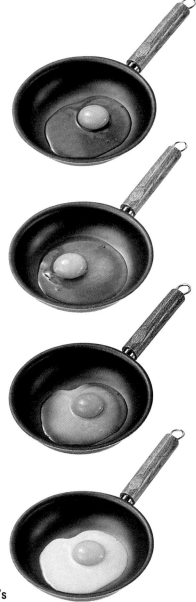

Notice how an egg's appearance changes as the protein in the egg coagulates.

What Makes Meringue Fluffy?

Do you enjoy meringue on a pie? This light, fluffy topping starts with egg whites.

Egg whites have a special property—they whip into foams. When you beat egg whites, you are whipping air into them. The egg whites increase in volume. As you continue to beat the foam, it becomes drier and firmer. Why? It's because beating an egg white produces almost the same changes as cooking does, just not carried so far.

The beating unwinds and elongates the proteins in an egg white and allows them to begin to clump together. The proteins coagulate and form a protective, stable coat around the air bubbles that you've whipped into the egg white. The result is a stiff foam that forms the meringue for pies. Beaten egg whites are also mixed into a soufflé to make it light and fluffy and into a mousse to lighten the texture.

Sugar interferes with the coagulation of the egg proteins, so add sugar at the end of the beating. Also, be sure no yolk mixes with the white. Even a little yolk may keep the white from reaching full volume. Egg yolk is about 35 percent fat, and fats prevent the egg whites from foaming.

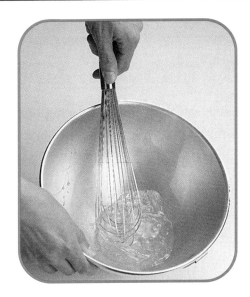

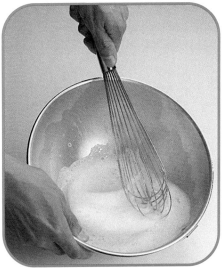

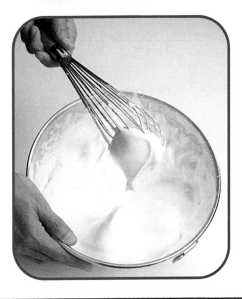

Metal bowls, especially copper, make it easier to whip egg whites into a foam. You can also save time if you start with the eggs at room temperature. A room-temperature egg will whip faster and produce a larger volume of foam than a cooler one.

The Science of Salads

Take some raw spinach leaves, chopped carrots, and a tomato or two. Add some sliced onions and perhaps some mushrooms. Toss it all together and you have a salad—a powerhouse dish full of nutrients. You also have what a scientist would call a mixture.

SCIENCE CONCEPT:
Mixtures

A **mixture** is *a material consisting of two or more kinds of matter, each retaining its characteristic properties.* When you toss a salad together, you are making a mixture. The spinach, carrots, tomatoes, and other ingredients mix together, but each retains its own color, flavor, and texture.

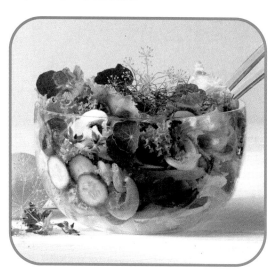

Why is a salad a mixture?

Why Do Some Dressings Separate?

For some people, a salad is not complete until they add the dressing. One basic, yet tasty, salad dressing is made from oil and vinegar. If you shake the two together vigorously, the oil will divide into many small particles distributed

evenly throughout the vinegar. However, if the mixture sits for a short time, the oil and vinegar will separate. If you wish to mix these two liquids more permanently, you must form an emulsion.

SCIENCE CONCEPT:
Emulsions

An **emulsion** is *a mixture of two liquids— such as oil and water—whose droplets do not normally blend with each other.* An emulsion contains a third substance, known as an emulsifier, that coats the droplets of one liquid so that they can remain mixed in another liquid. Fats and oils, for example, do not stay mixed with water unless they are emulsified.

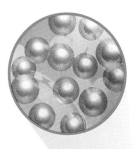

The oil in mayonnaise is dispersed throughout the vinegar. The egg yolk acts as the emulsifier.

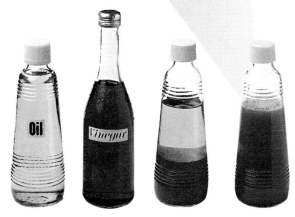

You can mix oil and vinegar together with egg yolk to form a familiar emulsion—mayonnaise. In mayonnaise, oil droplets are scattered throughout the vinegar, with the egg yolk serving as the emulsifier. The egg yolk sticks to the surface of the oil droplets, keeping them separated and evenly scattered throughout the vinegar.

Some emulsions, such as mayonnaise, salad dressings, sauces, gravies, and cream soups, are prepared. Others, such as whole milk, occur naturally. Foods that act as emulsifiers include egg yolk and egg white, starches, gelatin, and fine powders such as mustard powder.

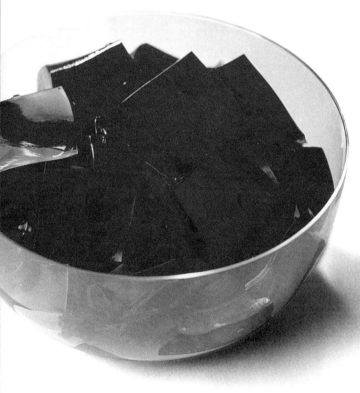

Links between protein molecules make gelatin firm enough to hold its shape.

Activity: Experiment with mixing vinegar and oil with and without egg yolk. Compare results.

What Makes Gelatin Firm?

To make a gelatin salad, you act a bit like a magician. Mix a tablespoon of gelatin with a cup or two of water. Add heat and stir. Then pour into a mold and let chill, and poof! You've just turned a liquid into a gelatin. You've also made an example of colloidal dispersion.

SCIENCE CONCEPT:
Colloidal Dispersion

A colloidal dispersion is a mixture in which the particles don't dissolve the way particles do in a solution. The particles, called colloids, are distributed, or dispersed, throughout the other substance. In gelatin, protein molecules are distributed throughout the water rather than dissolved in it. Egg white and jelly are other common food colloidal dispersions.

Just how does gelatin become firm after being heated and then cooled? The first step in getting gelatin to form a gel is to mix it with water. Gelatin is a protein that usually comes from the connective tissue of animals. A small amount of this protein can bind a large amount of water. When gelatin binds water, the gelatin granules swell up to about ten times their original size, trapping water molecules in the process.

The gelatin mixture is then heated. The protein molecules separate from one another and bind more water. As this liquid mixture cools, the gelatin molecules link together, and a rigid, firm gel is formed.

Raw pineapple, papaya, and some other fruits contain enzymes that will keep gelatin from setting. Recall that enzymes are special proteins that help chemical reactions happen. The enzymes in fruits such as pineapple digest the gelatin molecules and prevent the gel from becoming solid. Your gelatin salad will remain a liquid. If you'd like that pineapple taste in a gelatin salad, you can use canned or cooked pineapple. Cooking stops the enzyme from working.

The Science of Thickened Foods

Sauces and gravies can add zest and interest to a meal. Who can imagine a turkey dinner without the gravy, or macaroni and cheese without the cheese sauce?

One step in making a sauce is to thicken it. There are several ways to do this. One method uses evaporation. As a liquid boils, water turns into vapor and evaporates from the sauce, producing a thicker, more concentrated sauce. Chefs call this method "reduction" because the liquid is being reduced to one-half or less of its original volume.

Another method for thickening sauce is to mix a small amount of solids, such as pureed vegetables, into the sauce. Still another method is to add a starchy ingredient such as flour or cornstarch.

How Do Starches Thicken Foods?

Starches are used to thicken sauces, gravies, soups, salad dressings, and desserts. The most common sources of starch are cereal grains (corn, wheat, and rice) and tubers (potatoes and cassava).

To thicken a food, you heat a starch such as wheat flour or cornstarch in water. *The starch molecules absorb water in a process* called **gelatinization**.

Activity: Bring recipes of different kinds of sauces and gravies to class. Identify the thickening agent in each. Prepare one recipe and describe the results.

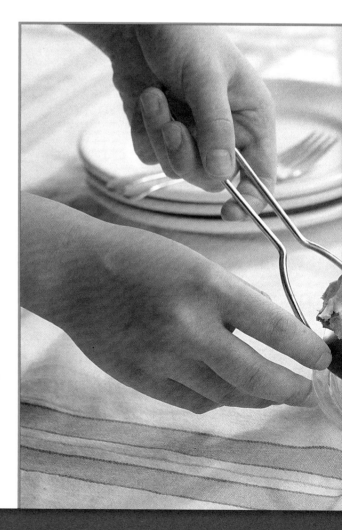

Cornstarch will thicken a lemon filling to make a taste-tempting lemon pie.

Gelatinization

Starch molecules do not dissolve in water because they are too large. However, when starches are cooked in water, the energy from the water molecules loosens the bonds between the starch molecules. Clusters of starch called granules then absorb water and swell in a process called gelatinization.

As you cook a starch and water mixture, more and more water enters each granule and is bound by the starch. There is now less liquid outside the granule. This causes the liquid to become thick.

Once a starch mixture is thickened, or gelatinized, and begins to cool, the starch can become rigid, forming a gel. A gel can be cut with a knife and will not spread out to take the shape of the container it is in. You see this in the cornstarch-thickened lemon filling of a lemon meringue pie. When the filling cools, it becomes firm—the starch has gelled.

What Makes Gravy Lumpy?

One problem with using starch to thicken liquids is its tendency to form clumps. Try adding a spoonful of flour to a hot liquid such as chicken soup. Instead of a smooth liquid, you'll get lumps! The starch granules around each lump of flour have swelled and formed a water-proof gel surrounding the lump. The granules inside the lump stay dry, so their thickening power is lost. The soup stays thin.

You can avoid lumpy soups, gravies, and sauces by dispersing the starch granules *before* you put them in hot water. One trick is to put the flour (or other starch) in a small bottle with ¼ cup (50 mL) of cold water, and shake well. This scatters the granules throughout the water. Then pour the starch mixture into your soup, sauce, or gravy. The result? A thick, smooth liquid.

Emphasize: If a gravy results in some lumps, you can minimize them by putting the gravy through a strainer or blender. Then reheat the mixture, stirring constantly.

The Science of Baking

To bake a loaf of bread, you mix the ingredients, knead the dough, and set it aside to rise. As you bake the dough, the aroma of baking bread fills the room. The dough rises and expands still more. The result is a light, tasty loaf. Have you ever wondered why these changes occur? Baked goods such as breads, cakes, and muffins rise as a result of physical and chemical changes.

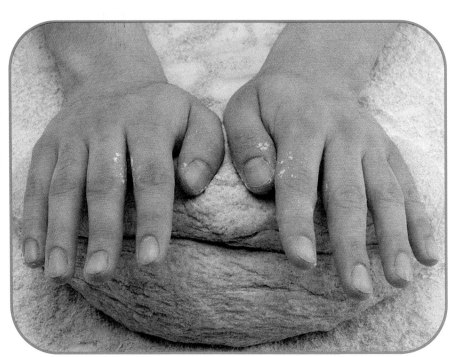

Kneading this bread dough adds air, which acts as a leavening agent.

What Makes Baked Goods Rise?

Baked goods rise because of leavening. To **leaven** means *to make light and porous*. In baked goods, leavening involves producing a gas that expands as the batter or dough is heated, leaving holes as the batter or dough sets during baking.

All baked goods are leavened in part by air and steam. Air is mixed in when you work a dough—when you mix, beat, or knead it—and when you cream fat and sugar together. Steam, or water vapor, is produced when the dough is placed in a hot oven. Water in the dough quickly vaporizes to steam, which takes up much more room than water. The steam expands the dough and causes it to rise.

Some baked products are also leavened by carbon dioxide. This gas is produced by leavening agents such as baking soda, baking powder, and yeast.

Activity: Create a cartoon that explains how baked goods are leavened by air and steam and by carbon dioxide. Display completed cartoons and evaluate the accuracy.

How Baking Soda Leavens

Baking soda is a chemical agent for producing carbon dioxide. Baking soda is a base. When it is mixed with an acid, a chemical reaction occurs:

Baking soda + Acid + Heat =
        Carbon dioxide + Water

SCIENCE CONCEPT:
Acids and Bases

Acid is the name for a group of chemicals that share certain characteristics. Weak acids taste sour. The acetic acid in vinegar and the citric acid in fruits such as oranges and lemons give these foods their sour taste.

Base is the name for another group of chemicals that reacts with acids. Bases are the chemical opposite of acids.

These acids can be used with baking soda to produce the chemical reaction that releases carbon dioxide.

More About Baking Powder: Baking powder needs to be stored in a cool, dry place and used before the expiration date. To test the freshness of baking powder, mix 1 tsp. of baking powder with ⅓ cup of hot water. If usable, the solution bubbles quickly.

When a recipe calls for baking soda, an acidic food such as vinegar, buttermilk, molasses, honey, fruit juice, or yogurt is also added. Together, the base and the acid react to give off carbon dioxide. The carbon dioxide leavens the baked good.

Many recipes call for baking powder. Baking powder is a convenience food used in recipes that do not have an acidic ingredient. Baking powder is baking soda plus a powdered acid (cream of tartar) and cornstarch.

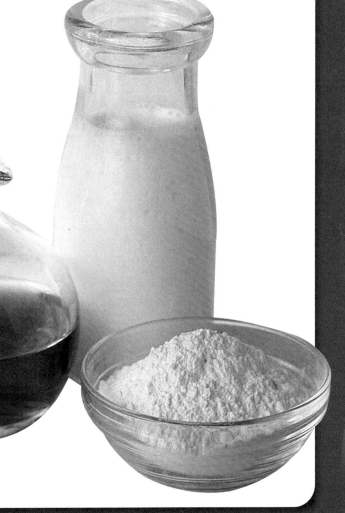

How Yeast Leavens

Yeast is *a one-celled fungus that will multiply rapidly, given the right conditions.* Yeast leavens bread because it ferments the carbohydrates naturally present in the flour.

SCIENCE CONCEPT:
Fermentation

Fermentation is a chemical reaction that breaks down large molecules into smaller ones. Usually fermentation involves breaking down sugars into carbon dioxide and alcohol.

When you add yeast to bread dough, it feeds on simple sugars in the flour, giving off carbon dioxide and alcohol. (The alcohol evaporates during baking.) Proteins in the flour trap the carbon dioxide bubbles in the bread dough. The dough rises and becomes lighter. Besides leavening dough, yeast gives bread its characteristic aroma and flavor.

Most breads are leavened solely by yeast. However, sourdough breads are leavened by yeast *and* by bacteria that produce carbon dioxide. The bacteria produce flavorful acidic by-products that give the characteristic sour taste to these breads.

Critical Thinking: Why is it important to mix flour and liquid ingredients as long as the recipe calls for?

What Does Gluten Do?

Wheat flour is used for yeast bread because of its special properties. When wheat flour is mixed with water and then kneaded, two proteins of wheat bond to form a stretchy, elastic network called gluten. Gluten forms a three-dimensional structure that holds the dough together. It is also elastic, so that the dough can expand. The dough becomes smooth and stretchy.

When the yeast in the bread produces carbon dioxide, the cell walls of the gluten stretch. The gluten traps the carbon dioxide, forming small holes in the dough. You can still see these holes in baked bread, because the heat coagulates the gluten, causing it to become solid.

Bubbles are trapped in the bread as it bakes.

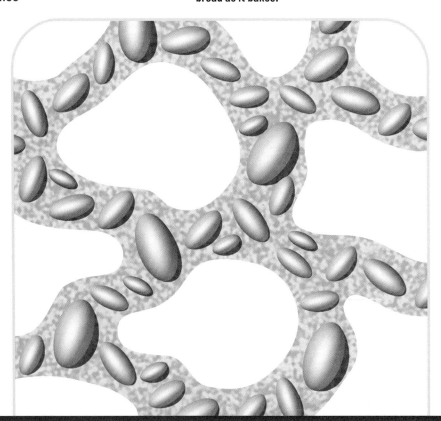

Coagulation

Coagulation occurs when a liquid is changed into a soft semisolid or solid mass. The gluten begins to coagulate when the protein molecules unwind and collide with one another. As the temperature rises, they bond and form into a solid. The bread is baked.

Without gluten, yeast-leavened breads would be next to impossible to prepare. They would expand as a result of the steam and carbon dioxide gases and then fall back down on themselves. Even yeast breads made with flours such as rye or oat must still have some wheat flour to stay firm.

Carbon dioxide in a wheat dough causes the gluten cells to rise and expand. These holes remain after the bread is baked.

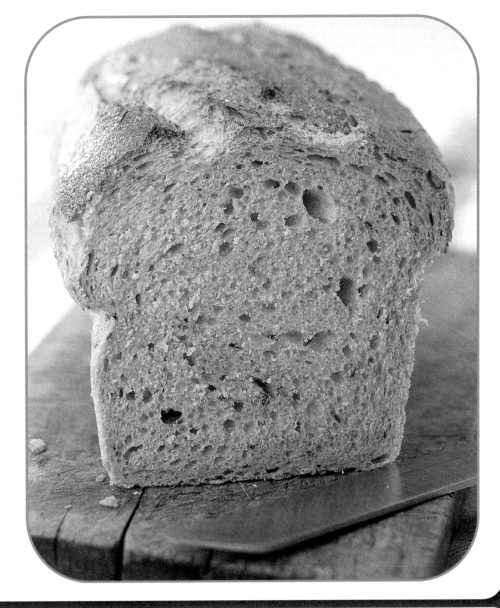

Review & Activities

LOOKING BACK

- All foods are made up of chemicals.
- During cooking, heat energy is transferred to or within food.
- When food is prepared, physical and chemical changes can take place. Understanding these changes can help you better manage food preparation.
- You've learned about changes that involve the starches in grain products and gravies; the pigments in fruits and vegetables; the proteins in dairy foods, eggs, and gelatin; the muscle and connective tissue of meat; the oil in salad dressings; and the leavening and gluten in baked goods, among others.

UNDERSTANDING KEY IDEAS

1. Describe each of the four basic chemical building blocks of food.
2. Contrast three types of heat transfer.
3. What causes pasta to become sticky after cooking? How can this be avoided?
4. Which vegetables and fruits get their color from flavonoids? How is this color affected by cooking?
5. What does coagulation mean? Give at least three examples of how protein coagulation can occur during food preparation.
6. What chemical reaction is involved in making yogurt? Explain what occurs.
7. What are enzymes? How do they play a role in tenderizing meat?
8. How is beating an egg white into a stiff foam similar to cooking an egg?
9. What is needed in order for oil and water to stay mixed together? Give an example.
10. In scientific terms, what type of mixture is gelatin? Describe its characteristics.
11. What process allows starch to be used as a thickener? How does it work?
12. What is gluten? How does it work together with leavening agents to make bread rise?

DEVELOPING LIFE SKILLS

1. **Critical Thinking:** "Learning about food science can help you select and prepare healthful, tasty foods." What evidence can you offer in support of this statement?
2. **Communication:** In what ways might it be important for a food scientist to have good communication skills?

Wellness Challenge

When their parents aren't home, Marcus and Jenessa would rather order out for dinner than try to cook. They have been discouraged by their previous attempts at cooking, which resulted in sticky spaghetti, dull green vegetables, and dry, tough chicken breast.

1. Why might Jenessa and Marcus get these results when they cook?
2. What can Marcus and Jenessa do to prevent these cooking problems?

APPLYING YOUR LEARNING

1. **Baking Soda Test:** Combine small amounts of baking soda and lemon juice. Observe what happens. What properties of the two substances explain the reaction? What is produced as a result? How does this relate to food preparation? Repeat the experiment with other liquids. Share your findings in class.

2. **Recipe Analysis:** Collect at least ten recipes for soups, gravies, sauces, salad dressings, or desserts that require the use of starchy ingredients as a thickener. How and when does each recipe instruct you to add the ingredient? Do you think the starch will get lumpy if you follow the directions as they are written? Why or why not?

EXPLORING FURTHER

1. **Go Sour:** Learn what makes sauerkraut sour. What other food mentioned in Part 4 undergoes a similar process? Present your findings to the class.

2. **Sweet Vegetables:** Find out why carrots, sweet peppers, and onions seem to become sweeter when cooked, even when sugar isn't added in the cooking process. Report to the class.

Making CONNECTIONS

1. **Science:** Does milk really curdle when it's overheated? Plan and carry out an experiment to find out. Write a report that includes your hypothesis, procedure, observations, and conclusions. Include information on the scientific principle of coagulation.

2. **Math:** Investigate the math knowledge and skills needed by a food scientist. What college math courses are required? What courses are recommended in high school? How might the concepts you are learning in math classes now be useful for a career as a food scientist?

FOODS LAB

Cut an apple into two pieces. Leave one piece plain, and sprinkle the other piece with lemon or orange juice. After half an hour, compare the color of each piece. What can you conclude about enzymatic browning?

PART 5

The Art of Preparing Food

SECTION 5-1
Meals with Appeal

SECTION 5-2
Creative Cooking

SECTION 5-3
Easy Entertaining

PART 5 REVIEW

Objectives

After studying pages 537-549, you will be able to:

- Explain ways to use variety, presentation, and garnishes to make meals appealing.

- Discuss ways to enjoy food preparation as a hobby.

- Describe how to use herbs, spices, and other flavorings.

- Give guidelines for successful entertaining.

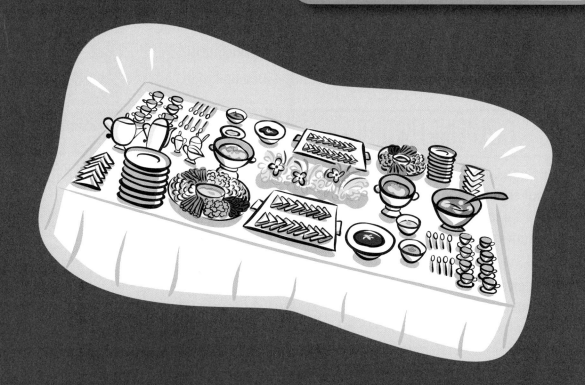

Meals with Appeal

Preparing and serving an appealing meal involves not only skill and science, but art. With the foods you choose, the way you arrange them, and the special touches you add, your meals can go from "ho-hum" to "wow!" What will you create as your next masterpiece?

Variety on the Plate

As you know, eating a variety of foods is one of the best paths to good nutrition. Variety is a key to making meals appealing, too. Just as an artist uses different paints to create a picture, you can create enticing meals with...

Variety in colors! Think of a rainbow when you plan a meal. Add color contrasts with bright fruits, vivid vegetables, and the soothing hues of other foods. For visual appeal, try not to repeat colors on the plate.

Variety in textures! Crisp or chewy, smooth or chunky—different textures make a meal more interesting. Remember, the way you prepare food can change its texture. Cooking makes crisp vegetables softer, and whirling fruit in a blender makes it smooth.

Variety in flavors! Use mild foods to balance strong flavors—such as garlic, onions, or hot peppers—so they don't overpower your meal. Try not to repeat a food in the meal. If your salad has apples, consider peach cobbler for dessert rather than apple pie.

Variety in temperatures! For interesting meals, try to include both hot and cold foods. A chilled fruit salad and cold milk contrast well with steaming hot stew. Serving foods at the proper temperature makes them taste better— and it's an important rule of food safety.

Variety in shapes and sizes! If your main dish is round meatballs, long green beans add more eye appeal than peas. Think of ways to add variety by using your cutting board and knife, too. You can cut bell peppers in strips or rings, or chop them finely. How might you cut up a tomato?

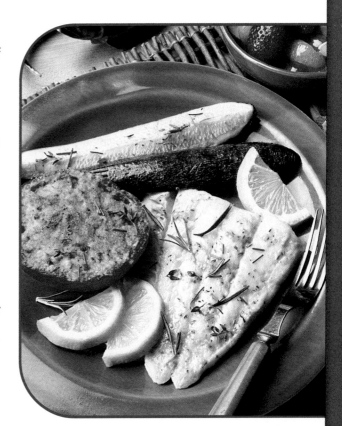

A variety of colors, textures, flavors, temperatures, and shapes are combined beautifully in this meal. If you were preparing a baked chicken dinner, what other foods would you add to make a balanced and attractive meal?

Food with a Flair

Create a feast for the eyes! If artistry is your goal, consider serving the meal "plate style"— arranging food on individual plates before bringing them to the table. Rather than just plop food on the plate, take cues from the many beautiful photos of food in cookbooks and magazines or the ways that TV chefs display their dishes.

Pick a plate—or two. Start by deciding whether you need more than one plate per person. Some foods, such as beets, need a small bowl so their juices won't run all over. If your main course is hot, serve chilled foods, such as gelatin salad, on a side plate to keep them cold.

Know the basic rules. As a general rule, avoid overcrowding a plate. Remember to use tongs or other utensils to arrange food, not your fingers!

Use your imagination. Arranging an attractive plate of food requires thought, but not necessarily much extra time. Try these quick, easy ways—or let them spark your own creativity.

- Serve salad mixtures on a bed of shredded lettuce, diced colorful bell peppers, or crunchy Chinese noodles.
- Cut vegetables such as zucchini into long, thin pieces. Fan them out alongside the main dish.
- Try edible containers, such as chicken salad served in a melon half.
- Use cookie cutters to cut cheese, deli meat, bread, or sandwiches into fun or fancy shapes.
- Create designs with a **decorating tube**—*a tool for squeezing soft foods through a shaped tube.* It can help you turn mashed potatoes into a work of art!
- Try putting sauces under or alongside foods instead of on top. For an extra special touch, use a squeeze bottle to make swirls or other patterns on the plate.
- Decorate the plate by sprinkling finely-chopped parsley or other fresh herbs around the rim.

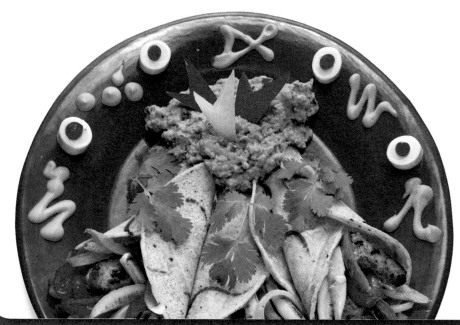

Attractive presentation isn't only for restaurant meals. With some simple attention to detail, you can serve a meal of which you'll be proud. Either write a description or draw a picture of an attractive meal you could serve your family.

Discuss: Think of a restaurant or a person who has a flair for making food look appealing on a plate. Discuss techniques the restaurant or person uses.

Garnishes—The Finishing Touch

A **garnish,** or *edible decoration*, adds a festive touch to make food more enjoyable. As you garnish, remember the guidelines for meals with appeal (page 537). Use garnishes as a way to add contrasts of color, texture, flavor, temperature, and shape. As for size, keep garnishes small and simple. They should enhance your food, not overpower it. Sometimes less is more! You don't need special skills to garnish food.

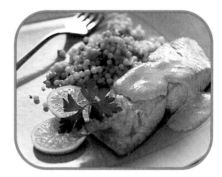

A garnish can be as simple as:
- Carrot shreds on a green salad.
- Grated orange rind or crunchy slivered almonds on grilled chicken.
- Garlic croutons or plain, air-popped popcorn on tomato-barley soup.
- Citrus slices or a few small berries beside broiled fish.
- A sprig of a fresh herb on almost any main dish.
- Edible flowers on salads, appetizers, or desserts. For food safety, use only those sold in the produce department and labeled "edible flowers."

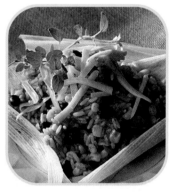

Garnishes can turn a simple meal into an artistic one. What contrasts do these garnishes add to these dishes?

When you have more time and skill, you might try fancier garnishes. Some creative cooks carve fruits and vegetables. You might like to try these:

Lemon twists. First cut the lemon into slices. Then cut from the center of each slice through the peel. Hold each side of the cut and twist in opposite directions.

Cucumber slices. Use a fork to score a cucumber. Then cut it into slices.

Carrot curls. Make thin strips of carrot with a vegetable peeler. Roll them up and use toothpicks to secure them. Chill them in ice water so they'll hold their shape, then remove the toothpicks.

Activity: Create your own garnish—one that is not listed in the text. Share your idea with the class or present a food using the garnish.

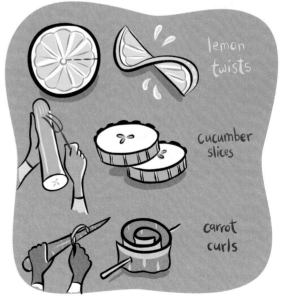

lemon twists

cucumber slices

carrot curls

Creative Cooking

Look *for these* **TERMS**

fusion cuisine   rub

herbs   condiments

spices

Everyone can benefit by learning how to prepare quick, easy, nutritious meals. The possibilities don't end there, however. In fact, that's just the beginning!

Cooking for Pleasure

Many people consider food their hobby and their creative outlet. If you're one of them—or would like to be—try expanding the roles that food preparation plays in your life.

Cook for the fun of it. Even if quick meals are the rule most days, you and your family might enjoy more leisurely food preparation when you have time. Preparing a special Sunday brunch, baking a loaf of cinnamon bread, or cooking a pot of savory vegetable soup can be a great way to unwind. Sharing talk and laughter as you work in the kitchen is fun, too!

Feast your senses. Take time to really notice and appreciate the wonderful colors, textures, flavors, and aromas of food. Have you ever browsed in the produce department or a farmer's market just for the fun of it? Try it sometime—and while you're at it, choose something new to buy and enjoy!

Learn new skills. Is your grandmother's lasagna the best you've ever had? Ask if she'll show you how to make it sometime. Grandparents, parents, and friends can be a great source of recipes and other ideas. You can pick up new skills from books, magazines, TV cooking shows, and web sites, too. Perhaps a nearby kitchen store or gourmet shop offers cooking classes.

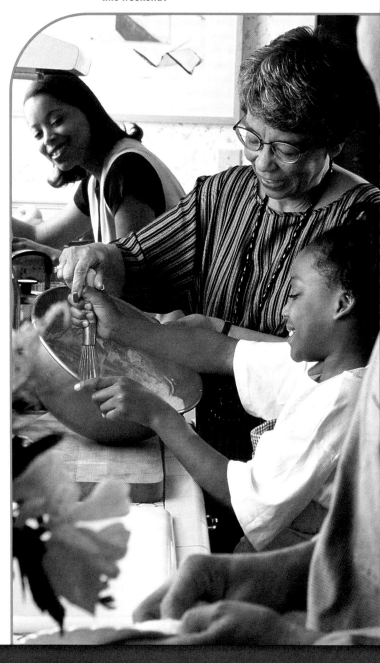

Cooking can be a fun family activity. What meals could your family prepare together this weekend?

Teach new skills. **Share what you've learned with others. Perhaps you could show a foreign student how to prepare your favorite American dish, or teach a kindergartner how to make instant pudding. You and a friend or neighbor might share your favorite recipes.**

Sample many cuisines. **As you learn and experiment, explore the cuisine of other countries. You might even try your hand at fusion cuisine**—*cooking that combines different cultural food traditions in one dish.*

Create your own recipes. **Many chefs experiment to come up with new dishes. When making a familiar recipe, they may add or delete an ingredient or two. You, too, can add your own special touches to remake recipes and create dishes that are truly your own.**

Give the gift of food. **What makes a better present than food you made yourself? You might give mini loaves of quick bread, a pretty bottle of herbed vinegar, or homemade trail mix. Besides birthdays and holidays, think of giving a food gift when you're a guest at someone's home, or to cheer someone who's housebound. These thoughtful gifts show you care.**

Discuss: What are some foods you have tasted that combined different cultural foods in one dish?

For a new twist on tacos, give them an Asian flavor with tuna and ginger. What other fusion dishes might you create?

Explore food as a business. **Why not make gift baskets to sell to others? You don't need to cook anything. Just put together your own combinations—perhaps uncooked rice with herbs, a colorful mixture of dry beans for soup, or a package of pasta with a jar of convenience sauce. Add value with your special packaging. You could arrange the items in an attractive basket, add a festive ribbon, and tuck your own recipe inside. If gift baskets aren't your style, you might hire yourself out as a kitchen helper to assist people when they entertain. What else could your business offer?**

INFOLINK

Check out the ideas for making recipe changes in Chapter 14, pages 196–198, and Chapter 32, page 427.

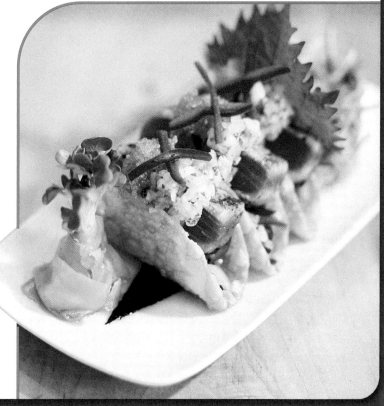

Using Herbs and Spices

One way to be a creative cook is to season foods your own way. You can give your dishes lots of pizzazz without adding salt or sugar. How? Learn how to use a wide variety of herbs and spices.

- **Herbs** are *fragrant, edible leaves used for seasoning food.* You can use them either fresh or dried.
- **Spices** are *seasonings that come from the bark, buds, seeds, roots, or stems of different plants and trees.* They are usually dried.

Improvising with herbs and spices. The more you use herbs and spices, the better you'll know how their flavors and aromas blend with foods. Then you can adapt recipes by substituting or adding herbs and spices to your taste. To get started, use the chart on page 543 as a guide.

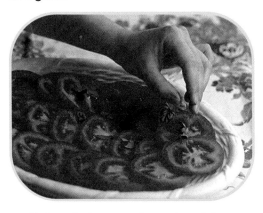

Herbs and spices open the way to a whole new taste experience. Choose a recipe and describe how you might alter the seasonings.

Substituting fresh and dried herbs. Dried herbs are stronger and more concentrated than fresh. When substituting dried herbs for fresh, divide the amount called for by three. Multiply by three when substituting fresh for dried. You can always adjust amounts if needed.

Releasing the full flavor. For the best flavor, add herbs and spices to soups and stews toward the end of cooking time. With chilled foods, such as dips, add seasonings several hours before serving so the flavors can blend. To release the flavor of dry herbs, crumble them between your fingers. Chop fresh herbs finely.

Using seasoning blends. You can buy herb and spice blends or make your own. For instance, to make an Italian blend, mix dried basil, marjoram, and oregano. When you're grilling, add zip with a **rub**—*an herb or spice mixture applied to tender meat, poultry, or fish before cooking.*

Storing herbs and spices. To keep dried herbs and spices at their peak of flavor for about a year, store them in airtight containers in a cool, dry place. Herbs and spices stored near the range lose their flavor more quickly. You can keep fresh herbs for a few days in the refrigerator. Wrap them in a damp paper towel and place them in an airtight plastic bag.

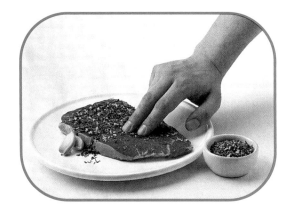

A rub can be any combination of fresh or dried herbs and spices you like. For a stronger flavor, apply a rub several hours ahead. Then cover and refrigerate the meat until it's time to cook it. Using the Herb and Spice chart on the next page, invent your own rub.

Activity: Start an herb garden. The seeds are inexpensive, and the plants can be grown indoors easily.

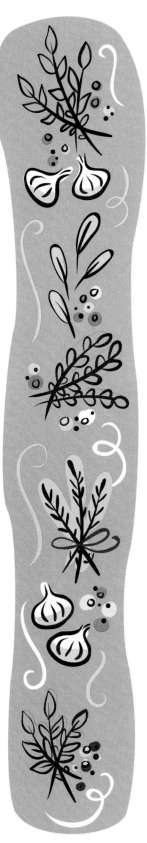

Herb and Spice Guide

Herb or Spice	Forms Available	Tastes Good With
Basil	Dried or fresh leaves, ground	All tomato dishes, peas, green beans, eggplant, zucchini, soups, eggs
Black pepper	Whole pepper-corns, ground	Vegetables, stews, meat, poultry, fish, soups, salads
Celery seed	Dried	Potato, egg, and tuna salads; soups; sauces; fish; vegetables
Chili powder	Ground	Mexican-style dishes, barbecue sauce, meat loaf, stews
Cinnamon	Ground, stick, with sugar, in blends such as pumpkin pie spice	Baked goods such as cakes, buns, breads, pies, and cookies; apples; hot chocolate
Cloves	Whole, ground	Whole ham, roast pork, stews, pickled fruit, baked goods, chocolate desserts, sweet vegetables
Garlic	Cloves, powdered, minced, salt	Meat dishes, sauces, dressings, vegetables, butter spread, salads
Ginger	Fresh, ground	Baked goods, stews, chicken, carrots, squash, sweet potatoes, pears, stir-fries, beverages
Nutmeg	Whole, ground	Baked goods, custard, puddings, apples, carrots, squash, eggnog
Oregano	Fresh and dried leaves, ground	Tomato dishes, Italian and Mexican foods, lamb, pork, poultry, peas, green beans, onions, zucchini
Paprika	Ground	Salads, cream sauces for vegetables, potatoes, eggs, poultry
Parsley	Fresh or dried flakes	Soups, salads, slaws, meat, fish, poultry, all vegetables, sauces, omelets, rice
Rosemary	Fresh or dried	Beef, lamb, and chicken dishes; fruits
Sage	Fresh or dried whole leaves, rubbed, ground	All pork dishes, meat, fish, poultry stuffings, consommé, cream soups, fish chowder, salad dressing
Thyme	Fresh or dried	Eggs, fish, stews, salads, tomato sauces, legumes, vegetables

Condiments

Besides using herbs and spices, you can flavor foods with a variety of **condiments**—*flavorful accompaniments to food.* Ketchup and mustard are well-known condiments, but there are many more to try.

Salsa is usually a mixture of chopped tomatoes, onion, peppers, and herbs. You can buy it in mild, medium, and hot versions or make your own. Try salsa with poultry, fish, and meat dishes; on baked potatoes; tossed with cooked rice or cooked pasta; or as a dip for raw vegetables.

Chutney is a mixture of fruit (or sometimes tomatoes), vinegar, sugar, and spices that you can make or buy. It can be mild, spicy, or sweet. You can serve chutney alongside meat, poultry, or fish; as a spread for bread or sandwiches; or with cheese as an appetizer.

Vinegar adds tartness to foods. Flavorful varieties include apple cider vinegar, balsamic vinegar (made from white grape juice), raspberry vinegar, or rice vinegar (a staple in Asian cooking). Herb vinegars are made by adding fresh herbs to any vinegar.

Pesto is a finely chopped mixture of basil, garlic, pine nuts, cheese, and olive oil. It's most often served with pasta. You may find variations made with other ingredients.

Other condiments include barbecue sauce, soy sauce, tamari sauce (similar to soy sauce), and Worcestershire (WOOS-tuhr-shuhr) sauce. The next time you're shopping for food, see how many varieties of these and other condiments you can find.

Other Flavor Boosters

Other ingredients with intense flavors can add spark to your dishes. Try these ideas:

Sun-dried tomatoes have a rich, intense flavor and chewy texture. You can buy them in their dry form or packed in oil. Try using them on pizza crust or in pasta dishes, salads, or soups.

Chili peppers range from mild to very hot. You can buy them fresh, dried, canned, pickled, or packed in oil. Be very careful when handling chili peppers—they contain a compound that can burn your eyes and skin. Wash your hands thoroughly with soap and water afterward.

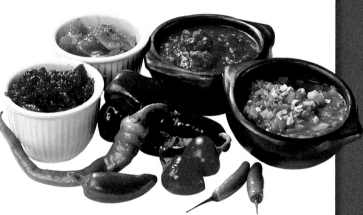

Check out the supermarket for these and other ways to flavor your recipes. What's your favorite way to spark up a recipe?

Citrus zest—the grated outer rind of citrus fruits—gives a fresh taste to many dishes. Try adding it to herb blends and rubs, too.

Flavoring extracts, such as vanilla extract or almond extract, are often used in baked goods such as cakes and cookies. Just a small amount of these liquids is enough to flavor the finished product.

Easy Entertaining

Whenever people gather to share an activity, celebrate a special occasion, or just enjoy one another's company, food is almost sure to play a part. Whether the gathering is casual or fancy, make it special with planning and a creative touch.

Planning a Get-Together

When you're the host, planning and organization are your keys to success. The more you plan and prepare ahead, the smoother everything will go. You'll be more relaxed, too, knowing that you're well prepared. That means you *and* your guests will enjoy yourselves! These are some things you'll need to plan:

What's the theme? Some gatherings have a built-in theme, such as a graduation party or a holiday celebration. You also can invent a theme of your own. How about a make-your-own pizza party or a backyard volleyball party? Not every gathering needs a theme, but having one can help you make some of your other decisions.

When will the gathering take place? Choose a date and time that's convenient for you, other family members, and your guests.

What will you serve? The theme, date, and time may affect what foods you choose. Are you having a brunch, a picnic, or a formal dinner party? No matter what the occasion, try to choose foods that are easy to prepare. Perhaps some can be made ahead of time. For food safety, think about how you'll keep hot foods hot and cold foods cold. To avoid unpleasant surprises, choose recipes that you've prepared before—or try out new ones in advance.

Who's coming? Decide how many people you can serve comfortably, then plan the guest list. Consider whether the people you invite will enjoy each other's company and have things to talk about together. They don't need to know each other to have fun.

Critical Thinking: What factors should you consider when deciding what food to serve at a party?

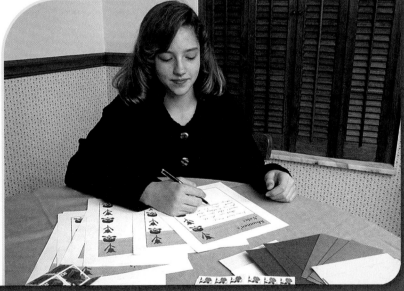

Send invitations two to four weeks in advance to allow your guests time to plan their schedules. What extra steps might you take when sending invitations to a surprise party?

How will you invite them? Invite your guests a few days or weeks in advance so that they can make plans to come. You might invite them in person, on the telephone, or in writing. Tell them all the basic information: the date, time, place, occasion, whether food will be served, and that you're the host. Ask them to let you know by a certain date whether they're coming. On a written invitation, you might use the initials **R.S.V.P.**, which come from a French phrase that means *"please reply."* Include your phone number or other way for them to contact you.

Party decorations add a festive touch. If you were going to give a party this month, how would you decorate? Is there a holiday coming up around which you could plan a theme?

How will you decorate? Think about how you'll create a pleasant atmosphere with tableware, a tablecloth or placemats, and a centerpiece. Depending on the occasion, you might want other decorations, too, such as balloons and streamers. Be inventive as you plan decorations to go with your theme.

How will you get ready? While you're planning, make lists of everything you'll need to do to prepare. Group tasks according to the earliest time they can be done: the week before, the day before, early in the day, and at the last minute. Plan to do as much ahead as possible. Then follow your plan, crossing off tasks as you accomplish them. Remember the final tasks— thanking your guests for coming, and cleaning up after they leave!

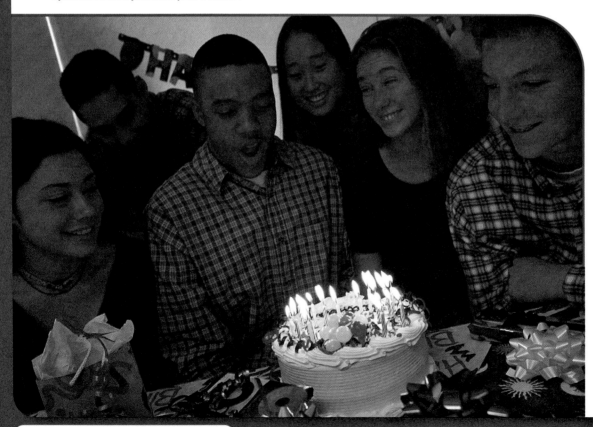

Buffet Service

Buffet service is an easy entertaining option, especially for a crowd. With this kind of setup, platters and serving dishes of food are arranged on a table. Guests walk up to the table, serve themselves, then sit or stand elsewhere while they eat.

Here are some tips for setting up a buffet table:

- If people will be eating from plates in their lap or while standing, choose foods that are easy to manage. Finger foods are a good choice. For example, you might serve raw vegetables with a dip, small meatballs on toothpicks, and cheese cubes with crackers.

- Plan the traffic flow so that people approaching the buffet table aren't in the way of those who've just served themselves. For a large group, consider setting up two buffet lines—one on each side of the table.

- Arrange items on the buffet table in an order that's easy for guests. Place a stack of plates at one end as the starting point, then the food. Flatware goes at the other end of the table—perhaps rolled in a napkin so it's easy to pick up. Place filled beverage cups at the end of the table, or on a separate table.

- If the buffet table will be set up for a while, take steps to keep hot foods hot and cold foods cold. Set out only some of each food at first, keeping the rest hot or cold in the kitchen. Refill the serving dishes as needed. You can also use warming trays, slow cookers, beds of ice, or insulated serving dishes to keep foods hot or cold on the buffet table. Remember the two-hour rule for food safety.

Activity: Sketch an arrangement for a buffet table. Share in class, explaining the reasons for the arrangement.

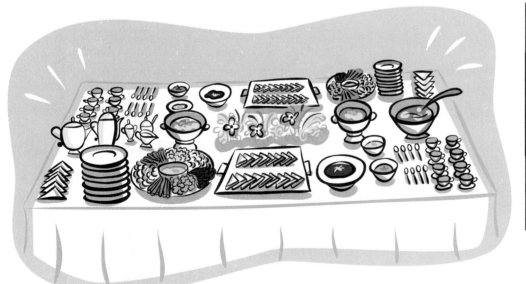

Set up a buffet table in a way that makes it easy for guests to serve themselves. Describe the types of food you might serve at a buffet.

INFOLINK

To learn about other styles of serving meals, see Chapter 2, page 40. Review the food safety guidelines in Part 1 of the Food Preparation Handbook.

LOOKING BACK

- Use variety, presentation, and garnishes to make meals appealing.
- You can enjoy food preparation as a hobby by expanding the roles it plays in your life.
- Herbs, spices, condiments, and other flavorful ingredients can add spark to your dishes.
- Planning and organization are the keys to successful entertaining.
- Buffet service is an easy entertaining option, especially for serving food to a large group of people.

UNDERSTANDING KEY IDEAS

1. How could you make meals appealing with variety in colors? In textures? In flavors?
2. What are the basic guidelines for presenting an appealing plate of food?
3. What are some ways to enjoy food preparation as a hobby?
4. Describe how and when you would add dried rosemary to a beef stew to get the best flavor. What would you do if the recipe called for fresh rosemary and you had only the dried version?
5. Besides ketchup and mustard, what other condiments add flavor to foods? Describe how you might use each one.
6. If you wanted to have a party, what might you do to prepare?

DEVELOPING LIFE SKILLS

1. **Creative Thinking:** If you were the cafeteria supervisor at an elementary school, how could you make the meals appealing for the children? What special touches might you add for holidays or changes of season?

2. **Leadership:** Many people value the creative and pleasurable aspects of food preparation. What are some ways in which older family members might pass these values down to younger generations? How might you pass an appreciation for enjoying food on to younger siblings or cousins?

Wellness Challenge

Brandon is a member of a community choir. This year the choir has decided to put on a winter holiday performance at the local senior center. The choir members plan to follow the show with refreshments, including fresh fruit, muffins, and hot cocoa. Brandon has volunteered for the planning committee.
1. In what ways will this holiday performance contribute to the wellness of senior center residents?
2. What might Brandon suggest to make the refreshments appealing and to add a special touch?
3. In what ways might the committee members decorate for the event?

APPLYING YOUR LEARNING

1. **Food Photos:** Food and home magazines often show examples of creative cooking. Find five photographs of dishes that appeal to you. How did the food stylist make the dishes look appealing? How might you adapt these techniques to other foods?

2. **Meal Makeovers:** Think about three meals that you have eaten recently. How could they have been made more appealing? How might herbs, spices, or other flavorings have been used to add pizzazz? Using a two-column chart, describe the three original meals and the suggested improvements.

EXPLORING FURTHER

1. **Growing Herbs:** Find out how you can grow your own fresh herbs in a garden or on a windowsill. Which ones would you choose to grow and why? Next learn how you can successfully dry your own fresh herbs. How do you think the cost of home-grown herbs compares to the cost of purchasing them in a grocery store?

2. **Fusion Cooking:** Find or create a recipe for a fusion dish. How does it combine food traditions from different cultures? Share your findings with the class.

Making CONNECTIONS

1. **Science:** Choose two fruit or vegetable garnishes. Plan and carry out an experiment to find out how moisture content affects their crispness and appeal. Write a report that includes your hypothesis, procedure, observations, and conclusions.

2. **Career Connections Experience:** Make arrangements to observe a local caterer or other food service professional in a job-shadowing experience. Report on what this experience has taught you about the art of preparing food.

FOODS LAB

Prepare five simple garnishes made from fruits or vegetables. You may use the suggestions given in the text as well as others that you find in cookbooks or other resources. Describe what foods you might enhance with each garnish.

Appendix

······································

Pyramid Serving Sizes

Bread, Cereal, Rice, & Pasta Group

One serving equals:

1 slice enriched or whole grain bread

1 6-inch (15-cm) tortilla

½ burger bun, bagel, pita, or English muffin

1 ounce (28 g) ready-to-eat cereal

½ cup (125 mL) cooked cereal, pasta, rice, or other cooked grain

1 4-inch (10-cm) pancake or waffle

3 to 4 small crackers

1 ounce (28 g) pretzels

Vegetable Group

One serving equals:

1 cup (250 mL) raw leafy greens

½ cup (125 mL) cooked or chopped raw vegetables

½ cup (125 mL) cooked dry beans, peas, or lentils*

1 small potato

¾ cup (175 mL) vegetable juice

Fruit Group

One serving equals:

1 medium whole apple, pear, orange, or banana

½ of a grapefruit, mango, or papaya

½ cup (125 mL) berries or cut-up, canned, frozen, or cooked fruit

¾ cup (175 mL) fruit juice

¼ cup (50 mL) dried fruit

Milk, Yogurt, & Cheese Group

One serving equals:

1 cup (250 mL) milk, buttermilk, yogurt, or pudding

1½ ounces (42 g) natural cheese, such as cheddar, Swiss, Monterey Jack, or mozzarella

2 ounces (56 g) process cheese, such as American

Other amounts:

½ cup (125 mL) cottage cheese = ¼ serving

½ cup (125 mL) frozen yogurt = ½ serving

½ cup (125 mL) ice cream = ⅓ serving

Meat, Poultry, Fish, Dry Beans, Eggs, & Nuts Group

One serving equals:

2 to 3 ounces (56 to 85 g) cooked lean meat, poultry, or fish

The following count as 1 ounce (28 g) of meat:

½ cup (125 mL) cooked dry beans, peas, or lentils*

1 egg

2 tablespoons (30 mL) peanut butter

¼ cup (50 mL) egg substitute

⅓ cup (75 mL) nuts

4 ounces (112 g) tofu

*Count dry beans, peas, or lentils toward a serving from either the Vegetable Group or the Meat, Poultry, Fish, Dry Beans, Eggs, and Nuts Group—but not both.

Daily Values and DRIs for Teens

The Daily Values are standard values developed by the Food and Drug Administration (FDA) for use on food labels. Dietary Reference Intakes (DRIs) are used by nutrition professionals. They give nutrient reference amounts for specific ages and genders. Only the amounts for teens are included here. You may find it interesting to compare the DRIs for your age and gender to the Daily Values.

The DRIs include four types of nutrient reference values. Most of the values listed below are Recommended Dietary Allowances (RDAs). An RDA is the daily amount of a nutrient that will meet the needs of nearly all healthy people. For some nutrients, there is not yet enough data to establish an RDA. In that case, the value listed is an Adequate Intake (AI), an amount believed to be adequate.

Nutrient	Daily Value	Dietary Reference Intake (RDA or AI)			
		Males 9-13	Males 14-18	Females 9-13	Females 14-18
Protein	50 g**	34 g	52 g	34 g	46 g
Carbohydrate (total)	300 g**	130 g	130 g	130 g	130 g
Fiber	25 g	31 g	38 g	26 g	36 g
Fat (total)	65 g**	*	*	*	*
Saturated fat	20 g**	*	*	*	*
Cholesterol	300 mg	*	*	*	*
Vitamin A	5,000 IU (875 µg RE)	600 µg RAE	900 µg RAE	600 µg RAE	700 µg RAE
Thiamin	1.5 mg	0.9 mg	1.2 mg	0.9 mg	1.0 mg
Riboflavin	1.7 mg	0.9 mg	1.3 mg	0.9 mg	1.0 mg
Niacin	20 mg NE	12 mg NE	16 mg NE	12 mg NE	14 mg NE
Vitamin B$_6$	2 mg	1.0 mg	1.3 mg	1.0 mg	1.2 mg
Vitamin B$_{12}$	6 µg	1.8 µg	2.4 µg	1.8 µg	2.4 µg
Folate	400 µg	300 µg DFE	400 µg DFE	300 µg DFE	400 µg DFE
Biotin	300 µg	20 µg	25 µg	20 µg	25 µg
Pantothenic acid	10 mg	4 mg	5 mg	4 mg	5 mg
Vitamin C	60 mg	45 mg	75 mg	45 mg	65 mg
Vitamin D	400 IU (6.5 µg)	5 µg	5 µg	5 µg	5 µg
Vitamin E	30 IU (9 mg α-TE)	11 mg α-TE	15 mg α-TE	11 mg α-TE	15 mg α-TE
Vitamin K	*	60 µg	75 µg	60 µg	75 µg
Calcium	1,000 mg	1,300 mg	1,300 mg	1,300 mg	1,300 mg
Copper	2 mg	700 µg	890 µg	700 µg	890 µg
Iodine	150 µg	120 µg	150 µg	120 µg	150 µg
Iron	18 mg	8 mg	11 mg	8 mg	15 mg
Magnesium	400 mg	240 mg	410 mg	240 mg	360 mg
Phosphorus	1,000 mg	1,250 mg	1,250 mg	1,250 mg	1,250 mg
Potassium	3,500 mg	*	*	*	*
Selenium	70 µg	40 µg	55 µg	45 µg	55 µg
Sodium	2,400 mg	*	*	*	*
Zinc	15 mg	8 mg	11 mg	8 mg	9 mg

* No value established   **Based on a diet of 2,000 calories per day

Key to nutrient measures

g	gram
mg	milligram (1000 mg = 1 g)
µg	microgram (1000 µg = 1 mg; 1,000,000 µg = 1 g)
IU	International Unit (an old measure of vitamin activity)
RAE	retinol activity equivalents (a measure of Vitamin A activity)
NE	niacin equivalents (a measure of niacin activity)
DFE	dietary folate equivalents (a measure of folate activity)
α-TE	alpha-tocopherol equivalents (a measure of Vitamin E activity)

551

Nutritive Value of Foods

Nutrients in Indicated Quantity

Item No.	Food Description	Approximate Measure	Weight	Food energy	Protein	Fat	Cholesterol	Calcium	Iron	Sodium	Vitamin A value* Retinol equivalents	Vitamin C
			Grams	Calories	Grams	Grams	Milligrams	Milligrams	Milligrams	Milligrams		Milligrams
Beverages												
9	Club soda	12 fl oz	355	0	0	0	0	18	Tr	78	0	0
10	Regular cola	12 fl oz	369	160	0	0	0	11	0.2	18	0	0
11	Diet, artificially sweetened cola	12 fl oz	355	Tr	0	0	0	14	0.2	32	0	0
20	Fruit punch drink	6 fl oz	190	85	Tr	0	0	15	0.4	15	2	61
Dairy Products												
Natural Cheese:												
32	Cheddar, cut pieces	1 oz	28	115	7	9	30	204	0.2	176	86	0
38	Cottage cheese, lowfat (2%)	1 cup	226	205	31	4	19	155	0.4	918	45	Tr
43	Mozzarella, part skim milk	1 oz	28	80	8	5	15	207	0.1	150	54	0
46	Parmesan, grated	1 tbsp	5	25	2	2	4	69	Tr	93	9	0
52	Pasteurized process American cheese	1 oz	28	105	6	9	27	174	0.1	406	82	0
Milk, fluid:												
78	Whole (3.3% fat)	1 cup	244	150	8	8	33	291	0.1	120	76	2
79	Reduced fat (2%)	1 cup	244	120	8	5	18	297	0.1	122	139	2
83	Nonfat (skim)	1 cup	245	85	8	Tr	4	302	0.1	126	149	2
85	Buttermilk	1 cup	245	100	8	2	9	285	0.1	257	20	2
88	Evaporated skim milk	1 cup	255	200	19	1	9	738	0.7	293	298	3
91	Dried, nonfat, instantized	1 cup	68	245	24	Tr	12	837	0.2	373	483	4
Milk beverages:												
94	Chocolate milk, low-fat (1%)	1 cup	250	160	8	3	7	287	0.6	152	148	2
105	Shakes, thick: Vanilla	10 oz	283	315	11	9	33	413	0.3	270	79	0
Milk desserts, frozen:												
Ice cream, vanilla, regular (about 11% fat):												
107	Hardened	1 cup	133	270	5	14	59	176	0.1	116	133	1
109	Soft serve (frozen custard)	1 cup	173	375	7	23	153	236	0.4	153	199	1
Ice cream, vanilla, low-fat:												
113	Hardened (about 4% fat)	1 cup	131	185	5	6	18	176	0.2	105	52	1
116	Sherbet (about 2% fat)	1 cup	193	270	2	4	14	103	0.3	88	39	4
Yogurt, made with low-fat milk:												
117	Fruit-flavored	8 oz	227	230	10	2	10	345	0.2	133	25	1
118	Plain	8 oz	227	145	12	4	14	415	0.2	159	36	2

Eggs

Eggs, large (24 oz. per dozen):

Item	Food	Measure	Grams	Food energy (Cal)	Protein (g)	Fat (g)	Cholesterol (mg)	Calcium (mg)	Iron (mg)	Sodium (mg)	Vitamin A	Vitamin C (mg)
124	Fried in margarine	1 egg	46	90	6	7	211	25	0.7	162	114	0
125	Hard-cooked, shell removed	1 egg	50	75	6	5	213	25	0.6	62	84	0

Fats and Oils

Item	Food	Measure	Grams	Food energy (Cal)	Protein (g)	Fat (g)	Cholesterol (mg)	Calcium (mg)	Iron (mg)	Sodium (mg)	Vitamin A	Vitamin C (mg)
129	Butter (4 sticks per lb) (⅛ stick)	1 tbsp	14	100	Tr	11	31	3	Tr	116	106	0
138	Margarine (⅛ stick)	1 tbsp	14	100	Tr	11	0	4	Tr	132	139	Tr
147	Corn oil	1 cup	218	1,925	0	218	0	0	0.0	0	0	0

Salad dressings, commercial:

Item	Food	Measure	Grams	Food energy (Cal)	Protein (g)	Fat (g)	Cholesterol (mg)	Calcium (mg)	Iron (mg)	Sodium (mg)	Vitamin A	Vitamin C (mg)
162	French, Regular	1 tbsp	16	85	Tr	9	0	2	Tr	188	Tr	Tr
163	French, Low calorie	1 tbsp	16	25	Tr	2	0	6	Tr	306	Tr	Tr

Fish and Shellfish

Item	Food	Measure	Grams	Food energy (Cal)	Protein (g)	Fat (g)	Cholesterol (mg)	Calcium (mg)	Iron (mg)	Sodium (mg)	Vitamin A	Vitamin C (mg)
177	Fish sticks, frozen, reheated (stock, 4 by 1 by ½ in.)	1 fish stick	28	70	6	3	26	11	0.3	53	5	0
181	Haddock, breaded, fried	3 oz	85	175	17	9	75	34	1.0	123	20	0
182	Halibut, broiled, with butter and lemon juice	3 oz	85	140	20	6	62	14	0.7	103	174	1
195	Tuna, canned, oil pack, chunk light	3 oz	85	165	24	7	55	7	1.6	303	20	0
196	Tuna, canned, water pack, solid white	3 oz	85	135	30	1	48	17	0.6	468	32	0

Fruits and Fruit Juices

Item	Food	Measure	Grams	Food energy (Cal)	Protein (g)	Fat (g)	Cholesterol (mg)	Calcium (mg)	Iron (mg)	Sodium (mg)	Vitamin A	Vitamin C (mg)
198	Apples, raw, unpeeled, 2¾-in. diam.	1 apple	138	80	Tr	Tr	0	10	0.2	Tr	7	8
202	Apple juice, bottled or canned	1 cup	248	115	Tr	Tr	0	17	0.9	7	Tr	2
204	Applesauce, canned, unsweetened	1 cup	244	105	Tr	Tr	0	7	0.3	5	7	3
215	Bananas, raw, without peel, whole	1 banana	114	105	1	1	0	7	0.4	1	9	10
229	Fruit cocktail, canned, juice pack	1 cup	248	115	1	Tr	0	20	0.5	10	76	7
230	Grapefruit, raw, without peel, 3¾-in. diam.	½ grapefruit	120	40	1	Tr	0	14	0.1	Tr	1	41
233	Grapefruit juice, canned, unsweetened	1 cup	247	95	1	Tr	0	17	0.5	2	2	72
237	Grapes, Thompson Seedless	10 grapes	50	35	Tr	Tr	0	6	0.1	1	4	5
239	Grape juice, canned or bottled	1 cup	253	155	1	Tr	0	23	0.6	8	2	Tr
242	Kiwifruit, raw, without skin	1 kiwifruit	76	45	1	Tr	0	20	0.3	4	13	74
250	Mangos, raw, without skin and seed	1 mango	207	135	1	1	0	21	0.3	4	806	57
251	Cantaloupe, orange-fleshed, 5-in. diam.	½ melon	267	95	2	1	0	29	0.6	24	861	113
253	Nectarines, raw, without pits	1 nectarine	136	65	1	Tr	0	7	0.2	Tr	100	7
254	Oranges, raw, whole	1 orange	131	60	1	Tr	0	52	0.1	Tr	27	70
260	Orange juice, frozen concentrate, diluted	1 cup	249	110	2	Tr	0	22	0.2	2	19	97
262	Papayas, raw, ½-in. cubes	1 cup	140	65	1	Tr	0	35	0.3	9	40	92
263	Peaches, raw, whole, 2½-in. diam.	1 peach	87	35	1	Tr	0	4	0.1	Tr	47	6
273	Pears, raw, with skin, cored, Bartlett, 2½-in. diam.	1 pear	166	100	1	1	0	18	0.4	Tr	3	7
283	Pineapple, chunks or tidbits, juice pack	1 cup	250	150	1	Tr	0	35	0.7	3	10	24
287	Plantains, without peel, cooked, boiled, sliced	1 cup	154	180	1	Tr	0	3	0.9	8	140	17
288	Plums, raw, 2⅛-in. diam.	1 plum	66	35	Tr	1	0	3	0.1	Tr	21	6
297	Raisins, seedless, cup, not pressed down	1 cup	145	435	5	1	0	71	3.0	17	1	5

Nutrients in Indicated Quantity

Item No.	Food Description	Approximate Measure	Weight (Grams)	Food energy (Calories)	Protein (Grams)	Fat (Grams)	Cholesterol (Milligrams)	Calcium (Milligrams)	Iron (Milligrams)	Sodium (Milligrams)	Vitamin A value* Retinol equivalents	Vitamin C (Milligrams)
303	Strawberries, raw, capped, whole	1 cup	149	45	1	1	0	21	0.6	1	4	84
309	Watermelon, 4 by 8 in. wedge	1 piece	482	155	3	2	0	39	0.8	10	176	46

Grain Products

Item No.	Food Description	Approximate Measure	Weight (Grams)	Food energy (Calories)	Protein (Grams)	Fat (Grams)	Cholesterol (Milligrams)	Calcium (Milligrams)	Iron (Milligrams)	Sodium (Milligrams)	Vitamin A value* Retinol equivalents	Vitamin C (Milligrams)
311	Bagels, plain or water, enriched	1 bagel	68	200	7	2	0	29	1.8	245	0	0
314	Biscuits, from mix, 2 in. diameter	1 biscuit	28	95	2	3	Tr	58	0.7	262	4	Tr
Breads:												
319	Cracked-wheat bread (18 per loaf)	1 slice	25	65	2	1	0	16	0.7	106	Tr	Tr
332	Pita bread, enriched, white, 6½-in. diam.	1 pita	60	165	6	1	0	49	1.4	339	0	0
346	White bread, enriched (18 per loaf)	1 slice	25	65	2	1	0	32	0.7	129	Tr	Tr
353	Whole-wheat bread (16 per loaf)	1 slice	28	70	3	1	0	20	1.0	180	Tr	Tr
355	Bread stuffing, dry type, from mix	1 cup	140	500	9	31	0	92	2.2	1,254	273	0
Breakfast cereals:												
359	Cream of Wheat®, cooked	1 cup	244	140	4	Tr	0	54	10.9	5	0	0
367	Cheerios®	1 oz	28	110	4	2	0	48	4.5	307	375	15
368	Kellogg's® Corn Flakes	1 oz	28	110	2	Tr	0	1	1.8	351	375	15
383	Shredded Wheat	1 oz	28	100	3	1	0	11	1.2	3	0	0
386	Sugar Frosted Flakes, Kellogg's®	1 oz	28	110	1	Tr	0	1	1.8	230	375	15
390	Wheaties®	1 oz	28	100	3	Tr	0	43	4.5	354	375	15
Cakes prepared from cake mixes:												
394	Angelfood, 1/12 of cake	1 piece	53	125	3	Tr	0	44	0.2	269	0	0
396	Coffeecake, crumb, 1/6 of cake	1 piece	72	230	5	7	47	44	1.2	310	32	Tr
398	Devil's food with chocolate frosting, 1/16 of cake	1 piece	69	235	3	8	37	41	1.4	181	31	Tr
Cookies, commercial:												
424	Brownies with nuts and frosting	1 brownie	25	100	1	4	14	13	0.6	59	18	Tr
426	Chocolate chip, 2¼ in. diam.	4 cookies	42	180	2	9	5	13	0.8	140	15	Tr
429	Fig bars, square, 1⅝ in. square	4 cookies	56	210	2	4	27	40	1.4	180	6	Tr
430	Oatmeal with raisins, 2⅝-in. diam.	4 cookies	52	245	3	10	2	18	1.1	148	12	0
437	Corn chips	1-oz pkg.	28	155	2	9	0	35	0.5	233	11	1
Crackers:												
444	Graham, plain, 2½ in. square	2 crackers	14	60	1	1	0	6	0.4	86	0	0
448	Snack-type, standard	1 cracker	3	15	Tr	1	0	3	0.1	30	Tr	0
449	Wheat, thin	4 crackers	8	35	1	1	0	3	0.3	69	Tr	0
Doughnuts, made with enriched flour:												
456	Cake type, plain, 3¼-in. diam.	1 doughnut	50	210	3	12	20	22	1.0	192	5	Tr
457	Yeast-leavened, glazed, 3¾-in. diam.	1 doughnut	60	235	4	13	21	17	1.4	222	Tr	0

458	English muffins, plain, enriched	1 muffin	57	140	5	1	0	96	1.7	378	0	0
461	Macaroni, enriched, cooked	1 cup	130	190	7	1	0	14	2.1	1	0	0
	Muffins, 2½-in. diam., commercial mix:											
467	Blueberry	1 muffin	45	140	3	5	45	15	0.9	225	11	Tr
468	Bran	1 muffin	45	140	3	4	28	27	1.7	385	14	0
470	Noodles (egg noodles), enriched, cooked	1 cup	160	200	7	2	50	16	2.6	3	34	0
	Pancakes, 4-in. diam.:											
474	Plain, from mix (with enriched flour), egg, milk, and oil added	1 pancake	27	60	2	2	16	36	0.7	160	7	Tr
	Pies, 9-in. diam:											
478	Apple, ⅙ of pie	1 piece	158	405	3	18	0	13	1.6	476	5	2
488	Lemon meringue, ⅙ of pie	1 piece	140	355	5	14	143	20	1.4	395	66	4
494	Pumpkin, ⅙ of pie	1 piece	152	320	6	17	109	78	1.4	325	416	0
	Popcorn, popped:											
497	Air-popped, unsalted	1 cup	8	30	1	Tr	0	1	0.2	Tr	1	0
498	Popped in vegetable oil, salted	1 cup	11	55	1	3	0	3	0.3	86	2	0
499	Sugar syrup coated	1 cup	35	135	2	1	0	2	0.5	Tr	3	0
500	Pretzels, stick, 2¼ in. long	10 pretzels	3	10	Tr	Tr	0	1	0.1	48	0	0
	Rice:											
503	Brown, cooked, served hot	1 cup	195	230	5	1	0	23	1.0	0	0	0
505	White, enriched, cooked, served hot	1 cup	205	225	4	Tr	0	21	1.8	0	0	0
	Rolls, enriched, commercial:											
509	Dinner, 2½-in. diam.	1 roll	28	85	2	2	Tr	33	0.8	155	Tr	Tr
510	Frankfurter and hamburger	1 roll	40	115	3	2	Tr	54	1.2	241	Tr	Tr
514	Spaghetti, enriched, cooked	1 cup	130	190	7	1	0	14	2.0	1	0	0
	Legumes, Nuts, and Seeds											
526	Almonds, shelled, whole	1 oz	28	165	6	15	0	75	1.0	3	0	Tr
	Beans, dry, cooked, drained:											
527	Black	1 cup	171	225	15	1	0	47	2.9	1	Tr	0
528	Great Northern	1 cup	180	210	14	1	0	90	4.9	13	0	0
531	Pinto	1 cup	180	265	15	1	0	86	5.4	3	Tr	0
536	Black-eyed peas, dry, cooked (with cooking liquid)	1 cup	250	190	13	1	0	43	3.3	20	3	0
544	Chickpeas, cooked, drained	1 cup	163	270	15	4	0	80	4.9	11	Tr	0
550	Lentils, dry, cooked, with peanuts	1 cup	200	215	16	1	0	50	4.2	26	4	0
553	Mixed nuts, dry roasted, salted	1 oz	28	170	5	15	0	20	1.0	190	Tr	0
555	Peanuts, roasted in oil, salted	1 cup	145	840	39	71	0	125	2.8	626	0	0
557	Peanut butter	1 tbsp	16	95	5	8	0	5	0.3	75	0	0
564	Refried beans, canned	1 cup	290	295	18	3	0	141	5.1	1,228	0	17
	Soy products:											
567	Miso	1 cup	276	470	29	13	0	188	4.7	8,142	11	0
568	Tofu, piece 2¼ by 2¾ by 1 in.	1 piece	120	85	9	5	0	108	2.3	8	0	0
569	Sunflower seeds, dry, hulled	1 oz	28	160	6	14	0	33	1.9	1	1	Tr
570	Tahini	1 tbsp	15	90	3	8	0	21	0.7	5	1	1

Meat and Meat Products

Item No.	Food Description	Approximate Measure	Weight Grams	Food energy Calories	Protein Grams	Fat Grams	Cholesterol Milligrams	Calcium Milligrams	Iron Milligrams	Sodium Milligrams	Vitamin A value* Retinol equivalents	Vitamin C Milligrams
Beef, cooked:												
Braised or pot roasted:												
575	Chuck blade, lean and fat, piece	3 oz	85	325	22	26	87	11	2.5	53	Tr	0
577	Round, bottom, lean and fat, piece	3 oz	85	220	25	13	81	5	2.8	43	Tr	0
578	Lean only from item 577	2.8 oz	78	175	25	8	75	4	2.7	40	Tr	0
580	Ground beef, regular, broiled, patty	3 oz	85	245	20	18	76	9	2.1	70	Tr	0
585	Round, eye of, lean and fat, roasted	3 oz	85	205	23	12	62	5	1.6	50	Tr	0
587	Sirloin, steak, broiled, lean and fat	3 oz	85	240	23	15	77	9	2.6	53	Tr	0
590	Beef, dried, chipped	2.5 oz	72	145	24	4	46	14	2.3	3,053	Tr	0
Lamb:												
593	Chops, loin, broiled, lean and fat	2.8 oz	80	235	22	16	78	16	1.4	62	Tr	0
Pork, cured, cooked:												
599	Bacon, regular	3 slices	19	110	6	9	16	2	0.3	303	0	6
601	Ham, light cure, roasted, lean and fat	3 oz	85	205	18	14	53	6	0.7	1,009	0	0
Luncheon meat:												
605	Chopped ham (8 slices per 6 oz pkg)	2 slices	42	95	7	7	2	3	0.3	576	0	8
Pork, fresh, cooked:												
610	Chop, loin, pan fried, lean and fat	3.1 oz	89	335	21	27	92	4	0.7	64	3	Tr
614	Rib, roasted, lean and fat	3 oz	85	270	21	20	69	9	0.8	37	3	Tr
Sausages:												
618	Bologna, slice (8 per 8-oz pkg)	2 slices	57	180	7	16	31	7	0.9	581	0	12
620	Brown and serve, browned	1 link	13	50	2	5	9	1	0.1	105	0	0
621	Frankfurter, cooked (reheated)	1	45	145	5	13	23	5	0.5	504	0	12

Mixed Dishes and Fast Foods

Item No.	Food Description	Approximate Measure	Weight Grams	Food energy Calories	Protein Grams	Fat Grams	Cholesterol Milligrams	Calcium Milligrams	Iron Milligrams	Sodium Milligrams	Vitamin A value* Retinol equivalents	Vitamin C Milligrams
Mixed dishes:												
629	Beef and vegetable stew, home recipe	1 cup	245	220	16	11	71	29	2.9	292	568	17
631	Chicken à la king, home recipe	1 cup	245	470	27	34	221	127	2.5	760	272	12
642	Spaghetti in tomato sauce with cheese, home recipe	1 cup	250	260	9	9	8	80	2.3	955	140	13
Fast food entrees:												
645	Cheeseburger, regular	1 sandwich	112	300	15	15	44	135	2.3	672	65	1
648	English muffin, egg, cheese, bacon	1 sandwich	138	360	18	18	213	197	3.1	832	160	1
649	Fish sandwich, regular, with cheese	1 sandwich	140	420	16	23	56	132	1.8	667	25	2
651	Hamburger, regular	1 sandwich	98	245	12	11	32	56	2.2	463	14	1
653	Pizza, cheese, ⅛ of 15-in. diam.	1 slice	120	290	15	9	56	220	1.6	699	106	2
654	Roast beef sandwich	1 sandwich	150	345	22	13	55	60	4.0	757	32	2
655	Taco	1 taco	81	195	9	11	21	109	1.2	456	57	1

Poultry and Poultry Products

Chicken:

Fried, flesh, with skin and bones:

No.	Food	Measure	Grams									
656	Breast, ½ breast, batter dipped	4.9 oz	140	365	35	18	119	28	1.8	385	28	0
657	Drumstick, batter dipped	2.5 oz	72	195	16	11	62	12	1.0	194	19	0

Roasted, flesh only:

660	Breast, ½ breast	3.0 oz	86	140	27	3	73	13	0.9	64	5	0
662	Stewed, flesh only, light and dark meat	1 cup	140	250	38	9	116	20	1.6	98	21	0

Turkey, roasted, flesh only:

665	Dark meat, piece, 2½ by 1⅝ by ½ in.	4 pieces	85	160	24	6	72	27	2.0	67	0	0
666	Light meat, piece, 4 by 2 by ¼ in.	2 pieces	85	135	25	3	59	16	1.1	54	0	0
667	Chopped or diced	1 cup	140	240	41	7	106	35	2.5	98	0	0

Soups, Sauces, and Gravies

Soups, condensed:

Canned, prepared with milk:

679	Cream of mushroom	1 cup	248	205	6	14	20	179	0.6	1,076	37	2
680	Tomato	1 cup	248	160	6	6	17	159	1.8	932	109	68

Canned, prepared with water:

681	Bean with bacon	1 cup	253	170	8	6	3	81	2.0	951	89	2
682	Beef broth, bouillon, consomme	1 cup	240	15	3	1	Tr	14	0.4	782	0	0
684	Chicken noodle	1 cup	241	75	4	2	7	17	0.8	1,106	71	Tr
693	Vegetarian	1 cup	241	70	2	2	0	22	1.1	822	301	1

Dehydrated, prepared with water:

697	Onion	1 pkt (6-fl-oz)	184	20	1	Tr	0	9	0.1	635	Tr	Tr

Sauces, ready to serve:

703	Barbecue	1 tbsp	16	10	Tr	Tr	0	3	0.1	130	14	1
704	Soy	1 tbsp	18	10	2	0	0	3	0.5	1,029	0	0

Gravies:

708	Brown, from dry mix	1 cup	261	80	3	2	2	66	0.2	1,147	0	0
709	Chicken, from dry mix	1 cup	260	85	3	2	3	39	0.3	1,134	0	3

Sugars and Sweets

Candy:

711	Chocolate, milk, plain	1 oz	28	145	2	9	6	50	0.4	23	10	Tr
712	Chocolate, milk, with almonds	1 oz	28	150	3	10	5	65	0.5	23	8	Tr
717	Fondant, uncoated (mints, other)	1 oz	28	105	Tr	0	0	2	0.1	57	0	0
720	Hard candy	1 oz	28	110	0	0	0	Tr	0.1	7	0	0
723	Custard, baked	1 cup	265	305	14	15	278	297	1.1	209	146	1
724	Gelatin dessert	½ cup	120	70	2	0	0	1	Tr	55	0	0
726	Honey, strained or extracted	1 tbsp	21	65	Tr	0	0	1	0.1	1	0	0
727	Jams and preserves	1 tbsp	20	55	Tr	Tr	0	4	0.2	2	Tr	Tr
739	Pudding, vanilla, instant	½ cup	130	150	4	4	15	129	0.1	375	33	1

Nutrients in Indicated Quantity

Item No.	Food Description	Approximate Measure	Weight (Grams)	Food energy (Calories)	Protein (Grams)	Fat (Grams)	Cholesterol (Milligrams)	Calcium (Milligrams)	Iron (Milligrams)	Sodium (Milligrams)	Vitamin A value* Retinol equivalents	Vitamin C (Milligrams)
Sugars:												
741	Brown, pressed down	1 cup	220	820	0	0	0	187	4.8	97	0	0
742	White, granulated	1 tbsp	12	45	0	0	0	Tr	Tr	Tr	0	0
745	White, powdered, sifted	1 cup	100	385	0	0	0	1	Tr	2	0	0
Syrups:												
748	Molasses, cane, blackstrap	2 tbsp	40	85	0	0	0	274	10.1	38	0	0
749	Table syrup (corn and maple)	2 tbsp	42	122	0	0	0	1	Tr	19	0	0
Vegetables and Vegetable Products												
750	Alfalfa seeds, sprouted, raw	1 cup	33	10	1	Tr	0	11	0.3	2	5	3
	Beans, snap, cooked, drained:											
761	From frozen (cut)	1 cup	135	35	2	Tr	0	61	1.1	18	71	11
	Broccoli:											
771	Raw	1 spear	151	40	4	1	0	72	1.3	41	233	141
772	Cooked	1 spear	180	50	5	1	0	82	2.1	20	254	113
	Cabbage, common varieties:											
778	Raw, coarsely shredded or sliced	1 cup	70	15	1	Tr	0	33	0.4	13	9	33
	Cabbage, Chinese:											
780	Pak-choi, cooked, drained	1 cup	170	20	3	Tr	0	158	1.8	58	437	44
	Carrots:											
784	Whole, 7½ by 1⅛ in.	1 carrot	72	30	1	Tr	0	19	0.4	25	2,025	7
786	Cooked, sliced, drained, from raw	1 cup	156	70	2	Tr	0	48	1.0	103	3,830	4
	Celery, pascal type, raw:											
792	Stalk, large outer, 8 by 1½ in.	1 stalk	40	5	Tr	Tr	0	14	0.2	35	5	3
	Collards, cooked, drained:											
795	From frozen (chopped)	1 cup	170	60	5	1	0	357	1.9	85	1,017	45
	Corn, sweet:											
	Cooked, drained:											
796	From raw, ear 5 by 1¾ in.	1 ear	77	85	3	1	0	2	0.5	13	17	5
798	From frozen kernels	1 cup	165	135	5	Tr	0	3	0.5	8	41	4
	Canned:											
799	Cream style	1 cup	256	185	4	1	0	8	1.0	730	25	12
800	Whole kernel, vacuum pack	1 cup	210	165	5	1	0	11	0.9	571	51	17
801	Cucumber, with peel, slices ⅛ in. thick, 2⅛-in. diam.	6 slices	28	5	Tr	Tr	0	4	0.1	1	1	1
806	Kale, cooked, drained, from raw	1 cup	130	40	2	1	0	94	1.2	30	962	53

#	Food	Measure										
Lettuce, raw:												
813	Crisp head, as iceberg, chopped	1 cup	55	5	1	Tr	0	10	0.3	5	18	2
814	Loose leaf, chopped or shredded	1 cup	56	10	1	Tr	0	38	0.8	5	106	10
830	Peas, green, frozen, cooked, drained	1 cup	160	125	8	Tr	0	38	2.5	139	107	16
832	Peppers, sweet, raw	1 pepper	74	20	1	Tr	0	4	0.9	2	39	95
Potatoes, cooked:												
834	Baked, with skin	1 potato	202	220	5	Tr	0	20	2.7	16	0	26
French fried, strip, frozen:												
838	Oven heated	10 strips	50	110	2	4	0	5	0.7	16	0	5
839	Fried in vegetable oil	10 strips	50	160	2	8	0	10	0.4	108	0	5
849	Potato chips	10 chips	20	105	1	7	0	5	0.2	94	0	8
852	Radishes, raw	4 radishes	18	5	Tr	Tr	0	4	0.1	4	Tr	4
Spinach:												
856	Raw, chopped	1 cup	55	10	2	Tr	0	54	1.5	43	369	15
858	Cooked, drained, from frozen (leaf)	1 cup	190	55	6	Tr	0	277	2.9	163	1,479	23
Squash, cooked:												
861	Summer, sliced, drained	1 cup	180	35	2	1	0	49	0.6	2	52	10
862	Winter, baked, cubes	1 cup	205	80	2	1	0	29	0.7	2	729	20
863	Sweet potatoes, baked in skin, peeled	1 potato	114	115	2	Tr	0	32	0.5	11	2,488	28
Tomatoes:												
868	Raw, 2⅗-in. diam.	1 tomato	123	25	1	Tr	0	9	0.6	10	139	22
869	Canned, solids and liquid	1 cup	240	50	2	1	0	62	1.5	391	145	36
870	Tomato juice, canned	1 cup	244	40	2	Tr	0	22	1.4	881	136	45
877	Vegetable juice cocktail, canned	1 cup	242	45	2	Tr	0	27	1.0	883	283	67
Miscellaneous Items												
885	Catsup	1 cup	273	290	5	1	0	60	2.2	2,845	382	41
894	Mustard, prepared, yellow	1 tsp	5	5	Tr	Tr	0	4	0.1	63	0	Tr
895	Olives, canned, green, medium	4	13	15	Tr	2	0	8	0.2	312	4	0
Pickles, cucumber:												
901	Dill, medium, whole, 3¾in.	1 pickle	65	5	Tr	Tr	0	17	0.7	928	7	4
903	Sweet, small, whole, 2½ in. long	1 pickle	15	20	Tr	Tr	0	2	0.2	107	1	1

* 1 RE = 3.33 IU from animal foods or 1 mcg retinol.
  1 RE = 10 IU from plant foods or 6 mcg beta carotene.
  Tr = Trace amount.

Source: USDA Home and Garden Bulletin No. 72, "Nutritive Value of Foods"

NOTE: Nutritive values of most packaged foods may be obtained from the "Nutrition Facts" panel on the container.

Glossary

A

acids. Water-soluble and sour chemicals that in solution share certain characteristics. (Handbook 4-4)

action plan. A step-by-step approach to identifying and reaching your goals. (Ch. 1)

additive. A substance added to foods during processing to make them safer, more appealing, or more nutritious. (Ch. 4)

aerobic activity. An activity that works your heart and lungs. (Ch. 17)

a la carte (ah-lah-CART). On a restaurant menu, describes items that are served separately, without side dishes. (Ch. 15)

al dente (ahl-DEN-tay). Used to describe pasta that is tender, but slightly firm in the center. (Ch. 21)

amino acids. The many small units that make up protein. (Ch. 6)

antioxidants. A substance that helps to protect your body from cell damage that can lead to health problems. (Ch. 6)

appetite. A psychological desire to eat. (Ch. 2)

appetizer. A small portion of food usually served at the start of a meal. (Ch. 12)

B

basal metabolic rate (BMR). The amount of energy used for automatic body functions such as breathing. (Ch. 5)

base. Chemical opposite of an acid. (Handbook 4-4)

batter. A flour mixture that is thin enough to pour or drop from a bowl or spoon. *See also* dough. (Ch. 30)

bisque (bisk). A thick, rich cream soup made with finely mashed or ground seafood, poultry, or vegetables. (Ch. 28)

body mass index (BMI). A tool for identifying appropriate weight that looks at weight in relation to height. (Ch. 20)

bran. The coarse outer layer of a grain that supplies fiber, B vitamins, and minerals. (Ch. 21)

broth. Seasoned, strained liquid from cooking meat, fish, or vegetables. Also called stock. (Ch. 28)

C

calorie. A unit used to measure the energy used by the body and the energy that food supplies to the body. (Ch. 5)

carbohydrate. An essential nutrient that is the body's main source of energy; includes sugars and starches. (Ch. 6)

carbohydrate loading. A way of training and eating several days before an athletic event; involves decreasing training while increasing carbohydrate intake. (Ch. 19)

cardiorespiratory endurance. How well your heart and lungs can keep up with your physical activity. (Ch. 17)

casserole. A mixture of several foods baked and served in the same dish. (Ch. 29)

chemical reaction. A process in which substances become new and different substances. (Handbook 4-1)

chiffon cake. A cake that includes oil or other fat, egg yolks, and both beaten egg whites and baking powder for leavening. (Ch. 32)

cholesterol. A waxy substance that is part of every cell of your body. (Ch. 6)

chowder. A thick, chunky soup made with vegetables and/or seafood. (Ch. 28)

citrus fruits. Fruits such as oranges, tangerines, and grapefruits. (Ch. 23)

coagulation. Process of changing a liquid into a soft semisolid or solid mass. (Handbook 4-5)

cobbler. A cooked fruit dessert with a sweetened biscuit-dough topping. (Ch. 32)

combination food. A food mixture of several ingredients that belongs in two or more food groups. (Ch. 8)

complete protein. A protein source that supplies all the essential amino acids needed by the body; examples include meat, poultry, fish, eggs, and dairy products. (Ch. 6)

complex carbohydrates. Starches; carbohydrates made of many sugars attached together. (Ch. 6)

condensed soup. A soup from which some of the water has been removed in processing. (Ch. 28)

condiment. A flavorful accompaniment to food. (Handbook 5-2)

convenience foods. Foods that are partly prepared or ready-to-eat. (Ch. 14)

cookware. Pots and pans used for cooking and baking. (Handbook 2-2)

CPR (cardiopulmonary resuscitation). A first aid technique to use when someone's breathing and heartbeat have stopped. (Handbook 1-5)

cross-contamination. The result of harmful bacteria being transferred from one food to another. (Handbook 1-3)

cuisine (kwi-ZEEN). Typical foods and ways of cooking associated with a group of people. (Ch. 3)

culture. The shared beliefs, values, and behavior of a large group of people, such as a nation, race, or religious group. (Ch. 1)

custard. A cooked mixture of milk and eggs prepared on the range top or baked in the oven. (Ch. 32)

customary measurement system. The system of measurement most commonly used in the U.S. (Handbook 3-1)

cut (also called retail cut). A section of meat that has been divided into sizes that are purchased by the consumer. (Ch. 25)

D

Daily Values. Nutrient reference amounts shown on the nutrition panel of food labels. Consumers can quickly compare the amount of calories and nutrients in the food with the Daily Values. (Ch. 5)

danger zone. The temperature range in which bacteria grow fastest—between 40 and 140°F (4 and 60°C). (Handbook 1-1)

decorating tube. A tool for squeezing soft foods through a shaped tip. (Handbook 5-1)

diabetes. A condition in which the body cannot control levels of sugar in the blood properly. (Ch. 10)

diet. A method for choosing everything you eat and drink; also called an eating plan. (Ch. 7)

dietary fiber. Plant material that can't be digested. (Ch. 6)

Dietary Guidelines for Americans. A set of guidelines about food choices developed by the U.S. government. (Ch. 7)

dietary supplement. Nutrients people take in addition to those that are in the food they eat; usually in the form of pills, capsules, liquid, or powder. (Ch. 6)

dough. A flour mixture that is stiff enough to be molded by hand, kneaded, or rolled on a board. *See also* batter. (Ch. 30)

dovetailing. The process of keeping two tasks going at the same time. (Handbook 3-7)

dry heat. Methods of cooking food uncovered without added liquid. (Ch. 14)

E

eating disorder. Extreme unhealthy behavior relating to food, eating, and weight. (Ch. 10)

eating plan. A method of choosing everything you eat and drink. Also called a diet. (Ch. 7)

egg substitute. A product made from egg whites that contains very little fat and no cholesterol. (Ch. 26)

electrolytes. Sodium, chloride, and potassium, which work together to help maintain your body's fluid balance. (Ch. 19)

emulsion. A mixture of two liquids—such as oil and water—whose droplets do not normally blend with each other. (Handbook 4-8)

endosperm. The inner part of the grain that is ground into white flour. (Ch. 21)

endurance. The ability to keep working your muscles without becoming overly tired. (Ch. 17)

energy balance. The point at which the energy from the food you eat equals the energy your body uses. (Ch. 20)

enrichment. Adding nutrients to a product to replace those lost in processing. (Ch. 4)

entree (AHN-tray). The main course in a meal. (Ch. 15)

enzyme. A special protein that helps chemical reactions happen. (Handbook 4-4)

ethnic foods. Foods and food traditions belonging to a cultural group based on a common heritage. (Ch. 3)

etiquette (EH-tih-kit). Polite conduct that shows respect and consideration for others. (Ch. 2)

F

fad diets. Weight-loss plans, often based on misinformation, that are popular for a short time. (Ch. 20)

fat. A nutrient that supplies energy, promotes healthy skin and growth, and carries certain vitamins in the body. (Ch. 6)

fermentation. A chemical reaction that splits complex compounds into simpler substances. (Handbook 4-5)

fetus. An unborn baby. (Ch. 9)

fiber. *See* dietary fiber.

finfish. Fish with fins, backbones, and gills. (Ch. 25)

flat bread. A bread that is made with little or no leavening agent. (Ch. 30)

flatware. The knives, forks, and spoons used when eating. (Ch. 2)

flavor. The combination of a food's taste, smell, and texture. (Ch. 2)

flexibility. The ability to move your muscles and joints through their full range of motion. (Ch. 17)

foam cake. A cake that does not include butter, shortening, or oil and uses beaten egg whites as the main leavening agent. (Ch. 32)

food allergy. A condition in which a sensitivity to food causes the body's immune system to react. (Ch. 10)

foodborne illness. Sickness resulting from eating food that is not safe to eat. (Handbook 1-1)

food budget. The amount you plan to spend on food. (Ch. 13)

Food Guide Pyramid. A guide developed by the U.S. government for healthful eating. It divides food into five food groups plus a Fats, Oils, and Sweets category, and indicates a range of the number of servings needed daily from each group. (Ch. 8)

food intolerance. A condition in which the body has trouble digesting or handling a component of food. (Ch. 10)

food jag. A state of wanting just one food for a while. (Ch. 9)

food processing. Methods of preparing and handling food for safety, nutrition, convenience, and appeal. (Ch. 4)

food science. The study of how food is produced, processed, prepared, and used. (Handbook 4-1)

fortification. Adding a nutrient that isn't naturally present to make a food more nutritious. (Ch. 4)

freezer burn. The changes in color, flavor, and texture that result when food loses moisture in the freezer. (Handbook 1-2)

fruit concentrate. Fruit juice with most of the water removed. (Ch. 23)

fruit nectar. A thick, sugar-sweetened beverage of fruit juice and pulp. (Ch. 23)

frying. Cooking food in fat. (Ch. 14)

fusion cuisine. Combining different cultural food traditions in one dish. (Handbook 5-2)

G H

garnish. An edible decoration. (Handbook 5-1)

gelatinization. The process of a liquid forming a gel, such as when starch molecules absorb water. (Handbook 4-9)

germ. The part at the base of a seed that sprouts when it's planted. (Ch. 21)

health fraud. False and possibly harmful approaches to personal health care. (Ch. 11)

Heimlich maneuver. A first aid technique for choking. (Handbook 1-5)

herb. A fragrant, edible leaf of a plant used to season food. (Handbook 5-2)

homogenize. To process milk so that the fat is evenly distributed. (Ch. 24)

hunger. A physical need to eat. (Ch. 2)

I J K

incomplete protein. A protein source that lacks one or more of the essential amino acids the body needs; examples include dry beans and peas, nuts, and grain products. (Ch. 6)

in season. Refers to a time of year when a particular type of vegetable or fruit is highest in quality, most plentiful, and lowest in cost. (Ch. 22)

instant-read thermometer. A thermometer that gives a quick reading of a food's temperature. (Handbook 1-4)

intensity. The speed and power of movement during physical activities. (Ch. 18)

irradiation. Passing food through radiant energy, such as X-rays, to increase shelf life and kill harmful microorganisms. (Ch. 4)

knead. To work and press dough with the hands. (Ch. 30)

L

lacto-ovo-vegetarian. A vegetarian who eats dairy foods and eggs in addition to foods from plant sources. (Ch. 16)

lactose. A natural sugar found in milk and milk products. (Ch. 24)

lactose intolerance. A condition in which the body is unable to adequately digest lactose. (Ch. 10)

lacto-vegetarian. A vegetarian who eats dairy foods in addition to foods from plant sources. (Ch. 16)

lean meat. Meat that has less total fat, saturated fat, and cholesterol. (Ch. 25)

leaven. To make light and porous. (Handbook 4-10)

leavening agent. Any substance that makes a baked product rise by causing pockets of gas to expand in the batter or dough as it bakes. (Ch. 30)

legumes (leg-yooms). Edible seeds that grow in pods. (Ch. 26)

life cycle. The various stages of life a person passes through from before birth through adulthood. (Ch. 9)

lifestyle. How you live your life and all the things you do. (Ch. 1)

M

malnutrition. Serious health problems caused by a lack of nutrients over a long period of time. (Ch. 5)

marbling. The thin streaks and flecks of fat visible in uncooked meat. (Ch. 25)

marinade. A flavorful liquid in which to soak meat, poultry, or fish before cooking. (Ch. 25)

menu. All foods served at a meal or for the whole day's meals and snacks. (Ch. 12)

metric system. The system of measurement, based on multiples of 10, used in most countries. (Handbook 3-1)

microorganism. A tiny living creature that can be seen only with a microscope. (Handbook 1-1)

minerals. Nutrients such as calcium, iron, and zinc; some regulate body processes, while others become part of body tissues. (Ch. 6)

mixture. A material consisting of two or more kinds of matter, each retaining its characteristic properties. (Handbook 4-8)

moist heat. Methods of cooking food using liquid or steam. (Ch. 14)

N

nutrient deficiency. A severe shortage of a nutrient which can cause illness or interfere with normal growth and development. (Ch. 5)

nutrient dense. A term used to describe food that contributes a significant amount of several nutrients compared with the food energy, or calories, it contains. (Ch. 8)

nutrients. The chemicals found in food that nourish your body. (Ch. 1)

nutrition. The study of nutrients in food and how they are used by your body. (Ch. 1)

Nutrition Facts panel. The section of a food label listing the calories, nutrients, cholesterol, and fiber in one serving. (Ch. 13)

O

omelet (ahm-let). A dish made by cooking beaten eggs without stirring. (Ch. 26)

open dating. Printing a date on a food package that consumers can understand, such as a "sell by" date or an expiration date. (Ch. 13)

open-face sandwich. A sandwich that has only a bottom slice of bread. (Ch. 31)

osteoporosis (AH-stee-oh-por-OH-sis). A condition in which bones become porous and can break easily. (Ch. 6)

ovo-vegetarian. A vegetarian who eats eggs in addition to foods from plant sources. (Ch. 16)

P Q

papillae. The tiny bumps on the upper surface of the tongue; they contain the taste buds. (Ch. 2)

pasteurize. To heat-treat milk to destroy bacteria that could cause disease or spoil the milk. (Ch. 24)

pastry dough. A blend of flour, fat, salt, and liquid. (Ch. 32)

perishable. Refers to foods that keep their peak quality for a short time and may spoil quickly. (Ch. 13)

physical activity. An action that uses your muscles to move your body. (Ch. 17)

physical change. A change in a food that does not change its basic chemical nature. (Handbook 4-1)

physical fitness. The condition of having the energy and ability to do everything you want and need to do in your daily life. (Ch. 17)

place setting. The dishes, flatware, glasses, and linens needed by one person to eat a meal. (Ch. 2)

prenatal. The period of time between conception and birth. (Ch. 9)

process cheese. A pasteurized blend of two or more ripened or unripened cheeses. (Ch. 24)

produce. A category of food that includes fresh vegetables, fruits, and herbs. (Ch. 22)

protein. An essential nutrient that helps your body grow, repair itself, and fight disease; can also provide energy if needed. (Ch. 6)

puree (pyu-RAY). To finely mash or grind cooked food. (Ch. 28)

Pyramid serving. A specific measured amount of food that counts as one serving in the Food Guide Pyramid. (Ch. 8)

quacks. People who promote a particular food, diet, or supplement by making false health claims. (Ch. 11)

quick bread. A bread in which the leavening agent is baking powder or baking soda. (Ch. 30)

R

recipe. A list of ingredients and a complete set of instructions for preparing a certain dish. (Ch. 14)

regional foods. Foods that are special to a geographic area. (Ch. 3)

resources. Objects and qualities such as time, money, equipment, skills, and personal energy that help you reach a goal or complete a task. (Ch. 1)

ripe. A term to describe fruit that is full of flavor and color and ready to be eaten. (Ch. 23)

risk factor. A condition that increases your chances of having health problems such as heart disease and cancer. (Ch. 7)

R.S.V.P. An abbreviation on a written invitation that means "please reply." (Handbook 5-2)

rub. A mixture of herbs and spices applied to tender meat, poultry, or fish before cooking. (Handbook 5-2)

S

salad greens. The edible leaves of vegetable plants. (Ch. 27)

sanitation. Actions to prevent illness through cleanliness. (Handbook 1-3)

saturated fat. A fat that is hard at room temperature, such as the fat in meat, poultry skin, and whole milk dairy products. It increases blood cholesterol levels and the risk for heart problems. (Ch. 6)

scratch cooking. Preparing a homemade dish from unprepared foods. (Ch. 14)

sedentary. Being physically inactive. (Ch. 18)

serrated. Sawtooth. (Handbook 2-1)

shelf life. The length of time a food can be stored and remain safe and appealing to eat. (Ch. 4)

shellfish. Fish that have a shell instead of bones and fins. (Ch. 25)

shortened cake. A cake that includes a fat such as butter or shortening and uses baking powder or baking soda as the main leavening agent. (Ch. 32)

shortening. A solid fat made from vegetable oil. (Ch. 30)

simple carbohydrates. Sugars; carbohydrates made of one or two sugar units. (Ch. 6)

solution. A mixture in which one substance is dissolved in another. (Handbook 4-2)

speed-scratch cooking. Preparing a homemade dish using partly prepared foods. (Ch. 14)

spice. A seasoning that comes from the bark, buds, seeds, roots, or stems of plants and trees. (Handbook 5-2)

standing time. The period during which a food continues to cook after being taken out of a microwave oven. (Handbook 3-5)

staples. Food items your family keeps on hand, such as milk, rice, or flour. (Ch. 13)

stock. Seasoned, strained liquid from cooking meat, fish, or vegetables. Also called broth. (Ch. 28)

strength. The power to work your muscles against resistance. (Ch. 17)

TUV

tender-crisp. A term to describe vegetables cooked to the point of being tender but still firm and slightly crisp. (Ch. 22)

tofu (TOE-foo). Soybean curd. (Ch. 16)

trade-off. An exchange in which you give up one thing so that you can have something else. (Ch.12)

unit price. The cost per ounce, quart, pound or other unit of measurement. (Ch. 13)

unsaturated fat. A fat that is liquid at room temperature, such as the fat in vegetable oils, nuts, and olives. (Ch. 6)

UPC symbol (Universal Product Code). A bar code on food labels and other products; it carries coded information, such as the price, that can be "read" by a scanner. (Ch. 13)

vegan (VEE-gun). A vegetarian who eats only foods from plant sources. (Ch. 16)

vinaigrette (vin-ih-GRET). A mixture of oil, vinegar, and seasonings. (Ch. 27)

vitamins. Nutrients that don't provide energy or build body tissue, but help regulate these and other body processes. (Ch. 6)

W

wellness. Reaching for your personal best level of health. (Ch. 1)

whole grain. Term used to describe a product made from the entire grain kernel, including the endosperm, germ, and bran. (Ch. 21)

wok (walk). A special pan, with a narrow, round bottom and a wide top, designed for stir-fry cooking. (Ch. 29)

work center. An area of the kitchen devoted to a specific task. (Handbook 2-4)

work plan. A list of all the steps required to prepare a food. (Handbook 3-7)

wrap. A flat bread rolled around a filling. (Ch. 31)

XYZ

yeast. A one-celled fungus that multiplies rapidly, given the right conditions. (Handbook 4-10)

yeast bread. A bread in which the leavening agent is yeast. (Ch. 30)

yield. The amount a recipe makes. (Handbook 3-1)

Credits

● ●

COVER/INTERIOR DESIGN
Bill SMITH STUDIO

COVER PHOTO
Superstock

ILLUSTRATION CREDITS
Tim Alt, 508, 509, 511, 512, 513, 515, 519, 526, 532
Paul Breeden, 282
Dave Foster, 181, 339, 344, 470, 474 b., 507
Olivia, 120, 122, 440, 441, 462, 467, 468, 469
Tony Persiani, 83, 463, 464, 465, 466, 472, 473, 474 t., 485, 486, 487, 495, 496, 497,
Juan Velasco, 60, 79, 265, 266
Tracey Wood, 110, 133, 207, 336, 438, 449, 450-451, 456, 475, 478, 483, 484, 488, 489, 490, 498, 499, 536, 539, 543, 547

PHOTO CREDITS
Age Fotostock
 Kathy Murphy, 311
 Ripp, 367
Steven Cohen, 102, 154, 155, 390, 539
Corbis
 94 Mug Shots, 92
 David Ball, 388, 396
 Peggy & Ron Barnett, 282
 Arthur Beck, 382
 Bojan Brecelj, 150
 C/B Productions, 51, 131
 Bryn Colton, 224
 George Diebold, 166
 Jack Fields, 71
 Owen Franken, 224
 Michael Freeman, 360, 363
 Michelle Garrett, 150
 Chris Hamilton, 23

Andrew Holbrook, 49
Jeremy Horner, 71
Dave G. Houser, 435
Japack Photo Library, 362
Wolfgang Kaehler, 332
Ronnie Kaufman, 80
Earl & Nazima Kowal, 151
Steve Lupton, 287
Robert Maass, 360
Don Mason, 326, 247, 432
Gabe Palmer, 114
Jose L. Pelaez, 77, 86, 127
Caroline Penn, 274
Reuters NewMedia, 362-363
Janez Skok, 277
Ted Spiegal, 70
Gerhard Steiner, 224
David Stoecklein, 10, 236, 396
James A. Sugar, 151
Ron Watts, 362
Corel, 94, 95, 118, 282
Jim Cummins Studio, Inc., 230
John Curry, 374
Mary Kate Denny, 139
Envision
 Andre Baranowski, 276, 420, 426
 David Bishop, 219
 Ed Bishop, 316
 Kenneth Chen, 541
 Peter Johansky, 46
 Henry T. Kaiser, 352
 Michael Major, 162
 Kam Mak, 361
 George Mattei, 108, 112
 Steven Morris, 72
 Steven Needham, 70, 107, 130, 151, 209, 215, 222, 278, 283, 322, 350, 369, 380, 425, 501, 527, 539
 Osetoski & Zoda, 262, 272
 Overseas, 280

Paul Poplis, 381
Guy Power, 12, 338
Amy Reichman, 73
Agence Top, 301
Brooks Walker, 433
Foodpix
 James Bairgrie, 361
 Matt Bowman, 88
 Burke/Triolo Productions, 538
 John Burwell, 190
 Steve Cohen, 70, 258
 Eisenhut & Mayer, 70
 Benjamin F. Fink Jr, 115
 Gibson & Smith, 268
 Brian Hagiwara, 106, 227
 Tim Hawley, 12, 416
 Rusty Hill, 342
 Brian Leatart, 208, 212, 327, 523
 Maximilian Stock Ltd., 526
 Keith Seaman, 61
Getty Images, 307
 Tony Arruza, 20
 Bruce Ayres, 24
 James Baigrie, 153
 Phil Banko, 20, 74, 154, 228, 278, 364
 Christopher Bissell, 27
 C Squared Studios, 225, 226
 Peter Cade, 96
 Paul Chesley, 73
 Davies & Starr Inc., 516
 Thomas Del Brase, 312
 Digital Vision, 145
 Michael Dunning, 433
 Chris Everard, 152
 Jules Frazier, 225
 Larry Dale Gordan, 455
 Bernard Grilly, 153
 Brian Hagiwara, 7, 121
 Walter Hodges, 540
 Nicole Katano, 24
 John Lawlor, 42

ACKNOWLEDGEMENTS

Helen Barrett /Alva Newsgram, Helena, OK, 199
Go Girls, NEDA, Seattle, WA, 237
Eleanor Keppler, Lawrence Central High School, Indianapolis, IN, 314
Nancy Mayer of Mayer/Myers Design, Philadelphia, PA, 123
Project LEAN, San Gabriel, CA, 85
Linda Valiga, Waukesha South High School, Waukesha, WI, 43

Index